Evidence Based Pathology and Laboratory Medicine

Alberto M. Marchevsky • Mark R. Wick
Editors

Evidence Based Pathology and Laboratory Medicine

Springer

Editors
Alberto M. Marchevsky, MD
Director, Pulmonary and Mediastinal Pathology
Department of Pathology and Laboratory Medicine
Cedars-Sinai Medical Center
and
Clinical Professor of Pathology
David Geffen School of Medicine
University of California
Los Angeles, CA, USA
marchevsky@cshs.org

Mark R. Wick, MD
Professor and Associate Director of Surgical Pathology
Department of Pathology
University of Virginia Medical School
Charlottesville, VA, USA
MRW9C@hscmail.mcc.virginia.edu

ISBN 978-1-4419-1029-5 e-ISBN 978-1-4419-1030-1
DOI 10.1007/978-1-4419-1030-1
Springer New York Dordrecht Heidelberg London

Library of Congress Control Number: 2011925569

Printed on acid-free paper

Springer is part of Springer Science+Business Media (www.springer.com)

Preface

Pathology and laboratory medicine are currently experiencing paradigm shifts that are likely to influence how our specialty is practiced in the not-too-distant future. Technical innovations in immunohistochemistry, molecular pathology, and pathology informatics are driving the acquisition of many new and exciting data. That phenomenon may well increase the quality and scope of the diagnostic information being provided by laboratory assays. Simultaneously, however, as new technologies invariably increase the cost of medical testing, considerable pressure has accrued concerning financial containment. Thus far, advocates of "the most, the newest, and the best, regardless of cost" have largely prevailed. Nonetheless, it is likely that in the near future, there will be considerable movement toward a strict, cost-effective utilization of laboratory resources that is centered on clinical value and direct applicability of test results in regard to individual patient care.

As practicing pathologists, it has been our impression that there is a great interest in the generation of new data and the exploration of clinical applications for new technologies. At the same time, as a group, we do not often pause to consider how well we are performing certain tasks, and how well we fulfill our charges as members of clinical teams that care for individual patients. Residency education in pathology and laboratory medicine tends to emphasize the acquisition of morphology-based diagnostic skills and information on various laboratory tests. Nonetheless, interest has been limited in teaching future pathologists to understand the pros and cons of various diagnostic models; critically evaluate the contents of medical publications; sift through apparently conflicting information; integrate data from divergent sources; effectively combine the medical literature with personal experience; and practice pathology in a cost-effective manner that does not compromise quality or waste resources.

Internal medicine and other medical specialties have confronted similar issues. They have supported the development of an analytical approach to the evaluation and use of medical information, under the rubric of *evidence-based medicine* (EBM). That term is somewhat fustian, because it appears to imply that other modes of medical practice are not "evidence-based" or objective. Advocates of EBM have explored the advantages and disadvantages of differing study designs; emphasized the advantages of gathering data through randomized clinical trials; classified medical data in terms of evidence-levels; advocated the use of standardized guidelines for clinical care; and stressed the use of a patient-centered approach to diagnosis and treatment. Some of those concepts have generated considerable resistance from the medical community at large, in part because EBM tends to deride case reports or small case series as anecdotal or inferior. Opponents of EBM have suggested that it leads to "cookbook medicine" and de-emphasizes clinical experience and the art of medicine. They have also pointed to the practical limitations of randomized clinical trials as a gold standard for the collection of medical information.

A debate continues between advocates of EBM and other physicians who favor more individualized case-based approaches to medical practice. However, regardless of that schism, the current trend toward EBM has provided a valuable service by emphasizing the importance of reliably produced data and suggesting how to best apply it to individual patient care.

In this volume, we explore the application of selected EBM concepts to anatomic pathology and laboratory medicine, embodied in a model that we have dubbed as *evidence-based pathology* (EBP). This book is unusual in the specialty of pathology, because it is not designed to provide readers with the means to diagnose specific lesions in biopsies or interpret particular laboratory tests. Rather, its intent is to discuss a variety of epistemological and practical issues, and to stimulate thoughts on how well we are doing in practicing truly scientific medicine as pathologists. Another focus is the contrast between rapidly accruing new technologies and health system-related pressures for cost containment.

This monograph addresses two general topics. One concerns a description of problems that occur in applying EBM to laboratory medicine, and the other considers available resources and possible modes of implementing EBP. The first section of the book includes chapters discussing evidence levels, best evidence, and other basic EBM concepts. This is followed by other material that concerns statistics. It does not attempt to teach the intricacies of various statistical tests, but instead is intended to familiarize readers with the basis of the probabilistic thinking that underlies the specific applications of such analyses. The use and misuse of pathological data for prognostication and prediction in anatomic pathology is discussed in detail, and the technique of meta-analysis is also summarized. The statistical discussion in this book is followed by three chapters that discuss the principles of classification and diagnosis in anatomic pathology, the general evaluation of oncopathological studies, and medical decision-making.

The second section of the book includes various solutions to problems in anatomic pathology and laboratory medicine that are offered by EBP. It includes chapters concerning evaluation of the medical literature; a discussion of how EBP might help advance histopathology in the future; an evaluation of diagnostic errors; the use of meta-analysis to investigate unusual diseases and select immunohistochemical tests; a consideration of the use of molecular tests in hospital practice, the application of tools for decision analysis in laboratory medicine; cost-benefit analysis in the hospital laboratory; and medicolegal aspects of EBP.

We sincerely thank all of our contributors for their willingness to participate in this project, and we hope that readers will be stimulated by the concepts that are discussed in this book. It is our wish that greater awareness of the value of EBP will engender more comprehensive and explicit guidelines for publications in pathology. EBM also has the ability to improve education in pathology; stimulate the future development of objective and reproducible guidelines for the practice of pathology; and further the longstanding identity of pathologists as physicians who provide intellectual leadership for their colleagues.

Los Angeles, CA — Alberto M. Marchevsky, MD
Charlottesville, VA — Mark R. Wick, MD

Contents

Contributors

Bonnie Balzer, MD, PhD Department of Pathology and Laboratory Medicine, Cedars-Sinai Medical Center, Los Angeles, CA, USA

David W. Bates, MD, MSc Department of Medicine, Division of General Internal Medicine and Primary Care, Brigham and Women's Hospital, Boston, MA, USA; Clinical and Quality Analysis, Partners HealthCare System, Inc., Boston, MA, USA; Department of Medicine, Harvard Medical School, Boston, MA, USA

José Costa, MD Department of Pathology, Yale School of Medicine, New Haven, CT, USA

Kenneth A. Fleming, MA (Oxon), DPhil, FRCPath, FRCP, MBChB Director, Oxford University Clinical Academic Graduate School, Associate Dean, Oxford Post Graduate Medicine and Dental Deanery, Oxford, UK

Elliott Foucar, MD Department of Pathology, University of New Mexico School of Medicine, Albuquerque, NM, USA

Wayne W. Grody, MD, PhD Divisions of Medical Genetics and Molecular Pathology, Departments of Pathology and Laboratory Medicine, Pediatrics, and Human Genetics, UCLA School of Medicine, Los Angeles, CA, USA

Ruta Gupta, MD Department of Anatomic Pathology, The Canberra Hospital, ACT Pathology, Garran, ACT, Australia

Michael Hendrickson, MD Department of Pathology, Stanford University Medical Center, Stanford, CA, USA

Ji Yeon Kim, MD, MPH Department of Pathology, Massachusetts General Hospital and Harvard Medical School, Boston, MA, USA

Kent B. Lewandrowski, MD Department of Pathology, Massachusetts General Hospital, Boston, MA, USA; Department of Pathology, Harvard Medical School, Boston, MA, USA

Alberto M. Marchevsky, MD Department of Pathology and Laboratory Medicine, Cedars-Sinai Medical Center, Los Angeles, CA, USA

Stacy E.F. Melanson, MD, PhD Brigham and Women's Hospital/ Massachusetts General Healthcare Center Laboratory, Harvard Medical School, Boston, MA, USA

Aileen P. Morrison, BS Department of Pathology, Clinical Laboratories Division, Brigham and Women's Hospital, Boston, MA, USA

Raouf E. Nakhleh, MD Department of Pathology, Mayo Clinic Florida, Jacksonville, FL, USA

Christopher N. Otis, MD Department of Pathology, Baystate Medical Center, Tufts University School of Medicine, Springfield, MA, USA

Peter J. Saunders, MD Department of Pathology, Baystate Medical Center, Tufts University School of Medicine, Springfield, MA, USA

Paul E. Swanson, MD Department of Pathology, University of Washington Medical Center, Seattle, WA, USA

Milenko J. Tanasijevic, MD, MBA Department of Pathology, Brigham and Women's Hospital and Dana Faber Cancer Institute, Harvard Medical School, Boston, MA, USA

Eleftherios C. Vamvakas, MD, PhD, MPH Department of Pathology and Laboratory Medicine, Cedars-Sinai Medical Center, Los Angeles, CA, USA

Elizabeth M. Van Cott, MD Department of Pathology, Massachusetts General Hospital and Harvard Medical School, Boston, MA, USA

Robin T. Vollmer, MD, MS Department of Laboratory Medicine, VA Medical Center, Durham, NC, USA

Jia-Perng Jennifer Wei, MD, PhD Ambry Genetics, Aliso Viejo, CA, USA

Sarah Whitaker, BA Department of Pathology, Yale School of Medicine, New Haven, CT, USA

Mark R. Wick, MD Department of Pathology, University of Virginia Medical School, Charlottesville, VA, USA

Part I

The Problem and Available Resources

Introduction to Evidence-Based Pathology and Laboratory Medicine

1

Alberto M. Marchevsky and Mark R. Wick

Keywords

Evidence-based medicine, definition • Evidence-based pathology and laboratory medicine • Pathology and laboratory medicine • Evidence • Search engines for evidence-based medicine

Evidence-based medicine (EBM) has been defined as "the conscientious, explicit, and judicious use of current best evidence in making decisions about the care of individual patients" or as "the integration of best research evidence with clinical expertise and patient values" [1–3]. It is an evolving discipline that applies analytical and quantitative methods to evaluate the validity of available medical information, with the overall goal of identifying scientifically sound data or "best evidence." This evidence is integrated to improve medical practice through clinical guidelines and other tools that are used for education, standardization of care, quality initiatives, and coverage decisions [4, 5]. The ideas of EBM have spread rapidly through medicine during the past decade and are recently eliciting a growing interest in Anatomic Pathology and Laboratory Medicine [6–8].

A.M. Marchevsky (✉)
Department of Pathology and Laboratory Medicine,
Cedars-Sinai Medical Center, Los Angeles, CA, USA
e-mail: marchevsky@chs.org

Environment that Created the Need for Evidence-Based Medicine

Traditional medical practice has been based on the fundamental assumption that physicians educated through rigorous medical school courses, postgraduate training programs, continuing education activities, journals, personal experiences, and interaction with colleagues are well equipped to consistently render correct diagnoses and do the right things for their patients. Individual physicians are expected to integrate complex information through "clinical judgment" or the "art of medicine" [6]. Decisions about the need for insurance coverage, medical necessity, and "standards of practice" are generally defined by the loose standard of "if the majority of physicians are doing it, it must be necessary, it should be covered and it is clinically useful" [9]. The use of more formal analytical methods and mathematical models to identify solutions to these questions has been mostly limited to research projects.

Research in the 1970s and 1980s documented several major flaws in these fundamental assumptions and stimulated an increasing focus on "technology assessment" [9]. For example, the United States Congressional Office of Technology

A.M. Marchevsky and M.R. Wick (eds.), *Evidence Based Pathology and Laboratory Medicine*,
DOI 10.1007/978-1-4419-1030-1_1, © Springer Science+Business Media, LLC 2011

Assessment of the Institute of Medicine emphasized as recently as the early 1980s the need to develop well-designed studies to evaluate technologies [10, 11]. Well-planned prospective randomized clinical trials (RCT) demonstrated that certain common practices, such as the use of anti-arrhythmic drugs to prevent heart attacks, lacked good evidence to support their usefulness and could be harmful to patients [12]. Few clinical guidelines were available at the time, but in the mid-1980s, an increasing interest in "outcomes research" led to the development of a large number of clinical trials and "evidence-based" guidelines that have recently grown into the thousands [13–16].

Medical data proliferate at an ever-increasing rate and often include a variety of features that are far too complex, uncertain, or even contradictory for analysis using simple "If–Then" logic. These problems have led to a deeper appreciation for the need to incorporate computer-based analytical methods that are more widely used in other disciplines such as epidemiology, engineering, and business [6, 17–21]. They include various analytical tools of Decision Analysis theory such as decision trees, utility theory, and Bayes theorem that can be used to estimate the validity of diagnostic tests, perform cost-effectiveness analysis, analyze with meta-analysis the effectiveness of various interventions, render more consistent and effective decisions that affect the welfare of individual patients, and evaluate the effectiveness of the various paradigms used in medical care [6, 18–21].

Evolution of Evidence-Based Medicine into a Well-Established Discipline

EBM evolved as a discipline in the United States, Canada and the UK in the 1990s and is already a well-established discipline that is now taught in many medical schools, through graduate programs, books, and other educational resources [5, 22, 23]. The American College of Physicians (ACP) developed the Clinical Efficacy Assessment Project in 1981 to promote the use of literature reviews and guidelines for various topics [24]. The American Cancer Society has sponsored the development of Evidence-Based Guidelines (EBG) for specific diseases using the following general concepts: "First there must be good evidence that each test or procedure recommended is medically effective in reducing morbidity or mortality; second, the medical benefits must outweigh the risks; third, the cost of each test or procedure must be reasonable compared to its expected benefits; and finally, the recommended actions must be practical and feasible" [6, 25–27]. Several centers have been dedicated to the development of medical practice guidelines based on "best evidence," such as the Cochrane collaboration in Oxford, the Centre for Evidence-Based Medicine at Oxford University, Cancer Care Ontario in Canada, the National Guideline Clearinghouse sponsored by the Agency for Healthcare Research and Quality (AHRQ), and others [16, 28, 29]. AHRQ has also promoted EBM-based research and policies and the development of Evidence-based Practice Centers to produce reports and technology assessments [28]. A wealth of books and other publications about EBM and its applications to a variety of subjects is available. For example, the *British Medical Journal* publishing group launched various journals available online: "Clinical Evidence," "Evidence Based Medicine," "Evidence Based Mental Health," "Evidence Based Nursing" to publish EBM type studies. The concepts of EBM have also spread beyond EBG into "evidence-based coverage," "evidence-based performance measures," and policies regarding quality improvement, medical necessity, and regulations.

Evidence-Based Medicine as a New Approach to Teaching the Practice of Medicine

The Evidence-based Medicine Working Group proposed in 1992 the use of EBM as a new approach to teaching the practice of Medicine [1–4, 12]. The emphasis was on individual physicians collecting computerized literature searches looking at the sensitivity and specificity of tests, selecting a test, assigning a pretest probability, calculating a posttest probability, and developing a management plan. The terminology of evidence-based individual decision-making or EBID has been proposed.

Basic Concepts of Evidence-Based Medicine

How is the Use of Medical Information Approached from the Standpoint of Evidence-Based Medicine?

EBM investigators attempt to identify the best current and relevant research information available for a particular problem and to integrate it into guidelines, rules, or other tools that will assist medical practitioners in their daily practice. Sackett and associates have suggested the use of five steps for the identification of "best evidence" and its integration with personal clinical expertise and values into guidelines, rules, or other protocols that can be used for the care of individual patients (Table 1.1) [1–4, 12]. Richard Gross summarizes the first four steps of Sacket et al., using the acronym "FRAP" – framing evidence-based questions, retrieving relevant evidence, appraising the quality and appropriateness of the evidence, and patient-based decision-making [22].

Table 1.1 Evidence-based medicine approach to the use and evaluation of information in daily practice

Formulation of specific questions regarding diagnosis, prognosis, causation, and/or treatment of any given clinical problem
Search for specific information in the scientific literature
Critical appraisal of the validity of the evidence, and its impact, applicability, and usefulness in clinical practice
Incorporation of "best evidence" from several "reliable" sources along with personal clinical experience, for the development of "Evidence-based" guidelines, rules, or other protocols
Evaluation of the effectiveness and efficiency of those recommendations

Basic Process for the Identification of Best Evidence and Its Integration into Guidelines, Rules, or Other Protocols

1. *Formulation of specific questions regarding the diagnosis, prognosis, causation, and/or treatment of a patient with a particular clinical problem*
   Evidence-based questions ideally attempt to address those issues that are most relevant to the materials being studied [1, 3–5]. These questions need to address a detailed query whose answer will provide useful and practical information for patient care. For example, if a pathologist is interested in comparing the results of the immunostains of a particular neoplasm, the summary of evidence from the literature would need to include specific questions such as: Which tissues were studied? What percentage of cells was used as a threshold for positive immunoreactivity? How where the changes quantitated or semiquantitated? What structures exhibited immunoreactivity? What antibodies were used? Did the study report the use of proper controls? What dilutions were used? What sensitivities and specificities were reported? Were the results compared with appropriate statistical tests? Did the study have sufficient power to detect significant differences in immunoreactivity? Table 1.2 lists examples

Table 1.2 Queries proposed for the assessment of "prognostic" information in the context of evidence-based medicine

Is the evidence valid?
Was the sample of patients assembled at the same point of the disease?
Can it be applied to individual patients?
Was the follow-up period sufficiently long and complete?
Were the results validated with a group of test (holdout) cases?
Is it important?
How likely are the outcomes over time?
How precise are the prognostic estimates?
Are the patients in the study being referred to similar to those of the physician using the evidence?
Will the evidence in hand have a significant impact in managing the disease in question?

of questions suggested by Sackett and colleagues to be considered in the assessment of studies that report "prognostic" information.

2. *Search for specific information in the scientific literature*
Hundreds of electronic bibliographic databases are currently available online. MEDLINE/PubMed is probably the database most familiar to pathologists, but it does not identify all known published RCT [30–32]. Other online databases include Cancerlit, Embase, "CENTRAL," developed by the Cochrane collaboration, MD Consult, UpToDate, Micromedex, STAT!Ref, SKOLAR MD, Australasian Medical Index, Chinese Biomedical Literature Database, Latin American Caribbean Health Sciences Literatures (LILACS), Japan Information Centre of Scientific and Technology File on Science, Technology and Medicine (JICST-E), AIDSLINE, SciSearch, TrailsCentral, and many others. Subscription-based lists of EBM-based guidelines such as EBMG and Web of Science are also available online (Figs. 1.1 and 1.2) [33–35].

Such a bewildering array of information sources has stimulated the development of better search engines that apply more advanced methods than simple Boolean searches based on the analysis of previously indexed information [36–39]. For example, the developers of the widely used web search engine Google have recently sponsored the development of Google Scholar to automatically analyze and extract citations from a variety of "scholarly"

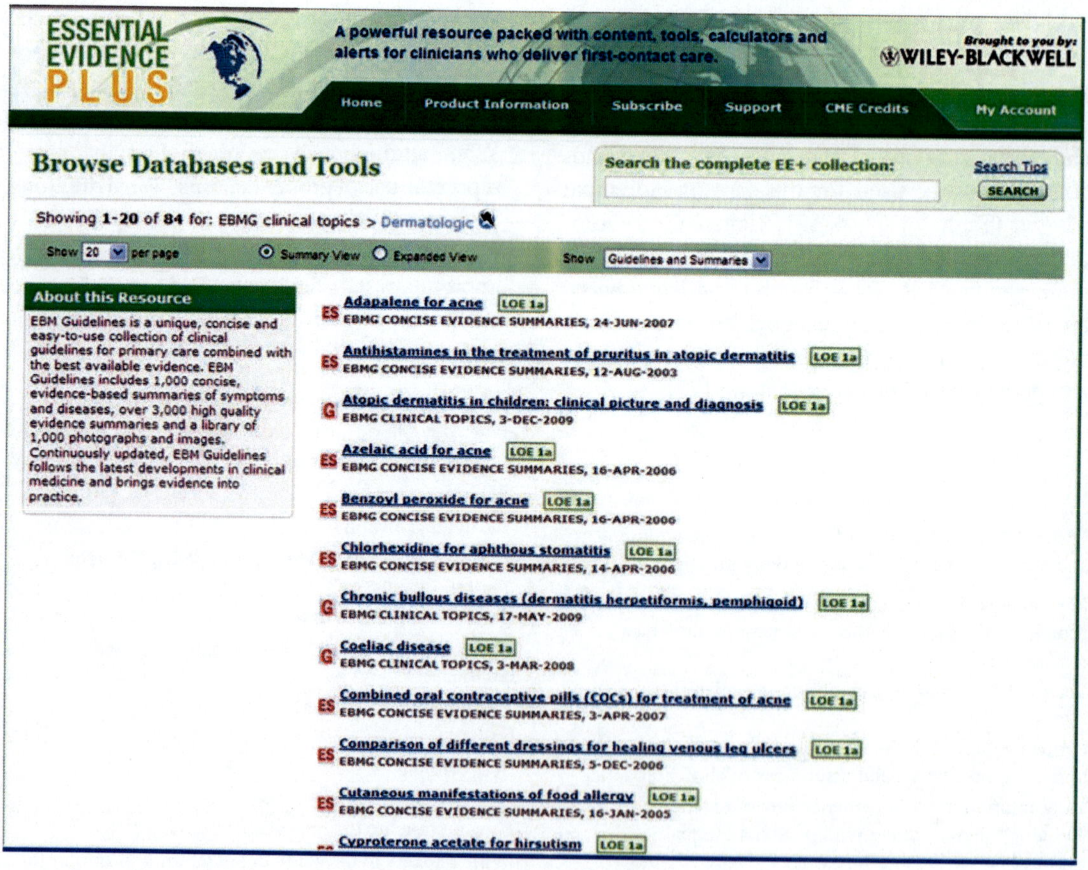

Fig. 1.1 Although pathologists are most familiar with the search engine Pubmed of the National Library of Medicine, there are other online services to retrieve scientific references. This figure shows the web page of Essential Evidence Plus, sponsored by a publisher, Wiley-Blackwell

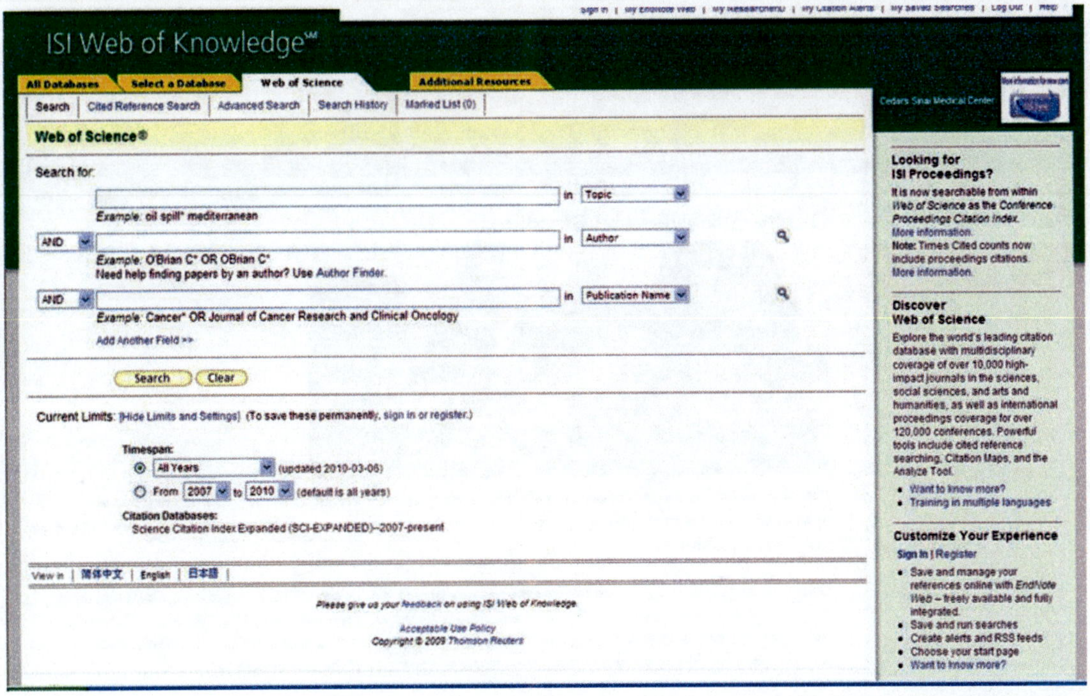

Fig. 1.2 Web page of another specialized search engine to retrieve scientific references, ISI Web of Knowledge. This search engine and the one shown in Fig. 1.1 are available only through individual or institutional subscriptions

literature and present them as separate results search even if the documents they refer to are not online [36–39]. The results of each query are organized by how relevant the information is to the query, using proprietary algorithms.

(a) *Best-evidence summaries*

Various formats have been proposed to summarize the "best evidence" into "evidence summaries" that include, in addition to the answers to the specific questions, information about the sources of the selected evidence, methods used for selection, estimates of precision and reliability, and other important details [5, 22]. Multiple Practice Guidelines and Evidence summaries have been developed by various organizations and are readily available online. For example, the web site of Cancer Care Ontario makes available a variety of Practice Guidelines and Evidence Summaries by disease site (Fig. 1.3) [40]. These documents generally list the dates of the original guidelines and subsequent updates, the guideline questions, the target population, description of methodology, recommendations, key evidence, related guidelines, and key contacts for further information. The Cochrane Collaboration also makes available online an EBM manual summarizing a variety of interesting topics and numerous guidelines published using a common format (Fig. 1.4) [41, 42]. To our knowledge, there are no such EBM-based Practice Guidelines and Evidence Summaries in Pathology. The Association of Directors of Anatomic and Surgical Pathology, the Cancer Committee of the CAP, and other groups have published "recommendations," "cancer protocols," and other documents that provide guidelines to practicing pathologists (Fig. 1.5) [43–46]. These documents have been developed by committees or other groups of experts, based on their experience and understanding of the "current state of the art," rather than the more analytical process followed by the proponents of EBM.

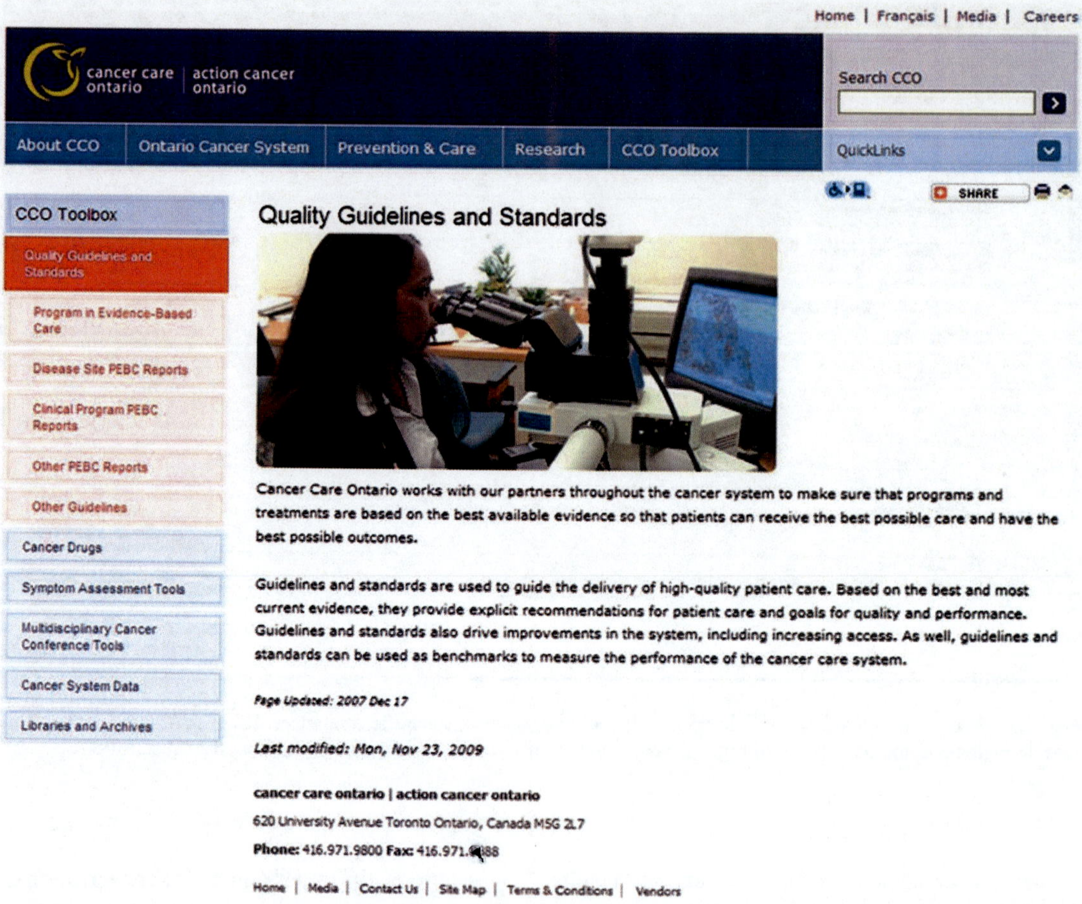

Fig. 1.3 Web site of Cancer Care Ontario showing the CCO toolbox with various practice guidelines. Other institutions in multiple countries offer similar evidence-based practice guidelines

(b) *Text data mining for the automated analysis of natural language texts*

A vast amount of information is available on the Web, textbooks, and other formats in unstructured text written in the natural language form [33–35, 39]. There is an increasing interest in computer science at developing tools to "mine" textual information with tools that can navigate text bases, creating summaries of documents, cluster them, and carry out semantic retrieval of information using neural network tools and other "intelligent" agents. Novel software tools such as TextAnalyst (Megaputer, Inc.), SAS TextMiners (SAS, Cary, NC), and others provide interesting tools for the future automated analysis of data available in pathology reports and other repositories of documents. Multiple online resources are available listing software, books, and other resources for text mining.

3. *Critical appraisal of the validity of the available evidence, and its impact, applicability, and usefulness in clinical practice*

(a) *Statistical significance: Type I and II statistical errors*

The quality and appropriateness of medical evidence is generally assessed with quantitative tools that are well known by clinical pathologists and some anatomic pathologists [47–51]. The purpose of most research projects is to search for "statistically significant" evidence that the value of a parameter in a population of interest is different from the value of this feature in a control group [6, 26].

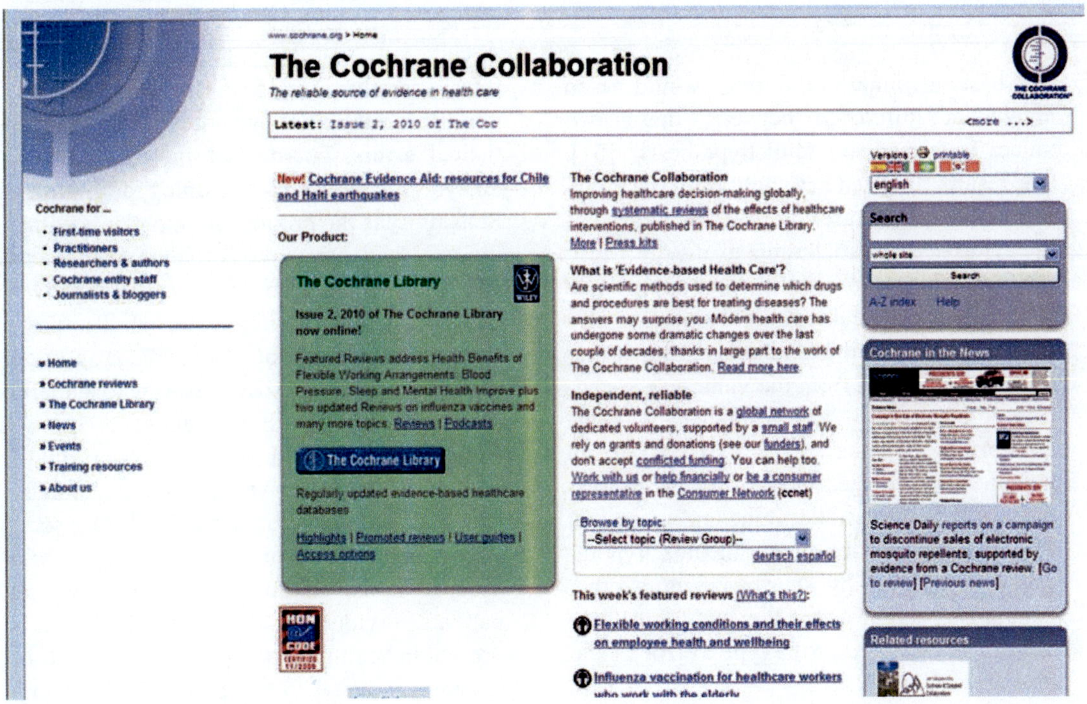

Fig. 1.4 Web site of the Cochrane collaboration, an international institution that has been a pioneer in the development of evidence-based guidelines

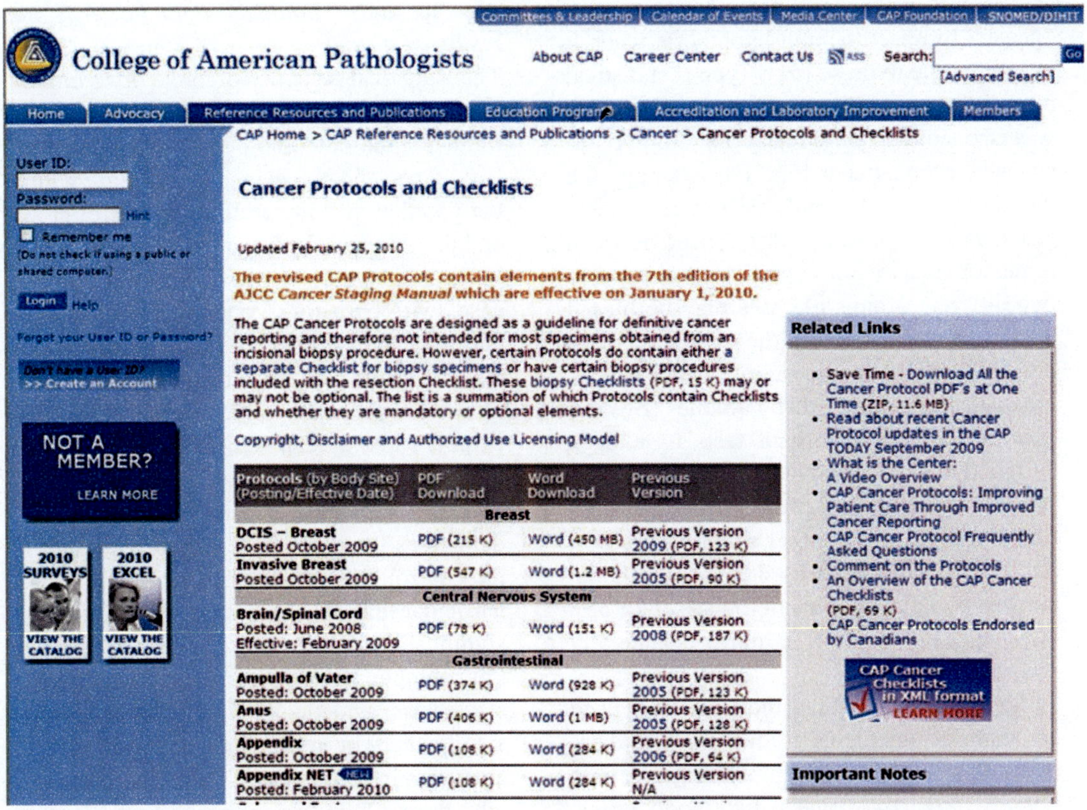

Fig. 1.5 The web site of the College of American Pathologists makes available numerous cancer protocols and checklists that are now being used in daily practice by most American pathologists

The basic assumption that there would be no significant difference between these two values is termed the "null hypothesis" [51]. The results collected in a study from the group of cases of interest are compared with those of the reference control group using the t-test, ANOVA, chi-square, and/or other appropriate descriptive statistical tests. If the p-value of a parameter measured from a study group is significantly different from the value in the control group by a p value smaller by some arbitrary cutoff value, such as $p<0.05$, the null hypothesis is rejected in favor of the alternative [6, 51]. A $p<0.05$ value indicates that there is a 5% probability that the null hypothesis was rejected by spurious factors other than those being tested in the study. This type of error is classified as the type I error in statistical textbooks.

An additional important potential source of error that is seldom given consideration in observational studies in pathology is whether the research study was designed with enough "power" to reject the null hypothesis when it is appropriate to do so [51]. Type II statistical error is the probability that the test in question will erroneously fail to reject the null hypothesis when the latter is true. For example, the fact that a particular study fails to establish a statistically significant difference between immunoreactivity for a particular epitope in two different groups of cases may be biased by the characteristics of the staining procedure, staining selection, sample size, variability of the data, and other variables. Several "power analysis" statistical tests have been designed to estimate for the probability of type II errors in scientific studies and are used routinely in RCT and in other scientific studies, but have seldom been used in observational studies by anatomic pathologists [52, 53]. A value of power=0.80 or higher is generally recommended.

Statistical calculations that have been used in laboratory medicine studies include measures of sensitivity, specificity, negative and positive predictive values, likelihood ratios, receiver-operator curves, misclassification rates, and others [54, 55]. These tests provide good information about potential type I statistical errors, but do not include "power" analysis to analyze for possible type II errors. Sensitivity is the proportion of patients with a disease who have a positive test, whereas specificity is the proportion of true negatives of all the negative samples tested. The positive predictive value of a test is the proportion of patients with a positive result who actually have the disease, while negative predictive value is represented by the proportion of patients with a negative test who are actually free of disease. Likelihood ratio (LR) associated with a positive test calculates the probability that the finding is seen in diseased patients, divided by the probability that is present in healthy people; the posttest odds of disease are equal to the pretest odds of disease multiplied by the LR.

(a) *Bayesian approach to the analysis of data: influence of prior probability of a finding and need to study "holdout" data to verify the results of a study*

The statistical tests listed above offer limited information about other features that can influence the outcome of observational studies, such as the prevalence of a disease within the population study and in the control group and the prior probability of a finding [56–60]. For example, the sensitivity of the AFB test in cases with caseating granulomas is probably better than in cases without granulomatous disease, as the pathologist is likely to examine more carefully the slides from cases that exhibit pathological findings that are known to be caused by mycobacteria. The prior probability of a finding can be simplistically defined as the probability that it is present in the control group. The prior probability for a particular finding can change dramatically the significance of the results of a particular study. For example, it is well known that lymph node status has a statistically significant prognostic significance in most patients with cancer. However, in patients with Stage IV neoplasms who have a high "prior probability" of dying from their disease, the prognostic value of the feature lymph node status is probably rather limited. Likewise, the value of certain immunophenotype for the determination of the site of origin of a neoplasm is also probably quite variable, dependent on what other clinico-pathologic information is available [61]. For example, an adenocarcinoma within a mediastinal lymph node that exhibits negative immunoreactivity for TTF-1 has, in our experience, a higher prior probability of representing a metastasis from a lung cancer than from an extrathoracic neoplasm with similar histological features. The "prior probability" of this assessment is probably a lot higher if the patient also has a single lung mass on chest imaging studies and a positron emission tomogram (PET) that shows only a positive lung mass. These considerations are intuitively used in daily practice by most pathologists, but there are few, if any, available EBG or other protocols that take into consideration the prevalence and prior probability of various findings into the selection and/or interpretation of immunostains or other ancillary tests in Anatomic Pathology.

Another consideration that has not been addressed in most observational studies in pathology is the need to divide the data into "training" or "testing" sets ("study" and "hold-out" cases) in observational studies attempting to derive classification or prognostic models [57, 59, 62]. Most clinico-pathological categorization has been based on data derived from analyzing the data from study groups and control groups with descriptive univariate, and less often multivariate, statistical methods. However, multiple studies using Bayesian methods have shown that models derived by the use of 100% of a dataset are not necessarily robust when applied to other datasets, as there is a certain element of "circular reasoning" in the modeling methodology. EBM emphasizes the value of RCT, of using prospective and retrospective data, and the need to compare the results from a study set with those of an "unknown" set that has not been used for the derivation of the classificatory model [1, 2, 15, 63, 64]. As discussed later on in this article, scientific papers using the latter methodology are given a higher value of credibility. To our knowledge, there have been few attempts to apply this methodology to most classification schema being used in Surgical Pathology and Cytopathology, perhaps providing an explanation for the high interobserver variability of certain diagnoses.

(b) *Interobserver variability: assessment with kappa statistics and effect on the interpretation of observational studies*
It is well known that the diagnosis of various neoplasms and nonneoplastic conditions using histopathology is subject to a certain degree of interobserver variability [65]. For example, lung pathologists can disagree in the classification of about 30% of certain neuroendocrine pulmonary neoplasms and 50% of poorly differentiated nonsmall cell lung carcinomas [65–67]. This variability can be measured with the so-called kappa statistics that estimate the proportion of chance versus expected agreements taking into consideration the fact that the raters and the samples are not independent from each other [68–72]. Kappa coefficients of 0.8 or higher are considered as good agreement rates. This methodology has been used mostly in cytopathology and in some surgical pathology and other studies.

However, little consideration has been generally given to the influence of interobserver variability in the assessment of the reproducibility of certain classification schema in Anatomic Pathology and the prognostic and predictive value of selected observations. For example, in a situation when pathologists have difficulties distinguishing small cell carcinoma, atypical carcinoid tumor, and nonsmall cell carcinomas of the lung in about a third of the cases, and the 5-year survival proportions for patients with these neoplasms vary from 0 to 50%, what would be the statistical "power" of a study needed to determine whether all these diagnostic categories have independent prognostic or predictive value? Could other stratification of the cases into categories such as "high-grade neuroendocrine carcinomas" and "atypical carcinoid" provide better discriminatory data? To our knowledge, there is no "best evidence" in the pathology literature to answer these questions. Another example could be a hypothetical situation where pathologists agree less than 100% of the time whether a resection margin is involved or not by a neoplasm and subsequent resection specimens detect residual tumor in a slightly smaller proportion of the patients who had negative margins than those with initially positive margins. How can we determine whether reexcision is a valuable procedure based on this "evidence"? How many cases would be needed to study this question with sufficient power? Could there be some definition of "positive" margin that would decrease the rate of interobserver variability, changing the parameters used for the evaluation of this problem? Future studies that address this type of practical problem with methodology that takes into account some of the analytical concepts being promoted by practitioners of EBM may improve the precision of specimen-derived data.

4. *Incorporation of "best evidence" from several reliable sources along with personal clinical experience into "evidence-based" guidelines, rules, or other protocols*

(a) *Evaluating the quality of published studies in the medical literature*

The medical literature includes many descriptive studies that include single case reports, large observational analyses involving many patients, and scientific studies in which a hypothesis is tested prospectively with appropriate controls [6, 26]. Observational studies are definitely valuable, but they suffer from biases owing to case selection, reporting methods, characteristics of control groups ("healthy cohort effect"), and other factors listed in Table 1.3 [1, 2, 4, 16, 73]. EBM studies also are influenced by "publication bias." Although pathologists frequently have a limited ability to control all these possible sources of bias in their observational studies, EBM does raise interesting questions about study design and interpretation of the data that could lead to better future approaches to the use of "specimen-based" data in improved diagnostic and prognostic models.

Table 1.3 Sources of bias in observational and other comparative studies

Selection bias (samples of convenience and others)
Sample size
Ratio between the number of observations and the number of variables
Characteristics of the control group (healthy cohort effect)
Performance bias
Attrition bias
Detection bias
Distribution of the data (normal vs. others)
Interpretation of the results
Lack of independent validation group
Publication bias

Ebell has proposed a system for classifying published medical evidence into four levels, with "grade I" being the best (most reliable) [23]. Grade I studies are those that include data validated with a "test" group that is from a different and distinct population from the "training" cohort. For example, a classification or a prognostic rule might be developed in one group of patients and validated in another. Grade II studies report data that are obtained from the same population, the members of which are divided into independent "training" and "validation" subsets and evaluated prospectively. Grade III analysis also include "training" and "validation" subsets from the same population, but data are collected contemporaneously rather than prospectively. Grade IV studies are those in which the "training" group is also used as the "validation group." According to this scheme, most studies in the pathology literature would probably be classified as Grade IV and are particularly vulnerable to the problems listed in Table 1.3.

(b) *Integration of "best evidence" from the literature with personal clinical experience into "evidence-based" guidelines, rules, or other protocols*

As mentioned earlier, advocates of EBM have attempted to organize "best evidence" from the scientific literature and their own experience into algorithms, protocols, guidelines, or "rules" that guide individual patient care by practitioners. Pathologists may benefit from emulating this approach, in future efforts at constructing "patient-based" prognostic and predictive models. For example, immunostains are most often used to distinguish between various neoplasms in a descriptive manner. Studies using immunostains in the pathology literature usually list the percentage of lesions that label for particular epitopes, as well as the sensitivity, specificity, and predictive values of such markers in narrow morphological contexts. However, few studies have assessed LR or other probabilistic measures as applied to *panels* of markers in selected differential diagnoses [60, 74] . At an even more basic level, the relative statistical values attending particular *morphological* findings have seldom been analyzed in the same fashion, to our knowledge.

In contrast, several prognostic scoring models or "rules" that integrate multivariate pathological, clinical, imaging, and other information are being developed by other specialists [75]. For example, Kattan and associates have developed pretreatment nomograms [76] that combine clinical and pathological data from prostate cancer patients and predict 5-year probability of metastasis .

5. *Evaluation of the effectiveness and efficiency of those "evidence-based" recommendations* The fact that a scientific study has been published in a peer-reviewed journal probably does not guarantee that the study design was methodologically sound, that the research was well conducted, the data analyzed correctly, and/or the results interpreted properly. Therefore, "evidence-based" information has become almost a "de rigueur" label in health care to convey a measure of credibility. However, as discussed recently by Steinberg and Luce, there is considerable variability in how information is been assembled, evaluated, and synthesized in different EBM type studies [77]. Different systems have been proposed for rating the stability and strength of medical evidence and are discussed in Chapter 13. [78] .

What Has Been the Impact of EBM in Improving the Quality of Medical Practices in the United States?

EBG have had a limited success at improving the overall quality of Medicine in the U.S and has elicited somewhat of a backlash from practitioners revolting against "cookbook medicine" [79–83]. Organizations sponsoring EBG have at times struggled to maintain these guidelines current. Research into the daily practices of physicians has demonstrated that the wide availability of new scientific data and/or clinical guidelines using "best evidence" has had a rather limited effect in changing the behavior of medical practitioners. Somewhat surprisingly, it can take years for physicians to incorporate new information into their practices and change their approach to the diagnosis and treatment of individual patients.

Pathology and Evidence-Based Medicine

Interestingly, pathology has not been an active participant in the EBM "movement" in spite of being considered as one of the more "scientific" branches of Medicine and a long and proud history of providing strong leadership among medical specialties in quality assurance and quality improvement issues [62]. Pathologists have faced to date limited scrutiny about the specificity and the cost-effectiveness of multiple practices. For example, although it is well documented that there can be considerable interobserver variability in the diagnosis of various disease entities with histopathology, there have been limited attempts at developing formal EBG or diagnostic algorithms to standardize these practices and proficiency testing programs to assess the effectiveness of these efforts. There is currently little consensus about "standard of practices" for the use and interpretation of immunostains and other ancillary studies for the diagnosis of various diseases and for the development of prognostic and predictive models for patients with various neoplasms and nonneoplastic conditions. Pathologists have had limited opportunities in the past to provide input into schema such as the TNM system developed by the American Joint Commission on Cancer (AJCC) [43]. Indeed, some of the current staging guidelines lack specific definitional detail that could help to decrease some of the variability in pathology practice. Most attempts at providing tools to improve the standardization of reporting information to practicing pathologists have been via published protocols developed by professional societies, such as the Cancer Protocols developed by the College of American Pathologists (CAP) or the Reporting Recommendations by the Association of Directors of Surgical Pathology and Anatomic Pathology (Fig. 1.6) [43]. Those documents have been written by groups of pathologists appointed by these organizations for their subspecialty or other experience and are based on the semisubjective "authoritative" interpretation of current practices and available information by these individuals. This approach may be effective, but it is based on opinion rather than on "best evidence" taken from a systematic analysis of data collected from controlled studies. Moreover, there have been to our knowledge few attempts at evaluating whether practicing pathologists are using the elements suggested in these guidelines in their daily practice and in estimating the effectiveness of these recommendations and protocols for the improvement of patient outcomes.

The College of American Pathologists (CAP) has also sponsored several multidisciplinary "consensus conferences," in which groups of specialists in different medical fields convened to perform systematic reviews of the literature, discussed salient problems, selected "best evidence," and proposed guidelines for their clinical management. These sessions have closely approximated the general idiom of EBM. More recently, the CAP has offered an EBM course at its annual meeting and the US and Canadian Academy of Pathology (USCAP) has sponsored a course on Evidence Based Pathology and Decision Analysis that is now available on line at http://www.uscap.org.

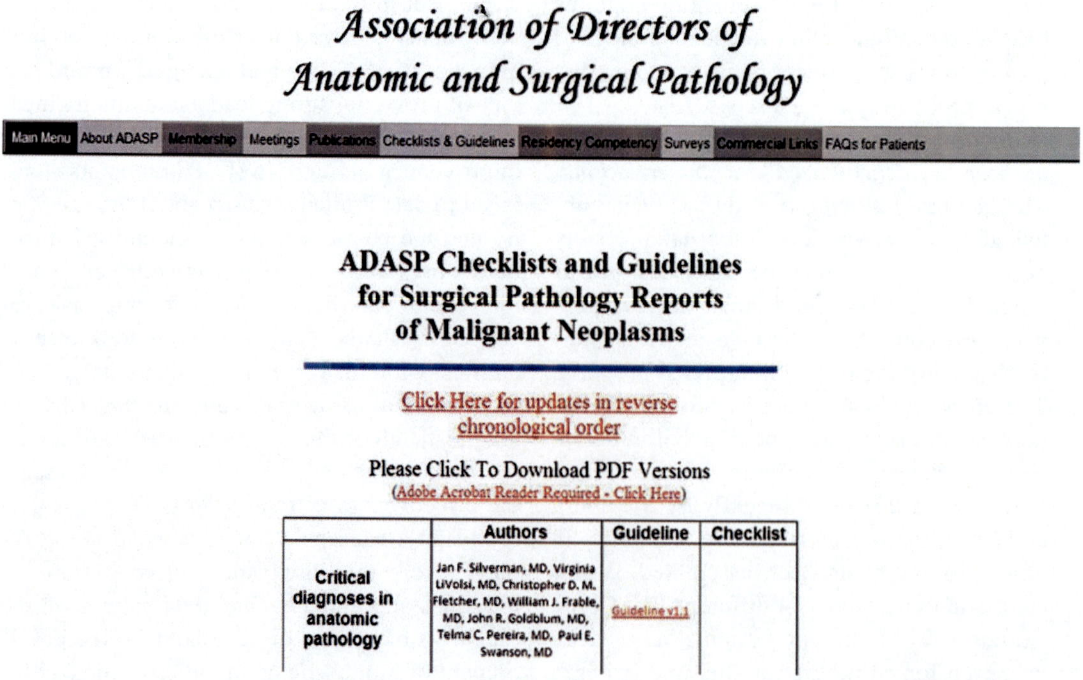

Fig. 1.6 The web site of the Association of Directors of Anatomic and Surgical Pathology (ADASP) also has multiple practice guidelines labeled as recommendations

Evidence-Based Medicine in the Future of Pathology

The increased interest in EBM through the healthcare environment poses risks for Pathology and Laboratory Medicine. Physicians and healthcare administrators familiar with the methodology being used for RCT and other studies that evaluate the efficacy and cost-effectiveness of selected procedures may decide that the utility provided by certain lab tests generated by either anatomic pathology or the clinical laboratory is not supported by "best evidence" and should not be reimbursed. EBM also offers an opportunity to use some of the concepts and methods described in this book to reassess the clinical effectiveness of classification schema being used by pathologists and to develop better diagnostic and prognostic models, more rational approaches for test selection, and better tools to evaluate the cost-effectiveness of various tests [25, 26, 84]. Examples of topics that could benefit from an EBM approach include evaluation of whether certain "pathologic entities" are based on "best evidence" and/or provide clinically valuable information, the development of EBG for the use and the interpretation of immunostains and other ancillary tests for specific differential diagnosis situations and for the selection and interpretation of laboratory tests in the context of specific clinical problems, evaluation of the effectiveness of selected practices such as the use of synoptic reports and checklists versus narrative reports, assessment of the effectiveness of various teaching activities, and others.

References

1. Sackett D. Evidence-based medicine. Lancet. 1995;346:1171.
2. Sackett DL, Rosenberg WM, Gray JA, et al. Evidence based medicine: what it is and what it isn't. BMJ. 1996;312:71–2.
3. Sackett DL. Evidence-based medicine. Semin Perinatol. 1997;21:3–5.
4. Straus SE, Sackett DL. Bringing evidence to the clinic. Arch Dermatol. 1998;134:1519–20.
5. Straus SE, Richardson WS, Glasziou P, et al. Evidence-based medicine. How to practice and teach EBM. New York, NY: Elsevier; 2005.
6. Marchevsky AM, Wick MR. Evidence-based medicine, medical decision analysis, and pathology. Hum Pathol. 2004;35:1179–88.
7. Fleming KA. Evidence-based pathology. J Pathol. 1996;179:127–8.
8. Costa J. Reflections about evidence-based pathology. Int J Surg Pathol. 2007;15:230–2.
9. U.S. Department of Health and Human Services Agency for Healthcare Research and Quality. Technology assessment. 2010.
10. Steinberg EP, Graziano S. Integrating technology assessment and medical practice evaluation into hospital operations. QRB Qual Rev Bull. 1990;16:218–22.
11. Steinberg EP. Health care technology assessment. Med Sect Proc. 1986;53–63.
12. Sackett DL, Rosenberg WM. The need for evidence-based medicine. J R Soc Med. 1995;88:620–4.
13. Carson SS. Outcomes research: methods and implications. Semin Respir Crit Care Med. 2010;31:3–12.
14. Carter BS. A new era of outcomes research. Neurosurgery. 2009;64:N15.
15. Krumholz HM. Outcomes research: myths and realities. Circ Cardiovasc Qual Outcomes. 2009;2:1–3.
16. Tanjong-Ghogomu E, Tugwell P, Welch V. Evidence-based medicine and the Cochrane Collaboration. Bull NYU Hosp Jt Dis. 2009;67:198–205.
17. Peirolo R, Scalerandi M. Markovian model of growth and histologic progression in prostate cancer. Phys Rev E Stat Nonlin Soft Matter Phys. 2004;70:011902.
18. Brown AW, Malec JF, McClelland RL, et al. Clinical elements that predict outcome after traumatic brain injury: a prospective multicenter recursive partitioning (decision-tree) analysis. J Neurotrauma. 2005;22:1040–51.
19. Galligan DT, Ramberg C, Curtis C, et al. Application of portfolio theory in decision tree analysis. J Dairy Sci. 1991;74:2138–44.
20. Hui L, Liping G. Statistical estimation of diagnosis with genetic markers based on decision tree analysis of complex disease. Comput Biol Med. 2009;39:989–92.
21. Link RE, Allaf ME, Pili R, et al. Modeling the cost of management options for stage I nonseminomatous germ cell tumors: a decision tree analysis. J Clin Oncol. 2005;23:5762–73.
22. Gross R. Decisions and evidence in medical practice. St. Louis, MO: Mosby; 2001.
23. Ebell MH. Evidence-based diagnosis. New York, NY: Springer; 2001.
24. American College of Physicians. Clinical efficacy assessment project. Internet Communication. 2010.
25. Marchevsky AM. The application of special technologies in diagnostic anatomic pathology: is it consistent with the principles of evidence-based medicine? Semin Diagn Pathol. 2005;22:156–66.

26. Marchevsky AM. Evidence-based medicine in pathology: an introduction. Semin Diagn Pathol. 2005;22:105–15.
27. American Cancer Society. Treatment decision tools. Internet Communication. 2010.
28. Agency for Healthcare Research and Quality (AHRQ). National guideline clearinghouse. Internet Communication. 2010.
29. Clarke M. The Cochrane Collaboration and the Cochrane Library. Otolaryngol Head Neck Surg. 2007;137:S52–4.
30. Chen TH, Li L, Kochen MM. A systematic review: how to choose appropriate health-related quality of life (HRQOL) measures in routine general practice? J Zhejiang Univ Sci B. 2005;6:936–40.
31. Deenadayalan Y, Grimmer-Somers K, Prior M, et al. How to run an effective journal club: a systematic review. J Eval Clin Pract. 2008;14:898–911.
32. Hunt DL, Haynes RB. How to read a systematic review. Indian J Pediatr. 2000;67:63–6.
33. Vanhecke TE, Barnes MA, Zimmerman J, et al. PubMed vs. HighWire Press: a head-to-head comparison of two medical literature search engines. Comput Biol Med. 2007;37:1252–8.
34. Booth A. Mapping the evidence base of pathology. J Pathol. 1999;188:344–50.
35. Rapport RL, Lancaster FW, Penry JK. Critical evaluation of a computer-based medical literature search and retrieval system. Postgrad Med. 1972;51:47–50.
36. Bakkalbasi N, Bauer K, Glover J, et al. Three options for citation tracking: Google Scholar, Scopus and Web of Science. Biomed Digit Libr. 2006;3:7.
37. Freeman MK, Lauderdale SA, Kendrach MG, et al. Google Scholar versus PubMed in locating primary literature to answer drug-related questions. Ann Pharmacother. 2009;43:478–84.
38. Kulkarni AV, Aziz B, Shams I, et al. Comparisons of citations in Web of Science, Scopus, and Google Scholar for articles published in general medical journals. JAMA. 2009;302:1092–6.
39. Shultz M. Comparing test searches in PubMed and Google Scholar. J Med Libr Assoc. 2007;95:442–5.
40. Cancer Care Ontario. Cancer Care Ontario. Internet Communication. 2010.
41. Anonymous. What does the Cochrane Collaboration say about adherence to evidence-based practice recommendations? Physiother Can. 2009;61:116.
42. Winkelstein Jr W. The remarkable Archie: origins of the Cochrane Collaboration. Epidemiology. 2009;20:779.
43. Amin MB. The 2009 version of the cancer protocols of the college of American pathologists. Arch Pathol Lab Med. 2010;134:326–30.
44. Amin MB. Key issues in reporting common cancer specimen findings using the College of American Pathologists cancer protocols. Arch Pathol Lab Med. 2006;130:284–6.
45. Fechner RE. Selected topics from ADASP. Am J Clin Pathol. 1996;106:S1–2.
46. Simpson PR, Tschang TP. ADASP recommendations: consultations in surgical pathology. Association of Directors of Anatomic and Surgical Pathology. Hum Pathol. 1993;24:1382.
47. Vollmer RT. Primary lung cancer vs metastatic breast cancer: a probabilistic approach. Am J Clin Pathol. 2009;132:391–5.
48. Multivariate statistical analysis for anatomic pathology. Part II: failure time analysis. Am J Clin Pathol. 1996;106:522–34.
49. Multivariate statistical analysis for pathologist. Part I, The logistic model. Am J Clin Pathol. 1996;105: 115–26.
50. Vollmer RT. Twin concordance: a set theoretic and probability theory approach. J Theor Biol. 1972;36:367–78.
51. Snedecor GW, Cochran WG. Statistical methods. Ames, IA: The Iowa State University Press; 1980.
52. Connelly LM. Research considerations: power analysis and effect size. Medsurg Nurs. 2008;17:41–2.
53. Zodpey SP. Sample size and power analysis in medical research. Indian J Dermatol Venereol Leprol. 2004;70:123–8.
54. Giard RW, Hermans J. The diagnostic information of tests for the detection of cancer: the usefulness of the likelihood ratio concept. Eur J Cancer. 1996;32A: 2042–8.
55. Hara M, Kanemitsu Y, Hirai T, et al. Negative serum carcinoembryonic antigen has insufficient accuracy for excluding recurrence from patients with Dukes C colorectal cancer: analysis with likelihood ratio and posttest probability in a follow-up study. Dis Colon Rectum. 2008;51:1675–80.
56. Gupta R, Dastane AM, McKenna Jr R, et al. The predictive value of epidermal growth factor receptor tests in patients with pulmonary adenocarcinoma: review of current "best evidence" with meta-analysis. Hum Pathol. 2009;40:356–65.
57. Gupta R, Dastane A, McKenna Jr RJ, et al. What can we learn from the errors in the frozen section diagnosis of pulmonary carcinoid tumors? An evidence-based approach. Hum Pathol. 2009;40:1–9.
58. Gupta R, McKenna Jr R, Marchevsky AM. Lessons learned from mistakes and deferrals in the frozen section diagnosis of bronchioloalveolar carcinoma and well-differentiated pulmonary adenocarcinoma: an evidence-based pathology approach. Am J Clin Pathol. 2008;130:11–20.
59. Herbst J, Jenders R, McKenna R, et al. Evidence-based criteria to help distinguish metastatic breast cancer from primary lung adenocarcinoma on thoracic frozen section. Am J Clin Pathol. 2009; 131:122–8.
60. Westfall DE, Fan X, Marchevsky AM. Evidence-based guidelines to optimize the selection of antibody panels in cytopathology: pleural effusions with malignant epithelioid cells. Diagn Cytopathol. 2010; 38:9–14.
61. Marchevsky AM, Gupta R, Balzer B. Diagnosis of metastatic neoplasms: a clinicopathologic and morphologic approach. Arch Pathol Lab Med. 2010;134:194–206.

62. Marchevsky AM, Wick MR. Evidence levels for publications in pathology and laboratory medicine. Am J Clin Pathol. 2010;133:366–7.
63. Cundiff DK. Evidence-based medicine and the Cochrane Collaboration on trial. MedGenMed. 2007; 9:56.
64. Overman VP. The Cochrane collaboration. Int J Dent Hyg. 2007;5:62.
65. Travis WD, Gal AA, Colby TV, et al. Reproducibility of neuroendocrine lung tumor classification. Hum Pathol. 1998;29:272–9.
66. Hirsch FR, Matthews MJ, Yesner R. Histopathologic classification of small cell carcinoma of the lung: comments based on an interobserver examination. Cancer. 1982;50:1360–6.
67. Roggli VL, Vollmer RT, Greenberg SD, et al. Lung cancer heterogeneity: a blinded and randomized study of 100 consecutive cases. Hum Pathol. 1985;16:569–79.
68. Cross SS. Kappa statistics as indicators of quality assurance in histopathology and cytopathology. J Clin Pathol. 1996;49:597–9.
69. Jensen P, Krogsgaard MR, Christiansen J, et al. Observer variability in the assessment of type and dysplasia of colorectal adenomas, analyzed using kappa statistics. Dis Colon Rectum. 1995;38: 195–8.
70. Malpica A, Matisic JP, Niekirk DV, et al. Kappa statistics to measure interrater and intrarater agreement for 1790 cervical biopsy specimens among twelve pathologists: qualitative histopathologic analysis and methodologic issues. Gynecol Oncol. 2005; 99:S38–52.
71. Tezuka F, Namiki T, Higashiiwai H. Observer variability in endometrial cytology using kappa statistics. J Clin Pathol. 1992;45:292–4.
72. Venkataraman G, Ananthanarayanan V, Paner GP. Accessible calculation of multirater kappa statistics for pathologists. Virchows Arch. 2006;449:272.
73. Summerskill W. Cochrane Collaboration and the evolution of evidence. Lancet. 2005;366:1760.
74. Marchevsky AM, Wick MR. Evidence-based guidelines for the utilization of immunostains in diagnostic pathology: pulmonary adenocarcinoma versus mesothelioma. Appl Immunohistochem Mol Morphol. 2007;15:140–4.
75. Moussa AS, Kattan MW, Berglund R, et al. A nomogram for predicting upgrading in patients with low- and intermediate-grade prostate cancer in the era of extended prostate sampling. BJU Int. 2010;105:352–8.
76. Kattan MW. Do we need more nomograms for predicting outcomes in patients with prostate cancer? Nat Clin Pract Urol. 2008;5:366–7.
77. Steinberg EP, Luce BR. Evidence based? Caveat emptor! Health Aff (Millwood). 2005;24:80–92.
78. Treadwell JR, Tregear SJ, Reston JT, et al. A system for rating the stability and strength of medical evidence. BMC Med Res Methodol. 2006;6:52.
79. Guerette PH. Managed care: cookbook medicine, or quality, cost-effective care? Can Nurse. 1995;91:16.
80. Holm RP. Cookbook medicine. S D Med. 2009; 62:371.
81. Leape L. Are practice guidelines cookbook medicine? J Ark Med Soc. 1989;86:73–5.
82. Parmley WW. Practice guidelines and cookbook medicine–who are the cooks? J Am Coll Cardiol. 1994;24:567–8.
83. Steinberg KE. Cookbook medicine: recipe for disaster? J Am Med Dir Assoc. 2006;7:470–2.
84. Wick MR, Bourne TD, Patterson JW, et al. Evidence-based principles and practices in pathology: selected problem areas. Semin Diagn Pathol. 2005;22:116–25.

Evidence-Based Pathology: A Stable Set of Principles for a Rapidly Evolving Specialty

2

José Costa and Sarah Whitaker

Keywords
Evidence-based pathology • Diagnostic pathology • Immunohistochemistry and evidence-based medicine • Molecular medicine and evidence-based medicine • Patient–physician relationship and evidence-based medicine

Of all the specialties in medicine, pathology, particularly diagnostic anatomical pathology, has been relatively slow in embracing the practice and principles of evidence-based medicine (EBM). Two reasons for this are as follows. First, pathology has been regarded for a long time as "the evidence" with respect to clinical inference. The classic clinico-pathological-correlation would finish with the pathologist lifting the veil from the hidden truth and providing the last word, often followed by a scholarly discussion of the science behind the disease. Second, pathologists involved in clinical care – particularly surgical pathologists – are expected to render a clear-cut diagnosis that will provide the basis for a therapeutic decision. Thus, there is a decisive moment in the clinic when there is little room for doubt, and it is easy to see why the processes of EBM – which, to a great extent, consist in managing uncertainty by using evidence of high quality – have not been readily embraced by the surgical pathologist. This initial reluctance is, however, slowly transforming into acceptance: it is hard to claim that pathology is an essential part of the medical practice, but that it is off-limits to the critical analysis driven by the EBM proponents. Practice guidelines have progressively been introduced in the diagnostic work-up of tissue samples, and technological innovation has significantly altered diagnostic methods. New technologies being applied to cytological and tissue specimens demand EBM not only at many points in the course of their development but also in their final application to the analysis of clinical samples.

EBM, a discipline that in part had its beginnings in technology assessment, evolved by adopting methodologies common in other domains of medicine such as epidemiology, but also by learning from the more remote fields of economics, business, and engineering. As it has matured, EBM has been incorporated into medical school curricula, and its principles, constantly refined, are used in the elaboration of widely used practice guidelines and consensus statements.

In this chapter, we consider how the recent advances in science and technology, as well as changes in cultural and social trends, act as powerful forces that argue in favor of the incorporation of the tenets of EBM into the rapidly changing

J. Costa (✉)
Department of Pathology, Yale School of Medicine, New Haven, CT, USA
e-mail: Jose.costa@yale.edu

A.M. Marchevsky and M.R. Wick (eds.), *Evidence Based Pathology and Laboratory Medicine*,
DOI 10.1007/978-1-4419-1030-1_2, © Springer Science+Business Media, LLC 2011

discipline of diagnostic pathology. We also consider some of the arguments of those who are critical of integrating EBM in the mainstream of pathology.

The Socio-Economical Context of the Changing Technological Landscape

Since the middle of the twentieth century, the pace of technical evolution in the medical sciences has accelerated. The consequences of this have been wide reaching. The practice of almost every single specialty of medicine today has been drastically affected by the technological innovation resulting from the unprecedented convergence of the progress made in each of several unrelated disciplines. The complexity of practicing medicine increased and required constant adaptation of the healthcare delivery models. Studies undertaken in the 1970s began to show that there was room for improvement in the way medicine was being practiced. Both academics and public interest groups began to question the efficiency of the medical system [1, 2].

Coming hand in hand with the rapid therapeutic and technological advances of the 1960s was a significant increase in the intrinsic cost of treating illness. An increase in diagnostic procedures and means to establish the cause of disease multiplied the cost of health care. Thus from a purely practical standpoint, the need emerged to critically evaluate all new technologies before they would be widely adopted. In 1973, as a consequence of the first oil crisis, the economic burden imposed by the cost of medical care was underscored further as the crisis revealed how vulnerable national economies were to perturbation and how the subsequent destabilization of the economy and inflation affected medicine. Both the cost of health care and the cost of medical research increased. Those bearing the cost of health care, whether governments, nonprofit or private enterprise, began to seek ways to actively manage the resources needed to provide health care. Thus by the last quarter of the twentieth century, it became clear there was a need for a framework through which to look at the objective evidence that was the basis of medical practice.

Finally, through globalization, the industrialized nations realized how much the improvement of the health and life chances of the neediest impacted on the wealthiest. Effective therapies and diagnostic technologies available to the developed nations have not been and are still not yet available to the poor. As a consequence, many of the components of the medico-industrial complex have intensified their engagement in generating robust and cheap diagnostic technologies and therapies suitably adapted to be deployed in the developing world and among underserved populations. As these new tools are created and used in the clinic, each requires a rigorous evidence-based analysis of its precision and efficacy.

Recent Forces Reshaping the Practice of Pathology

At the core of EBM is the question of how we handle information that serves to support medical intervention. What value we decide to place on the information, how we go about obtaining new information, and how we compile existing knowledge are all crucial processes of EBM. And of paramount importance is how we obtain the information pertinent to the diagnosis and management of a single patient.

In recent years, pathology, and more specifically diagnostic pathology, has undergone profound change due to the rapid accumulation of basic knowledge and due to the rapid, almost vertiginous, development of technologies that expand the possibilities of tissue and cell analysis. New information, which is not necessarily clinically worthwhile, is accumulating so fast that it is difficult to distinguish the truly important content from the noise. This proliferation of available information is another reason why the principles of evaluating the value of the evidence are becoming ever more crucial for both the general practitioner and the academician.

In laboratory medicine, two types of information are used in medical decision-making: (1) laboratory values and (2) anatomical pathology diagnoses and values. Each of these two subdisciplines has its specific challenges and is moving toward EBM at a different speed. Because of its interpretative nature, however, anatomical pathology tends to remain anchored in "eminence-based medicine" mode rather than relying on strong grades of evidence. It is precisely here, in the realm of tissue analysis, that modern technologies are opening inroads and calling for the rigorous use of evidence-based tools. The tissue samples interrogated under the microscope are now amenable to a workup that provides resolutive answers to the questions raised by the diagnostic pathologist. The question is not only what kind of disease, process, or lesion are we confronting but also what is the best and most efficient therapy and what response is to be anticipated.

The first tissue analysis technology to make an impact in diagnostic surgical pathology was immunohistochemistry (IHC), and it has served as an effective vehicle for the adoption of EBM. For example, IHC not only provided evidence for a diagnosis but it also began to introduce quantitative histopathology by enumerating cells expressing a given antigenic determinant. Where the quantitative approaches of morphometry had failed to impact daily diagnostic practice, IHC changed it by storm and brought the rigor of the laboratorian to histopathology, creating best practices, practice algorithms, and practice standards [3].

Yet one of the most profound developments to affect the practice of medicine in the last 20 years has unquestionably been the emergence of the field of molecular medicine. Molecular medicine has brought unprecedented knowledge about the pathogenesis of many diseases and served as a rational basis for therapy design. Molecular technologies have brought and continue to bring constant innovation to all branches of laboratory medicine, and with that, a quantum leap in the volume of information to be managed. The ability to extract tissue components such as proteins or nucleic acids from tissues and subject them to a comprehensive analysis has provided us with high-density data sets ("omics") that can be mined by artificial intelligence [4]. The general strategy is to reduce these large assemblies of data to a few features that can then be turned into a clinically applicable test in the laboratory. In other instances, PCR-based approaches applied to a micro-dissected sample enable the pathologist to detect with specificity an infectious agent or a genetic lesion and thus diagnose with precision the etiology of a lesion.

The modern tools of molecular diagnostics allow us to obtain information from a patient with unprecedented precision and breadth. Two tumors arising in the same organ and histologically similar can now be sorted out by analyzing which signal transduction pathway is preferentially and differentially activated in each one of them or what specific mutational spectrum is present in each one of the tumors [5–7]. The molecular alterations found in each tumor may dictate specific targeted therapies. This type of characterization of a lesion is the basis for personalized medicine, "the right treatment for the right person at the right time," and the cornerstone for predictive medicine: the ability to predict the response of an individual patient to a specific therapy. The crucial characteristics of this type of evidence are (1) its objective precision inherent in modern molecular analytical techniques and (2) the fact that in most instances the molecular alteration is causally linked to the pathophysiology of the disease. When present, the causal nature of the link established by experimental studies and refined by observational and therapeutic studies in the human constitutes the highest quality of evidence upon which to base a targeted therapy for an individual patient.

With the availability of reliable, fast, and economic sequencing technologies, the individual genome is becoming a reality, and it has been argued that the requirements for the recovery of clinically useful insights from an individual's genome are different from those of traditional cohort-based medical knowledge.

Since evidence rules must be applied to the singularity of the individual (her or his unique sequence), we ought to consider how the traditional tenets of EBM will be applied to specific information only valid for a single patient. The case is being made for an alternative approach based on translational engineering and intelligence (biointelligence) for interpreting the genomic information from an individual patient [8]. The ability to sequence the 1–2% of a patient's genome that encodes for structural proteins of the cell can enable the detection of disease causing mutations in a single patient. For example, the detailed examination of the DNA of a single patient suffering from Bartter syndrome revealed a novel mutation in the gene coding for a protein responsible for the absorption of water and salt in the intestine. Not only was the case of the index patient resolved, but when other infants with a presumptive diagnosis of Bartter syndrome were examined, five more mutations were identified in the transporter protein [9]. These results illustrate how the new technologies, in this case exon capture and sequencing, generate clinically useful results.

In parallel to the advances in biomedical technologies, there have been advances in information processing, acquisition, and display that have allowed the pathologist to continue as the physician-integrator of information. The capacity of an individual to apprehend and integrate different streams of general evidence and information about a given patient has been progressively taxed. Fortunately, information technology and computational science have come along at the right time, expanding our capacities to display, analyze, and integrate complex and rich streams of data. It is now possible to enlist computational power to carry out the integration of thousands of features and select a small subset of parameters that solve the question (diagnostic, prognostic, predictive). Statistical methods can then be used to test thousands of features for predictive power and select the most powerful ones (feature reduction) to generate a test that can be validated. Modern machine vision technologies that use segmentation, object identification, and topology can derive thousands of objective reproducible features from a tissue section and then proceed to overlay specific molecular markers on the segmented image to produce a "quantitative functional histopathology," thus creating a powerful and precise diagnostic tool [10, 11].

A task once done by a master diagnostician, who, however, was informed by many fewer elementary features, can now reach every single patient and be performed in a reproducible manner. When done by artificial intelligence as opposed to an unaided human mind, the processing will be repeated without error 100% of the time.

From Precision Medicine to Efficient Medicine

With the advent of precision technologies that identify and measure one or several components in a clinical specimen with high specificity and sensitivity or reveal a submolecular alteration, the science of diagnostics enters the realm of "precision medicine." The evidence obtained is objective and precise, and the principles of EBM can then be turned to the task of refining precision medicine into efficient medicine. Efficiency is to be considered with the patient in mind: Are we subjecting the person to the minimal number of tests necessary to best identify and treat the problem? Are we using the best combination of drugs for that particular patient? EBM offers the optimal path to define the most economical way to deliver the personalized precision medicine that we can provide today. It is important to keep in mind that "economical" is used in the sense of the most benefit for the resources used and not necessarily the cheapest.

In our current climate, the cost of medical resources is a major concern. At a time when the cost of health care is becoming prohibitive for industrialized nations (U.S. health expenditures are projected to reach 20% of the GNP by 2020), the tenets of EBM are being used to base policy and resolve debate. Right-thinking people may come to different conclusions based on the available evidence, but to oppose someone's evidence-based stance does not require invective, rather facts and logical argument. Many government funding research in healthcare quality are banking on the power of EBM to decrease the rising share of the national economies taken by healthcare expenditures. Costs can be brought down by encouraging efficient medicine and by discouraging ineffective medical practices, but only with the acceptance of the EBM process can we arrive at a consensus concerning what is medically efficient and what is ineffective. In the U.S., Comparative Effectiveness Research (CER), a broad initiative sponsored by the Agency for Health Care Research and Quality, funds a wide spectrum of research ranging from meta-analyses of trials, to methods of behavior modification, to methods for formulating health policy. Whereas traditionally the evidence has been produced by studies designed specifically to generate the data to support a statement or recommendation, the widespread application of information technology to medical practice is enabling the collection and aggregation of data from the routine medical "day to day" practice [12].

Anatomical Pathology has been a low-cost discipline, a highly efficient one considering the value it contributes, but with the increase in the use of sophisticated technologies and methods the question of efficiency will surface more often. Let us not ignore that pathology tests will become the gatekeepers of expensive therapies as personalized medicine gains momentum.

Evidence-Based Medicine Must Take the Patient into Account: Participatory Medicine

One of the interesting aspects of the real-world approach in gathering data is taking into account the patient–physician relationship as one crucial component of the system to be analyzed. In fact, we have little detailed evidence of how natural phenomena such as disease interact with a social construct such as a health system [13].

The present emphasis on patient's choices *de facto* introduces the patient into the process of generating data. With the information revolution in full gear, much of the knowledge that was exclusive to physicians and other trained health personnel is now accessible to the lay public. Information is read and absorbed with avidity by those facing the distressing but motivating condition of being a patient. Through the aggregation of many patients' personal experiences, new communities are organized around the commonality of shared medical circumstance, such as physical illness or genetic condition. The formation of virtual communities or support networks, a phenomenon for which Rabinow has proposed the concept of "biosociality" [14], has the potential of becoming an active contributing factor to data sets that can be further mined using computational tools. It does not seem risky to predict that the communication revolution will enable observations made and rigorously recorded by lay individuals to be admitted as "evidence" and form the basis for future observational studies. In the near future, patients will be contributing to shape, in many ways, the evidence with which the EBM methods will generate the "best practice standards."

Is There Evidence to Support the Need for Evidence-Based Medicine in Pathology?

The overarching argument we have put forth is that the best way to handle the vertiginous changes affecting pathology, particularly diagnostic pathology, is to adhere to the tenets of EBM. Critics of this argument will present a number of objections. They will hasten to point out that there is no robust body of evidence to support our position; that time and resources are limited and are less and less available to busy practitioners; that EBM will require training in additional skills to search for the available information and evaluate the strength of the available evidence; that EBM is "cookbook medicine" and "takes the art out of diagnostic clinical medicine"; that it will threaten current standards of therapeutic excellence as initiatives of the CER type use EBM to cut costs without regard for the quality of care [15].

It is certainly true that *stricto sensu* there is no formal evidence to support EBM. A randomization study of traditional style versus EBM practice style in diagnostic pathology is practically impossible and would very likely be unethical. The fact is, however, that pathologists, because of the nature of their practice, have operated *close* to EBM standards for a long time and have more often than not recorded their diagnostic outcomes in observational studies involving case series or, more recently, in studies coupled to clinical trials. The leap to formalizing the principles of EBM in the practice of pathology is not great. As a discipline, pathology has traditionally been seen as providing "the evidence," and yet pathologists and clinicians have come to realize that appearances can be deceiving and that very similar if not identical morphologies can have very different clinical behaviors that demand different therapeutic strategies. Not knowing how to distinguish the mimics from the authentic lesion constitutes individual ignorance that can be repaired by acquiring the knowledge to make the distinction. By contrast, being confronted by lesions that are identical and thus indistinguishable but with a very different behavior constitutes collective ignorance. Two prominent examples presenting a dilemma rooted in this type of ignorance are intraductal low-grade breast cancers and prostate cancers with a Gleason grade of 6 or less. Both are early cancers often found in asymptomatic patients at screening, and their therapy ranges from watch-and-wait surveillance to aggressive intervention designed to eradicate the tumor. We are just beginning to learn how to make such distinctions, making appeal to objective tools such as the ones used in systems pathology. Conclusive evidence upon which to base a distinction and rational therapy will hopefully be validated in the near future.

The paradox is that the same diagnosticians who have acquired new powerful tools must now seek additional evidence to support their reasons for saying what they say, for diagnosing what they diagnose, and for recommending what they recommend. In other words, pathologists have transitioned from embodying the evidence to having the tools to uncover it and having to justify the use of these tools. The principles of EBM may not be perfect, but they are probably the best for the evaluation of technologies, codifying their use in practice, and assessing their cost and effectiveness. The accuracy, value, and efficacy of these new ways must be methodically documented, ideally by randomized trials that compare a new diagnostic or predictive modality to the conventional approach used to solve a specific clinical problem. It behooves the practitioner working on a specific case to follow the well-defined steps involved in the practice of EBM: (1) convert information needs into answerable questions, (2) track down the best evidence with which to answer these questions, (3) critically appraise the evidence for its validity and importance, (4) integrate this appraisal with clinical expertise and patient values to apply the result in clinical practice, (5) evaluate performance. Adherence to these tenets will go a long way to manage uncertainty in clinical practice.

Objections to EBM, on the basis of the increasingly limited time and resources available to busy practitioners and on the perceived additional burden of developing the skills necessary to search for the available information and evaluate the strength of the available evidence, raise legitimate concerns. Fortunately, however, the IT revolution has gone a long way to mitigate these factors. The skills necessary to access information can be learned at any stage of clinical training and are now taught to medical students in most medical schools. More articles of the "systematic review" type are appearing in general, not just in subspecialty journals, and brief summaries of evidence relevant to common clinical questions can be accessed at the point of care.

Many of the objections articulated by opponents of EBM are based more on misperception than on substance. Two of the major arguments of opponents to EBM are that "it is cookbook medicine" and that "it takes the art out of clinical medicine." Following the principles of EBM does by no means exclude creativity. The best clinicians are the ones capable of making cognitive connections between facts and rules. That is the product of a creative process – a process that, if grounded on the rules of evidence, will be able to be taught, learned, and constantly perfected.

It is also a misperception that EBM is used by initiatives of the CER type simply to cut costs without regard for therapeutic standards or the quality of care. Those who feel uncomfortable with EBM argue that the use of the findings will not be geared to the benefit of the patient, but to the rationing of health care [12]. As noted earlier, many aspects of EBM lead directly to more effective patient care.

EBM is not designed to answer philosophical questions about the values and priorities of a society and therefore cannot pretend to. But one can strive for a democratically based transparent process that, after informed dialog and debate, will generate a consensus that accommodates the values and priorities of the vast majority of peoples and interests.

Conclusion

Modern technologies and ever more incisive methods of tissue analysis are providing increasing accuracy, resolution, and effectiveness to modern diagnostic sciences. We are immersed in a rapidly evolving world where disruptive technologies come at such speed and information is generated in such abundance that EBM becomes an essential philosophical and practical factor of stability. It behooves all of us in pathology to establish EBM as the linkage of technological innovation and research to the resolution of patient illness and problems in the delivery of care.

References

1. Hardy A, Tansy EM. Medical enterprise and global response, 1945–2000. In: The Western medical tradition 1800–2000. Cambridge: Cambridge University Press; 2006.
2. Office of Technology Assessment. Assessing the efficacy and safety of medical technologies (OTA-H-75). Washington, DC: OTHA; 1978.
3. Wolff AC et al. American Society of Clinical Oncology/College of American Pathologists guideline recommendations for human epidermal growth factor receptor 2 testing in breast cancer. Arch Pathol Lab Med. 2007;131:18–43.
4. Costa J. Systems approach to the practice of pathology: a new role for the pathologist. Arch Pathol Lab Med. 2009;133:524–6.
5. Hayden EC. Personalized cancer therapy gets closer. Nature. 2009;458:131–2.
6. Brown RE. Morphoproteomics: exposing protein circuitries in tumors to identify potential therapeutic targets in cancer patients. Expert Rev Proteomics. 2005;2:337–48.
7. Lievre A, Blons H, Laurent-Puig P. Oncogenic mutations as predictive factors in colorectal cancer. Oncogene. 2010;29:3033–43.
8. Mousses S et al. Using biointelligence to search the cancer genome: an epistemological perspective on knowledge recovery strategies to enable precision medical genomics. Oncogene. 2008;Suppl 2:S-58–66.
9. Choi M et al. Genetic diagnosis by whole exome capture and massively parallel DNA sequencing. Proc Natl Acad Sci USA. 2009;106:19096–101.
10. Donovan MJ et al. Personalized prediction of tumor response and cancer progression on prostate needle biopsy. J Urol. 2009;182:125–32.
11. Donovan MJ et al. A systems pathology model for predicting overall survival in patients with refractory, advanced non-small-cell lung cancer treated with gefitinib. Eur J Cancer. 2009;45:1518–26.
12. Topol EJ. Transforming medicine via digital innovation. Sci Transl Med. 2010;2:16.
13. Liu J et al. Complexity of coupled human and natural systems. Science. 2007;317:1513–6.
14. Rabinow P. Artificiality and enlightenment. From sociobiology to biosociality. In: Essays on the anthropology of reason. Princeton: Princeton University Press; 1996.
15. Straus SE, McAlister FA. Evidence-based medicine: a commentary on common criticisms. CMAJ. 2000;163:837–41.

What Is Best Evidence in Pathology?

3

Peter J. Saunders and Christopher N. Otis

Keywords
Evidence-based medicine in pathology • Best evidence, defined • Evidence evaluation • Internal validity of evidence

What is Evidence?

With the advent of evidence-based medicine (EBM), the word and concept "evidence" needs to be explored. The concept of evidence is the crux of what is attractive (or controversial) about the practice of evidence-based medicine. Webster's dictionary defines evidence as "something that furnishes truth" or "an outward sign" [1]. The former definition embraces the idea of objectivity and has a great deal of purpose to it. The latter seems to equate evidence with an observation that gives insight into an occult process and makes no judgment of how likely said process is to occur. In this context, evidence is an indication, not proof. By including these two definitions, Merriam-Webster's English dictionary comments on the heterogeneity of the worth of evidence. In other words, evidence is of variable quality. Merriam-Webster's Legal dictionary also embraces this ambiguity by including an element of doubt when it comes to the merit of evidence, defining it as "something that furnishes or tends to furnish proof" [2]. Something that *tends* to achieve a certain goal is obviously not completely efficacious. If we consider these definitions to be equally valid, we arrive at the conclusion that in a linguistic or legal environment, evidence is recognized to be neither completely specific nor completely sensitive. In the spirit of incomplete sensitivity and specificity, we might define evidence as something that tends to furnish proof. Of interest are the lack of entries for "evidence" and "evidence based medicine" in the 28th and most recent edition of Stedman's Medical Dictionary, published in 2006.

C.N. Otis (✉)
Department of Pathology, Baystate
Medical Center, Tufts University
School of Medicine, Springfield, MA, USA
e-mail: Christopher.otis@bhs.org

Best Evidence: Where Did the Term Come from?

The term "best evidence" first appeared in accounts of English legal proceedings dating to the mid-eighteenth century. It was born of the idea that some types of legal evidence are better than others which are nevertheless useful and admissible in court if no other evidence is available. It was codified into law in the UK soon after the case in which the principle made its first appearance was decided [3] and subsequently in the United States in 1975 [4]. According to

A.M. Marchevsky and M.R. Wick (eds.), *Evidence Based Pathology and Laboratory Medicine*,
DOI 10.1007/978-1-4419-1030-1_3, © Springer Science+Business Media, LLC 2011

Webster's New World Law Dictionary, the best evidence rule is defined as: "The rule that, to prove the contents of a writing, recording, or photograph, the original is required unless it is not available for some reason other than the serious fault of the party trying to prove the contents thereof. If the original is unavailable, the testimony of the person who created the original or the person who read it (if a writing), listened to it (if a recording), or saw it (if a photograph) may testify to its content. However, modern evidentiary rules usually permit the use of mechanical, electronic, or other similar copy instead of the original" [2].

Thus, in the legal arena, "best evidence" may be interpreted as "best *available* evidence," rather than "the best *type* of evidence." Physicians desire to provide the best for patients, but are intimately aware of the real-life constraints that make for suboptimal solutions. Perhaps practitioners of medicine might take a cue from the legal profession and regard "best evidence" as something that is the best that can be done at a given point in time (that is, the best that is available), and subsequently something that may be improved upon (something that may be bested).

How Is the Quality of Evidence Evaluated in Evidence-Based Medicine?

Study quality is synonymous with study internal validity. Internal validity is generally defined as how well a study measures what it is designed to measure. A study without design flaws that is executed properly and is not subject to unexpected environmental influences will not yield poor-quality data, and vice versa: a poorly conceived, executed, and storm-tossed study will not yield good quality data. Thus, quality of evidence is evaluated by evaluating the study from which it is derived. Study quality is currently evaluated using different criteria for different kinds of studies. This is to say that a meta-analysis and a case–control study must meet different criteria to be deemed of high quality. There are multiple different bodies across the globe that create criteria in order to perform this function, and as one might expect, the criteria differ from one organization to the next. Overall, the decision of which criteria to include and which to exclude appears fairly subjective.

What Is Internal Validity?

The Center for Evidence Based Medicine (CEBM) defines validity and internal validity as follows:

The extent to which a variable or intervention measures what it is supposed to measure or accomplishes what it is supposed to accomplish. The internal validity of a study refers to the integrity of the experimental design [5].

The U.S. Preventive Services Task Force (USPTF), an offshoot of the Agency for Healthcare Research and Quality and a part of the U.S. Department of Health and Human Services, is the CEBM's American counterpart. The USPTF refers to internal validity as "strength of study design" [6]. The USPTF uses a ranking system for assessing the internal validity of evidence at an individual study level. The hierarchy of this ranking system is as follows:

I. Properly powered and conducted randomized controlled trial (RCT); well-conducted systematic review or meta-analysis of homogeneous RCTs

II-1. Well-designed controlled trial without randomization

II-2. Well-designed cohort or case–control analytic study

II-3. Multiple time series with or without the intervention; dramatic results from uncontrolled experiments

III. Opinions of respected authorities, based on clinical experience; descriptive studies or case reports; reports of expert committees [7]

The USPFT uses sets of criteria that are specific to study type to determine whether a study possesses "good," "fair," or "poor" internal validity. For example, systematic reviews are checked to determine whether or not they meet the following criteria that have been deemed critical for minimal internal validity:

- Comprehensiveness of sources considered/search strategy used.
- Standard appraisal of included studies.

- Validity of conclusions.
- Recency and relevance are especially important for systematic reviews [7].

A good study is described as a "recent, relevant review with comprehensive sources and search strategies; explicit and relevant selection criteria; standard appraisal of included studies; and valid conclusions" [7]. A fair study is described as a "recent, relevant review that is not clearly biased but lacks comprehensive sources and search strategies" [7]. A poor study is described as "outdated, irrelevant, or biased review without systematic search for studies, explicit selection criteria, or standard appraisal of studies" [7].

Good internal validity is the result of good study design. An appraisal of the design of a study under consideration might include searching for evidence of the above types, as well as answering the following questions:

- Is the question properly defined?
- Are inclusion and exclusion criteria stated?
- Is the sample size large enough?
- Are the units of analysis well defined? Are they independent of each other?
- Are measurements made in the same way (same time, same conditions, etc.) for all?
- Is the scale of measurement objective? [8]

What Statistics Are Generally Used to Analyze Data in Studies? How Should Their Results be Interpreted to Determine the Internal Validity of the Studies?

Before proceeding, it might be prudent to review the basic concepts of sensitivity, specificity, positive likelihood ratio, and positive predictive value (PPV). Sensitivity is perhaps best viewed as the true positive rate. It is the number of times that a test is deemed positive divided by the number of times that the test *should* be positive if the assay were to detect all cases of the condition under investigation: TP/(TP+FN). Otto von Bismarck, Germany's first Chancellor, is reputed to have said "it is better that ten innocent men suffer than one guilty man escape" [9]. This is an example of high sensitivity for guilt at the cost of specificity. Specificity can analogously be viewed as the true negative rate. It is the number of true negatives divided by the number of times the test is *initially* thought to be negative: TN/(TN+FP). Blackstone's formulation, named for English jurist William Blackstone and later echoed by Benjamin Franklin, states that it is "better that ten guilty persons escape than that one innocent man suffer" [10]. This is an example of high specificity (for guilt) at the cost of sensitivity. The positive likelihood ratio (+LR) is a very powerful tool that determines how much pretest probability increases due to the procurement of a positive test result. The positive likelihood ratio changes as the threshold for positivity changes, as do the sensitivity and specificity of a given test type. This can be demonstrated graphically as the derivative of the slope of a plot of sensitivity versus 1-specificity (the receiver operating characteristic (ROC) curve, to be discussed in more depth later in this chapter). Positive predictive value (PPV) is the proportion of patients with positive test results who are correctly diagnosed, that is to say the number of true positives divided by the number of all results *initially* considered positive (including those that are later determined to be false positives): TP/(TP+FP). An interesting attribute of PPV is that with this concept we are beginning to venture into the realm of creating a denominator that is not one group (like all the patients who have a disease), but rather comprises parts of two groups (some of the patients who have a disease and some of the patients who do not have the disease). This results in a situation in which the population from which the sample size is derived can drastically affect the outcome of a test. Specifically, two populations with different prevalences of a certain disease will yield two different PPVs so that clinical use of PPV should be restricted to populations in which the prevalence is the same as test population from which the results were derived [11].

Relative risk and absolute risk are frequently employed statistical tools that, when used together, unveil the degree of additional risk above a baseline. Odds ratio, the ratio of the odds of a given phenomenon occurring in two separate groups, is used to determine the differential risk for the two groups. The ROC curve is an underused statistical method of determining likelihood ratios, the approximate accuracy of a test, and for evaluating sensitivity and specificity at given diagnostic thresholds. Positive and negative predictive values are statistical tools that help determine how likely a positive or negative test is to represent the presence or absence of a condition within a given population.

There are other statistical functions within most studies that are included to showcase internal validity (a form of internal quality assessment), rather than to prove causation (the usual goal of studies investigating both therapeutic and diagnostic interventions). These include the confidence interval, the confidence level, the *p*-value, the funnel plot, and Cohen's kappa.

Confidence intervals are usually included after a measurement of probability (e.g., odds ratio), as an assessment of the reliability of the measurement. If a distribution is nonparametric (i.e., non-Gaussian), statistics like the odds ratio and relative risk do not accurately portray reality. For example, if there exists a bimodal distribution of events, one single odds ratio may spear the nadir between the two peaks which is misleading. Assuming something like this is not overlooked, a large confidence interval will result from a distribution with a flattened appearance graphically – the result of minimal correlation between supposed cause and effect. Large confidence intervals for multiple parameters indicate that a study may possess poor internal validity that is contributing to difficulty in determining accurate statistical estimates.

P-values are ubiquitous throughout medical trials. A *p*-value greater than 0.0X indicates the probability that the results of a study were achieved with less than X% likelihood that this is due to chance. Simply put, the *p*-value is the percent chance that the null hypothesis explains the results obtained. The preferred *p*-value for the majority of studies is 0.05 or 5%. The concept that the results of a given test resulted from serendipity (a 1 in 20 chance) is somewhat arbitrary. Nevertheless, it functions such that there is a statistical standard. The *p*-value can be looked upon as a statistical gauge of internal validity: studies with large *p*-values are more likely to falsely connect cause and effects, and thus more likely to be designed in a way that does not isolate and exclude the mechanism by which chance may lead to seemingly significant results. The lower the *p*-value, the greater is the likelihood that the study has good internal validity.

Cohen's kappa is a powerful tool for internal quality assessment of a study and relates specifically to how often multiple detectors arrive at the same conclusion for the same reasons as each other. It is a way of determining inter-rater agreement that does not occur by chance (e.g., how often two pathologists agree on the same diagnosis other than the times they agree for divergent reasons). Cohen's kappa is calculated by dividing the rate of nonrandom agreement (total agreement minus chance agreement) by the percent of occurrences that something other than chance agreement occurs (1-rate of chance agreement). The rate of nonrandom agreement is calculated by summing the product of the positive result rate from two detectors and the product of the negative result rate from the two detectors. For example, if pathologists A and B are given 50 cases and they agree on a positive diagnosis 20 times (or 40% of the time) and they agree on a negative diagnosis 15 times (or 30% of the time), then the total agreement is 70% of the time, or 0.70. Now assume that pathologist A makes a positive diagnosis 50% of the time and negative diagnosis 50% of the time, while pathologist B makes a positive diagnosis 60% of the time and a negative diagnosis 40% of the time. This last piece of data can be used to determine how frequently the two pathologists agree by chance: the hypothetical probability of chance agreement is calculated by multiplying the rates of both pathologists' positive diagnoses ($0.5 \times 0.6 = 0.3$), multiplying the rates of both pathologists' negative diagnoses ($0.5 \times 0.4 = 0.2$), and summing them ($0.3 + 0.2 = 0.5$). In this example, a kappa of 0.4 is generated by applying these elements to the kappa function defined above ($[0.7 - 0.5]/[1 - 0.5]$). Generally, kappa values of less than 0 represent no agreement, 0–0.2 slight agreement, 0.21–0.40 fair agreement, 0.41–0.60 moderate agreement, 0.61–0.80 substantial agreement, and 0.81–1.00 almost perfect agreement.

When attempting to determine the internal validity of a meta-analysis, it is imperative to determine whether or not as many individual studies as possible have been incorporated. Unfortunately, not all studies that are conducted are published. Frequently, this is due to effect size lying outside (too high or too low) a desired target, which is often the result of studying a population larger or smaller than that which might yield a significant result. A funnel plot is a plot of study size against a marker of treatment effect (e.g., mean standard error), which can uncover silencing of results due to unwanted results derived from large or small studies. If publication bias is absent, the points plotted on the funnel plot will take the form of an inverted funnel. Inclusion of a funnel plot that has this inverted-funnel shape is reassuring that publication bias is not impeding the flow of such studies into the information pool.

Besides the above statistical tests that one should expect to see in a given study (and the absence of which might raise questions about the rigor of the study), there are other more complicated manipulations, the inclusion of which should prompt careful critique of the study. Per Dr. Trisha Greenhalgh, professor of primary care at University College, London "The number of possible statistical tests sometimes seems infinite. In fact, most statisticians could survive with a formulary of about a dozen" [12]. These critical statistical tests include: the *t*-test; the Mann–Whitney *U*-test; the Wilcoxon matched pairs test; the one-way analysis of variance (*F*) test; the Kruskal–Wallis one-way analysis of variance; the two-way analysis of variance; the c^2 test; Fisher's exact test; Pearson's *r*; Spearman's rank correlation coefficient; regression by least squares method; nonparametric regression [12]; and the ROC curve. Of course, just because a test not mentioned above is employed does not mean that it is part of an attempt to make the data fit at all costs, but the more complicated the function the less useful the resulting trends are to everyday diagnosis or intervention. Per Dr. Greenhalgh's comments on the statistical tests other than those listed above, "The rest should generally be reserved for special indications. If the paper you are reading seems to describe a standard set of data which have been collected in a standard way, but the test used has an unpronounceable name and is not listed in a basic statistics textbook, you should smell a rat. The authors should, in such circumstances, state why they have used this test, and give a reference (with page numbers) for a definitive description of it" [12].

The Receiver Operating Characteristic Curve: A Special Tool

This is a statistical tool that first saw use during World War II by the Royal Air Force. It was used to optimize radar operators' level of suspicion regarding the identification of objects in the airspace off the English coast. It was crucial to the survival of the United Kingdom that the appearance of phosphorescence on an oscilloscope accurately alerted operators to incoming enemy aircraft. An operator's threshold was adjusted by plotting a graph of the percent of the time he or she identified enemy aircraft correctly (true positive rate) against the percentage of the time he or she identified other entities (clouds, birds, etc.) incorrectly (the false positive rate). As true positive rate is equal to sensitivity and false positive rate is equal to 1-specificity, this is also a plot of sensitivity versus 1-specificity. The curve that is generated is known as the Receiver Operating Characteristic (ROC) curve. As with all curves, the derivative and the integral provide interesting information. The derivative, that is to say the slope of the curve, equates to the positive likelihood ratio (+LR). The integral, i.e., the area under the curve (AUC), is approximately equivalent to the accuracy of the test (it is not absolute accuracy because it does not take into account values that have fallen under the curve due to chance, but this is accepted to be a small proportion of the total measurements and can be addressed with a correcting factor if need be). It would be fairly easy to generate ROC curves (using the true positive rate and the false positive rate) for a number of studies and to determine which ones generated the maximal +LRs and AUCs. These values could be averaged over multiple studies of the same type and then compared with other study types in order to determine which study type was optimal.

Although the ROC curve is a powerful tool, statistical methods like the ROC curve do not eliminate the biases that exist in a poorly designed study, and in fact, may be misleading by generating inaccurate assessments of the intervention as they may not reveal the internal biases in studies.

What is External Validity?

The CEBM defines external validity in reference to a study as "The appropriateness by which its results can be applied to non-study patients or populations" [5]. The USPTF refers to external validity as "applicability" [13] and "generalizability" [14].

What Role Does External Validity Play in the Evaluation of Evidence Quality?

External validity is important in determining whether or not evidence should be incorporated into a specific recommendation and the strength (or the grade) associated with the recommendation. Applicability, or lack thereof, has nothing to do with how good the study is at answering a particular question. It is a mistake to confuse the trueness of an answer with how useful that answer will be in a given situation. The CEBM's levels of evidence are grouped into "grades of recommendation" denoted A, B, C, and D. The groupings are not based upon the quality (internal validity) of the evidence, but the clinical applicability of the study (external validity) which is influenced by such factors as "cost, ease of implementation (of treatment, diagnostic test ,etc.), and importance of the disease" [15].

Study Designs: How Are They Used to Rank the Quality of Studies?

This is a critical concept and one that the individual pathologist (or any other physician) must consider. Ranking one study or one set of diagnostic criteria over another is the pathologist's bread and butter. It might seem that this should have been well fleshed out by now. However, the ranking systems seem to contain important contradictions. For example, the University of Oxford CEBM, a body consulted by the U.K.'s National Health Service, includes only systematic reviews in its highest stratum of evidence-generating studies even if the individual studies are not RCTs. It is difficult to imagine that there exists evidence to prove that a single large, well-conducted RCT generates lower quality data than a systematic review of multiple small RCTs, each with its own microcosm of variables.

Internal validity alone cannot be used to rank studies. For example, consider a common diagnostic dilemma encountered in pathology: The distinction of mesothelioma from mimics such as reactive mesothelium and adenocarcinoma. It would be very helpful to the pathologist if an immunohistochemical (IHC) stain was available to identify neoplastic mesothelial cells. A well-developed study would be prospective, randomized, blinded, and controlled. Such a study, if conducted in concordance with these principles, would be said to be internally valid. However, such a study would be extremely difficult to construct in the everyday environment of pathology practice. The closest study likely to be conducted would be a retrospective review of known cases of mesothelioma and compared to cases of known mesothelioma mimics, employing a novel antibody hypothesized to discriminate between the two groups. This typical study conducted in pathology is at perhaps level III according to USPFT criteria. Obviously, such common pathology studies do not reach the upper levels of best evidence. Even though both studies might have excellent internal validity, the RCT is deemed to have generated better evidence because the design is intrinsically better.

What Is the "Evidence Pyramid"?

This leads to the concept of evidence stratification based upon the quality of various study designs. The evidence pyramid is a simple graphical way of representing relative quality of evidence generated by different study types. Many versions of the evidence pyramid exist. For our purposes, we refer to the following evidence pyramid:

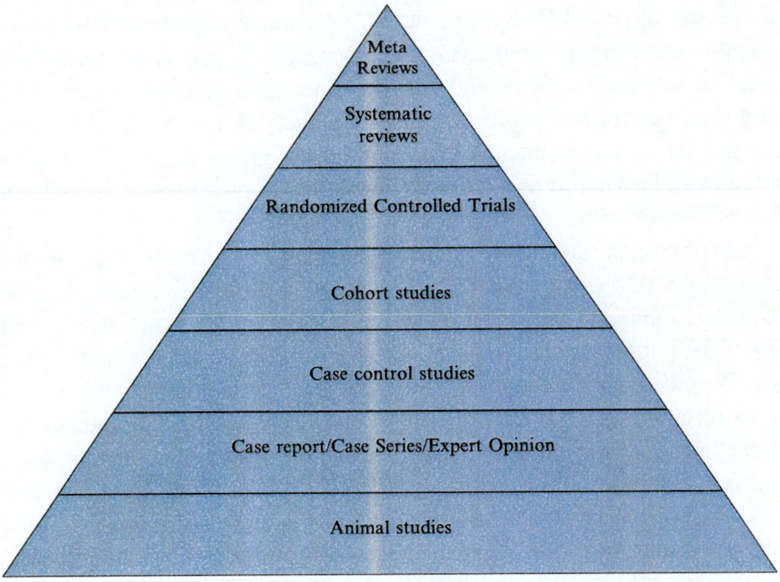

The differences in the relative sizes of the pyramid levels represent the approximate number of each kind of study in existence. The location with regard to superior and inferior is relative to the quality of evidence that each type of study generates: the type of study generating the highest quality data (meta-analysis) is at the top of the pyramid, and the type of study generating the lowest quality data (animal study) is at the base.

Many charts similar to this one have been generated for the new discipline of evidence-based medicine, which has frequently been concerned with treatment, and less so with diagnosis. It can be readily appreciated from a chart of evidence stratification like the CEBM's [16] (essentially a deconstructed evidence pyramid) that the relative value of a particular study type changes with respect to whether diagnosis, intervention, or some other parameter is being evaluated. Although the stratification of evidence quality seen in the EBM pyramid is fairly subjective, pathologists must not simply adopt this pyramid without some investigation into the possibility that diagnostic tests may require a differently organized algorithm. For example, the pyramid above is slightly different from those seen in EBM in that it incorporates a level of the pyramid for case report/case series/expert opinion. We choose to rate this as better evidence than animal studies, but inferior to controlled studies. It seems logical that these human-based endeavors should yield evidence of better quality than nonhuman-based studies if we are dealing with diagnosing and treating humans (the astute reader might point out that this is an external validity problem, not an internal validity problem, which would be a valid argument). Expert opinion is included in this tier by default: it is not controlled in any formal way, but again, it is, after all, presumably based on human data. If an expert has personally scrutinized many cases of a pathologic entity and taken a strong interest in many cases representing the entity with knowledge of clinical outcome, the expert's opinion may be significantly better than second-to-bottom tier level evidence. The time-honored expert opinion in pathology may yet represent good evidence, although proving this point remains difficult.

Study Designs Providing "Best Evidence" in Clinical Medicine: Systematic Reviews and Meta-Analysis

A systematic review is "an article in which the authors have systematically searched for, appraised, and summarized all of the medical literature for a specific topic" [17]. Systematic reviews are compilations of multiple individual studies performed in attempt to overcome the problem of low power. Low power is principally due to small sample sizes of individual studies. A systematic review can be viewed as a study in which the "subjects" are a number of other studies. Systematic reviews can be qualitative where the results of the primary studies are summarized but not statistically combined, or quantitative where the results of the primary studies are statistically combined. Quantitative systematic reviews are also known as meta-analyses [17]. The term "overview" is sometimes used to denote a systematic review, whether qualitative or quantitative [17]. Summaries of research that lack explicit descriptions of systematic methods are often called narrative reviews [18]. Both the USPTF and the CEBM rank systematic reviews and meta-analyses as the highest level of evidence. Numerous other textbooks on evidence-based medicine laud systemic analysis, and specifically meta-analysis, as generating the best quality of evidence. Of course, the validity of a systematic study is only as strong as the individual studies that it comprises. Additionally, as for any study type, the validity may suffer if the design of the review itself is poor. Two important statistical tools used in meta-analysis are subgroup analysis and meta-regression (a type of regression analysis).

What Is Subgroup Analysis?

Subgroup analysis compares smaller groups within the test group and the control group in order to determine if heterogeneity within these groups skews the data derived from the trial. This is a subjective, nonmathematical endeavor.

What Is Meta-Regression Analysis?

While the mathematical details of regression analysis are beyond the scope of this chapter, suffice it to say that regression analysis is an extremely powerful tool for modeling systems with many variables, some of which may not be quantifiable. These unquantifiable variables do, however, have effects on the dependent variables (that which we are measuring and are most interested in) creating "wobble" in the dependent variable. The idea behind regression analysis is to create equations in terms of quantifiable variables to represent the unquantifiable variables, thus accounting for the "wobble". This is most important when the results of different studies are aggregated in meta-analyses: the "wobble" in the final values being compared (e.g., relative risk, PPVs, or other values used to compare studies in meta-analyses) needs to be explained mathematically so that an equation can be developed to describe the collective environment of the studies. The commonly employed types of regression analysis are linear regression (dependent variable solutions fall along a straight line, seen in system without "wobble"), fixed meta-regression (which uses effect size as a constant, and therefore cannot be used to compare across studies, only within a single study), and random meta-regression (which does not set the effect size, and so can be used to compare different studies that have different effect sizes).

What Is More Commonly Employed to Evaluate the Significance of Results Generated by Meta-Analysis, Subgroup Analysis or Meta-Regression?

Unfortunately, meta-regression, the most objective tool that we have to help generate the highest level of evidence, is difficult to employ due to its complexity. Per the Cochrane Collaboration, an international initiative that produces and disseminates systematic reviews of healthcare interventions, "Meta-regression is rarely performed in Cochrane reviews and not an available option in Cochrane software, so should you have strong reason to include a meta-regression in your review, you will need the help of a statistician" [18]. As physicians, we need to educate ourselves about how statistical tools such as meta-regression function and then to advocate for their use if we expect to receive the highest quality data.

So Is the Final Meta-Analysis Really Used to Make Clinical Decisions?

The Cochrane Collaboration has received recent attention regarding breast cancer screening guidelines. The USPTF has recommended that women receive mammograms starting at age 50, and at 2 years intervals (as opposed to annually screening starting at age 40, as previously recommended) [19]. A 1993 review of annual screening mammography estimated that it reduced breast cancer-related mortality by 20–30% [20]. However, a 2005 Cochrane review estimated that the relative risk reduction was 15%, the absolute reduction of risk was 0.05%, and that mammography may do more harm than good [21]. This Cochrane Collaboration systematic review from 2005 is being cited as evidence in favor of the recent suggested changes in mammographic screening. In order to determine which review generated the best quality evidence, we have to explore how to critically assess the designs of the studies.

How to Tell a Good Systematic Review from a Bad One

For systematic reviews, Oxford's CEBM provides a checklist of questions to help with this process [22]. In the first step, the question "What question did the systematic review address?" is asked. This is aimed at determining the basic parameters of study design: the nature of the test population; the intervention; what was compared; and what outcome resulted. The second question, "Is it unlikely that important, relevant studies were missed?," is posed to help determine whether or not the creators of the meta-analysis found most of the studies on the topic. This should include a search of major bibliographic databases, a search of reference lists from relevant studies, and contact with experts to inquire about unpublished studies. The search "should not be limited to the English language and should include medical subject heading (MeSH) terms and text words." The third question, "Were the criteria used to select articles for inclusion appropriate?," involves determining whether the studies selected by the creators are of good quality. In a good systematic review, the inclusion and exclusion criteria of the individual studies "should be clearly defined a priori, and the eligibility criteria used should specify the patients, interventions, or exposures and outcomes of interest." In many cases, the type of study design will also be a key component of the eligibility criteria. The fourth question "Were the included studies sufficiently [internally] valid for the type of question asked?" attempts to uncover systemic reviews that are based on poor-quality data. The fifth question "Were the results similar from study to study?" deals with determining if the results of the individual studies are similar enough to combine.

As noted previously, the USPTF uses the following criteria when determining the internal validity of an individual systematic review:

- Comprehensiveness of sources considered/search strategy used.
- Standard appraisal of included studies.
- Validity of conclusions.
- Recency and relevance are especially important for systematic reviews [7].

Typically, What Types of Studies Generate the Best Evidence?

The sine qua non of scientific study is the prospective, randomized, controlled, double-blind (PRCDB) study, a type of RCT. A PubMed search for "randomized controlled" yields 358,053 articles. The oldest of these is an article titled *Interactions between pharmacodynamic and placebo effect in drug evaluations in man* by Modell and Garrett, published in the February 1960 edition of *Nature*. The idea behind the PRCDB design is simply that a group of subjects is intervened upon and that the group is compared to a group not receiving intervention in an environment free from tampering (intentional or otherwise). The prospective, double-blind, and randomization design of such studies attempts to minimize subjectivity. Retrospective studies are plagued by problems related to data retrieval, incomplete records, and internal biases. Studies that are not blinded may be led astray by unintended (and often unconscious) interpretation biases. Nonrandomized studies may generate evidence that is reflective of the patient characteristics rather than by the intervention imposed on the test and nontest groups. A great deal of time and effort may be dedicated to minimizing these confounding variables that disturb and obscure the primary purpose of the study, to determine the effect of the imposed intervention.

Are There Any More Comprehensive Evidence-Level Tables in Existence?

The University of Oxford Centre for Evidence-based Medicine (CEBM) is a body that was assembled to promote evidence-based health care in the United Kingdom. One of its roles is to stratify the quality of evidence coming from various study types. The CEBM has published a comprehensive table which stratifies evidence into ten levels (the rows of the table): 1a–c, 2a–c, 3a–b, 4, and 5 [16]. There are five columns, each representing a different parameter of patient care for which a physician may seek guiding evidence. These correspond to: therapy/prevention, etiology/harm; prognosis; diagnosis; differential diagnosis/symptom prevalence study; and economic/decision analysis. The study type that is assigned to each level varies by column. For example, for the highest level of evidence for guiding therapy/prevention, etiology/harm is listed as the systematic review of randomized controlled trials. The highest level of evidence for differential diagnosis/symptom prevalence study is the systematic review of prospective cohort studies. There are 50 individual fields in the chart and 41 different study types assigned to the fields.

The part of the chart most useful to pathologists is the column corresponding to diagnostic studies. Within this category, level 1a is systematic review of studies (with homogeneity) as well as the clinical decision rule involving 1b studies from different clinical courses. Level 1b is the validating cohort study with good reference standards or the clinical decision rule tested within one clinical center. Level 1c encompasses tests that exhibit specificity so great that a positive result rules a diagnosis in, or sensitivity so great that a negative test rules a diagnosis out. Level 2a is a homogenous systematic review of diagnostic studies that are level 2 or higher. Level 2b is an exploratory cohort study with good reference standards or a clinical decision rule. Level 3a is the homogenous systematic review of studies determined to be level 3b or better. Level 3b is the nonconsecutive study or a study without consistently applied reference standards. Level 4 is the case–control study with a poor or nonindependent reference standard. Level 5 is the expert opinion without explicit critical appraisal, or based on physiology, bench research or "first principles" [16]. This is illustrated more simply in the evidence pyramid described earlier.

Best Evidence in the Pathology Literature. How Good Is It?

Pathologists are at a distinct disadvantage regarding the quality of the evidence we rely upon. As a group, pathologists generally use data that are generated by studies that fall within the bottom reaches of the evidence pyramid. Pathologists are both aided and disadvantaged by large volumes of archived material: while this provides ample fodder for research, it means pathologists rely heavily on retrospective studies. Retrospective studies are universally accepted to generate evidence of lower quality than prospective studies due to the loss of data that inevitably occurs relative to prospective studies. Sometimes this is unavoidable. Some diseases are rare or progress very slowly to hinder accrual of significant number of cases or arrive at the final outcome. When especially uncommon diseases are encountered, it may be that there are not enough cases in existence to derive statistically significant results. This often leads to the generation of case studies and case series, which are considered by most to be of even lower quality evidence than retrospective studies.

Should Pathologists Concern Themselves with Understanding only the Studies that Exclusively Aim to Answer Questions Pertaining to Diagnosis?

In addition to deriving the best diagnosis, the pathologist is also responsible in part for directing the course of patient care. As the clinical colleagues of pathologists feel increasingly overwhelmed by mounting volumes of data, the pathologist is relied upon more heavily in this capacity. As per the concept described by Sinard and Morrow, the pathologist is at the center of receiving evidence from a multitude of sources and is responsible for integrating these elements into the best information in an effort to properly guide patient care [23]. In order to do this, the pathologist must be familiar with the literature of other branches of medicine as well as pathology. This is especially critical in the case of the expert. The best anatomic pathology data come from meta-analyses of cohort studies (randomized controlled trials are rare), and for this reason, the expert must be familiar with clinical literature (in which randomized controlled trials and meta-analyses of such trials are common). The expert should be familiar with the available literature and understand which studies have generated higher quality data and why this is the case.

Are Different Strata of Evidence Preferable for Different Applications in Pathology Research?

The standard of the PRCDB has historically been held above the rest. The PRCDB is not necessarily the best study type for many types of research questions. According to the guidelines published by the USPTF (which includes proper design with prospective and blinded characteristics), the highest quality data come from PRCDBs only when considering studies that examine the "benefits or harms of various interventions" [14]. The USPSTF notes that "RCTs cannot answer all questions" [14], which implies that studies other than RCTs are better employed to answer those questions. The CEBM's stratification strategy is another example of an algorithm that does not rank the RCT above all other studies. In fact, systematic reviews that do not include RCTs are ranked higher.

The PRCDB study is not the highest rated study type for determining diagnosis or prognosis (many systems rank it as the highest level of evidence only when the questions asked pertain to therapy or harm). It is difficult to understand why any study would benefit from not being randomized or controlled. However, real-world limitations may cause some researchers to abandon the PRCDB when investigating a diagnostic test when the potential harm to patients as a result of an incorrect diagnosis is considered. The aim of such studies is to determine the accuracy of a diagnostic test and a control group is essential to developing tests that accurately diagnose diseases. However, such studies may not be appropriate or justifiable if the potential harm of the diagnostic test in the test and control groups is considered.

A close approximation of a randomized, controlled, and blinded study in pathology may be constructed in the case of a hypothetical IHC assay being investigated to determine its usefulness in the diagnosis of mesothelioma. Pathologist "X" applies a current gold standard in identifying cases of mesothelioma as well as mimics such as reactive mesothelial hyperplasia. Pathologist "X" randomly separates them into two groups and applies the IHC stain to one group. Pathologist "X" gives pathologist "Y" slides of the two groups. Pathologist "Y" determines if mesothelioma or reactive mesothelial hyperplasia is present or absent. After pathologist "Y" records his answers, the diagnoses of pathologist "X" based upon the gold standard are compared to the interpretations of pathologist Y who applied the IHC assay. The result of this comparison measures, at least in part, the usefulness of the IHC assay in discriminating mesothelioma from reactive mesothelial hyperplasia.

How Can a Pathologist Distinguish a Good Case–Control Study from a Bad One

The USPFT uses the following criteria when evaluating the internal validity of case–control studies. These criteria apply to treatment studies that employ a diagnostic test and therefore assume a certain level of accuracy in the diagnostic test.

- Accurate ascertainment of cases.
- Nonbiased selection of cases/controls with exclusion criteria applied equally to both.
- Response rate.
- Diagnostic testing procedures applied equally to each group.
- Measurement of exposure accurate and applied equally to each group.
- Appropriate attention to potential confounding variables [7].

How Can a Pathologist Distinguish a Good Case Series from a Bad One

Criteria for determining a good case series from a bad case series might include: number of cases in the series; the similarity of the cases with regard to the disease process, case selection and manner of accrual (e.g., consultation file bias); and whether or not the patients are treated similarly. It would also be advantageous to know follow-up or outcome endpoints.

How Can a Pathologist Distinguish a Good Expert Opinion from a Great One

Determining a good expert opinion from a great one is highly subjective. Miriam-Webster defines "expert" as "having, involving, or displaying special skill or knowledge derived from training or experience" [1] and opinion as "belief stronger than impression and less strong than positive knowledge" [1]. Given this, one might want to know if the expert's opinions are skewed more towards knowledge or impression. The expert's reputation in the field may give a glimpse of how weak or strong others perceive to be the expert's reasoning and knowledge. It might be advantageous to ascertain how often the expert has been proven to be correct. This may be difficult or impossible, but in some instances may be based on prior experience relative to outcome in cases previously referred for expert opinion. An additional indicator may be how extensively the expert has published on the topic, the number of relevant cases involved in these publications, and if these publications are recent.

Summary

Most of the experience in evidence-based medicine has been derived from clinical medicine that seems more easily suited to the rigors of the higher tiers of quality. In pathology, it is difficult to apply many of the stringent requirements necessary to generate high quality. For example, there is some debate over what tests should be used to distinguish squamous cell carcinoma of the lung from other types of non-small cell carcinoma, as the former may be associated with severe pulmonary hemorrhage when treated with recently developed agents which inhibit angiogenesis [24]. Should the identification rely only on routine histologic criteria (keratinization and intercellular bridges), or should it include a group of IHC studies such as p63, TTF-1, and high molecular weight keratin antibodies without regard to the presence of morphologic features of squamous differentiation? Obviously, the patient selection for this new therapy differs depending on the diagnostic test. One manner to obtain best evidence regarding the diagnostic test would include two randomized groups of patients of similar characteristics selected but distinguished by how the carcinoma is characterized (by morphology alone or by the use of the IHC tests). The pathologist could be assigned to one study group only and blinded to the other group as well as outcome. The outcome would be the frequency of pulmonary hemorrhage in the two groups. Such a study is difficult to envision as a viable manner of determining which diagnostic criteria are best in predicting the outcome for both obvious, serious ethical as well as logistical reasons. On the other hand, it remains unknown if patients are unnecessarily excluded from receiving antiangiogenesis factors in the treatment of lung carcinoma based on the IHC studies without consideration of morphology. With the introduction of new therapies and diagnostic tests including molecular and cytogenetic assays, this scenario may become common place.

Nevertheless, there are effective strategies to improve the quality of evidence in pathology which have been illustrated in this chapter, building upon the cornerstones of observation and clinical correlation which have heretofore defined much of what we know as pathologists about disease and diagnosis.

References

1. Merriam-Webster's Online Dictionary, F.C. Mish, Editor. 2010. http://www.merriam-webster.com/dictionary/evidence.
2. Wild SE. Webster's new world law dictionary. Hoboken, NJ: Wiley; 2006. p. 320.
3. Lieberman D. The province of legislation determined: legal theory in eighteenth-century Britain. Cambridge: The Press Syndicate of the University of Cambridge; 1989. p. 312.
4. Rule 609. *Impeachment by evidence of conviction of crime.* 2010.
5. Center for Evidence Based Medicine. 2010. http://www.cebm.net/?o=1116.
6. McCrory DC, Samsa GP, Hamilton BB, et al. Treatment of pulmonary disease following cervical spinal cord injury: evidence report/technology assessment no. 27. Rockville, MD: Agency for Healthcare Research and Quality; 2001.
7. Appendix VII. Criteria for assessing internal validity of individual studies. 2010. http://www.ahrq.gov/clinic/uspstf08/methods/procmanualap7.htm.
8. Röhrig B, du Prel JB, Blettner M. Study design in medical research: part 2 of a series on the evaluation of scientific publications. Dtsch Arztebl Int. 2009;106(11):184–9.
9. Volokh A. *n Guilty Men.* Univ PA Law Rev. 1997; 146(1):173–216.
10. Trosset M. An introduction to statistical inference and its applications with R. Boca Raton, FL: Taylor and Francis Group LLC; 2009. p. 208.
11. Gunnarsson RK, Lanke J. The predictive value of microbiologic diagnostic tests if asymptomatic carriers are present. Stat Med. 2002;21(12):1773–85.
12. Greenhalgh T. How to read a paper: Statistics for the non-statistician. I: Different types of data need different statistical tests. Br Med J. 1997;315: 364–6.
13. Meenan RT, Saha S, Chou R, et al. Effectiveness and cost-effectiveness of echocardiography and carotid imaging in the management of stroke: evidence report/technology assessment no. 49. Rockville, MD: Agency for Healthcare Research and Quality; 2002.
14. Procedure Manual. Section 4: Evidence report development. 2010. http://www.ahrq.gov/clinic/uspstf08/methods/procmanual4.htm.
15. Levels of evidence. 2002. http://www.eboncall.org/content/levels.html.
16. Oxford Center for Evidence-based Medicine-Levels of Evidence (March 2009). http://www.cebm.net/index.aspx?o=1025. 2009.
17. Cook DJ, Mulrow CD, Haynes RB. Systematic reviews: synthesis of best evidence for clinical decisions. Ann Intern Med. 1997;126(5):376–80.
18. Garg AX, Hackam D, Tonelli M. Systematic review and meta-analysis: when one study is just not enough. Clin J Am Soc Nephrol. 2008;3:253–60.
19. The Cochrane Collaboration's open learning material. diversity and heterogeneity. http://www.cochrane-net.org/openlearning/HTML/mod13-5.htm. 2002.
20. From the U.S. Preventive Services Task Force, AfHRaQ, Rockville, Maryland. Screening for breast cancer: U.S. Preventive Services Task Force Recommendation Statement. Ann Intern Med. 2009; 10:716–26.
21. Elwood JM, Cox B, Richardson AK. The effectiveness of breast cancer screening by mammography in younger women. Online J Curr Clin Trials. 1993;Vol. 2.
22. Systematic Review Critical Appraisal Sheet. Critical appraisal sheets. http://www.cebm.net/index.aspx?o=1913. 2010.
23. Sinard JH, Morrow JS. Informatics and anatomic pathology: meeting challenges and charting the future. Hum Pathol. 2001;32:143–8.
24. Ricciardi S, Tomao S, de Marinis F. Toxicity of targeted therapy in non-small-cell lung cancer management. Clin Lung Cancer. 2009;10:28–35.

Biostatistics 101

4

Robin T. Vollmer

Keywords
Probability • Biostatistics in evidence-based medicine • Cox model • Hazard function • Log rank • Conditional probabilities • Receiver operator curve

Probability

The notion of probability began with questions regarding games of chance during the seventeenth century, so that the probability of an event can be defined as the chance of observing that event. In a more experimental mode, probability relates to the relative frequency of observing an outcome after many repeated trials. For example, suppose we perform an experiment and observe an outcome E. Now let us repeat the experiment n times and tally the number of times E occurs to be m. The probability of E, $P(E)$, would be estimated as m/n. In this manner, the probability of the outcome could be defined as the limit of m/n when n becomes infinite.

In the twentieth century, however, probability was redefined in set theoretic and mathematical terms. What follows is an abbreviated version of this mathematics. If we have a discrete set, S, of all possible observed events, then the probability of observing an event E is symbolized as $P(E)$. $P(E)$ must be a real number between 0 and 1. The probability of any event in S must be 1, that is, $P(S)=1$. The probability of no event in S is 0. If the event E does not happen, then this is also an event that is termed "not E" or sometimes symbolized as $\sim E$. The probability of $\sim E$ is given as:

$$P(\sim E) = 1 - P(E).$$

The odds of an event E is defined as the ratio of the probability of E divided by the probability of $\sim E$, or as:

$$\text{Odds (E)} = P(E)/(1 - P(E)).$$

Finally, if there are two events E_1 and E_2, the probability of observing either E_1 or E_2 is:

$$P(E_1 \text{or } E_2) = P(E_1) + P(E_2) - P(E_1 \text{ and } E_2).$$

Here, $P(E_1$ and $E_2)$ is the probability of observing both events. Two events, E_1 and E_2, are mutually exclusive if the probability of observing both is zero, i.e. $P(E_1$ and $E_2)=0$.

R.T. Vollmer (✉)
Department of Laboratory Medicine,
VA Medical Center, Durham, NC, USA
e-mail: Robin.Vollmer@va.gov

A.M. Marchevsky and M.R. Wick (eds.), *Evidence Based Pathology and Laboratory Medicine*,
DOI 10.1007/978-1-4419-1030-1_4,

Statistical Independence

Two events E_1 and E_2 are statistically independent if and only if the probability of observing both is the product of each of their separate probabilities, that is, if and only if:

$$P(E_1 \text{ and } E_2) = P(E_1) \times P(E_2).$$

This is the only true notion of statistical independence. When we read that variables like tumor stage and grade provided "independent" prognostic information, such conclusions and wordings are most often wrong, because variables important to survival are often codependent, not statistically independent. What they may provide is additive, not independent, information.

Conditional Probabilities

Conditional probabilities are of great importance in medicine, including pathology. For example, sensitivities, specificities, and positive predictive values are examples of conditional probabilities. Using a general approach, consider the two events E_1 and E_2. The probability of observing event E_2 given that E_1 has already been observed is the conditional probability $P(E_2 \mid E_1)$. If the two events are the presence of a positive laboratory test $T+$ and the presence of a particular diagnosis $D+$, then $100 \times P(T+ \mid D+)$ is the sensitivity of the test for the diagnosis (expressed here as a percent). In other words, the sensitivity of the test T is the conditional probability that T is +, given the presence of the diagnosis D. (In what follows, the 100× will be omitted, and the conditional probabilities will be expressed as fractions rather than percents.) Table 4.1 lists and defines several commonly used conditional probabilities for tests and diseases.

One can also form ratios of these conditional probabilities. For example, the relative risk is defined as the positive predictive value of the test divided by the probability of a false negative test or:

$$\text{Relative risk} = P(D+ \mid T+) / P(D+ \mid T-).$$

Table 4.1 Conditional probabilities in pathology

Sensitivity of test *T* for diagnosis *D*:	$P(T+ \mid D+)$
Specificity of test *T* for diagnosis *D*:	$P(T- \mid D-)$
Probability of false positive test *T*:	$P(T+ \mid D-)$ $= 1 - P(T- \mid D-)$
Probability of false negative test *T*:	$P(T- \mid D+)$ $= 1 - P(T+ \mid D+)$
Positive predictive value of test *T* for diagnosis *D*:	$P(D+ \mid T+)$
Negative predictive value of test *T* for diagnosis *D*:	$P(D- \mid T-)$

And the likelihood ratio is defined as the sensitivity divided by the probability of a false positive test or as:

$$\text{Likelihood ratio} = P(T+ \mid D+) / P(T+ \mid D-).$$

ROC Curves

A graphical tool that has been helpful for evaluating new tests in clinical medicine is the ROC curve. ROC stands for receiver operator curve, and it was used in World War II to evaluate the abilities of plane spotters to classify aircraft as either friendly or enemy. In medicine, the ROC is formed by plotting sensitivity against 1-specificity. In other words, the vertical axis is $P(T+ \mid D+)$ and the horizontal axis is $1 - P(T- \mid D-)$. Furthermore, 1-specificity is the same as the probability of a false positive test. Consequently, a perfect diagnostic test – one with sensitivity of 1 and a false positive probability of 0 – would appear as single point in the upper left corner of the ROC. An example of an ROC is the following plot, which demonstrates the value of serum PSA for the diagnosis of prostate cancer (Fig. 4.1).

The points on the curve (Brawer et al.'s data) and angles in the line (Catalona et al.'s data) are due to the use of different cutpoints in serum PSA for the diagnosis of prostate cancer [1, 2]. For example, locations on the ROC in the lower left side of the plot are for cutpoints at high values of serum PSA, where the sensitivity is low and the specificity high. Locations on the ROC in the upper right side of the plot are for cutpoints at low values of serum PSA, where the sensitivity is high and the specificity low. The straight line on the plot indicates ROC locations

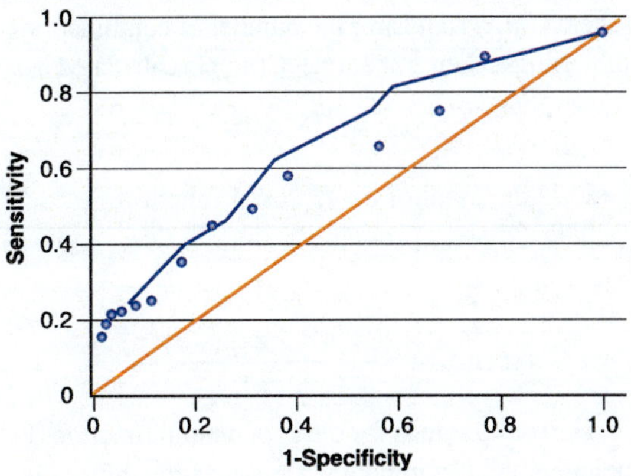

Fig. 4.1 ROC plot of sensitivity versus 1-specificity for serum PSA and the diagnosis of prostate cancer. The data come from studies by Brawer et al. (*points*) [1] and Catalona et al. (*curved line*) [2]. For each point and each angle in the curve, a different cutpoint in serum PSA was used. The straight line indicates the locations where tests are not helpful, that is, where sensitivity equals 1-specificity

for a test that is not diagnostically helpful, that is, where sensitivity equals 1-specificity. In fact, the further the curve lies above this line, the better will be the test. Higher ROC curves also imply larger areas under the ROC curve, and this area, which commonly ranges from 0.5 to 1.0, is often used as a measure of a good test.

Bayes Theorem or Rule

Thomas Bayes was a Presbyterian minister who lived in England in the eighteenth century, and he also was a mathematician with interests in calculus and numerical series. But he is best known for his formula. Although he developed the rule to solve a problem dealing with billiard tables, it is seen most clearly in set theoretic notation. What Bayes' rule allows us to do is to estimate the positive predictive value of a positive test *T+* for a diagnosis *D+* by using the sensitivity and underlying probabilities of *T+* and *D+* as follows:

$$P(D+ \mid T+) = \frac{P(T+ \mid D+) \times P(D+)}{P(T+)}.$$

Here, *P(D+)* is the a priori probability of the disease without consideration of the test *T*. The denominator *P(T+)* is the a priori probability of a positive test, and if there are just two possibilities, *D+* and *D–*, it can be calculated as:

$$\begin{aligned} P(T+) = {} & P(T+ \mid D+) \times P(D+) \\ & + P(T+ \mid D-) \times P(D-) \\ = {} & \text{sensitivity} \times \text{prevalence} \\ & + (1 - \text{specificity}) \times (1 - \text{prevalence}) \end{aligned}$$

Thus, if one knows the sensitivity and the specificity of a test and the prevalence or incidence of the disease, then one can estimate the positive predictive value of the test for the disease.

Random Variables

In the foregoing, we have talked of probability of events such as E_1, E_2, or of *T+* and D_x+, but in fact many events of interest are numerical. We call such numerical events random variables, and in what follows, we will use the symbol x to represent a generic random variable. Examples of random variables include the Gleason score for prostate cancer, the Breslow thickness for malignant melanoma, and the values of many clinical chemistry results such as serum PSA. Random variables can be classified as discrete or continuous. Discrete random variables include binary ones, which take just two values like 0 or 1, or yes or no. Discrete random variables can also be categorical and ordered, and an example is the Gleason score which takes the integer values of 2–10. Continuous random variables, by contrast, can have an infinite number of values, and examples include serum Na, serum creatinine, and serum PSA.

Probability Distributions for Discrete Random Variables

For a discrete random variable like the Gleason score, the probability that the Gleason score takes a particular numerical value is called its probability distribution, which we symbolize here as $f(x)$. In other words, the probability that x takes the value of α is written as:

$$P(x = \alpha) = f(\alpha).$$

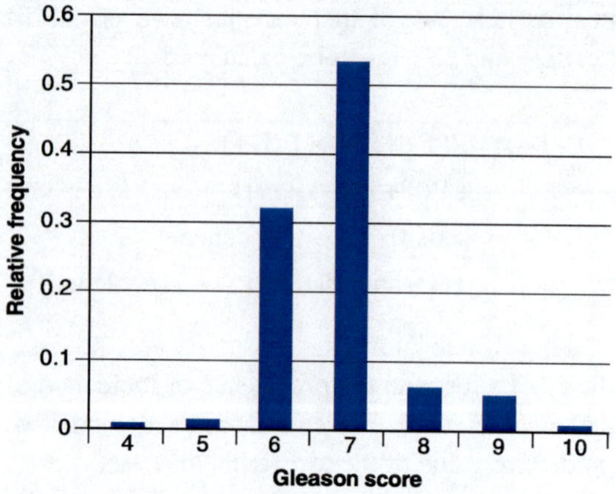

Fig. 4.2 Frequency distribution of cases of prostate cancer according to their Gleason grading scores (the author's data)

For a population of 891 tissue samples of prostate with cancer (data collected by the author), the probability distribution for the Gleason score *f*(Gleason score) took the follow values: $f(2) \sim 0, f(3) \sim 0, f(4)=0.002, f(5)=0.016, f(6)=0.32, f(7)=0.54, f(8)=0.063, f(9)=0.053$, and $f(10)=0.0067$. Notice that the values of *f*(Gleason score) sum to approximately 1. This distribution function is illustrated in the histogram in Fig. 4.2.

The Binomial and Poisson Probability Distributions for Counted Random Variables

Two mathematical forms appropriate for discrete random variables that are counted phenomena are the binomial and Poisson probability distribution functions. These are of special interest to pathologists, because both can deal with counts of cells. For example, if one counts *n* cells and observes that *x* number of these cells stain positive for an immunohistochemical marker, then the fraction of cells with staining would be estimated as *x*/*n*. If the underlying probability of observing a cell with staining is symbolized as θ, then the binomial distribution for the probability of observing *x* cells with staining is given as:

$$f(x;n,\theta) = c(n,x) \times \theta^{(x)} \times (1-\theta)^{(n-x)},$$

where C(*n*,*x*) stands for the number of combinations of *n* things taken *x* at a time. C(*n*,*x*) is calculated as:

$$C(n,x) = n!/\{x! \times (n-x)!\}$$

and ! is the symbol for factorial function.

The Poisson probability distribution is given as:

$$f(x;n,\theta) = \frac{(\theta \times n)^x \times \exp(-\theta \times n)}{x!}.$$

Here, exp stands for the exponential function. In practice, the binomial and Poisson probability distribution functions agree closely with one another, especially if *n* exceeds 20 and θ is less than 0.05. The Poisson function, however, can be applied to situations when the counts of *x* are expressed as number per area. An example comes from primary cutaneous melanoma for which the mitotic count is expressed as number per square millimeter. All one needs to do is to substitute area for *n* in the above equation.

Probability Distributions for Continuous Random Variables

If the random variable *x* is continuous, then it can take an infinite number of values, and its probability distribution must rely on calculus. Instead of writing the probability that *x* takes a certain value α as $P(x=\alpha)$, we are restricted to consider, for example, the probability that $x \leq \alpha$ which we write as an integral as follows:

$$P(x \leq \alpha) = \int f(x)\,dx.$$

Here, the limits of the integration are from $-\infty$ to α, and once again *f*(*x*) is the distribution function for *x*. Distribution functions commonly used for continuous random variables include the normal, the log-normal, the chi-square, and the exponential. The log-normal and exponential distribution functions are particularly suitable for continuous random variables used in pathology because they deal with random variables that always take positive values, and this is the case for many continuous variables in clinical medicine. For example, the following bar graph shows the observed

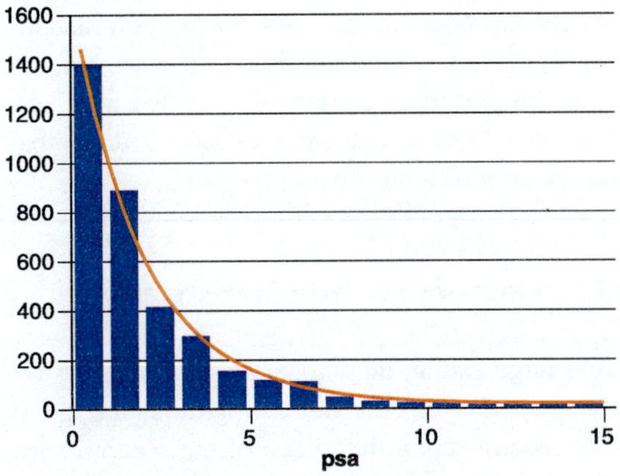

Fig. 4.3 Frequency distribution for values of serum PSA taken from data reported by Morgan et al. [3]. The smooth line is a superimposed fit obtained by using the exponential distribution function

frequency distribution for values of serum PSA taken from a study by Morgan et al. [3]. The smooth line is a superimposed fit obtained by using the exponential distribution function Fig. 4.3. This distribution demonstrates that for most men with negative biopsies, PSA is less than 5 ng/mL.

Distribution Functions of Two Random Variables and Statistical Independence

If there are two random variables, *x* and *y*, then the distribution function for observing both is symbolized as *f*(*x*,*y*). Following the same logic used for independent events, two random variables, *x* and *y*, are statistically independent of one another if and only if:

$$f(x, y) = f1(x) \times f2(y),$$

where f1(*x*) is the distribution function for *x* and f2(*y*) is for *y*.

Independent Samples

If we observe a random variable, *x*, on each patient in a study of *n* patients, we can symbolize the entire sample as x_1, x_2, x_3, … x_n. For such a sample to be a random sample, the joint probability distribution of observing $x_1, x_2, x_3, \ldots, x_n$ should be given as:

$$f(x_1, x_2, x_3, \ldots x_n) = \prod fi(xi).$$

(Here, $\prod$ is a symbol for product, and the index *i* goes from 1 to *n*.) In other words, to comprise a random sample, the joint distribution function should equal the product of all the individual distribution functions for the individual patients. In short, the patients and their random variables should be statistically independent from one another.

Statistics

Statistics are numerical summarizing measures of random variables taken from a (usually random) sample as described above. Examples of statistics include the mean, median, variance, standard deviation, the *t* statistic, the *F* statistic, and the chi-square statistic.

Statistical Hypothesis Testing

Statistical testing most commonly involves making what is called the null hypothesis. For example, if we have observed two random variables, *x* and *y*, and if we suspect that these two are related to one another, then we begin the process with the null hypothesis that there is no such relationship. Having made the null hypothesis, we then apply a statistical test or model to the data and calculate a statistic, *s*. Under conditions of the test or model, we obtain the probability of observing *s* if the null hypothesis is true. This probability is called the *p* value. If the *p* value is low (typically less than 0.05 or 0.01), we conclude that the null hypothesis is unlikely and reject it. In other words, we accept the alternative hypothesis, which in the above example is that *x* and *y* are related to one another. If there are multiple random variables involved in the study, then a multivariable model and analysis may yield multiple statistics and multiple *p* values.

The *p* value is also known as the probability of making a Type I error, which is defined as the error of rejecting a null hypothesis that is in fact true. Thus, many researchers choose low thresholds for the p value, such as 0.01, in order to make their Type I errors unlikely.

Type II Errors, Statistical Power, and Sample Sizes

If there is a Type I error, then there must be a Type II error, and it is defined as the error of rejecting the null hypothesis when in fact it is true. The probability of making a Type II error is often symbolized as β. Naturally, researchers desire to make β small. Statistical power equals $1-\beta$, but is often difficult to calculate. Researchers minimize β by choosing statistical tests that are naturally powerful and by increasing the number of cases or patients that they are studying, because the larger the sample size, the smaller will be the β. In general, numbers of cases or patients less than 100 are sufficient for exploratory analyses, but usually numbers in the 100s will be required for definitive results. Numbers in the 1,000s will allow statistical models to include multiple important random variables, and such models, if validated with new data, may then provide prognostic algorithms that can be applied to new patients.

Table 4.2 Features of commonly used statistical tests

Test	Application
Chi-square	Test for effects of two categorical variables on one another
Fisher exact	Test for effects of two categorical variables on one another
t test	Comparison of means of a continuous variable between two groups
Wilcoxon	Nonparametric comparison of means of a continuous variable between two groups
One-way AOV	Test for effects of one categorical variable on the mean of a continuous variable
Kruskal–Wallis	Nonparametric test for effects of one categorical variable on the mean of a continuous variable
Two-way AOV	Test for effects of two categorical variables on the mean of a continuous variable
Linear regression	Test for effects of one or more explanatory variables on a continuous-dependent variable
Logistic regression	Test for effects of one or more explanatory variables on a binary-dependent variable
Log-rank	Test for effects of a categorical variable on survival time
Cox model	Test for effects of one or more explanatory variables on survival time

Overview of Common Statistical Tests

To a large extent, the choice of statistical test we use for analyzing data and testing the null hypothesis depends upon the nature of the random variables in the data. For example, if there are two random variables and both are binary (i.e. they have just two values), then the chi-square or Fisher tests could be used. If there are two random variables, x and y, and if y is a dependent continuous variable and x is a categorical one, then the t test or one-way analysis of variance (AOV) would be appropriate so long as y was approximately normally distributed. If y were not normal, then nonparametric tests like the Wilcoxon or Kruskal–Wallis tests could be used. If y is a dependent continuous random variable and there are several continuous or categorical explanatory variables x_1, x_2, x_3, etc., then regression analysis is appropriate so long as the residual error measurements are approximately normally distributed. If y is a binary-dependent variable and there are several continuous or categorical explanatory variables x_1, x_2, x_3, etc., then logistic regression is appropriate. If y is a failure time and there are several continuous or categorical explanatory variables x_1, x_2, x_3, etc., then the Cox proportional hazard model is appropriate. Table 4.2 summarizes features for commonly used statistical tests.

Chi-Square Tests

The chi-square test has been the workhorse of medical statistics for decades. It most often deals with two binary random variables, x and y. The data are typically presented in a 2×2 table as follows:

		x	
		Negative	Positive
y	Negative	a	b
	Positive	c	d

Here, a is the count of patients negative for both x and y, b the count of those positive for

x and negative for y, c the count of those negative for x and positive for y, and d the count of those positive for both x and y. The null hypothesis for this test assumes that y and x are statistically independent, that is, that $P(y \mid x) = P(y)$ and $P(x \mid y) = P(x)$. Then the software estimates the probabilities $P(y)$ and $P(x)$ from the data and without regard to each other. Next, the test compares the number of observed results for each category of y and x with that expected from the pooled estimates of $P(y)$ and $P(x)$. Specifically, it forms ratios comprising the squared differences between observed and expected numbers divided by the expected number and sums these over the cells in the table to yield a statistic s as follows:

$$s = \sum (\text{no. observed} - \text{no. expected})^2 / \text{no. expected}.$$

Because under the null hypothesis, this s follows the chi-square distribution, the test is called the chi-square test, and it can also be used for categorical random variables with more than two results. If there are r categories or possible values of y and c or possible categories for x, then the total number of possible categories using both variables is $r \times c$; however, the numbers of observations in each combined category or cell should exceed 5. The product $(r-1) \times (c-1)$ is called the degrees of freedom. When the estimated chi-square is sufficiently large, then the deviations of observed from expected numbers are high, and the null hypothesis is rejected.

When the counts of cases in the cells of the table are smaller than 5, then the statistic does not follow a chi-square distribution, and one must use an alternative test such as the Fisher exact test, which relies on the geometric distribution.

Sometimes the categorical observations of y and x variables are paired. This could happen when one evaluates two immunohistochemical stains on a set of tumors, one tumor from each patient. In such a study, the routine chi-square test would be inappropriate and one must use the McNemar variant of the chi-square test. Its chi-square statistic relies on just the discordant results for each pair of staining results.

Another variant of the chi-square test applies when one questions whether the proportions of cases with a key result are the same across several studies. This issue commonly arises in meta-analyses. Before studies can be combined to produce an overall result, one must usually test if the studies are homogeneous in their design and in the way they recruited patients. For example, Table 4.3 lists observed probabilities that patients had cancer of the prostate given a PSA value ≥4 ng/mL. The data come from four different studies [1–4]. The probability is listed as ppv, and the total number of patients is listed as n.

Table 4.3 Observed probabilities that patients had cancer of the prostate given a PSA value ≥4 ng/mL

Study	n	ppv
Babaian	404	0.45
Catalona	750	0.34
Brawer	227	0.34
Morgan	5258	0.76

The data come from four different studies (Babaian et al. [4] Catalona et al. [2]; Brawer et al. [1]; and Morgan et al. [3]). The probability is listed as ppv, and the total number of patients is listed as n

Whereas the values of ppv in the first three studies appear reasonably close to one another, the value of 0.76 in the last study is approximately twice as high. Are these results significantly different from one another? The test of equality of proportions can provide an answer. First, a weighted estimate of the overall proportion positive is calculated. Then this estimate with its derived variance is used to once again calculate the difference between observed and expected values as above. The result gives another statistic with a chi-square distribution. In S-PLUS, this test is done with the call to *prop.test*, and for these data, it yielded a chi-square statistic of 358 ($p \sim 0$) for the null hypothesis that the observed proportions were the same. Thus, we can conclude that there were significant differences between these four studies, and in fact, the design for the first three differed from that of the fourth. Whereas the first three assayed serum PSA in men all of whom underwent biopsy of the prostate, the fourth collected PSA data from two populations, one selected because they had a positive biopsy for prostate cancer and a control group that included many who did not have biopsies done. Because the control groups in the first three studies included many men with BPH or other conditions which required biopsy, they also included many with elevated PSA but without cancer, and this had the effect of lowering the ppv in comparison with the fourth study.

Finally, the Mantel–Haenszel chi-square test is done to test for statistical independence between *y* and *x* when there is a third confounding variable present. The third variable could be the presence of another disease, a drug, or that the observations came from different institutions or overall categories. For example, Morgan et al. published the frequencies of patients with prostate cancer (*y* variable) versus PSA levels >=4 ng/mL (*x* variable), stratified by eight categories of age and race [3]. A Mantel–Haenszel test for the relationship between presence of cancer and PSA, while controlling for these eight categories, yielded a chi-square value of 2,519 and a *p* value of approximately 0, thus allowing one to reject the null hypothesis of no association between PSA and presence of cancer.

t Test

The *t* test is another long-used workhorse in statistical analysis of medical data. Although its popularity is now less than that for tests that can deal with multiple random variables, it continues to be used and has proven useful as a screening device for proteomic data. The *t* test is most commonly used to see if the means of a continuous random variable, *y*, are the same in two separate populations, and it requires that *y* be normally distributed and that its variance is the same in the two populations. Consider the following example.

In 2002, Petricoin et al. published a SELDI-TOF analysis of the serum proteome on 50 women with ovarian cancer and 50 women without ovarian cancer [5]. The data comprised mass spectral patterns of intensities versus mass/charge ratio (*M/Z*). Figure 4.4 plot shows a portion of the spectrum with the mean intensities for the two groups of women (two lines on the plot).

Where the lines separate, the higher line shows the means for women with ovarian cancer. The question is whether these sites of separation are significantly so. A series of *t* tests was applied

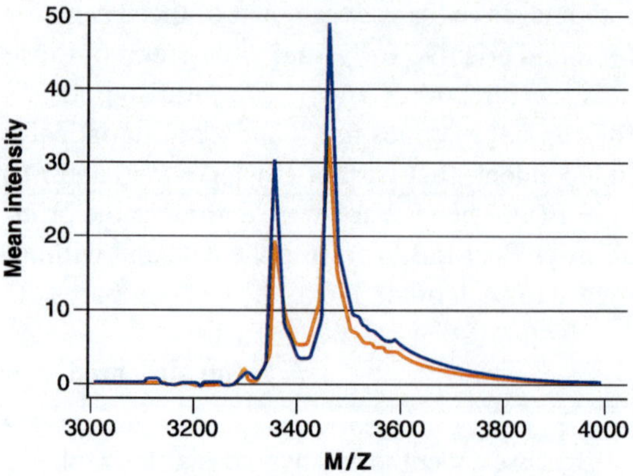

Fig. 4.4 A portion of mass spectral patterns of intensities versus mass/charge ratio (*M/Z*) for two groups of women (two lines on the plot), one with ovarian cancer (*upper line*) and one without cancer (*lower line*) (data from Petricoin et al. [5])

to the data, one for each value of *M/Z*, and the values for these *t* statistics appear in Fig. 4.5.

The graph now shows calculated values of the *t* statistic versus values of *M/Z*, and the upper and lower horizontal lines show thresholds for a *p* value of 0.01 in the *t* test. Consequently, in the region near *M/Z* values of 3,400, there were negative *t* values of such a magnitude that they fell beyond the $p=0.01$ threshold. This result then suggested that there were serum proteins in this *M/Z* range which were likely to differ between women with and without ovarian cancer.

The *t* test is also commonly applied to paired observations of a continuous random variable, which may arise when a continuous random variable is observed before and after some intervention. Furthermore, even when the original random variable is not normally distributed, the difference between the paired values may be at least approximately normal, and in this circumstance the prerequisites for the *t* test are satisfied.

Parametric Tests and Normally Distributed Random Variables

Tests designed to be used on normally distributed random variables are often described as "parametric" as opposed to "non-parametric". In general, these parametric tests will be more powerful than their nonparametric counterparts. In other words, the parametric tests will yield lower *p* values for the

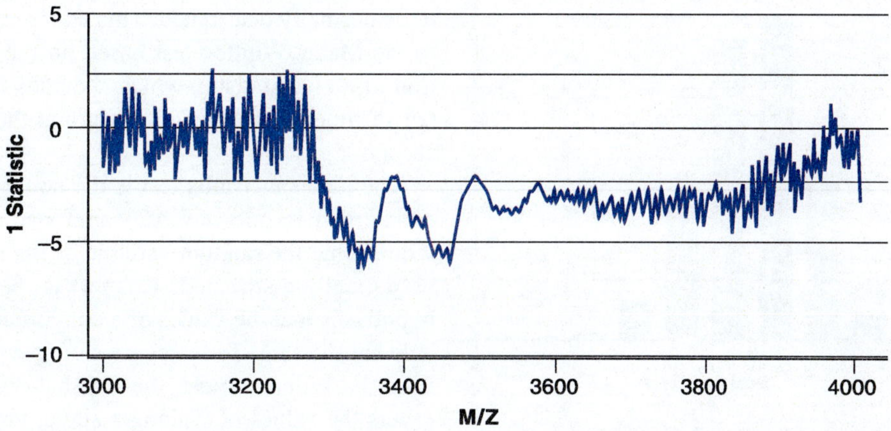

Fig. 4.5 Plot of *t* statistics versus *M/Z* for the portion of the *M/Z* spectrum in Fig. 4.4. The *t* statistic evaluates the difference in mean intensities between women with ovarian cancer and those without cancer, and this is done for each value of *M/Z* in the spectrum. The upper and lower lines on the plot show where values of *t* indicate significant differences in means for the two groups of women at a *p* value of 0.01

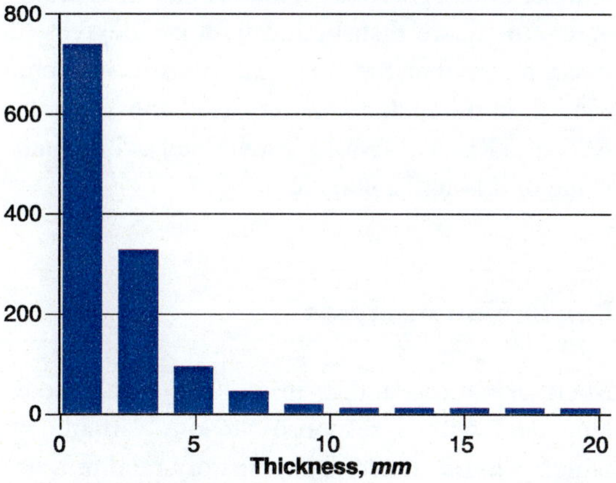

Fig. 4.6 Frequency distribution of tumor thickness in malignant melanoma (the author's data)

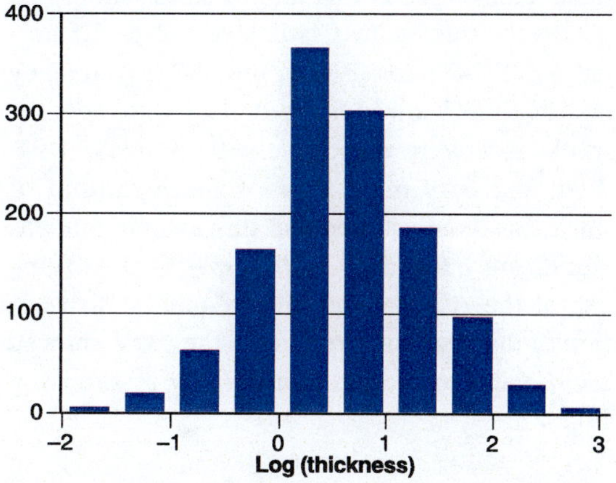

Fig. 4.7 Frequency distribution of natural logarithm (Log) of tumor thickness in malignant melanoma (the author's data)

null hypotheses and will require fewer data to do so. Nevertheless, before using parametric tests, one should at least attempt to see if the random variables or their residual errors are normally distributed. For a given continuous random variable, the easiest way to do this is to plot its frequency distribution, see if it is symmetric (versus skewed) with the peak in the middle of the range, and to see that it is neither too flat nor too narrow. If the frequency distribution does not appear normal, then some transformation of the variable, such as the logarithm or square root, may be normally distributed. In that case, the parametric tests can still be applied. For example, the Breslow thickness in over 1,000 cases of cutaneous melanoma has the following approximately skewed and exponential frequency distribution (Fig. 4.6).

Yet, using the natural logarithm converts tumor thickness to an approximately normally distributed as seen in Fig. 4.7.

In some tests like AOV and regression analyses, it is more important that the residual error values are normally distributed than to have the original dependent random variables be normal. Finally, in general, regression analyses do not require that the explanatory variables be normal.

One-Way Analysis of Variance

AOV provides a way to see if the means of a normally distributed random variable y are the same across several levels of a categorical variable x.

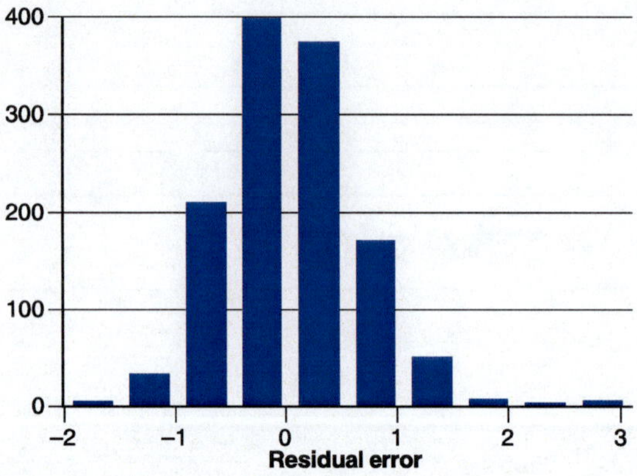

Fig. 4.8 Frequency distribution of residual error values from the AOV of logarithm of tumor thickness according to Clark levels in malignant melanoma (the author's data)

For example, common familiarity with cutaneous melanoma suggests that the thickness should be positively related to Clark levels 2–5. Examination of the cases used in the above frequency distributions showed that the mean thickness for levels 2–5 were respectively 0.46, 1.65, 1.94, 2.50, and 6.29 mm. AOV of the logarithm of thickness demonstrated that this association was significant (*F* statistic = 784, $p \sim 0$). Justifying use of the AOV model, the frequency distribution of the residual errors from the AOV showed a close approximation to normality as shown in Fig. 4.8:

Wilcoxon and Kruskal–Wallis Tests

The Wilcoxon test is the nonparametric counterpart to the *t* test. In other words, it is appropriate for the null hypothesis that a continuous variable, *y*, is the same for two groups of patients, and it can deal with paired or nonpaired data. Its analysis and results are based on ranks of *y* rather than the values of *y* directly, and it does not require *y* to be normally distributed. This test is equivalent to the Mann–Whitley test based on the calculation of a Uy2 statistic, which provides the number of times y is larger in one group than in the second.

The Kruskal–Wallis test is the nonparametric counterpart to one-way AOV and also does not require that the random variable or the residuals be normally distributed. This test is for the null hypothesis that the values of a continuous *y* variable are the same for categories of an *x* variable. Like the Wilcoxon test, the Kruskal–Wallis test orders the values of *y* along a single virtual row and then sums the ranks for each category of *x*. It then computes an H statistic based on the sum of squared values of these ranks divided by the number of patients in each *x* category. If k is the number of categories of *x*, then H has an approximate chi-square distribution with *k*-1 degrees of freedom, so that the final test statistic is a chi-square. In the melanoma data used above for the AOV, the Kruskal–Wallis test yielded a chi-square value of 434 and a *p* value of ~0.

Regression Analyses

Many statistical studies in pathology and medicine deal with a response random variable, *y*, which is to be related to explanatory random variables, $x_1, x_2, \ldots, x_n$. This is the domain of regression analyses. The *y* variable is the dependent one, and the *x* variables are usually called the independent variables, explanatory variables, or covariates. Examples of regression analyses include linear regression, general linear model analysis, logistic regression analysis, and the Cox proportional hazard model for survival time. In these examples, some function of *y*, *f*(*y*), is related to a linear combination of the *x* variables as follows:

$$f(y) = b_0 + b_1 \times x_1 + b_2 \times x_2 + b_3 \times x_3 + \ldots + b_n \times x_n + \text{error}.$$

Here, the b_0 is an intercept, and the $b_1, b_2, \ldots, b_n$ are coefficients to be multiplied times their respective *x* variables. The *x* variables can be binary (e.g., 0 vs. 1), categorical like Gleason grade, or continuous; and if continuous, they need not be normally distributed.

In linear regression, even some degree of nonlinearity can be accommodated. For example, one can use interaction terms that combine the effects of two or more explanatory variables. For example, adding a variable x_4 equal to the product $x_2 \times x_3$ would make it an interaction variable. Such an interaction might apply when $f(y)$ increases with positive x_2, increases with x_3, but does not increase as much when both x_2 and x_3 are positive. In this example, coefficients b_2 and b_3 would be positive, but the coefficient b_4 for the interaction variable x_4 would be negative. Second and third powers of explanatory variables can also be used to accommodate nonlinearity in the relationship between y and the explanatory variables.

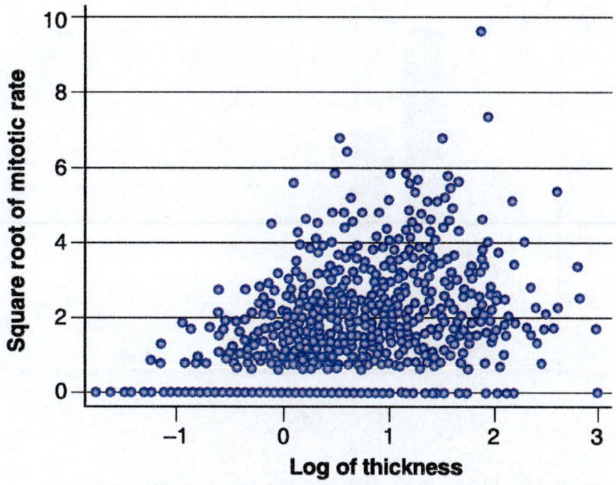

Fig. 4.9 Plot of square root of mitotic rate (number per square millimeter) versus logarithm of tumor thickness in malignant melanoma (the author's data)

Linear Regression Analysis

In linear regression, the dependent y variable is continuous and may be used as it is or transformed but it does not need to be normally distributed. By contrast, the error term must be approximately normally distributed, and in this circumstance, linear regression results in t statistics for the null hypotheses that the b coefficients in the regression equation are 0. Large values of the t statistics imply low p values, and then allow us to reject the null hypothesis of no association between y and the respective x variable. For example, consider the relationship between mitotic rate in cutaneous melanoma and tumor thickness. Mitotic rate in melanoma is usually expressed as number per square millimeter, and thickness as millimeters. A plot of square root of mitotic rate versus log(thickness) for over 1,000 patients with melanoma appears in Fig. 4.9, and in spite of scatter in the data, there is a hint of a positive relationship.

Linear regression analysis of this data uses the following equation:

$$\text{Sqrt(mitoses)} = b_0 + b_1 \times \log(\text{thickness}) + b_2 \times \text{ulcer} + \text{error},$$

where Sqrt symbolizes the square root transformation, log is the natural logarithm, and ulcer takes the values 0 or 1. Table 4.4 shows the results of the linear regression.

Table 4.4 Linear regression of square root of mitotic rate in melanoma

Variable	Coefficient	t	p Value
Intercept	0.989	24.3	~0
log(thickness)	0.568	12.0	~0
Ulceration	0.718	8.9	~0

These results, including the high values of t and low p values, demonstrate that mitotic rate is not independent of either thickness or ulceration. Examination of the residuals from the analysis shows an approximately normal distribution as shown in Fig. 4.10.

(A histogram of the error residuals should be routinely examined to see if the assumption of normally distributed residuals is justified.) The breadth of the residual histogram hints that the linear model explained a fraction of the scatter in the former plot, and the R^2 value from the

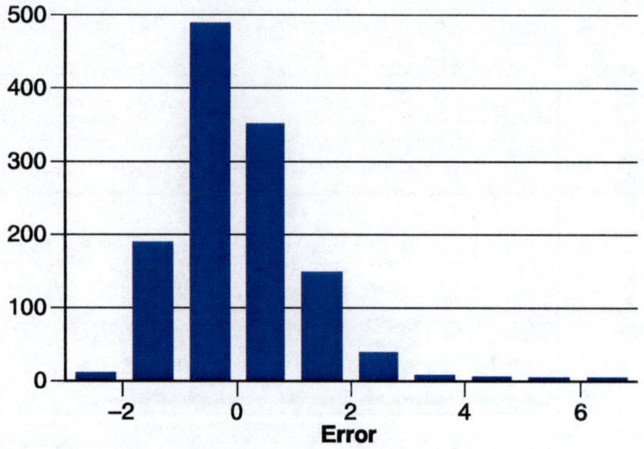

Fig. 4.10 Frequency distribution of residual error values from the linear regression analysis of how mitotic rate depends upon tumor thickness and ulceration in malignant melanoma (the author's data)

regression analysis tells us more specifically how much of the variance in the data was explained by the regression model. For this data, R^2 was 0.23 indicating that the model explained just 23% of the variance in the data.

General Linear Model (GLM)

The GLM is analogous to the linear regression model except that GLM does not assume that the residuals are normally distributed. Nevertheless, GLM does assume that the variance of the dependent random variable, *y*, is constant. The GLM has the same linear form as in linear regression:

$$f(y) = b_0 + b_1 \times x_1 + b_2 \times x_2 + b_3 \times x_3 + \ldots + b_n \times x_n + \text{error}.$$

The *y* variables may be either continuous or categorical. Instead of obtaining a least squares fit to the collected data of $\{y, x_1, x_2, \ldots\}$ as done in linear regression, the GLM obtains estimates of the *b* coefficients to maximize a likelihood function, *L*, or its natural logarithm ln(*L*). The exact form of *L* depends on the nature of *f*(*y*). GLM obtains its solutions for the *b* coefficients through an iterative fitting procedure. As in linear regression the null hypothesis is that the values for the *b* coefficients are 0, and when this is the case, a likelihood ratio statistic has a chi-square distribution with the number of degrees of freedom equal to the number of *x* variables used in the model. The result is termed the "likelihood ratio test" for testing the significance of one or more of the *x* variables. The next model to be discussed, the logistic model, provides an example. Others can be found in the McCullach and Nelder text [6].

The Logistic Regression Model

The logistic regression model deals with a dependent random variable, *y*, which is binary, that is, either 0 or 1. In other words, logistic regression is appropriate when we want to know which *x* variables increase, or decrease, the chance of a diagnosis or an important clinical outcome. In logistic regression, the transformation of *y*, which is considered linear, is the natural logarithm of the odds as follows:

$$f(y) = \log\{\text{odds } (y = 1)\} = b_0 + b_1 \times x_1 + b_2 \times x_2 + b_3 \times x_3 + \ldots + b_n \times x_n.$$

Because the odds ($y = 1$) is defined in terms of probability $P(y = 1)$ as:

$$\text{Odds } (y = 1) = P/(1 - P),$$

the probability *P* can also be written as:

$$P(y = 1) = 1/\{1 + \exp(-E)\}$$

with *E* given as:

$$E = b_0 + b_1 \times x_1 + b_2 \times x_2 + b_3 \times x_3 + \ldots + b_n \times x_n.$$

Once again the null hypothesis is that the coefficients *b* are equal to 0. Peduzzi et al. suggest that for the logistic analysis to produce reliable results, the data should include at least ten events for each *x* variable with event being defined as the smaller number of those with either $y = 1$ or $y = 0$ [7]. Because of the importance of this multivariable logistic model, three examples of its use on real data follow.

Logistic Regression Analysis of HPV DNA Testing in Women with ASCUS

Recently, Siddiqi et al. examined the results of hybrid capture two human papillomavirus DNA testing (HC2) in 8,195 women with atypical squamous cells of undetermined significance (ASCUS) in their liquid-based cervical samples.[8] The authors used the SurePath technique for 4,235 specimens and the ThinPrep technique for 3,960 specimens, and one of the goals of their study was to see if the technique affected a positive HC2 test. They stratified the women according to six age groups and demonstrated that age affected the probability of a positive HC2 test. Then they ran six chi-square tests – one for each age group – to see if the technique affected the probability of a positive HC2 test within the age groups. They found that only in the group of women under 19 years of age was the HC2 test dependent on the technique (the ThinPrep technique yielded more positive HC2 results).

The data from this study comprise a single binary-dependent variable – a positive HC2 test – and 2 explanatory variables: age of the patient and the technique for the liquid-based PAP processing. Consequently, the logistic regression model is ideal for this three variable data and has the advantage of analyzing all the data without breaking it into subsets or relying on multiple chi-square tests and multiple *p* values. Furthermore, when there is one variable that strongly affects the outcome – in this case age – it is important to control for its effect while analyzing the effect of the variable of interest – in this case, the liquid-based technique. Consider, for example, the following plot of the probability of a positive HC2 versus median patient age in authors' data (Fig. 4.11).

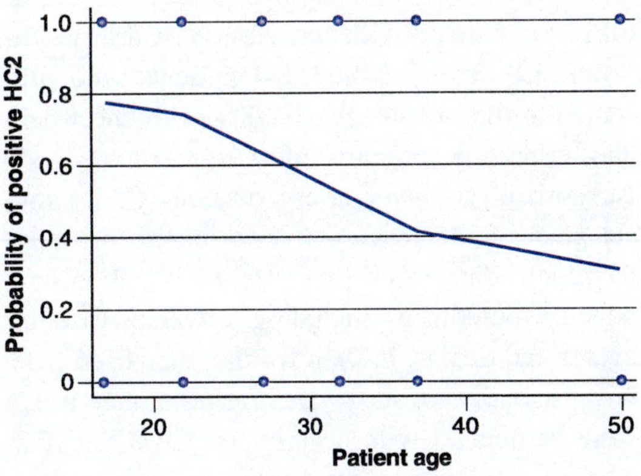

Fig. 4.11 A plot of the probability of a positive hybrid capture 2 human papillomavirus DNA testing (HC2) versus median patient age in the data reported by Siddiqi et al. [8]

The smooth line shows the relationship and demonstrates that the probability of a positive HC2 decreases smoothly with increase in age. This plot also suggests that age should be used as a continuous variable, rather than categorized into six groups. Logistic regression analysis can deal with continuous variables like age, and for this data, the logistic regression analysis yielded the following results.

Variable	Coefficient	*p* Value
Age	–0.0707	~0
ThinPrep technique	0.0548	0.03

The negative coefficient of –0.0707 for age demonstrates that increased age was associated with decreased probability of a positive HC2, as the above plot shows, and the *p* value of approximately zero indicates that age was strongly associated with the HC2 result. The positive coefficient of 0.0548 indicates that after controlling for the age effect, the ThinPrep technique resulted in more positive HC2 tests than did the SurePath technique, and that this difference was significant at a *p* value of 0.03. Thus, unlike the multiple chi-square tests done by the authors, the multivariable logistic model was able to demonstrate a significant overall effect of technique on the probability of a positive HC2 test.

Logistic Regression Analysis of Antiphospholipid Antibodies in Acute Coronary Artery Syndrome

To further illustrate the logistic regression model, consider the data published by Greco et al. regarding the importance of antiphospholipid antibodies (aPL's) in patients with acute coronary artery syndrome [9]. They studied 334 patients who presented to their acute care facility with chest pain and suspected coronary artery syndromes. They categorized coronary artery disease (CAD) into six grades of increasing severity based on catheterization data, and they recorded subsequent adverse outcomes, including adverse vascular events and deaths. In their results, they used pairwise statistical tests to demonstrate that aPL's were associated with severity of CAD and that adverse outcomes were associated with aPL's, with severity of CAD, and with aPL's within some categories of CAD. But logistic regression analysis offers the advantage of one statistical analysis of all the data to see how the binary event of adverse outcome depends on both aPL's as well as CAD grade. For the analysis, severity of CAD was collapsed into 4 levels of a single variable coded (0–III, IV, V and VI), because just one adverse event occurred in the 0–III group. Presence of aPL was coded as absent (0) versus positive (1). The results appear in the following table.

Variable	Coefficient	*p* Value
CAD	1.03	$5.2 \times 10-8$
aPL	1.3	$6.9 \times 10-4$

The very low *p* values demonstrate first that these two, related variables can provide additive information about the probability of an adverse outcome. After controlling for the information that CAD provides, the logistic model results demonstrate that aPL's provide additional helpful information. The positive coefficients demonstrate that both CAD as well as presence of aPL's imply increased probability of an adverse outcome.

Finally, the coefficients of the logistic regression can be used to form a predictive model to be used for new patients as follows. Using the model's intercept value, which was found to be –4.04, *E* can be calculated as

$$E = -4.04 + 1.03 \times CAD + 1.30 \times aPL$$

and the probability *P* of an adverse outcome for a new patient's values of CAD and aPL can then be estimated as:

$$P(\text{adverse event}) = \frac{1}{1 + \exp(-E)}$$

(The intercept value may need to be adjusted to reflect the local prevalence of adverse events.)

Logistic Regression Analysis of Atypical Epithelium in the Prostate

A third example of logistic regression analysis comes from studies of atypical small glands (ASAP) and high-grade prostatic intraepithelial neoplasia (HGPIN) in needle biopsies of the prostate. In 2005, Schlesinger et al. published their experience with 336 men who had either HGPIN or ASAP in an initial set of biopsies of the prostate and who subsequently had follow-up biopsies [10]. Importantly, there was not a control group of men with follow-up biopsies, but who had neither HGPIN nor ASAP. The question to consider is whether HGPIN adds information to the presence of ASAP regarding the outcome of cancer in the follow-up biopsies. A logistic regression analysis on their published data yielded the following results:

Variable	Coefficient	*p* Value
ASAP	0.512	0.012
HGPIN	–0.16	0.65

The results suggest that in this restricted situation where all men had either HGPIN or ASAP, the presence of ASAP was associated with cancer in the follow-up biopsy, but HGPIN was not.

In their publication, Schlesinger et al. summarized prior studies of HGPIN and ASAP, and in their summary, they demonstrated that the probability of cancer in the follow-up biopsy decreased with the time of the study [10]. The following plot shows the fraction of positive follow-up biopsies on the vertical axis versus the median study year on the horizontal axis, and the line for the trend in the data demonstrates that the probability of a positive follow-up biopsy decreased with time of the study (Fig. 4.12).

Thus, in the overall analysis, three variables seemed to be important: ASAP, HGPIN, and the time of the study cases. Because the logistic regression model can easily accommodate continuous variables such as time of study and easily accommodate three explanatory variables, I applied it to this summarizing data. (To do this, one must form a composite response variable that

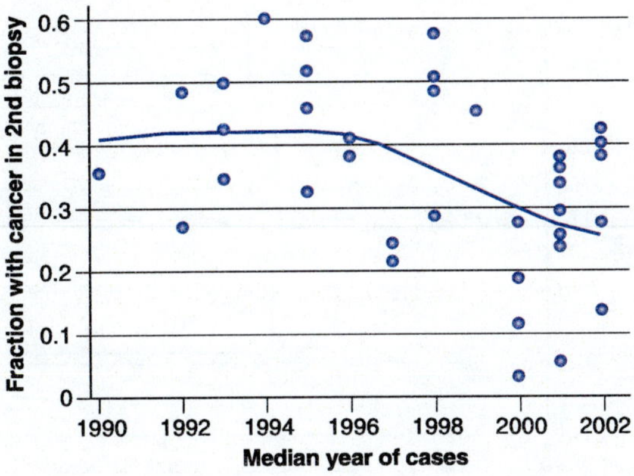

Fig. 4.12 Plot of the probability of prostate cancer in a second, follow-up biopsy of the prostate versus the median year of cases in studies summarized in the study by Schlesinger et al. [10]

combines the number of cases with cancer in the follow-up biopsy and the number of cases without cancer.) This analysis yielded the following results:

Variable	Coefficient	p Value
Median year	−0.0639	~0
ASAP	0.726	~0
HGPIN	0.0577	0.77

Once again, logistic regression demonstrated that after controlling for the important variables of year of study and presence of ASAP, HGPIN was not related to a positive follow-up biopsy. This example also demonstrates how helpful the logistic model can be in meta-analyses of prior studies.

Introduction to Survival Analysis

Whereas logistic regression deals with a binary outcome, survival analysis deals with two outcomes: a binary failure event like death and the time to the occurrence of that event. Survival data thus comprise the following categories:

Failure event: 1 if it occurred at the last observed time, 0 if it had not

Time of last observation: T

Explanatory regression variables: $x_1, x_2, \ldots, x_n$

The most commonly studied failure event in medicine is death, but other binary failure events can be analyzed, such as tumor recurrence, metastasis, and diagnosis of malignancy. Furthermore, the failure events need not be what we normally perceive as failures. For example, the event could be the achieving of a cure, the ending of symptoms, or the return to normal levels of some laboratory test. Similarly, the time variable need not be time. Other positive, continuous variables can be used such as the value of serum PSA.

If the patient has failed by the last observed time, then the value of the event is 1, and the patient is said to be uncensored. If the patient has not failed at the last time, then the value of event is 0, and the patient is said to be censored at the last time. One of the great strengths of survival analysis is its ability to deal with censored patients, but there is a cost. In general, most of the results come from the uncensored patients. Data rich in censored patients provide few helpful results, and Concato and Peduzzi et al. suggest that there should be at least ten uncensored patients for every explanatory variable [7].

The Survival Plot

Survival probability $S(t)$ is defined as the probability that survival time exceeds t. The most common way to illustrate $S(t)$ is the Kaplan–Meier plot, which plots $S(t)$ on the vertical axis versus time on the horizontal axis. For each time, the Kaplan–Meier method considers the number of persons at risk and the number of persons who fail. Times of observed failures cause vertical drops in the plot, and times when patients are censored are often illustrated with short vertical lines. As an example, consider two studies of pleomorphic liposarcoma published by Gebhard et al. and by Hornick et al. [11, 12]. Altogether, these two studies comprised 98 patients with follow-up. Forty were observed to die (uncensored), and 58 were living at last follow-up (censored). The Kaplan–Meier plot of all 98 appears as seen in Fig. 4.13.

The short vertical bars mark the times of last observation for the 58 censored patients, and the stair-step drops in the curve mark the times of death for the 40 uncensored patients. The faint lines above and below the curve indicate the estimates of 95% confidence limits.

As time t increases in Kaplan–Meier plots, there are fewer patients available for the analysis, because most have been either censored or died.

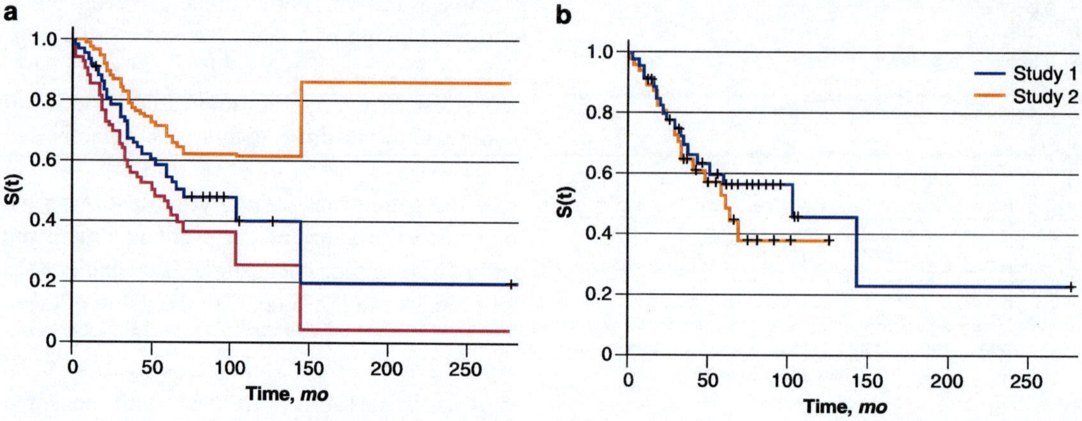

Fig. 4.13 (**a**, **b**) Plot of probability of survival versus time of follow-up in patients with pleomorphic liposarcoma reported by Gebhard et al. (study 1) and by Hornick et al. (study 2) [13, 14]

For example, in these two studies, less than 25% of the patients were observed past 64 months. What limited follow-up times does is to decrease the denominator of patients at risk for later times. Consequently, any deaths at these times cause steep drops in $S(t)$. This is also why the 95% confidence lines widen.

The Log-Rank Test for Equality of Survival Plots

In the above example of pleomorphic liposarcoma, 48 patients were studied in France (the Gebhard et al. study) [11], and the remaining 50 were studied in either England or the USA (the Hornick et al. study) [12]. Before combining data from both studies, one needs to test to see if the study affected survival. For example, study biases of potential importance could include how different pathologists in different countries defined and graded liposarcomas. The Kaplan–Meier plot can help by displaying survival curves for each study on the same graph as Fig. 4.13b: This plot shows that the survival curves for the two studies are quite close.

To statistically test the null hypothesis that there is no difference between these survival curves, we use the log-rank test, which is based on comparisons of observed versus expected deaths at the various times for the two studies. The expected deaths are formed by assuming there is no difference between the studies, so that their results can be combined into a multinomial table. Then, comparisons of observed versus expected numbers of deaths yield a chi-square statistic. For these two studies, the log-rank test yielded a chi-square value of 0.7 and a p value of 0.4 suggesting that the null hypothesis of no difference is true.

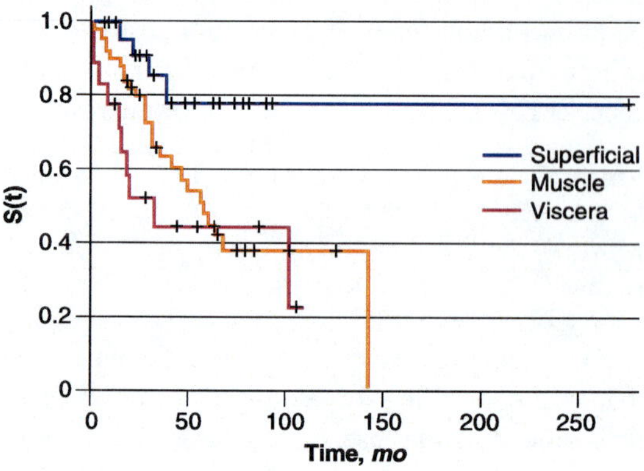

Fig. 4.14 Plot of probability of survival versus time of follow-up in patients with pleomorphic liposarcoma reported by Gebhard et al. and by Hornick et al. with survival broken into groups according to the level of tissue involved by tumor [13, 14]

Both studies of pleomorphic liposarcoma also classified the tumors into three levels: superficial (skin or subcutaneous), deep skeletal muscle, or internal viscera. The Fig. 4.14 survival plot demonstrates how these levels affected survival.

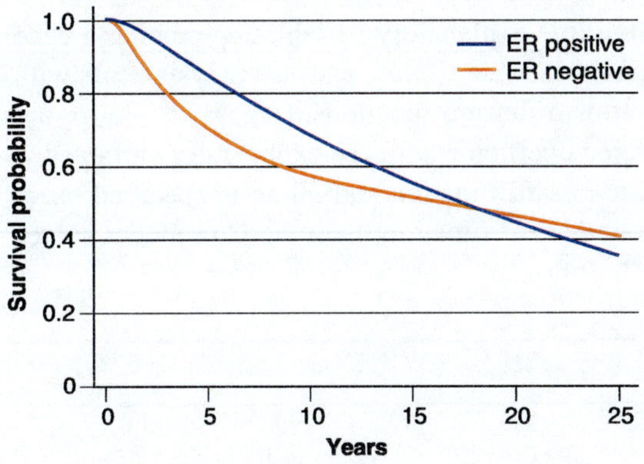

Fig. 4.15 Plot of probability of survival versus time of follow-up in patients with invasive ductal carcinoma of the breast and broken into estrogen receptor (ER) positive and negative status. The plots were obtained from digitization of the data reported by Pestalozzi et al. [14]

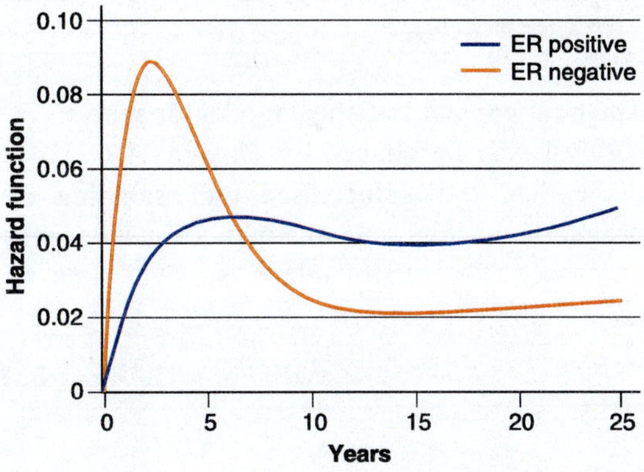

Fig. 4.16 Plot of hazard function versus time of follow-up in patients with invasive ductal carcinoma of the breast and broken into estrogen receptor (ER) positive and negative status. The hazard functions were obtained from curve fitting analysis of the survival curves in Fig. 4.15 and using the foregoing equation as well as gamma functions to model the hazard functions. The accuracy of the hazard functions was then checked by showing that they regenerated the survival curves of Fig. 4.15 accurately

The plots suggest that pleomorphic liposarcomas located in skin and subcutaneous tissues have the best prognosis, that those located in deep viscera have the worst prognosis, and that those located in deep skeletal muscle have an intermediate prognosis. The way to test if these differences in survival are significant is to once again use the log-rank test, which yielded a chi-square value of 8.5 ($p=0.01$). Thus, the combined data from the two studies validate the notion that the tissue level of origin for these sarcomas affected overall survival.

The Hazard Function

Next, consider the following survival plots of women with invasive ductal carcinoma of the breast sorted into two groups according to estrogen receptor (ER) status (Fig. 4.15).

The data come from Pestalozzi et al.'s collection of over 9,000 patients with invasive ductal carcinoma of the breast [13]. Although the two curves are close to one another and have similar shapes, the ER-positive patients have higher survival probabilities in the first 10 years of follow-up time. The slopes of these survival curves relate closely to something called the hazard function, $h(t)$, which sometimes is called the force of mortality. We define the hazard function as follows:

$$h(t) = -d\ln[s(t)]/dt,$$

where ln stands for the natural logarithm (ln) and the right side of the equation is the derivative of $\ln[S(t)]$ with respect to time. The minus sign implies that when the survival probability drops, the hazard function $h(t)$ is positive. In other words, the higher and more positive the hazard function is, the faster the survival plot should drop. One can see this effect if one plots the hazard functions for the women with ER-positive and -negative tumors as follows (Fig. 4.16):

The hazard function for ER-negative patients is much higher than that for the ER-positive patients in the first 5 years after diagnosis. After that period, the hazard for ER-negative patients drops suggesting that if a woman with ER-negative tumor survives 5 years, then her survival will improve. For ER-positive tumors, the hazard steadily increases in the first 5 years and then becomes nearly stable. In this way, the hazard function tells us much about the dynamics of survival after the diagnosis of breast cancer.

The Cox Model

The most popular statistical model for analysis of survival was introduced by Cox in 1972 [14]. Since then it has increased understanding of prognostic factors and treatments for all forms of cancer. The model relates survival time to multiple explanatory variables, symbolized once again as $x_1, x_2, \ldots, x_n$, and its analysis deals with ratios of hazard functions. If $b_1, b_2, b_3, \ldots, b_n$ are fixed coefficients for the explanatory variables, h the hazard function and $h0$ an unspecified baseline hazard function, then the Cox model solves the following regression equation:

$$\log(h / h_0) = b_1 \times x_1 + b_2 \times x_2 + b_3 \times x_3 + \ldots + b_n \times x_n.$$

Because the baseline hazard function, h_0, is left unspecified, the Cox model is semiparametric. The Cox model requires that hazard function ratios do not change with time – an assumption that can be checked, and it obtains solutions for $b_1, b_2, b_3, \ldots, b_n$ through an iterative process that maximizes a partial likelihood function. As with other regression analyses, the null hypothesis is that the b coefficients are 0. In practice, the Cox model has been found to be robust, and its iterative solution is completed within seconds on desk-top computers.

As an example, consider men with advanced prostate cancer. Whereas most men with prostate cancer die of other causes, a fraction have tumors that progress to eventually become refractory to hormonal therapy. At this stage, these men have rising values of serum PSA while on hormonal treatment, and most have boney metastases. One of the most important prognostic variables for this group of men is their clinical performance status (PS), which can be classified as 0 for normal, 1 for fatigue but without decrease in daily activities, and 2 for fatigue with impairment of daily activity but with less than 50% time in bed. In a group of 575 men with hormone refractory prostate cancer studied by the author, the performance status was significantly associated with subsequent survival ($p \sim 0$ by log-rank test). However, other factors such as serum PSA are important, and before testing new therapies for advanced stage of prostate cancer, it is important to control for all prognostic variables. The Cox model is ideal for this multivariable analyses. In three Cancer and Leukemia Group B (CALGB) studies, Cox model analysis yielded the following results [15–17].

Variable	Coefficient(b)	Exp(b)	p Value
PS	0.497	1.64	$5.5 \times 10-12$
Log PSA	0.0942	1.10	0.0011
Log hemoglobin	−1.27	0.281	0.00067
Study No. 2	−0.191	0.826	0.036

Log indicates that serum PSA and hemoglobin were both transformed into natural logarithms, and exp(b) symbolizes the function of natural exponentiation, i.e., 2.718 raised to the exponent b. The low p values for these four variables indicated that each provided additive information about survival. Furthermore, the lower the p value, the more important the variable. Thus, clinical performance status was most important, followed by serum hemoglobin, serum PSA, and finally study number 2. The positive values of the coefficients for performance and serum PSA indicate that the hazard increased with increased performance status and PSA, that is, survival time shortened. The negative coefficient for hemoglobin indicates that the hazard was lower with higher values of serum hemoglobin, and survival time lengthened. The negative coefficient for study number 2 indicates that after controlling for the effects of performance, serum PSA and serum hemoglobin, those on this study had a lower hazard and survived longer.

The effect of each variable on the hazard ratio is given in the column labeled exp(b), which provides the hazard ratios. For example, each increase in performance category raised the hazard by a multiplicative factor of 1.64, and each unit increase in log(PSA) raised the hazard by a multiplicative factor of 1.1. By contrast, each unit increase in log(hemoglobin) decreased the hazard to approximately 0.281 of what it was, and presence of a patient on study number 2 decreased the hazard to approximately 0.826 of what it was for the other two CALGB studies.

Using the Cox Model to Form a Hazard Score

Graphical nomograms and other prognostic models have become popular for several cancers including prostate cancer. These models combine information from several prognostic variables to attain a hazard score (HS), which then can be related to survival time. When these models have been derived from a Cox model analysis, the hazard score can be calculated from the coefficients of the Cox model. For example, a hazard score for men with hormone refractory prostate cancer and using just PS, PSA, and hemoglobin (Hgb) and the above Cox model results would be formed as follows:

$$HS = 0.497 \times PS + 0.0942 \times \log(PSA) - 1.27 \times \log(Hgb).$$

In a graphical nomogram, the value of HS corresponds to the sum of the individual variable scores. The final survival probability then comes from whatever survival model and corresponding software is used to estimate both the baseline hazard as well as the hazard ratio.

For example, for men with hormone refractory prostate cancer, the following plot (Fig. 4.17) demonstrates how expected survival probability at 2 years and 5 years depends upon the HS. (The values of HS are less than zero, because the range of HS in the CALGB patients was from –3 to approximately 0.)

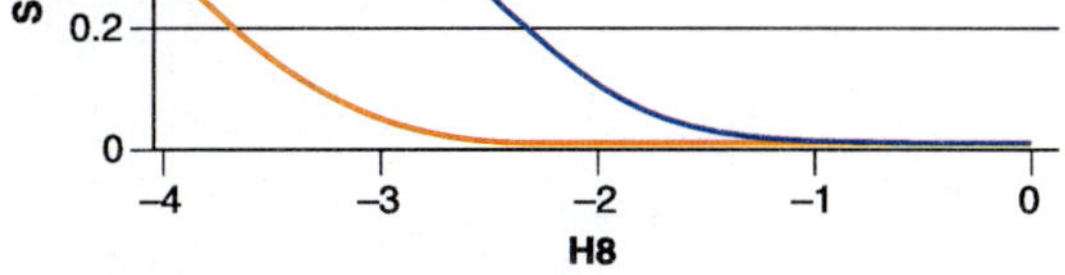

Fig. 4.17 Plots of the probability of survival at 2 and 5 years versus hazard score (HS) in men with hormone refractory prostate cancer. The plots were obtained with use of a Weibull parametric survival model

References

1. Brawer MK, Aramburu EAG, Chen GL, et al. The inability of prostate specific antigen to enhance the predictive value of prostate specific antigen in the diagnosis of prostatic carcinoma. J Urol. 1993; 150:369–73.
2. Catalona WJ, Hudson MA, Scardino PT, et al. Selection of optimal prostate specific antigen cutoffs for early detection of prostate cancer: receiver operating characteristic curves. J Urol. 1994;152:2037–42.
3. Morgan TO, Jacobsen SJ, McCarthy WF, et al. Age-specific reference ranges for serum prostate-specific antigen in Black men. N Engl J Med. 1996;335: 304–10.
4. Babaian RJ, Mettlin C, Kane R, et al. The relationship of prostate-specific antigen to digital rectal examination and transrectal ultrasonography. Cancer. 1992;69:1195–200.
5. Petricoin EF, Ardekani AM, Hitt BA, et al. Use of proteomic patterns in serum to identify ovarian cancer. Lancet. 2002;158:1491–502.
6. McCullagh P, Nelder JA. Generalized linear models. 2nd ed. London: Chapman & Hall; 1989.
7. Peduzzi P, Concato J, Kemper E, Holford TR, Feinstein AR. A simulation study of the number of events per variable in logistic regression analysis. J Clin Epidemiol. 1996;49:1373–9.
8. Siddiqi A, Spataro M, McIntire H, et al. Hybrid Capture 2 human papillomavirus DNA testing for women with atypical squamous cells of undetermined significance. Papanicolaou results in SurePath and ThinPrep specimens. Cancer Cytopathol. 2009;117:318–25.
9. Greco TP, Conti-Kelly AM, Creco Jr T, et al. Newer antiphospholipid antibodies predict adverse outcomes in patients with acute coronary syndrome. Am J Clin Pathol. 2009;132:613–20.
10. Schlesinger C, Bostwick DG, Iczkowski KA. High-grade prostatic intraepithelial neoplasia and atypical

small acinar proliferation. Predictive value for cancer in current practice. Am J Surg Pathol. 2005; 29:1201–7.
11. Gebhard S, Coindre CJ-M, Michels J-J, et al. Pleomorphic liposarcarcoma: clinicopathologic, immunohistochemical, and follow-up analysis of 63 cases. Am J Surg Pathol. 2002;26:601–16.
12. Hornick JL, Bosenbert MW, Mentzel T, et al. Pleomorphic liposarcoma. Clinicopathologic analysis of 57 cases. Am J Surg Pathol. 2004;28:1257–67.
13. Pestalozzi BC, Zahrieh D, Mallon E, et al. Distinct clinical and prognostic features of infiltrating lobular carcinoma of the breast: combined results of 15 International Breast Cancer Study Group Clinical Trails. J Clin Oncol. 2008;26:3006–14.
14. Cox DR. Regression models and life tables (with discussion). J R Stat Soc B. 1972;34:187–220.
15. D'Amico AV, Halabi S, Vollmer R, Loffredo M, McMahon E, Sanford B, et al. Cancer and Leukemia Group B. p53 protein expression status and recurrence in men treated with radiation and androgen suppression therapy for higher-risk prostate cancer: a prospective phase II Cancer and Leukemia Group B Study (CALGB 9682). Urology. 2008;71(5): 933–7.
16. D'Amico AV, Halabi S, Tempany C, Titelbaum D, Philips GK, Loffredo M, et al. Cancer and Leukemia Group B. Tumor volume changes on 1.5 tesla endorectal MRI during neoadjuvant androgen suppression therapy for higher-risk prostate cancer and recurrence in men treated using radiation therapy results of the phase II CALGB 9682 study. Int J Radiat Oncol Biol Phys. 2008;71(1):9–15.
17. Humphrey PA, Halabi S, Picus J, Sanford B, Vogelzang NJ, Small EJ, et al. Prognostic significance of plasma scatter factor/hepatocyte growth factor levels in patients with metastatic hormone – refractory prostate cancer: results from cancer and leukemia group B 150005/9480. Clin Genitourin Cancer. 2006;4(4):269–74.

Suggested Readings

Casella G, Berger RL. Statistical inference. 2nd ed. Pacific Grove, CA: Duxbury; 2002.

Venables WN, Ripley BD. Modern applied statistics with S-PLUS. 3rd ed. New York, NY: Springer; 1999.

Cox DR, Oakes D. Analysis of survival data. London: Chapman & Hall; 1984.

Therneau TM, Grambsch PM. Modeling survival data. Extending the Cox model. New York, NY: Springer; 2000.

Harrell Jr FE. Regression modeling strategies. With applications to linear models, logistic regression, and survival analysis. New York, NY: Springer; 2001.

Hosmer DW, Lemeshow S. Applied logistic regression. 2nd ed. New York, NY: Wiley; 2000.

Hosmer DW, Lemeshow S. Applied survival analysis. New York, NY: Wiley; 1999.

Miller I, Miller M, John E. Freund's mathematical statistics with applications. 7th ed. Upper Saddle River, NJ: Pearson Prentice Hall; 2004.

Vollmer RT, Kantoff PW, Dawson NA, Vogelzang NJ. Importance of serum hemoglobin in hormone refractory prostate cancer. Clin Cancer Res. 2002;8:1049–53.

Prognostication and Prediction in Anatomic Pathology: Carcinoma of the Breast as an Illustrative Model

5

Mark R. Wick, Paul E. Swanson, and Alberto M. Marchevsky

Keywords
Prediction in anatomic pathology • Breast cancer as model of prognostication • Prognostication in anatomic pathology • Anatomic pathology

Along with other physicians, pathologists have long been interested in how to forecast the future for patients with a variety of diseases. Common questions for anyone having an illness are the following:

1. How will this problem affect my life and how long will I live after today?
2. Which treatments could I receive for this problem?
3. What is the likelihood that therapy will be effective, and at what cost?

Such queries are particularly pointed for people with malignant neoplasms, or for clearly life-threatening non-neoplastic illnesses such as Wegener granulomatosis, usual interstitial pneumonitis, scleroderma, and others.

Intuitively, physicians learned long ago that marked anatomic or physiological deviations from the norm likely indicated a problem of unusual severity, and, therefore, a more guarded outlook for the patient. During the early part of the twentieth century, this awareness led doctors to develop schemes for the semiquantitation of adverse risk. *Histological grading* of malignant tumors was devised, as a reflection of progressively increasing visual differences from the images of corresponding normal tissues [3–12]. The higher the grade of a neoplasm, the less it was felt to resemble its non-neoplastic counterpart under the microscope.

The scope of tumor growth was also codified in tumor staging systems. Even before the current "primary tumor-lymph node-distant metastasis" (TNM) system for tumor staging was proposed in the mid-1940s [13], other effective paradigms were devised in reference to specific malignancies. For example, Dr. Cuthbert Dukes published an effective surgical staging system for colorectal adenocarcinoma in 1932 [14]. Once again, the underlying principle attached to increasing tumor stages is a progressive departure from the normal state. In other words, the farther a neoplasm grows from its anatomical origin, the more aggressive its behavior is felt to be.

As the natural history of malignant tumors was better understood using such tools, efforts at biological interdiction became more focused. For example, because axillary lymph nodes were often involved by metastatic carcinomas of the breast, *pro forma* removal of the nodes

M.R. Wick (✉)
Professor and Associate Director of Surgical Pathology, Department of Pathology, University of Virginia Medical School, Charlottesville, VA, USA
e-mail: MRW9C@hscmail.mcc.virginia.edu

A.M. Marchevsky and M.R. Wick (eds.), *Evidence Based Pathology and Laboratory Medicine*,
DOI 10.1007/978-1-4419-1030-1_5, © Springer Science+Business Media, LLC 2011

was incorporated into surgical treatment for mammary cancer [15]. After intraosseous "skip" lesions of bone sarcomas were characterized, limb amputation was employed more freely in the days before effective drug treatments were available [16]. The recognition that leukemia could use the central nervous system as a "haven" to escape the effects of chemotherapy prompted systematic irradiation of the neuraxis and the use of "Ommaya reservoirs" for drug delivery as prophylaxes against that phenomenon [17, 18]. The use of such preemptive measures in treating human malignancies continues to this day.

One can rightly conclude that two major goals exist for medical prognostication and prediction. One is forecasting the future for individual patients, and the other is choosing the most effective treatments for the types, grades, and stages of the illnesses they have. Pathologists have become important providers of measurable and seemingly objective "prognostic" information on diseases of all kinds, but with a particular focus on malignant neoplasms. This role is quite different than the one played by most laboratory-based physicians until the 1980s. Although pathological observations did play a definite role in medical forecasting in the past, as discussed above, the principal task of pathologists was the attainment of diagnostic certitude. Once they had recognized and properly classified an illness, the subsequent role of prognosticator was largely situated in the bailiwick of clinical physicians.

Roughly 30 years ago, the advent of diagnostic immunohistology altered that scenario drastically [19]. The latter technique allowed pathologists to "map" the protein chemistry of tissues and tumors in a theretofore-unparalleled fashion, quickly and reproducibly. For the first time, biological molecules with possibly determinative functions could be detected in situ in clinical specimens without the need for laborious and special tissue processing. A tidal wave of medical publications on "pathological prognostic factors" began in the late 1980s [20, 21] and has yet to abate.

To those who are naïve regarding the practice of laboratory medicine, it would seem that pathologists and oncologists have now reached the state of Hindu *Moksha*. Surely, neoplastic cells no longer can hold secrets unto themselves in the face of immunohistochemistry, in situ nucleic-acid hybridization, proteomics, and gene-sequencing. Nonetheless, in a real sense, that assumption is incorrect. Several obstacles continue to encumber the task of pathobiological prognostication, and this chapter aims to discuss them. We will review the definitions and basic concepts of risk, prognosis and prediction, and consider the important role of pathologists as assessors of "new" tests using current information about mammary carcinoma as an example.

Risk, Prognosis and Prediction

The terms *risk, prognosis* and *prediction* have been inconsistently and ambiguously used in the medical literature as indicators of the likely course of a disease and/or response to a particular treatment. The term risk is derived from a Greek word rizikon, literally meaning root but later on used in Latin for "cliff" [22]. It describes the deviation of one or more future events from their expected course, and usually focuses on the harm that may arise from such events. The term risk has been used in various disciplines, as health risk, economic risk, psychological risk, and others. It has been used variably as the probability of certain negative events or hazards or to describe future issues that should be avoided or mitigated. In Medicine and Epidemiology, risk is usually estimated simply as the probability of an event, based on past experience. In business and engineering, more complex mathematical risk models have been proposed, using functions that integrate the probability of a threat, the probability of various other vulnerabilities, and their potential impact to a business or product [23]. Risk has been distinguished semantically from uncertainty, the lack of complete certainty, resulting from the possibility of various possible outcomes for an event or situation [24]. Uncertainty is usually measured as sets of probabilities of the various possible events or outcomes. The term risk has been generally used in pathology to describe the probability that patients with certain findings will develop a future malignancy in an attempt to develop strategies that will prevent the development of cancer or lead to its early detection [25]. For example, patients with atypical adenomatous hyperplasia (ADH) and other conditions of the breast have a higher risk of developing breast cancer and are followed more carefully with mammography than patients without these findings, in efforts at detecting early breast cancer [26]. The term risk has also been used in a different context to describe the probability of detecting a malignancy in a subsequent specimen [27]. For example, various "risks" of finding a malignancy in a thyroidectomy specimen have been described for various findings detectable on fine needle aspirate specimens of the thyroid [28].

The term prognosis is also derived from a Greek work describing foreknowing or foreseeing and is used in Medicine to describe the likely outcome of a patient with a particular disease [29]. Prognostic estimates are usually calculated as percentages or other proportions and are generally variably accurate when applied to large populations of patients with a disease. Physicians since the time of Hippocrates have been interested in understanding the prognosis of various illnesses and have devised various prognostic models based on astrology or other theories [30]. For example, medieval physicians would use numerology to calculate a prognosis, using the Sphere of Petorisis, a circular chart designed by one of the founders of astrology, while modern medical informaticians currently propose the use of prognostic models based on data mining, multivariate numerical data, and various classification models based on decision trees, decision rules, logistic regression, artificial neural networks, and other computational models derived from probability theory [31, 32]. It is beyond the scope of this chapter to discuss the concept of prognosis and various methodologies used for its estimation in further detail, but it is important to consider that prognostic estimates are not static for a particular disease. For example, the prognosis of a patient with mammary carcinoma is dependent on the age of the individual, presence or absence of other medical conditions, time of diagnosis during the natural history of the disease, treatment effectiveness, and many other known and unknown variables [33]. It is also important to consider that prognostic estimates have been usually calculated for populations of patients with a particular disease. An individual patient may have a prognosis that varies considerably from the mean or median estimates for a population of individuals with the same disease.

The term prediction is based on Latin *pre* or before and *dicere* or say [34]. A prediction or forecast is used to estimate future events, usually but not always based on experience or knowledge. Predictions can be rendered as statements regarding the outcome that is expected, a probability of the occurrence of the expected event or as forecasts describing a range of possible events [35]. In Medicine, prediction has been used in the context of estimating the efficacy of specific therapeutic interventions [36]. However, the influence of various other variables that can affect the prognosis of a disease is frequently not considered as covariates in the forecasting models. Moreover, most predictive information in pathology is currently available for populations of patients with particular disease and treated with specific therapeutic agents. No generally used predictive models have been devised for estimating the future course of diseases after treatment in individual patients, a limitation that is important to consider in the era of "personalized medicine" [37]. As famously stated by Niels Bohr, "prediction is difficult, especially if it is about the future" [38].

Personalized Medicine: Current Environment for the Development of Prognostic and Predictive Laboratory Tests

Advances in molecular medicine and our understanding of the human genome have opened a new paradigm in Medicine, where new therapies will be developed based on the understanding of the molecular basis of neoplasms and other diseases and the treatment of patients will be individualized [39]. There is great hope and hype about the great potential of Personalized Medicine [40]. This paradigm is based on the availability of sensitive, specific and accurate prognostic and predictive laboratory tests, and of new effective drugs.

In a perfect world, one would be able to evaluate each prospective prognostic or predictive medical test (PPMT) on a large-scale, in a measured way, and with the use of proper statistical guidelines. Unfortunately, that ideal may never be realized. Pragmatic influences that hinder the process of medical research and development are basically threefold – financial factors, political imperatives, and test reproducibility and applicability to "routine" clinical specimens.

In order to understand the role of financial and political factors on PPMT development, one must look outside the realm of medicine and science to the fields of business administration and sociology. Projections for the cost of health care in the United States in the next 15 years are sobering [41]. Healthcare spending (HCS) already approximates 20% of the gross domestic product (GDP), and, if the system is unchanged, it will steadily climb ever-higher (Fig. 5.1). Because a sizable fraction of U.S. citizens comprises "baby boomers" in the 50-and-older age range, who are increasingly becoming eligible for Medicare health coverage, federal HCS could soon exceed 10% of the GDP. Most private health insurers have adopted practices that parallel those of Medicare. Thus, patients in their HCS plans confront the same patterns of medical practice and billing as the U.S. government does, albeit with a different, more capitalistic, business model. James Traficant, a business executive who underwent two liver transplants, has written the following about the cost of modern U.S. health care [42], using a currently popular television medical drama as a reference:

> Each week, a team of five doctors works around the clock and orders countless long-shot tests to diagnose a single patient suffering from an incredibly rare condition. That the American healthcare system doesn't [really] work this way isn't the issue. It's that everyone believes it *should,* when they're the ones in the hospital gowns.

Returning to the issue of PPMTs, patients with malignancies *are* the ones in the hospital gowns, and, being human, they want ever-more and better information about their personal medical outlooks. They also have a natural tendency to believe that any new treatment which is tied to a "cutting-edge" PPMT is the one they should get.

Technological medical entrepreneurs are all-too-ready to respond to this philosophical atmosphere. Some companies may exert not-so-subtle pressure on physicians who are testing their new products – both PPMTs and associated therapies – to give them "positive" information that can be used in successful marketing and sales

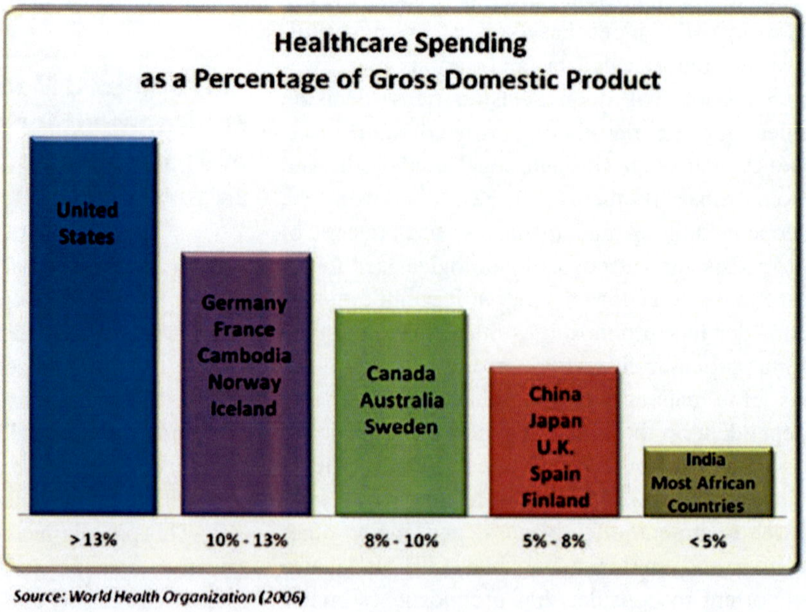

Fig. 5.1 Bar graph demonstrating relative international healthcare expenditures in 2006, as fractions of the gross domestic product. (From *The World Health Report 2006 – Working together for health*, http://www.who.int/whr/2006/en/, with permission from the World Health Organization)

campaigns. Such partnerships are scientifically unsound and also may be unethical. One can easily envision a situation in which a large, well-funded, well-connected medical development firm could effectively sell a marginally functional test or treatment, whereas a much smaller corporation could not so succeed, even if it had a clearly superior product.

Federal politicians are caught in a three-way vise between their constituents' demands for comprehensive health care, including few if any limits; the interests of local businesses in the regions they represent; and the exigencies of maintaining a balanced national budget for the general welfare of the country. Interestingly, the effects of lobby-pressure on this tri-cornered teeter-totter are not often mentioned. Over time, for example, the *sub rosa* financial influence of U.S. tobacco companies undeniably impeded medical advances in the control of smoking-related cancers, particularly lung carcinomas [43]. Now, many years later, American politicians must find the monetary support to treat the malignancies (and other disorders) that are related directly to their prior decisions. This situation includes the development of associated PPMTs.

What are the conclusions that one can draw from this information? First, the burden of overall health care will almost certainly curb the extravagant use of medical testing that is not cost-effective. Second, patients will have to undergo a "religious conversion" regarding their presumed entitlement to unlimited medical services. Third, politicians – and medical care-providers – will need to look past their fiduciary and personal interests to establish a truly evidence-based and effective system of health care for their patients and constituents. They will need the concerted help of laboratory professionals and other scientists to do that task properly.

As the U.S. Congressional Budget Office has stated:

> Two potentially complementary approaches to reducing spending on Medicare, Medicaid, and health care generally – rather than simply reallocating spending among different sectors of the economy – involve generating more information about the relative effectiveness of medical treatments [and testing, including PPMTs] and changing the incentives for providers and consumers in the supply and demand of health care … Medicare could tie its payment to providers to the cost of the most effective or most efficient treatment. If that payment was less than the cost of providing a more expensive service, then doctors and hospitals would probably elect not to provide it … Alternatively, enrollees could be required to pay for the additional costs of less effective procedures [41].

Out with the Old, in with the New?

In their excellent treatise on the vicissitudes of modern health care, entitled *Hope or Hype: the Obsession with Medical Advances and the High Cost of False Promises*, Deyo and Patrick address a common trait of both doctors and patients [44]. That is, both groups are extremely eager to dismiss "the old" in Medicine in favor of "the new." The latter statement applies to any number of contextual topics, such as the value of good physical diagnosis and history-taking, contrasted with data from reflexive barrages of laboratory testing and radiological studies; the relative diagnostic benefits of plain-film radiographs as compared with magnetic resonance-imaging or positron-emission tomography; support for a rational and humane use of hospice-care instead of heroic but pointless end-of-life medical intervention; and reliance on time-tested and proven PPMTs in pathology and laboratory medicine [45–47] as compared with wholesale dependence on genomics and proteomics [48, 49]. Medical advances have almost always been heralded initially as "breakthroughs," despite accrual of subsequent information – usually not shared with the public – that has debunked the efficacy of many of them [50].

Mammary Carcinoma as a Model to Discuss the Challenges of "Prognostication" and "Prediction"

In order to provide a tangible focus for discussion, we will use "usual" ductal adenocarcinoma (UDA) of the breast as a model to discuss the challenges associated with the development of various prognostic and predictive laboratory tests and integrating the information developed by these tests into daily clinical practice. The information on breast carcinoma that will be presented is certainly not identical to that associated with colon cancer, prostate cancer, lung cancer, or other human malignancies. Nevertheless, general *principles* are the same concerning the forecasting of outcomes for neoplastic diseases.

Breast cancer is the most common malignancy in American women, and the second-leading cause of death in that group. It has been predicted that in the year 2012, the annual prevalence of mammary carcinoma will be >950,000 cases in the U.S., and greater than four million cases worldwide. More than 210,000 new cases will accrue each year in this country, and >43,000 women will die of the disease [51]. In the face of those daunting figures, efforts have been redoubled to improve "forecasting" of individual breast cancer cases, and to match therapies with individual tumors in an optimal fashion.

In sorting through the statistics just listed, one must delve further to identify the most formidable challenge to the process of prognostication for UDA. Among the 194,300 new instances of breast carcinoma in the U.S. in 2009, 70% (136,000) were classified as UDAs pathologically, and 60% (81,600) of those patients had stage I tumors (localized to the breast) at diagnosis [52]. The latter subgroup is the crux of very pressing problems, the pertinent questions for which are – *how many new stage I breast cancers will resist therapy and threaten life, and how can they be identified prospectively*? Based on historical data, the answer to the first question would be approximately 24,500 [51]. An accurate response to the second query is much more difficult to formulate, as discussed subsequently.

For other UDAs that are stage ≥II at presentation, the biological attributes of the tumor (a relatively large size and/or metastatic involvement of regional lymph nodes) have already made it apparent that such lesions have aggressive potential (i.e., a relatively poorer prognosis) and must be treated accordingly. In reference to that cohort of patients, the likely clinical outlook is not quite as uncertain – especially with no further treatment – but the possible individual benefit of various therapeutic interventions is still problematic. In that context, it must be understood that forecasting a biological response of a tumor to any given treatment type is properly termed *prediction*, whereas foretelling the overall outcome of a case (life vs. death; short vs. long survival; low vs. high morbidity) is appropriately labeled as *prognostication*. The two terms must not, and cannot, be interchanged, for breast cancer or any other malignant neoplasm.

Forecasting the Prognosis of Mammary Carcinoma Patients

There are several "old" evaluations of mammary carcinoma, which not only still have value but also match or even out-perform newer methods as forecasting tools [53–57]. Moreover, these "old" procedures can be done by pathologists anywhere, with standard hematoxylin–eosin (H&E) stains and a microscope.

Effects of Tissue Sampling on Prognostication and Prediction

Before considering the specifics of prognostic and predictive factors for mammary carcinomas, one must attend to the issue of tissue sampling. In modern practice, a common modality for the surgical diagnosis of mass lesions uses cutting biopsy needles of variable diameters. These instruments commonly allow for a generic morphological diagnosis of malignancy to be made pathologically (Fig. 5.2),

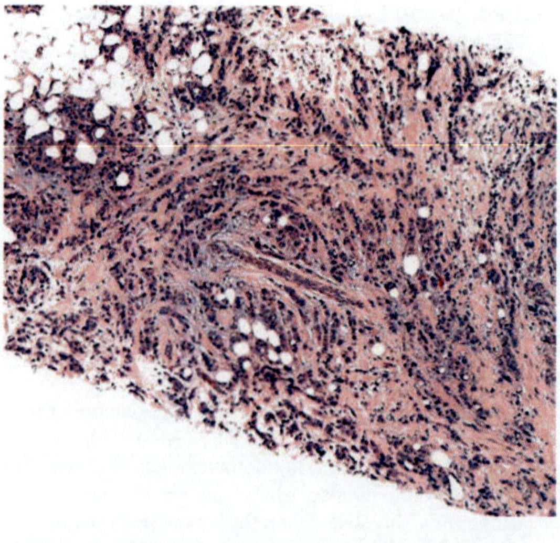

Fig. 5.2 Needle-core biopsy specimen of invasive breast carcinoma. Samples such as this may contain significant artifacts that impede prognostic and predictive studies

but there are real limitations to the use of needle biopsies for prognostic and predictive studies.

The latter statement is true because of two important factors [58–64]. The first is the distortion of tissue that may be seen in small, "closed" biopsy specimens, such that important histological details may be artifactually obscured. The second relates to the inherent spatial heterogeneity, which is a part of many human malignancies. In other words, if one samples several aspects of a tumor, several and conflicting data on prognosis may be obtained. Conversely, very limited sampling can produce artificial results that in fact do not represent the biological lesion as a whole.

As a result of those realities, our opinion is that cutting-needle or fine-needle aspiration biopsies of breast masses are best used for diagnostic purposes *only*. If additional information is requested of the pathologist – concerning tumor type, grade, or expression of various biochemical markers – a caveat should be included in the surgical pathology report on the possibly confounding effects of limited sampling methods.

Recognition of "Special" Histologic Breast Cancer Variants

The first of the established methods for prognostication of breast carcinoma concerns the accurate morphological and conceptual identification of its "special" variants [65–73]. These differ structurally and biologically from the most common form of mammary carcinoma, UDA, and these can be segregated into three groups, which relate to the relative behavioral characteristics of the tumors in question. They are group I – more favorable behavior than that of comparably sized UDA; group II – similar behavior to that of comparably sized UDA; and group III – more aggressive behavior than that of comparably sized UDA. These are segregated as follows, with the percentage fraction of all breast cancers they represent in parentheses:

Group I (Figs. 5.3–5.8) – "Pure" lobular carcinoma (10–15%); "pure" mucinous carcinoma (2%); "pure" tubular carcinoma and low-grade invasive cribriform carcinoma (1–2%); salivary gland-type carcinomas of the breast (adenoid cystic carcinoma, acinic cell carcinoma, mucoepidermoid carcinoma, low-grade adenosquamous carcinoma; malignant [adeno-]myoepithelioma) (1%); intracystic papillary carcinoma (1%); primary mammary "carcinoid" tumor (<1%); and "pure" medullary carcinoma (5%).

Group II (Figs. 5.9–5.11) – "Pure squamous cell carcinoma" (<1%); secretory adenocarcinoma (<1%); "pleomorphic" lobular carcinoma (<1%); and "atypical" or mixed medullary carcinoma (1–2%).

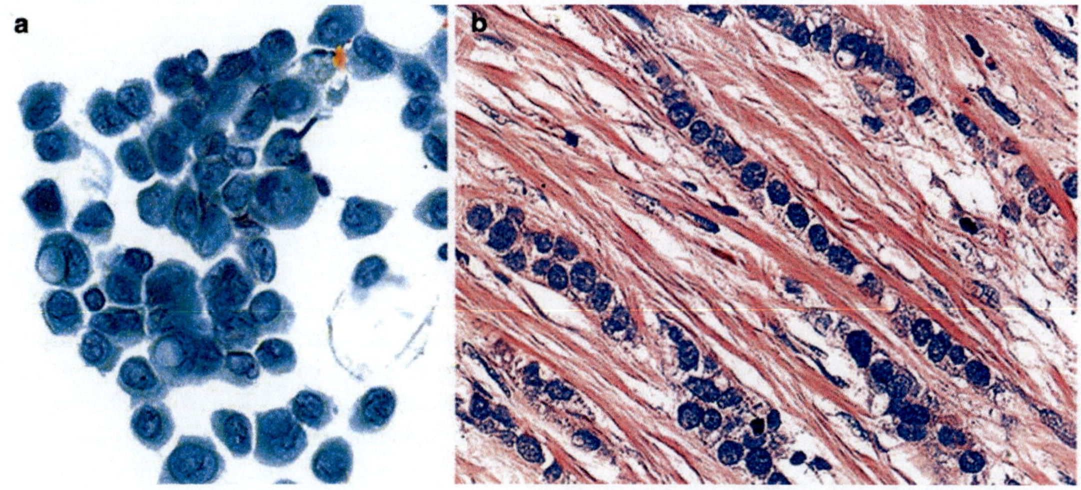

Fig. 5.3 (a) Fine-needle aspiration biopsy and (b) excisional biopsy specimen of "classical" invasive lobular carcinoma

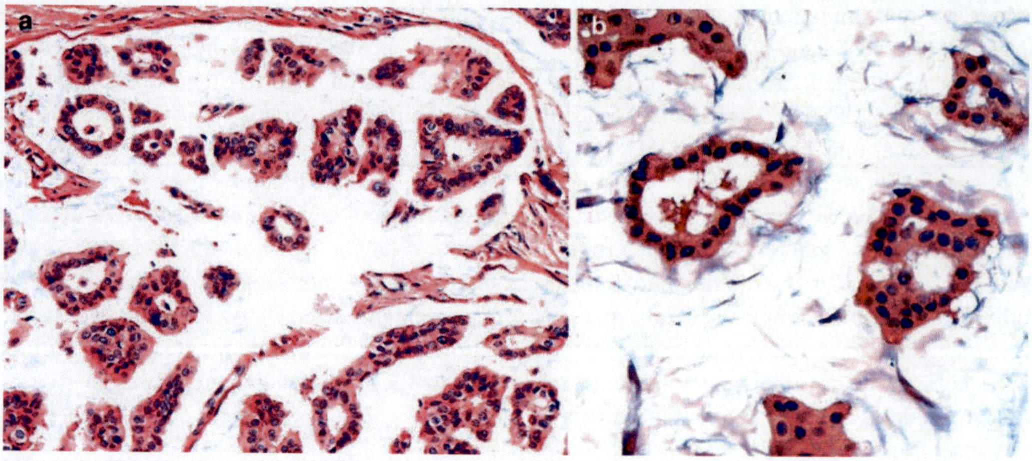

Fig. 5.4 (**a**, **b**) "Pure" mucinous adenocarcinoma of the breast, showing aggregates of rather bland tumor cells suspended in extracellular mucin

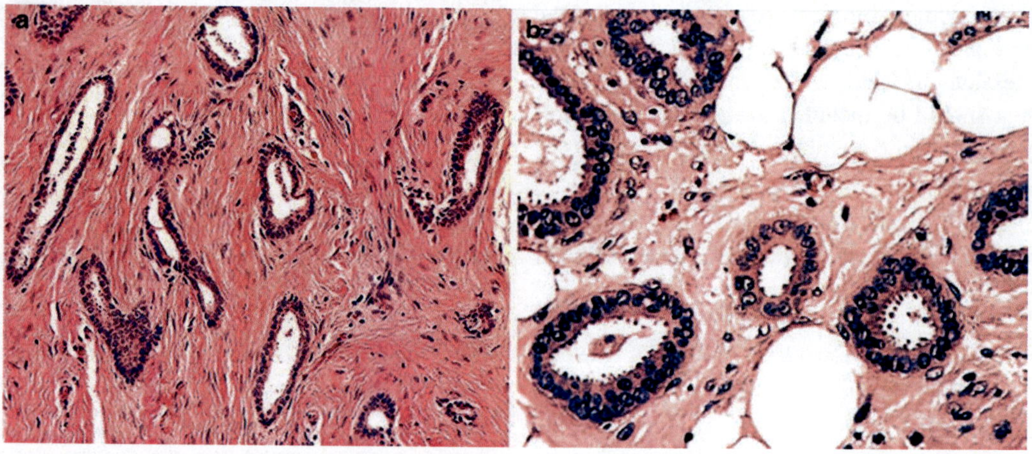

Fig. 5.5 (**a**, **b**) "Pure" tubular carcinoma of the breast, showing open tubular profiles that contain secretory "snouts"

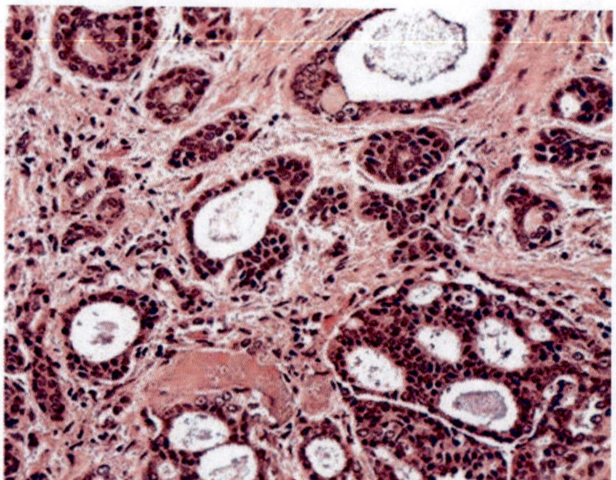

Fig. 5.6 Adenoid cystic carcinoma of the breast, comprising tubules and nests of monotonous basaloid cells

Group III (Figs. 5.12–5.15) – Metaplastic carcinoma (sarcomatoid carcinoma; spindle-cell carcinoma; "carcinosarcoma") (1%); neuroendocrine carcinoma (<1%); invasive micropapillary carcinoma (<1%); and undifferentiated carcinoma, not otherwise specified (<1%).

In current practice, the lamentable tendency of surgeons, radiotherapists, and medical oncologists is to adopt a "one size fits all" mentality in reference to breast carcinoma. In that approach, the histologically defined entities listed above are not distinguished conceptually from UDA. Studies for estrogen and progesterone receptor proteins, *HER-2* gene amplification, and other biochemical and genetic analytes are demanded *pro forma* [74], despite the fact that morphological

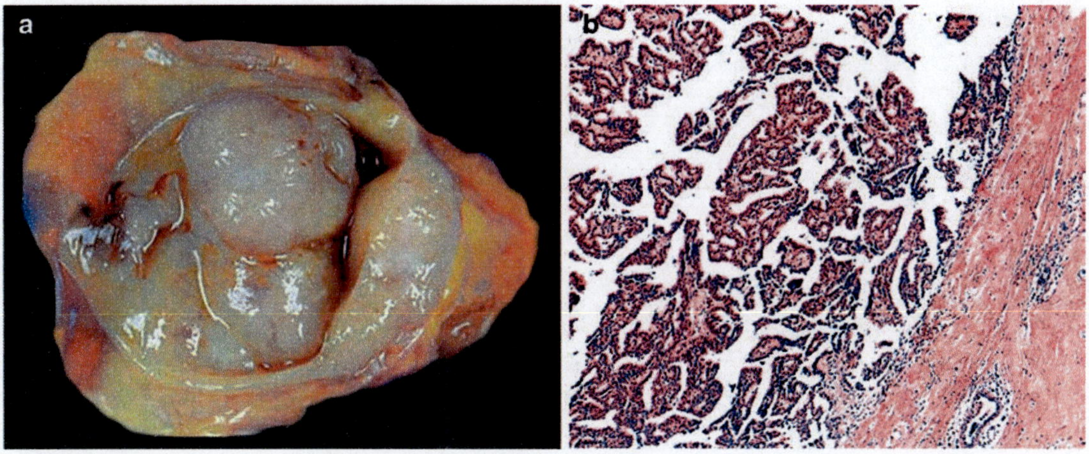

Fig. 5.7 (**a**) Gross and (**b**) microscopic photographs of intracystic papillary carcinoma of the breast. Numerous micropapillary structures, most of which lack fibrovascular cores, are present

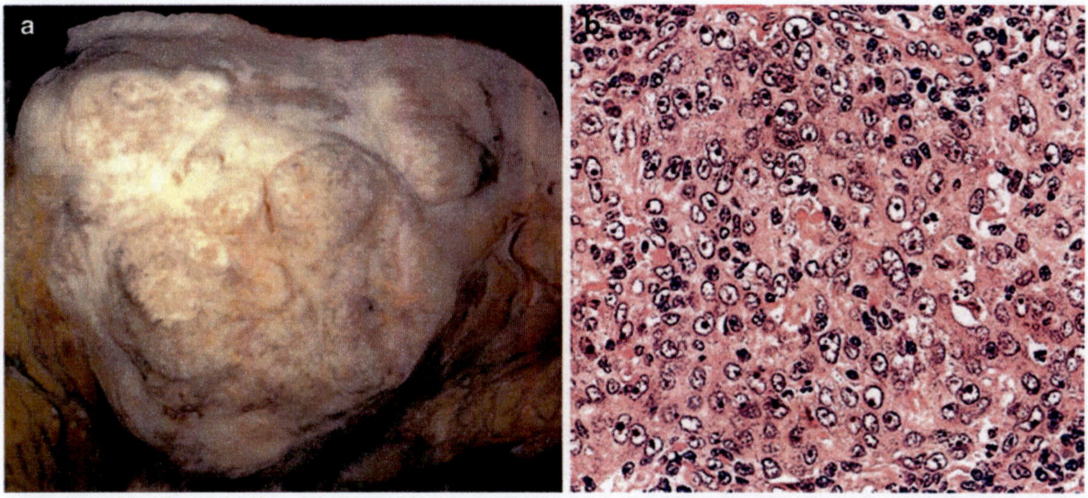

Fig. 5.8 (**a**) Gross and (**b**) microscopic images of medullary breast carcinoma. The "cerebroid" nature of the macroscopic tumor is apparent, and its histologic image features a syncytium of neoplastic cells with admixed lymphocytes

assignment alone clearly overrides the importance of those evaluations [65, 66].

In other words, histopathologic descriptors preceding the word "carcinoma" are regarded only with feeble interest and as having no practical significance. That attitude sets the stage for an uninformed and unscientific approach to management of the tumor types in question. In group I, all of the lesions (except, possibly, for medullary carcinoma) do not require anything more than local excision if they measure <3 cm. in maximal dimension [55]. The presence of larger masses should prompt a sentinel axillary lymph node biopsy, but, if it shows no metastasis, nothing further needs be done. Lesions in group II can be managed surgically in the same fashion as that used for UDAs, stage-for-stage. However, in the former of those cohorts, it should be understood that squamous cell carcinomas and medullary carcinomas almost always fail to show immunoreactivity for estrogen or progesterone receptor proteins (ERP/PRP), or to manifest amplification of the *HER-2* gene [65, 66]. Furthermore, they respond differently to conventional chemotherapy, as compared with UDAs. Finally, metaplastic carcinomas, small-cell

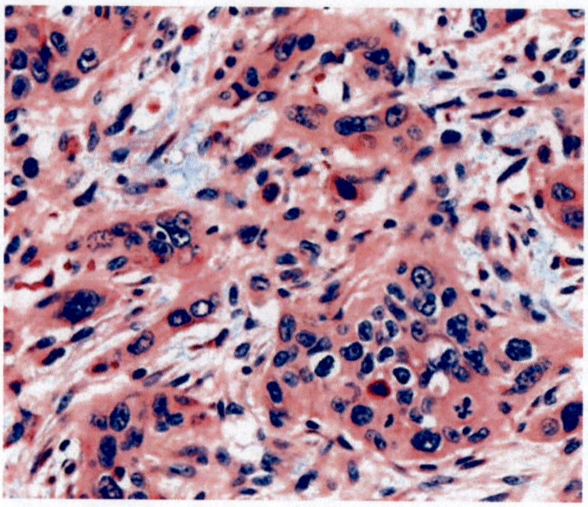

Fig. 5.9 Poorly differentiated "pure" squamous carcinoma of the breast, with notable cytoplasmic eosinophilia and individually dyskeratotic cells

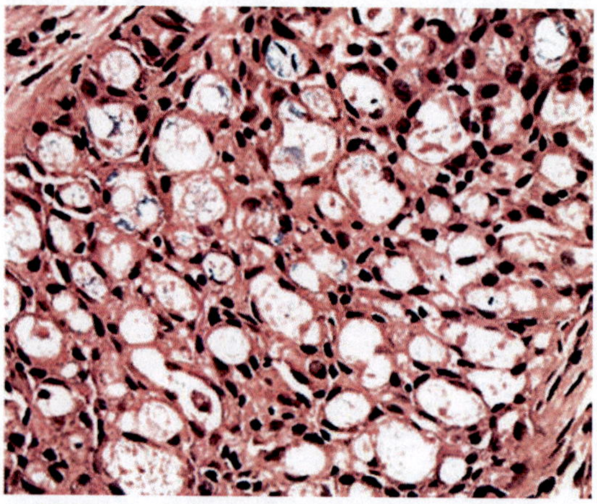

Fig. 5.10 "Secretory" adenocarcinoma of the breast, as seen in a 12-year-old girl. A lacework of epithelial tumor cells encloses eosinophilic secretory material

neuroendocrine carcinomas, invasive micropapillary carcinomas, and undifferentiated carcinomas of the breast in group III comprise a behaviorally aggressive subgroup and must be treated accordingly with a multimodal approach [71, 72, 75–82].

In summary, then, if one were to make no distinction between any of these pathologic-variant carcinomas and UDA, managing all breast cancers in the same fashion, the end result would be overtreatment (or, sometimes, undertreatment) of at least 10% of cases. That statistic may not seem critical, but it represents a sufficient number to

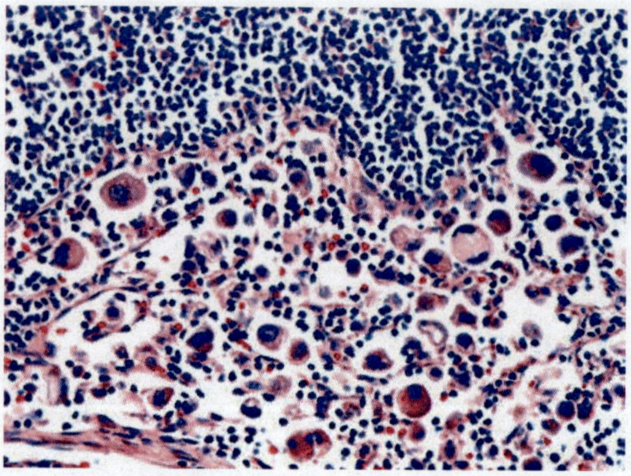

Fig. 5.11 Metastatic "pleomorphic" lobular mammary carcinoma in an axillary lymph node. There is much more cellular heterogeneity than that seen in the tumor in Fig. 5.3

falsely skew the results of a new treatment or a novel variation on an old one. With additional regard to the use of medical resources, automatic studies for ERP/PRP and *HER-2* are unnecessary in reference to many special breast tumor types. Lobular, tubular, invasive cribriform, mucinous, and papillary carcinoma are essentially *all* capable of expressing hormone receptors, and they all lack *HER-2* amplification [65, 66]. Medullary and metaplastic carcinomas consistently lack ERP/PRP, and, usually, *HER-2* abnormalities as well [71, 83, 84].

Accurate Measurement of Tumor Size

Tumor size is, by itself, a meaningful prognostic factor [85–88], and there are two probable explanations for that fact. The most likely one is that robust local growth of a primary malignancy indicates an overall dominance of tumor cell proliferation over the host's mechanisms for containing it [53]. That same supremacy applies in metastatic sites as well. A second explanation regarding the significance of primary tumor size is that large masses of replicating, clonal, malignant cells are prone to undergo additional mutational events that may increase their growth potential, viability, and capacity for metastasis [88, 89].

The greatest dimension of any given invasive breast cancer has usually been measured from the gross specimen in the pathology laboratory. That is still the best method, although it must be

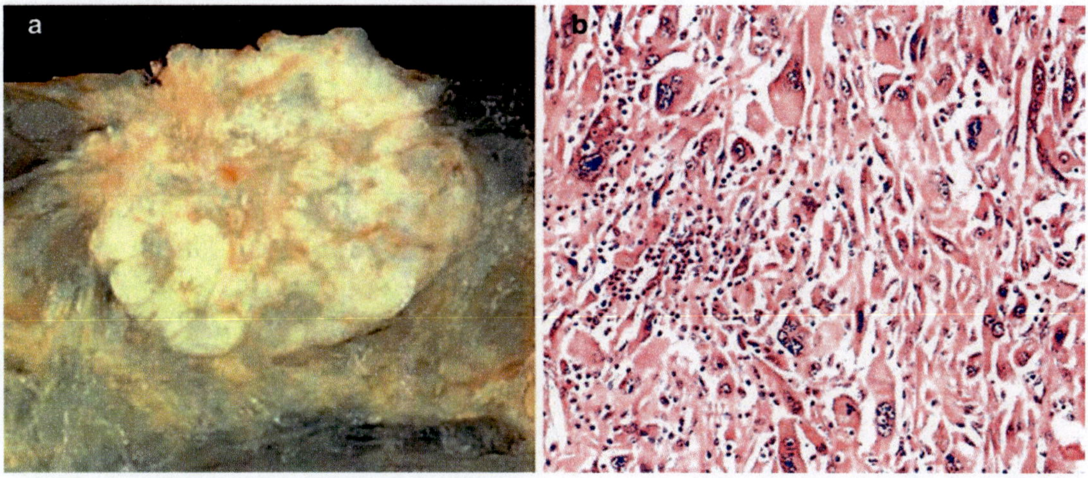

Fig. 5.12 (**a**) Gross and (**b**) microscopic images of "metaplastic" (sarcomatoid) breast carcinoma. The tumor is bulky macroscopically, and comprises fusiform and pleomorphic cells with no ductal structures

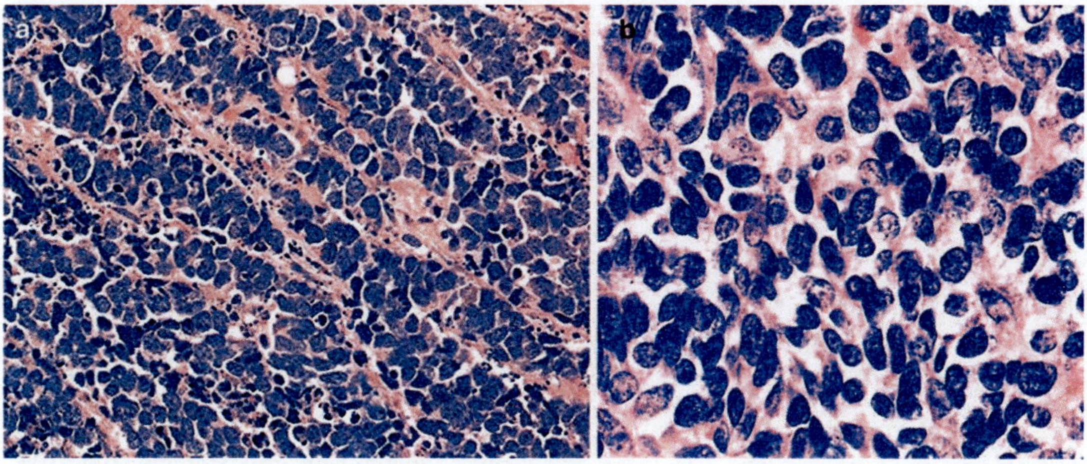

Fig. 5.13 (**a**, **b**) High-grade primary neuroendocrine carcinoma of the breast, showing dispersed nuclear chromatin, numerous mitotic figures, nuclear "molding," and abundant apoptosis

acknowledged that peritumoral desmoplasia may falsely increase the result somewhat. On the other hand, very small tumors (<0.5 cm) can be difficult to see well macroscopically, and their dimensions must then be taken from microscopic slides or radiological images [87, 89].

Histologic Grading of Invasive Breast Carcinoma

As stated earlier, iterations of histological schemes for the grading of malignant tumors have been extant for almost 100 years, but some have been more useful than others. With regard to breast cancer – and, in particular, UDA – Bloom and Richardson introduced an effective grading system in 1957 [90]. It was subsequently modified slightly by Scarff and Torloni in 1968 [91], and again by Le Doussal et al. in 1989 [92], and continues to be used today on a worldwide scale. Details of the Bloom–Scarff–Richardson (BSR) grading method are shown in Table 5.1.

Many publications have attested to the interobserver reproducibility and prognostic value of the BSR grade, when used by itself and in combination with other clinicopathologic observations [93–99]. For example, the Nottingham Prognostic

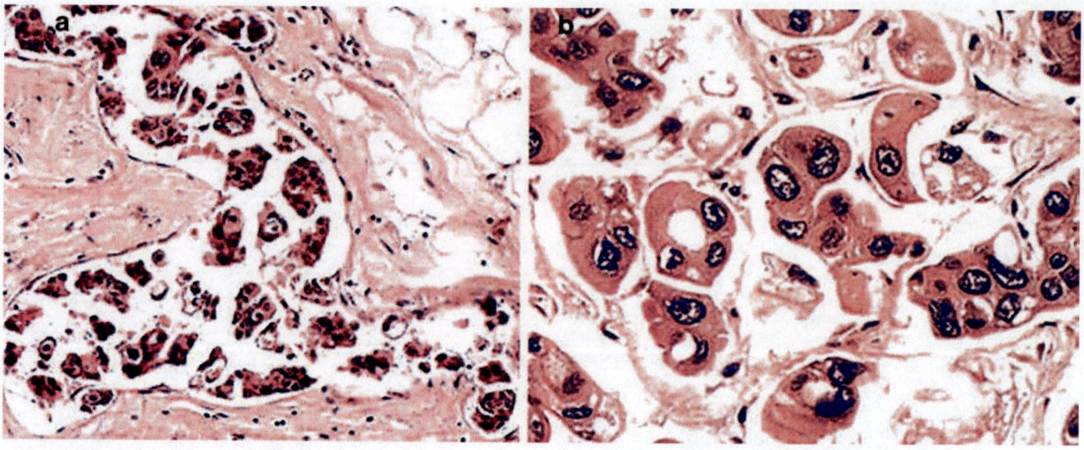

Fig. 5.14 (**a**) Extensive intramammary lymphatic involvement is present in this invasive micropapillary breast carcinoma. The tumor cells are variably pleomorphic (**b**); they form small tubules and micropapillae

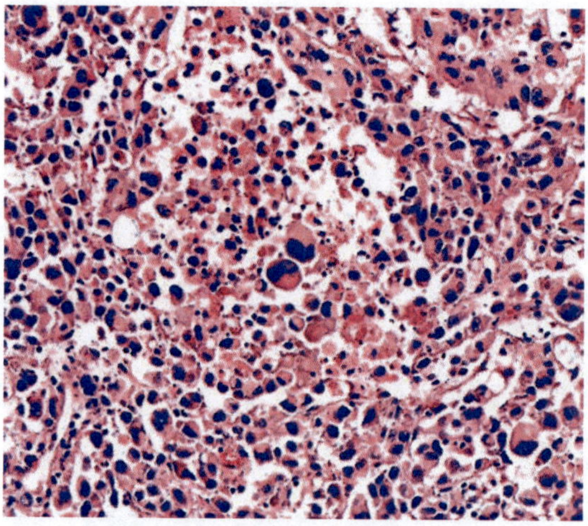

Fig. 5.15 Large-cell undifferentiated carcinoma of the breast, with "rhabdoid" features

Index (NPI) melds the BSR grade with the tumor stage, as defined by the system put forth by the American Joint Committee on Cancer (AJCC) [95]. The latter includes factors reflecting primary tumor size, lymph nodal involvement, and distant metastasis. Relative weights have been assessed for individual components of the BSR grade and the AJCC stage, as in the *modified* BSR (MBSR) system of Le Doussal and coworkers [92]. From those analyses, it would appear that the degree of nuclear atypia-pleomorphism, mitotic rate per 10 high-power (×400) microscopic fields, and metastatic involvement of regional lymph nodes are the principal contextual determinants of final case outcome.

The BSR and MBSR grading methods are best applied to UDAs, because the morphologic details of other nosological tumor types are so reproducible that they are also dispositive of grade. For example, tubular and invasive cribriform carcinomas are all grade I tumors, whereas medullary, neuroendocrine, and metaplastic carcinomas are all grade III lesions [53].

Lymph Node Status as a Prognosticator for Breast Cancer

Dr. William S. Halsted, the first chief of surgery at Johns Hopkins University Hospital [100, 101], had a lasting influence on the way in which physicians thought about breast cancer and its natural evolution. Up until 1882, the diagnosis of mammary carcinoma was usually a lethal one [102], and, owing to the lack of an effective treatment for that tumor, many cases had been observed from their initial manifestations through advanced stages of growth. Halsted recognized that "scirrhous" (invasive) breast cancers had a reproducible tendency for involvement of the skin and chest wall, and for metastasis to regional (axillary, intramammary, and supraclavicular) lymph nodes. He postulated that if those tissues were removed early, tumors could be blocked from exercising their ability for "in-line" growth from the primary intramammary lesion [101].

Table 5.1 Scarff–Bloom–Richardson grading scheme for invasive ductal breast carcinoma[a]

Tumor tubule formation		Score
>75% of tumor cells arranged in tubules		1
>10% and <75%		2
<10%		3
Number of mitoses		
Low power scanning (×100), find most mitotically tumor area, proceed to high power (×400)		
<10 mitoses in 10 high-power fields		1
>10 and <20 mitoses		2
>20 mitoses per 10 high power fields		3
Nuclear pleomorphism		
Cell nuclei are uniform in size and shape, relatively small, have dispersed chromatin patterns, and are without prominent nucleoli		1
Cell nuclei are somewhat pleomorphic, have nucleoli, and are intermediate size		2
Cell nuclei are relatively large, have prominent nucleoli or multiple nucleoli, coarse chromatin patterns, and vary in size and shape		3
Combined scores[b]	Differentiation/grade	
3, 4, 5	Well-differentiated (grade I)	
6, 7	Moderately differentiated (grade II)	
8, 9	Poorly differentiated (grade III)	

[a] The SBR grading scheme is based on three morphologic features: (1) degree of tumor tubule formation; (2) mitotic activity; and (3) degree of nuclear pleomorphism. Seven possible scores are condensed into three grades

[b] To obtain the final SBR score, one adds subscores from tubule formation, mitotic activity, and nuclear pleomorphism. The combined score yields the final grade

A logical extension of Halsted's concepts held that embolic tumor implants in lymph nodes were "way-station" sources of additional, distant metastases to deep structures such as the lungs, liver, brain, and bones. Hence, radical surgical excision of the breast, pectoralis muscles, and all accessible regional nodes was undertaken from the early 1880s onward – the so-called "radical" mastectomy or Halsted procedure. It was the therapy of choice for breast carcinoma through the late 1970s [102].

Even today, many surgeons believe that aggressive axillary lymphadenectomy has a curative purpose, hypothetically preventing the visceralization of mammary cancers. Nonetheless, that line of reasoning is fallacious. Malignant neoplasms with the ability to metastasize *at all* will exercise that capacity globally as soon as they acquire it. Metastases may first be *detected* in regional lymph nodes, but distant implants are also concurrently present in viscera with the capability of growing to attain clinical visibility at some time in the future [103]. Strong evidence in favor of that mechanistic construct was published in 1981 by Fisher et al. [104]. Those investigators randomized patients with clinically lymph-node-negative breast cancers to three groups. The first was treated with radical mastectomy, whereas the second underwent total mastectomy and thoraco-axillary irradiation, to "sterilize" any occult tumor deposits in axillary and internal mammary lymph nodes. The third group was managed with total mastectomy alone. Long-term surveillance showed no difference whatsoever in survival or rates of distant metastasis among the three groups [104].

Using those data, Fisher and coworkers rightly concluded that tumor implants in regional lymph nodes were *not* the source of visceral metastases. Instead, they were … *indicators of a host-tumor relationship which permits the development of metastases and…not important instigators of distant disease* [104]. Put another way, regional lymph node metastases are merely tangible proof that any given breast cancer can successfully spread from the mammary gland and grow in a secondary site. As such, in specific reference to UDAs, they are also markers for the presence of *systemic* disease [105].

Thus, it comes as no surprise that neoplastic implants in regional lymph nodes are, in fact, associated with a significant worsening of prognosis. How *much* it is lessened depends on the number and locations of nodes that are involved [106–108] – indirectly indicating the vigor of tumor proliferation in anatomically "foreign" sites – as well as markers of growth potential (especially mitotic rate) in the neoplastic population itself.

The latter comments have a direct bearing on a related topic – that is, the biological "meaning" of very few (Fig. 5.16) vs. very many tumor cells in a lymph node. Conflicting data have been recorded in reference to that subject [109]. However, our synthesis of them suggests that many other factors have a bearing on ultimate case outcomes besides tumor-cell-counting. Not all metastasizing neoplasms are the same behaviorally; some may have the capacity for angiolymphatic invasion and embolic spread to other sites, but they may lack the necessary metabolic machinery to *thrive* in those locations. A concrete example of that situation is illustrated by lymph node positivity in cases of "pure" tubular or invasive cribriform

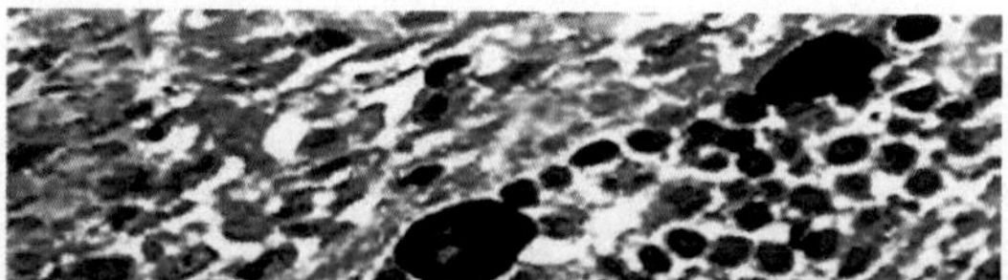

Fig. 5.16 Isolated tumor cells are seen in an axillary lymph node in a case of invasive ductal adenocarcinoma of the usual type, with this pankeratin immunostain. The prognostic significance of this finding is nil, and such nodes should be classified as "negative for tumor"

breast carcinoma, which empirically has been shown to have no association with a decrement in prognosis. Host immunity is also variable from case to case, but it represents another crucial part of the biological mix that determines whether metastatic cells can gain a foothold and flourish. In sum, we believe that "micrometastatic" tumor implants in lymph nodes (or viscera) reflect a lack of robustness in the neoplastic cell population in general, and we agree with recommendations that they be grouped with true "N0" lymph nodes for purposes of staging [110].

In light of these considerations, we cannot support the practice of reflexive immunohistochemical staining or "molecular assessment" [111, 112] of regional nodes for epithelial markers, with the aim of finding histologically occult, dispersed tumor cells. Moreover, we see no therapeutic purpose – beyond, perhaps, a small step in benefitting the local control of tumor growth – in doing extensive "completion lymphadenectomies" for UDAs with clearly positive axillary "sentinel" lymph node biopsies [113]. Those individuals have systemic disease, cannot be cured by the surgeon, and will all require adjuvant treatments of some type. Therefore, the "sentinel" node technique is a generic prognostic tool, *and*, if the node is involved by a UDA of the breast, it should drive the decision to employ an appropriate nonsurgical therapy [114].

Is There a Surrogate for Formal Lymph Node Substaging of Breast Cancer?

Interest has grown in recent years over the possibility that histological nuances of a primary breast carcinoma could obviate the need for formal lymph node substaging. In particular, a logical focus has been drawn on the presence of intramammary angiolymphatic invasion by tumor cells, as seen in H&E sections [115–119] or in immunostained preparations with D2-40 (Fig. 5.17), an antibody recognizing lymphatic endothelium [120–122]. In particular, de Mascarel et al. have shown that if lymphovascular tumor emboli (LTE) are seen in the breast, with an uninvolved zone of normal tissue between the primary carcinoma and the emboli, the likelihood of metastasis-free survival is significantly lessened

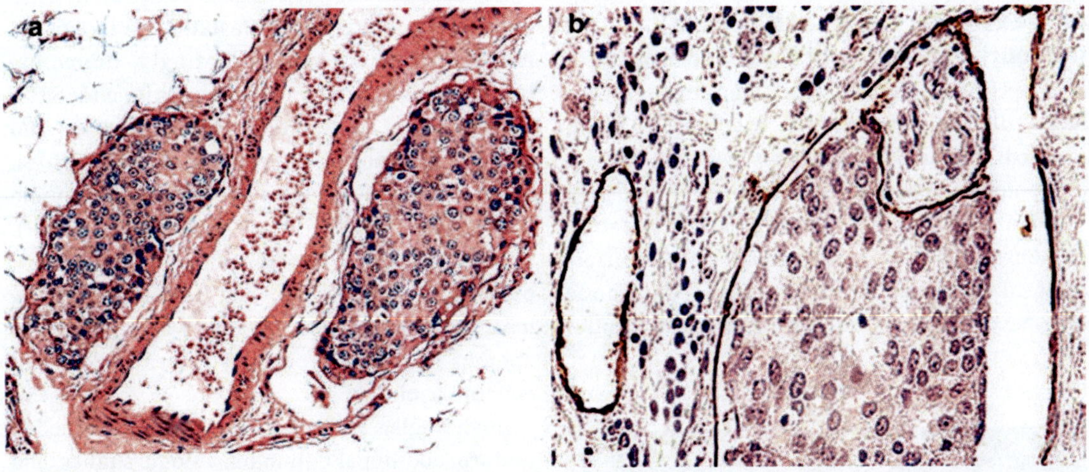

Fig. 5.17 Angiolymphatic invasion by breast carcinoma, as seen with in a hematoxylin and eosin-stained slide (**a**) and an immunostain for podoplanin (**b**) done with antibody "D2-40"

[120]. Moreover, Gurleyik and coworkers and Klar et al. demonstrated a strong correlation between the presence of LTE and metastasis to regional lymph nodes [115]. These findings are not unexpected, because acquisition of the ability for tumor cells to cross vascular basement membranes goes hand-in-hand with development of a metastasis-capable genotype and phenotype [123].

"New" Putatively Prognostic Analytes in Breast Carcinomas

In the wake of the worldwide "genome project" and the common use of comparative genomic hybridization, many candidate genes have been identified with possible behavioral importance for breast carcinomas. These include nm23, p53, *c-myc*, H-, K-, and N-*ras*, PS2, *c-erbB-2(HER-2/neu)* and *c-erbB-3 (HER-3)*, epidermal growth factor receptor-1, "heat shock" genes, *int-2/hst/bcl-1*, *RB1*, and many others [48, 49, 124–136]. Mutations or amplifications of such moieties have been correlated with allegedly worsened behavior of mammary cancers. In addition, "molecular" markers of cell replication, such as Ki-67/MIB-1, proliferating cell nuclear antigen (PCNA), and the cyclin family of proteins, have been studied as substitutes for, or adjuncts to, morphologic quantitation of mitotic activity in breast carcinomas [137, 138].

Assertions have been made that such analytes should replace morphology-based observations in the prognostication of malignant tumors of the breast and other organs [135–156]. The following sections address several problems, which are attached to those recommendations.

Heterogeneous Data Types Affecting Prognostic Factors

In any discipline, data exist in one of three basic forms. They are categorical (nominal), binary, or semiquantitative-quantitative [157]. An example of categorical data is represented by discrete, mutually exclusive, morphologically defined diseases or disease subsets, which must be inherently uniform internally. That type of information has formed the backbone of investigations in anatomic pathology. A common form of binary data is the positive/negative reporting format that pertains to many medical tests, defined by the presence or absence of a predefined analyte. Binary information has a tendency to be artificially delineated, because very few (if any) constituents of biological systems are either ubiquitous or undetectable in a mutually exclusive way. The semiquantitative-quantitative category is self-explanatory and best suited to measurements in biology and Medicine. It is also the most dependent of all data sets on methodological precision, reproducibility, and accuracy.

Case Example: Effects of Incorrect Categorical and Binary Data Generation

A 53-year-old woman detected a mass in her left axilla while bathing. It was confirmed on physical examination by her physician, and by computed tomography of the thorax (Fig. 5.18). Surgical excision and histological examination demonstrated a malignant, large-cell undifferentiated neoplasm in an axillary lymph node (Fig. 5.19). The morphological differential diagnosis centered on metastatic carcinoma vs. metastatic melanoma. Accordingly, immunostains were obtained for pankeratin and S100 protein; these were interpreted as negative and positive, respectively (*binary data generation*), and a final diagnosis of metastatic melanoma was made (*categorical data generation*). Reexamination of the skin showed no evidence of a pigmented lesion, but it was thought to have regressed. The patient was referred to another institution for entry into a melanoma-vaccine trial.

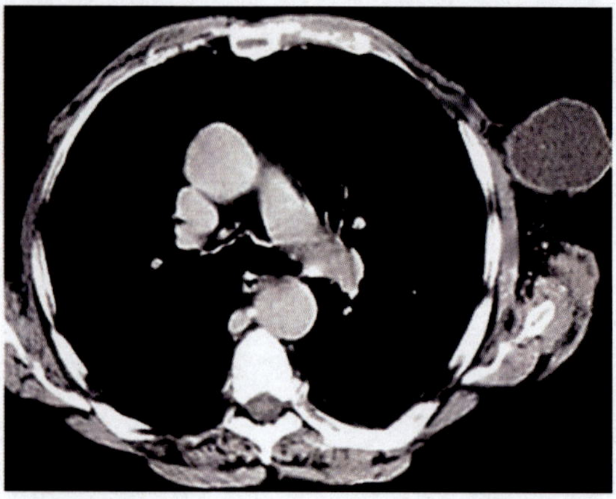

Fig. 5.18 Thoracic computed tomogram showing a large left axillary lymph node in a middle-aged woman

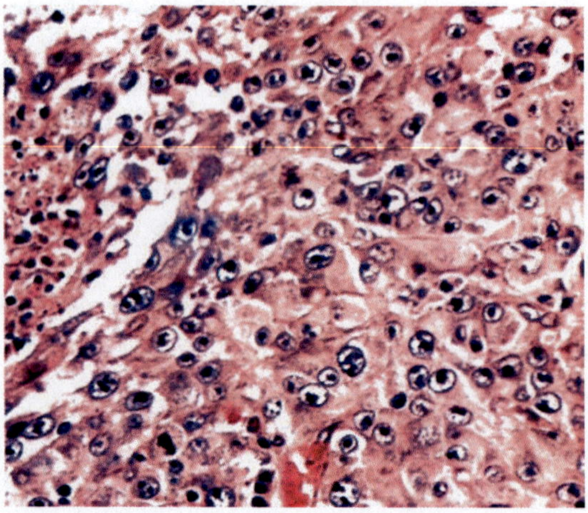

Fig. 5.19 Excision of the mass shown in the previous figure demonstrated a large-cell undifferentiated malignancy. The principal differential diagnosis was between carcinoma and melanoma

Pathologists at the second institution wished to perform additional immunohistologic studies, and they asked for the original paraffin blocks of tumor tissue. Immunostains for pankeratin and S100 protein were also repeated. This time, the tumor was found to be reactive for *both* keratin and S100 protein [158]; in addition, it lacked melan-A, tyrosinase, and PNL2, all of which are melanocytic markers [159]. Another stain for gross cystic disease fluid protein-15 (a breast epithelium-related analyte) [160] was positive (Fig. 5.20), establishing the diagnosis of metastatic breast carcinoma. Mammography then disclosed a mass in the left breast, a fine needle aspiration biopsy of which showed adenocarcinoma (Fig. 5.21). Subsequent discussion with the referring pathologists revealed that recommended epitope-retrieval methods were *not* used in doing pankeratin immunostains [161] at their institution, accounting for the false negativity of that analyte.

Had the original pathological data been used in prognostication and treatment planning, several derivative mistakes would have been made. Incorrect categorical information – which, in turn, was produced by incorrect binary data – would have put the patient in the wrong treatment "bin," "contaminating" accrued results of melanoma vaccine therapy at institution no. 2 and excluding the possibility of effective breast cancer-directed intervention. Parenthically, *predictive* markers for mammary cancers, including ERP/PRP and *HER-2*, also would not have been assessed. It is likewise probable that identification of the primary mammary tumor would have been delayed or not made at all.

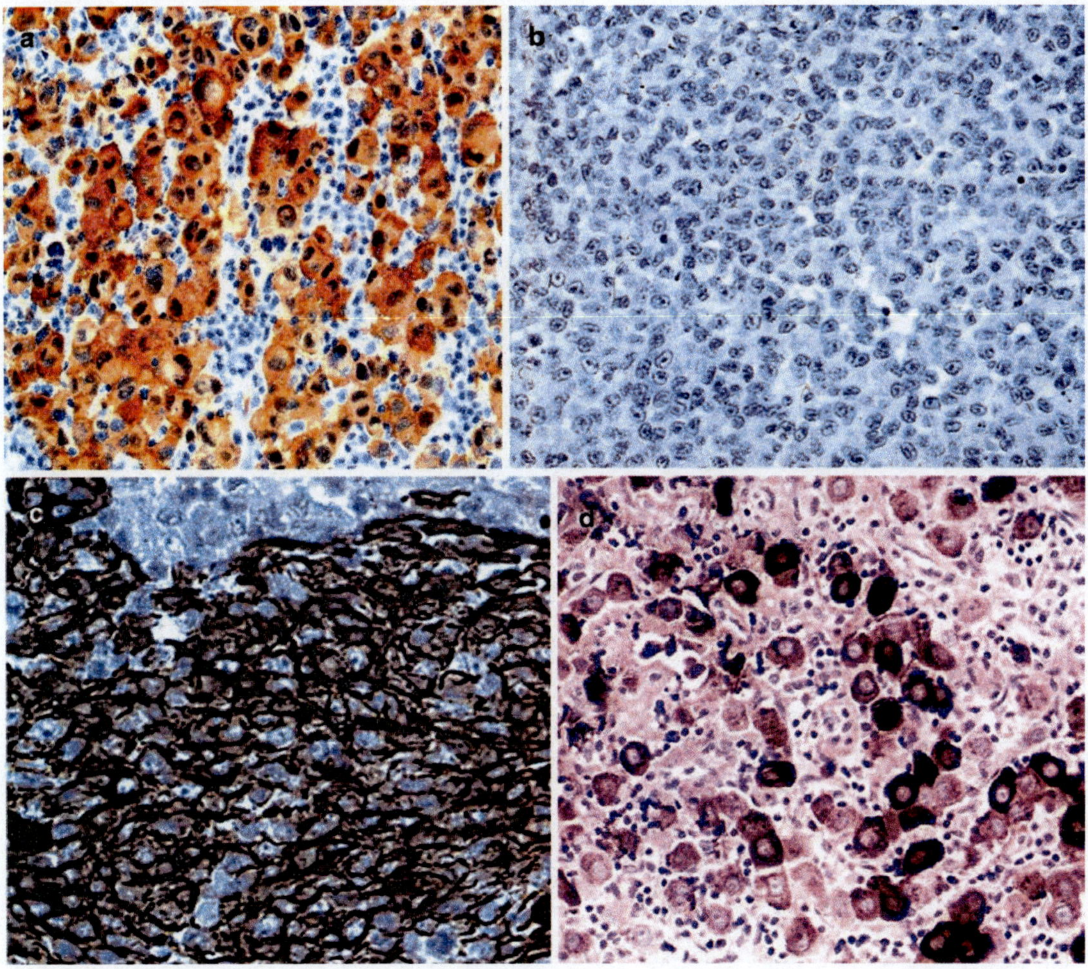

Fig. 5.20 (**a**) S100 protein-staining of the lesion shown in Fig. 5.19 produced positive results, and a pankeratin stain (**b**) was interpreted as negative. The tumor was therefore classified as a melanoma. However, repeated keratin immunostaining with proper epitope retrieval showed obvious positivity (**c**). An additional study showed gross cystic disease fluid protein-15 in the tumor cells (**d**). The final diagnosis was that of metastatic mammary adenocarcinoma

The particular danger that is tied to binary data is that they often are used in a contingent fashion for treatment planning. In other words, a "positive" result leads in one direction, a "negative" in another. Hence, mistakes in generating binary data can be crucial ones. Returning to the illustrative case, the only practical way for pathology laboratories to quality-control immunohistologic results is to utilize a combination of internal duplicate-testing and extramural validation by another reference laboratory [162–164] (see Chap. 16).

The situation is even more complicated if one attempts to substitute one binary test as a surrogate for another one, or to use a binary assay for multivariate targets. For example, several studies have shown that immunohistological assessment of *HER-2* gene amplification is an imperfect substitute for in-situ hybridization or polymerase chain reaction-based assays [165–177]. In other words, a "positive" *HER-2* immunostain may be unassociated with actual gene amplification in a sizable proportion of breast cancer cases. Similar comments apply to the relationship between "positive" immunostains for epidermal growth factor receptor (EGFR) and actual mutations in the EGFR gene, in reference to lung or colon carcinomas. Yet another example of the same hiatus is "positive" immunostaining for CD117 (*c-kit*),

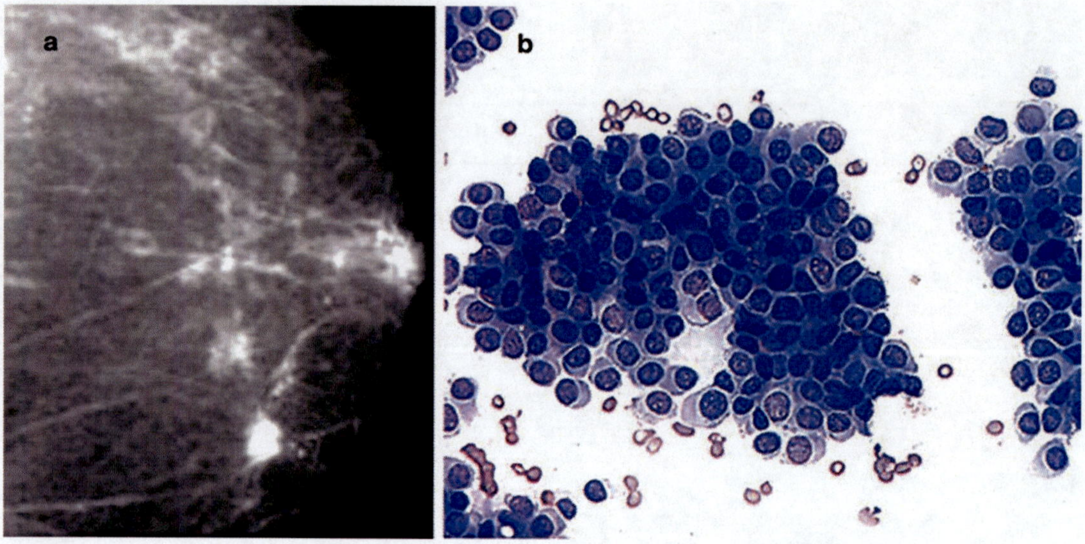

Fig. 5.21 Subsequent mammography of the left breast, in the case discussed in Figs. 5.19 and 5.20, showed a mass with the phenotype of carcinoma (**a**); that impression was confirmed by fine-needle aspiration biopsy (**b**)

but with no actual activating mutation in the CD117 gene [178, 179].

The outcome of all of those scenarios is again a likely misdirection of treatment. Biological agents that are inhibitors of *HER-2*, EGFR, or CD117 may be administered on the basis of "positive" respective immunostains, but there will be no clinical response because the surrogate "binary" tests are poor ones.

As considered elsewhere in this monograph, statistical methods also differ significantly for the evaluation of binary and semiquantitative or quantitative data of prognostic or predictive use. Binary information is often assessed using Bayesian techniques; nonbinary data require evaluations using receiver-operator-characteristic (ROC) curves; likelihood ratios, Wilcoxon analysis, Kruskal–Wallis testing, and other similar procedures [180].

Interpretative and decision-making applications of binary or categorical data can be facilitated by constructing partially redundant algorithms that are based on *constellations* of test results. An example is shown in Fig. 5.22, in reference to immunohistochemical identification of metastatic carcinomas of unknown origin. Nevertheless, such constructions cannot compensate for poor methodology.

Methodological Reproducibility and Cross-Validation

Methodological reproducibility is, sadly, rarely discussed in the practice of anatomic pathology [162, 164]. As an example, one could obtain biologically "proven," analyte-positive cases to use as "in-run" controls. In the context of immunostains in breast cancer cases, such specimens are exemplified by ERP-positive invasive carcinomas that are known to have responded clinically to hormonal therapy. Unfortunately, the latter portion of that requirement is typically ignored.

Cross-validation of methods (CVM: also known as interanalytical agreement) is also a cornerstone of proper testing for prognostic and predictive factors. In the realm of breast cancer evaluation, examples of CVM are represented by parallel evaluations of ERP content by dextran-coated charcoal assays and immunostaining, done on the same tissue specimens [181–183]; immunostaining for nuclear p53-reactivity (Fig. 5.23), compared with formal gene-sequence analysis to identify p53 mutations, again on the same tissue samples [184–189] (Fig. 5.24); and *HER-2* immunostaining compared with results of *in-situ* hybridization (ISH) using the same tissue substrate [168–177]. Again, the routine application of CVM is a sad rarity in the practice of surgical pathology.

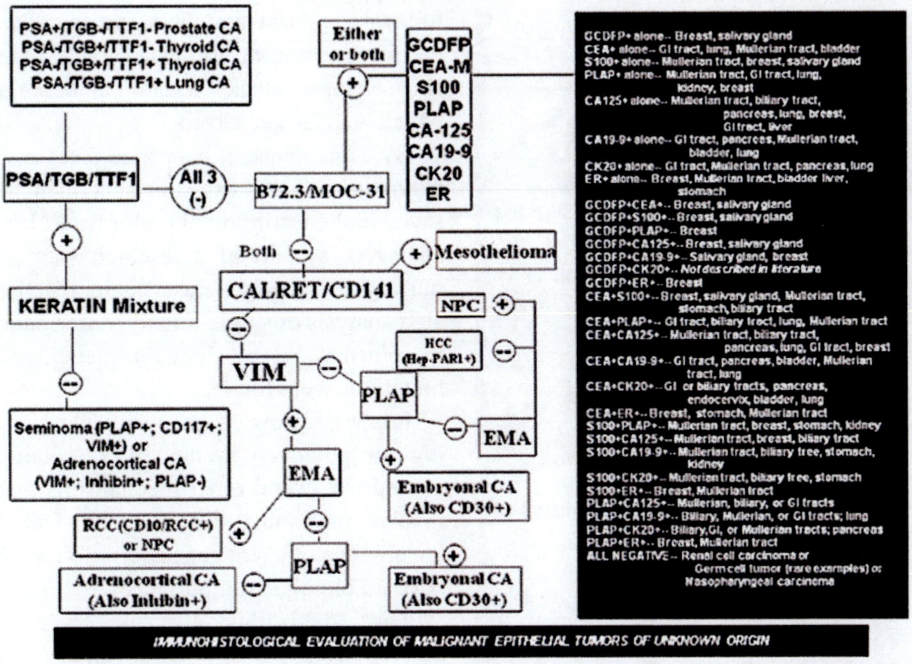

Fig. 5.22 Algorithm for the immunohistochemical identification of metastatic epithelioid malignancies. The inherent redundancy in this approach compensates, at least in part, for biological variation in this group of tumors

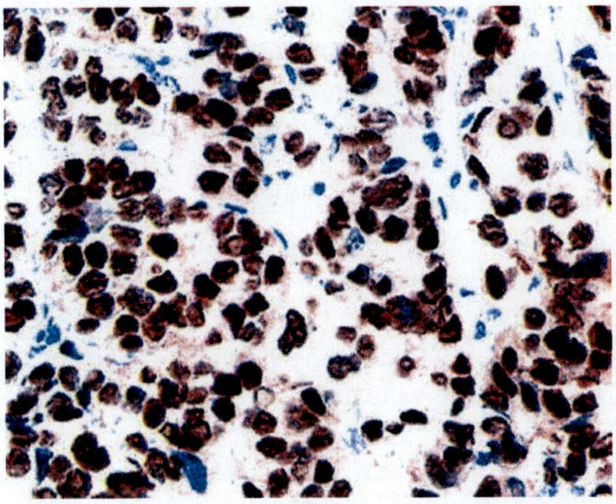

Fig. 5.23 Nuclear immunolabeling of ductal breast carcinoma for putatively mutant p53 protein

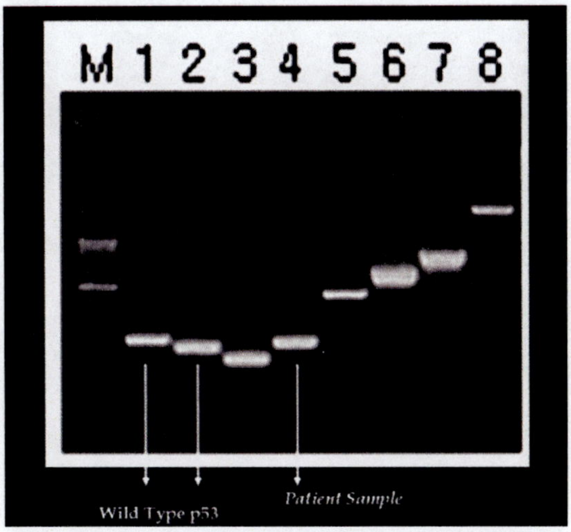

Fig. 5.24 Southern blot preparation for mutant p53, demonstrating a nonmutated patient sample as compared with "wild type" control tissues

Case Example: Effects of Omitting Cross-Validation of Methods

A 39-year-old woman found a mass in her right breast by monthly self-examination. The lesion was confirmed mammographically, and its image suggested a malignancy. Excision and pathological examination of the mass showed an invasive 1 cm, UDA of BSR grade II (Fig. 5.25). It exhibited no angiolymphatic invasion and had a low mitotic rate; all surgical margins were uninvolved by tumor. It was immunoreactive for ERP and PRP, and lacked *HER-2* amplification in ISH studies.

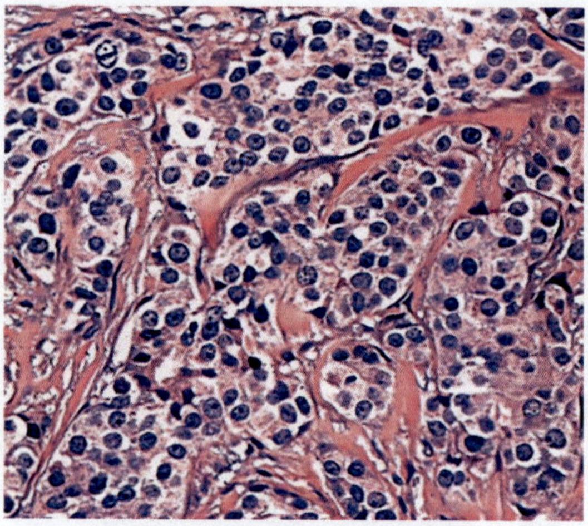

Fig. 5.25 Bloom–Scarff–Richardson grade II ductal adenocarcinoma, as seen in a 39-year-old woman

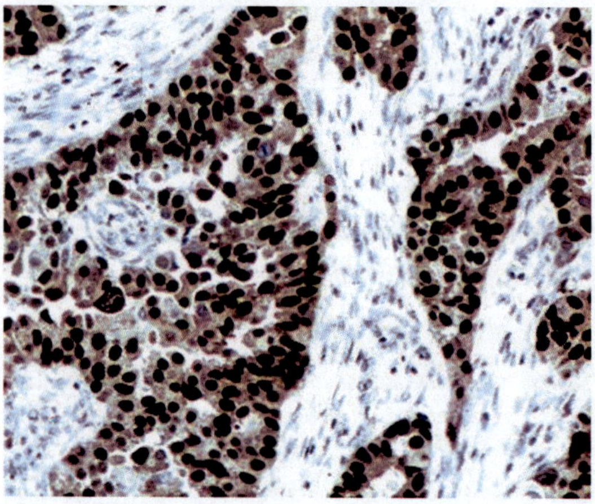

Fig. 5.26 The tumor in Fig. 5.25 unexpectedly immunolabeled for p53 protein, but no actual p53 mutations were found on subsequent blotting studies

The surgeon handling the case specifically requested that an immunostain for p53 be done, predicated on his recent perusal of literature on that analyte in breast cancer. Without asking about the use the surgeon intended for that result, the test was done by the pathologist. Unexpectedly, it showed significant nuclear reactivity for p53 (Fig. 5.26), which was reported in an addendum with no additional comments.

Based on that finding, the surgeon informed the patient that she had a poor-prognosis neoplasm. He recommended, and performed, a modified radical completion mastectomy (which demonstrated no residual tumor or lymph node involvement), followed by adjuvant chemotherapy. The patient had severe vomiting during her course of treatment and developed a local "seroma" at the surgical site, which gradually resolved.

By coincidence, it happened that frozen tissue from the original excision specimen had been saved in the institutional tumor bank. It was later analyzed, as part of a research study, for p53 mutations by polymerase chain reaction-mediated analysis of single-strand conformation polymorphisms and by direct sequencing. No p53 mutations were found.

It is well known that "positive" nuclear labeling for putatively mutant p53 protein can be caused by several other mechanisms that do not involve gene mutation [184, 185, 188, 189]. In the absence of a real gene aberration, such results have no biological importance.

Thus, in this illustrative case, several mistakes derived from the *failure to validate immunostaining results* by more sophisticated methods. First, a conceptual failing by the surgeon – that is, using an isolated test result to determine therapy – undeniably occurred in the face of morphological and supplementary laboratory information that was prognostically *favorable*. That misstep produced unnecessarily aggressive treatment with unwanted morbidity. Second, a failure of the pathologist to explain the limitations of p53 immunostaining in the surgical pathology report indirectly fostered incorrect decisions by the surgeon. If it is done at all in UDA cases, p53 immunostaining should be viewed as a screening procedure; "positive" results *must* be validated by additional studies.

Sources of Clinical Bias in Reference to New "Prognostic" Markers

Some pathologists pay little attention to medical publications in other specialty areas, including those that discuss new "prognostic" markers for breast carcinoma and other malignant tumors. That is an unfortunate oversight. Pathologists must be able to discern whether or not such clinical studies have been properly constructed and performed, in order to help their colleagues decide which new "prognostic" laboratory assays are worthy of implementation and which are not.

Reproducible mistakes exist in a substantial number of "forecast"-oriented clinical publications in oncology. The first is the inclusion of tumors of different histologic types, grades, and stages in the same cohort of cases. The second is the indiscriminate mixing of patients who have never before been treated for their malignancies, with others who have failed prior therapies, in the same study group. The third is represented by attempts to compare the outcomes of patients who have received a heterogeneous hodgepodge of treatments, but with focus on a single "prognostic" factor. Finally, there may be inattention to important and variable comorbid conditions in the study population. *Any one* of these flaws casts serious doubt on the validity of conclusions regarding "prognosis." Another problem concerns a failure to use "power analysis;" that is, predefined statistical construction of studies with sufficient case numbers and controls to yield valid information [190]. Those measures are necessary because "large groups" of study cases may, in fact, be inadequate to allow for definite conclusions about them. A study set of 50 prostatic leiomyosarcomas would seem huge to any given surgical pathologist because of the rarity of that tumor type, but, in fact, it would not allow for any truly meaningful studies on the prognosis of the lesion.

An additional pertinent issue is the definition of "outcomes." They may be binary (e.g., dead or alive; tumor-free or not), or qualified (overall survival vs. disease-free survival). These definitions have distinct implications for the estimation of prognosis. Some analytes may be prognostic in regard to one outcome measure, but not another. For example, factor "X" may correlate well with disease-free survival but not *overall* survival. Others may be prognostic for one patient subgroup, but not others (e.g., individuals with stage I breast cancers vs. those with nonstage I tumors).

Two truisms attach to these issues. First, *in any proper comparison of 2 or more prognostic factors that are derived from different patient-cohorts, the cohort compositions and measures of "outcome" must be the same.* Second, it must be understood that "surrogate" measures of outcome are not the same as "real" outcomes. Statements about surrogacy go as follows ... *factor "Z" forecasts well for lymph node metastasis, and lymph node metastasis correlates well with overall prognosis, so therefore factor "Z" also forecasts overall prognosis.* That form of logical construction often falls into the "true-true-unrelated" category and is therefore incorrect. Regrettably, surrogate outcome measures have become very common in the literature on anatomic pathology, because of modern difficulties in obtaining information from long-term surveillance of patients. Those problems stem from bureaucratic obstacles to follow up – principally derived from the U.S. Health Insurance Portability and Accountability Act of 1996 [191] – and also the fact that patients only uncommonly receive continuous care at any one medical center.

The McGuire Criteria: Template for Evaluation of "Prognostic" Tests

Dr. William L. McGuire was a professor and the division chief of Medical Oncology at the University of Texas-San Antonio for many years before his untimely death in 1992, and an internationally renowned researcher on breast cancer [192]. In the latter part of his career, Dr. McGuire wrote a landmark editorial on prognostic and predictive factors in oncology, as applied to breast carcinoma or any other malignant neoplasm [193]. That document described several characteristics of any effective test for clinical forecasting, which have since become known as the *McGuire criteria* (MC) (Fig. 5.27). They not only address the major laboratory problems that can

McGuire Criteria for Evaluation of Putative Prognostic Markers

1. Is there a presumptive biological effect caused by the analyte in question?
2. Is there a control population bias with regard to distribution of the analyte?
3. Has there been validation of the methodology used to evaluate the analyte?
4. Have optimized "cutoff values "for the analyte been determined by rigorous clinical testing?
5. Has the method used to evaluate the analyte demonstrated reproducibility?
6. Has the definitive clinical study been performed to determine efficacy of the analyte ?

Fig. 5.27 The McGuire criteria for evaluation of proposed prognostic and predictive tests in anatomic pathology and oncology be associated with tests for "forecasting" factors, but also require that proof of a true biological effect on tumor growth be supplied for each new marker. The final criterion centers on performing "definitive" clinical studies of prognostic and predictive markers. That stipulation touches on the problems with study-group composition and statistical analysis that were mentioned above.

In applying the MC to currently utilized PPMTs, where do we stand? Summaries are given for exemplary markers in Figs. 5.28–5.31. In examining the details, the reader will note that each of several common breast carcinoma-related markers – including ERP/PRP, p53, *HER-2*, and Ki-67 – still is plagued by clinicopathologic shortcomings vis-à-vis the MC.

HER-2 and Herceptin: An Historical Review

In 1987, Slamon and colleagues discovered a possible therapeutic target in some breast carcinomas [194]. Those tumors overexpressed the

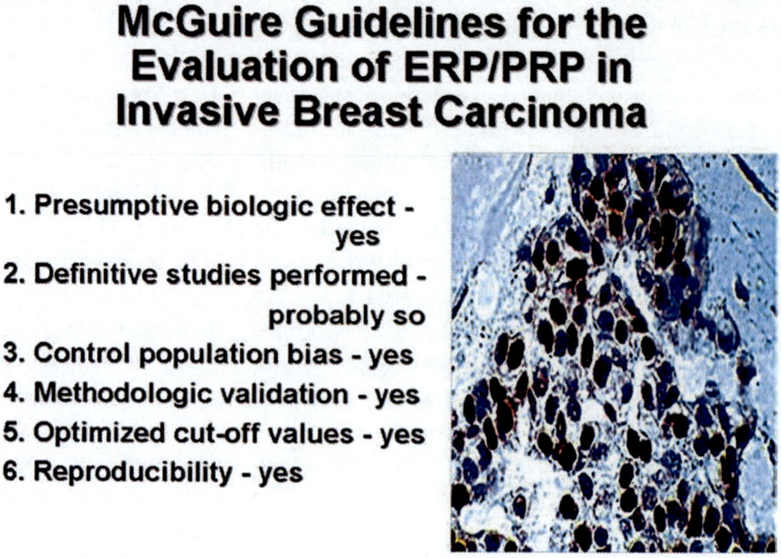

Fig. 5.28 The McGuire criteria, applied to estrogen receptor and progesterone receptor proteins as detected immunohistologically

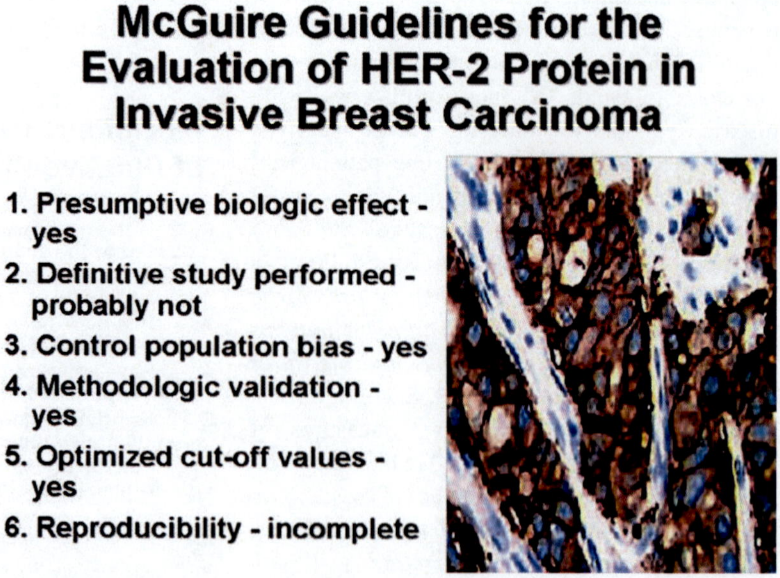

Fig. 5.29 The McGuire criteria, applied to *HER-2* protein as detected immunohistologically

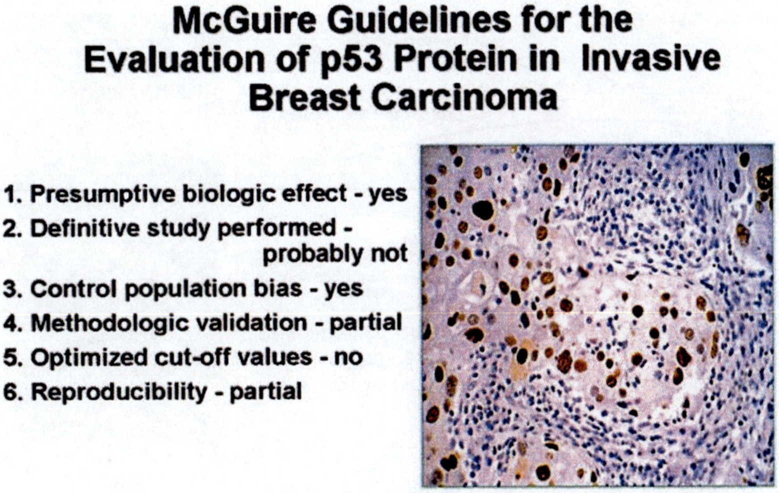

Fig. 5.30 The McGuire criteria, applied to mutant p53 protein as detected immunohistologically

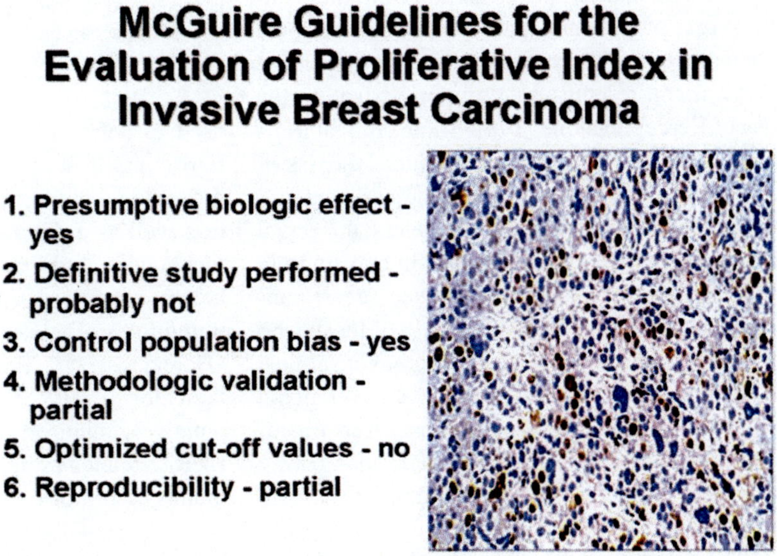

Fig. 5.31 The McGuire criteria, applied to Ki-67 (a proliferation marker) as detected immunohistologically

HER-2 gene, which codes for one of the epidermal growth factor receptors (*c-erbB-2)* with tyrosine kinase activity. Amplification of the *HER-2* gene and corresponding overexpression of the receptor protein were found to cause aberrant intracellular signaling and increased cell division; that abnormality was present in 20–30% of stage I UDAs.

Trastuzumab (Herceptin ©) is a humanized monoclonal antibody, developed by Genentech Co., which binds to the [195] extracellular segment of *HER-2* receptor, blocking its coupling with extracellular mitogens (Fig. 5.32). The result is growth arrest in the G1 phase of the cell cycle. Trastuzumab may suppress angiogenesis as well through unrelated mechanisms, and it may serve as the target for antibody-dependent cellular cytotoxicity by the host [137].

If it is determined that a breast cancer shows c-erbB2 amplification (*HER-2*+ status; see below), the patient is eligible for treatment with trastuzumab. Nevertheless, the actual rates of success with that agent are troubling; 70% of *HER-2*+ patients fail to respond, and resistance to trastuzumab is developed rapidly in virtually all cases that do show an initial benefit [196].

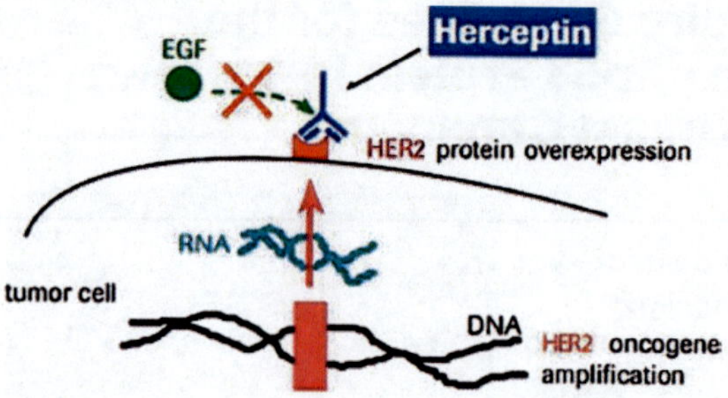

Fig. 5.32 Illustrative diagram depicting how the therapeutic biological agent, trastuzumab (Herceptin ©), is intended to block mitogens (growth factors) that bind to the *HER-2* receptor

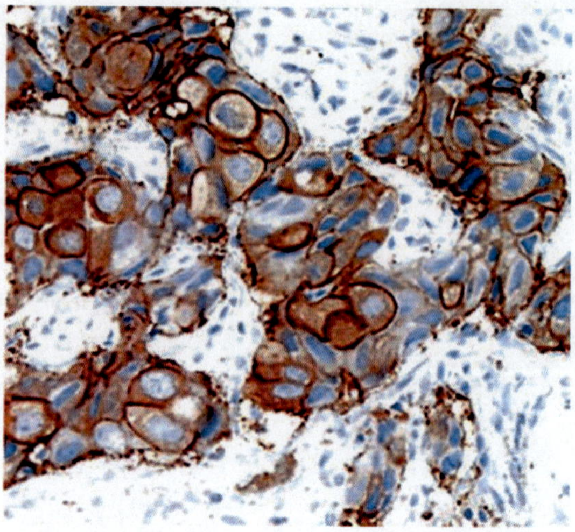

Fig. 5.33 Immunohistologic staining for *HER-2* protein is predicated on the premise that *HER-2* gene amplification in breast carcinoma will produce an excess of the cell membrane-bound protein target

Herceptin has been touted as having a "major impact in the treatment of HER2-positive metastatic breast cancer" [197]. In addition, the combination of trastuzumab with conventional chemotherapeutic agents has been said to increase survival and response rate, in comparison to the use of Herceptin alone [198]. Some clinical trials have concluded that Herceptin reduced the risk of relapse by 50% when given in the adjuvant setting for 1 year [199, 200]. Nonetheless, the actual case numbers are more sobering. In one study in England, 9.4% of Herceptin-treated breast cancers relapsed compared with 17.2% of those who were not given trastuzumab. Moreover, almost 85% of the patients would not have developed a recurrence whether or not they received trastuzumab, and roughly 10% relapsed *despite* getting the drug. Only 8% of cases showed a durable response to Herceptin [201].

The actual benefits of Herceptin are also not very impressive when viewed in terms of all-cause mortality. Large studies have shown that one must treat between 25 and 100 patients with breast cancer to prevent a single death during a follow-up period of 4 years [202, 203]. For each patient who benefits, 10–25 will develop Herceptin-mediated cardiomyopathy, and some of those individuals will die from congestive heart failure. Finally, it is worth taking special note that the average cost to the healthcare system of 1 years' treatment with trastuzumab is approximately $100,000 per patient [204–207].

Additional problems come to light when one considers the laboratory methods that have been used to define *HER-2* amplification [165–177]. Early on, it was realized that the humanized monoclonal antibody, trastuzumab, did not function well as a diagnostic reagent in immunohistochemical studies. Therefore, alternatively, heteroantisera to *HER-2* were utilized in an immunohistologic assay that was marketed as the "Herceptest ©." That evaluation is an indirect indicator of *HER-2* gene amplification, which is putatively manifest by causing a large amount of HER-2-related protein to accumulate in the membranes of tumor cells (Fig. 5.33). Problems that have been encountered with the Herceptest include fixation-related variation in sensitivity, suboptimal reproducibility between laboratories, a subjective threshold for interpreting the test as "positive," and imperfect correlation with ISH studies as a true marker of gene amplification [208–214]. As this chapter is being written in mid-2011 – 13 years after the introduction of Herceptin – position papers are still being published on the "optimal" way of detecting *HER-2* amplification in the laboratory [215–219].

Hence, we come to a denouement regarding the use of *HER-2* as a PPMT, and Herceptin, one of the most championed single treatments of all time. In the final analysis, *HER-2* gene amplification in breast carcinomas – which we believe is

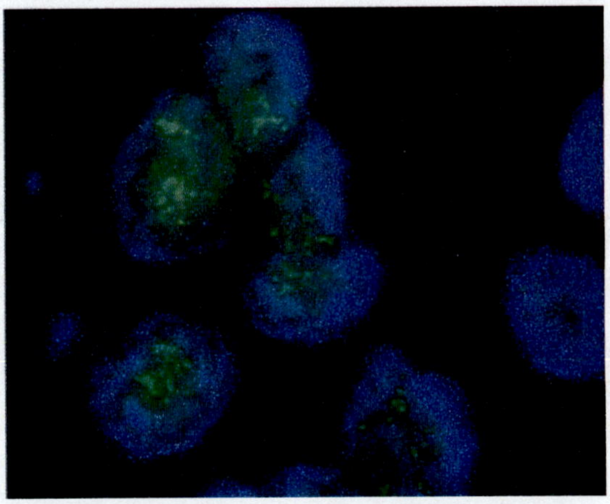

Fig. 5.34 Fluorescent in-situ hybridization preparation of ductal breast carcinoma, demonstrating several copies of the *HER-2* gene in each tumor cells and confirming the presence of gene amplification

best detected using ISH (Fig. 5.34), *not* the Herceptest – is treated with an agent that is very expensive, with long-term effectiveness in no more than 10% of cases and potentially lethal cardiotoxicity [51, 220–226]. Elkin et al. [227] have concluded that the healthcare system "gets a good deal" by supporting reflexive testing for *HER-2* amplification in all breast cancers. If that is done by ISH, with an average cost of $350 per assay, $73,500,000 would be expended yearly in testing the 195,000 new cases of mammary carcinoma in the U.S. [227]. Herceptin-related expenditures for the 25% of new UDAs that are *HER-2+*, with 1 full year of treatment, add $3,400,000,000 to the tally for an annual total of $3,473,500,000. With due respect, we are led to disagree with Elkin and coworkers regarding their opinions on this topic.

Conclusions

Despite strong assertions to the contrary – both in the lay press and in medical publications [204–207] – the current status of "new" PPMTs for human malignancies is a chaotic one with dubious cost-effectiveness. A lack of uniformity exists in how those tests are performed and interpreted, and their "meaning" is often obscured by poorly constructed and administrated clinical trials. This averral is not unique to the authors; indeed, the College of American Pathologists has convened two multidisciplinary meetings on the topic of PPMTs, with comparable conclusions to ours [228]. On the other hand, "old" PPMTs, when properly performed, are still extremely valuable and trustworthy with regard to clinical forecasting [53, 115]. In specific reference to breast carcinoma, these have been enumerated earlier in our discussion, including factors such as recognition of "special" histologic variants, accurate measurement of tumor size, BSR grade, mitotic rate, lymph node substage, and the presence of angiolymphatic invasion.

As laboratory methods are refined, and as novel, potentially highly effective biological treatments become available and are tailored to specific neoplasms (e.g., imatinib for gastrointestinal stromal tumors and chronic myelogenous leukemia [1, 2], this situation may well change). At the present time, however, pathologists must be systematic and critical in their assessments of new PPMTs, with a strict threshold for acceptance of those methods as "state-of-the-art" procedures. As explained in different chapters of this volume, the evidence-based process starts by formulating patient-related questions, such as: What are we trying to achieve with the new laboratory test? What are the specific indications of this new test, based on previous knowledge about a particular disease? Are the findings obtained with the new test going to be used by clinicians to select the treatment of a patient? Is the therapeutic intervention indicated by the information provided by the tests going to significantly affect the outcome of a disease, in terms of survival, quality of life, or other indicators? Are there other less expensive tests that could provide similar information? Application of "evidence-based" principles will be a crucial part of the process of realizing the full potential of the personalized medicine paradigm in a manner that optimizes the clinical applicability of all relevant available information, and discourages the use of laboratory tests and other diagnostic procedures that often add only inconvenience, morbidity, false hopes, confusion, and/or unnecessary cost to the treatment of patients with breast cancer and other diseases.

References

1. Waller CF. Imatinib mesylate. Recent Results Cancer Res. 2010;184:3–20.
2. Arifi S, El-Sayadi H, Dufresne A, et al. Imatinib and solid tumors. Bull Cancer. 2008;95:99–106.
3. Broders AC. Squamous cell epithelioma of the lip: a study of 537 cases. JAMA. 1920;74:656–64.
4. Edmundson WF. Microscopic grading of cancer and its practical implications. Arch Dermatol Syphilol. 1948;57:141–50.
5. Eker R, Weyde R. The significance of histological grading in the prognosis of carcinomas in the true oral cavity. Acta Pathol Microbiol Scand. 1949;26: 750–68.
6. Ringertz N. Grading of gliomas. Acta Pathol Microbiol Scand. 1950;27:51–64.
7. Goyanna R, Torres ET, Broders AC. Histological grading of malignant tumors; Broders' method. Hospital (Rio J). 1951;39:791–818.
8. Fahmy A. Histological grading of urinary bladder tumors: a study of 411 urinary bladder biopsies. Urol Int. 1963;15:358–77.
9. Pugh RC. The grading and staging of bladder tumors: the Institute of Urology classification. Br J Urol. 1957;29:222–5.
10. Graham JB. Histologic grading of cancer of the uterine cervix. Surg Gynecol Obstet. 1953;96:331–7.
11. Price CH. The grading of osteogenic sarcoma. Br J Cancer. 1952;6:46–68.
12. Broders AC, Hargrave R, Meyerding HW. Pathological features of soft tissue fibrosarcoma with special reference to the grading of its malignancy. Surg Gynecol Obstet. 1939;69:267–80.
13. Denoix PF. Enquate permanent dans les centres anticancereaux. Bull Inst Nat Hyg. 1946;1:70–5.
14. Dukes CE. The classification of cancer of the rectum. J Pathol Bacteriol. 1932;35:323–40.
15. Mathews FS. The ten-year survivors of radical mastectomy. Ann Surg. 1933;98:635–43.
16. Enneking WF, Kagan A. The implications of "skip" metastases in osteosarcoma. Clin Orthop Relat Res. 1975;111:33–41.
17. Kim TH, Nesbit ME, D'Angio GD, Levitt SH. The role of central nervous system irradiation in children with acute lymphoblastic leukemia. Radiology. 1972; 104:635–41.
18. Spiers AS, Booth AE, Firth JL. Subcutaneous cerebrospinal fluid reservoirs in patients with acute leukemia. Scand J Haematol. 1978;20:289–96.
19. Taylor CR. Immunoperoxidase techniques: practical and theoretical aspects. Arch Pathol Lab Med. 1978; 102:113–21.
20. Mori M, Ambe K, Adachi Y, et al. Prognostic value of immunohistochemically-identified CEA, SC, AFP, and S100 protein positive-cells in gastric carcinoma. Cancer. 1988;62:534–40.
21. Kluftinger AM, Robinson BW, Quenville NF, Finley RJ, Davis NL. Correlation of epidermal growth factor receptor and *c-erb*B-2 oncogene product to known prognostic indicators of colorectal cancer. Surg Oncol. 1992;1:97–105.
22. Rescher N. A philosophical introduction to the theory of risk evaluation and measurement. Washington: University Press of America; 1983.
23. Hubbard D. The failure of risk management: why it's broken and how to fix it. Baltimore: John Hopkins; 2009.
24. Risk and uncertainty. http://en.wikipedia.org/wiki/Risk.
25. Wolf DC, Mann PC. Confounders in interpreting pathology for safety and risk assessment. Toxicol Appl Pharmacol. 2005;202:302–8.
26. Carter BA, Page DL, O'Malley FP. Usual epithelial hyperplasia and atypical ductal hyperplasia. In: O'Malley FP, Pinder SE, editors. Foundations in diagnostic pathology – breast pathology. Churchill Livingstone: Elsevier; 2006. p. 164–8.
27. Marchevsky AM, Walts AE, Bose S, et al. Evidence-based evaluation of the risks of malignancy predicted by thyroid fine-needle aspiration biopsies. Diagn Cytopathol. 2010;38:252–9.
28. Cibas ES, Ali SZ. The Bethesda system for reporting thyroid cytopathology. Thyroid. 2009;19:1159–65.
29. Prognosis. http://en.wikipedia.org/wiki/Prognosis#References.
30. Hippocrates. http://en.wikipedia.org/wiki/Prognosis#References.
31. Petosiris. http://en.wikipedia.org/wiki/Petosiris_to_Nechepso.
32. Bellazzi R, Zupan B. Predictive data mining in clinical medicine: current issues and guidelines. Int J Med Inform. 2008;77:81–97.
33. Breast cancer prognosis. http://www.cancer.gov/cancertopics/pdq/treatment/breast/Patient.
34. Prediction. http://en.wikipedia.org/wiki/Prediction.
35. Copeland AH. Predictions and probabilities. Erkenntnis. 2007;6:1572–8420.
36. Pepe MS. Evaluating technologies for classification and prediction in medicine. Stat Med. 2005;24: 3687–96.
37. Mahapatra A. Lung cancer – genomics and personalized medicine. ACS Chem Biol. 2010;18:529–31.
38. Bohr. http://www.quotationspage.com/quote/26159.html.
39. Personalized Medicine. http://www.sciencedaily.com/news/health_medicine/personalized_medicine/.
40. Jain KK. Innovative diagnostic technologies and their significance for personalized medicine. Mol Diagn Ther. 2010;14:141–7.
41. U.S. Congressional Budget Office. The long-term outlook for health care spending. http://www.cbo.gov/ftpdocs/MainText.3.1.shtml. Accessed 12 June 2010.
42. Traficant J: What 2 liver transplants taught me about how to heal health care. http://www.foxnews.com/jim-traficant-healthcare. Accessed 12 June 2010.
43. Drew EB: The quiet victory of the cigarette lobby: how it found the best filter yet – Congress. Atlantic Monthly. September 1965.

44. Deyo RA, Patrick DL. Hope or hype: the obsession with medical advances and the high cost of false promises. New York: AMACOM; 2005.
45. Hanby AM. The pathology of breast cancer and the role of the histopathology laboratory. Clin Oncol. 2005;17:234–9.
46. Korkolis DP, Tsoli E, Fouskakis D, et al. Tumor histology and stage but not p53, Her2-neu, or cathepsin-D expression are independent prognostic factors in breast cancer patients. Anticancer Res. 2004;24:2061–8.
47. Bilous M, Ades C, Armes J, et al. Predicting the HER2 status of breast cancer from basic histopathology data: an analysis of 1500 breast cancers as part of the HER2000 International Study. Breast. 2003;12:92–8.
48. Kim C, Taniyama Y, Paik S. Gene-expression-based prognostic and predictive markers for breast cancer. Arch Pathol Lab Med. 2009;133:855–9.
49. Sandhu R, Parker JS, Jones WD, Livasy CA, Coleman WB. Microarray-based gene expression profiling for molecular classification of breast cancer and identification of new targets for therapy. Lab Med. 2010;41:364–72.
50. Rettig RA, Jacobson PD, Farquhar CM, Aubry WM. False hope: bone marrow transplantation for breast cancer. New York: Oxford University Press; 2007.
51. Gonzalez-Angulo AM, Morales-Vasquez F, Hortobagyi GN. Overview of resistance to systemic therapy in patients with breast cancer. Adv Exp Med Biol. 2007;608:1–22.
52. Anonymous. Cancer Statistics, 2009. Oklahoma City: American Cancer Society; 2009.
53. Page DL, Jensen RA, Simpson JF. Routinely-available indicators of prognosis in breast cancer. Breast Cancer Res Treat. 1998;51:195–208.
54. Klar M, Foeldi M, Markert S, Gitsch G, Stickeler E, Watermann D. Good prediction of the likelihood for sentinel lymph node metastasis by using the MSKCC nomogram in a German breast cancer population. Ann Surg Oncol. 2009;16:36–42.
55. Rosen PP, Groshen S, Kinne DW, Norton L. Factors influencing prognosis in node-negative breast carcinoma: analysis of 767 T1N0M0./T2N0M0 patients with long-term followup. J Clin Oncol. 1993;11:2090–100.
56. Scawn R, Shousha S. Morphologic spectrum of estrogen receptor-negative breast carcinoma. Arch Pathol Lab Med. 2002;126:325–30.
57. Robertson JF, Ellis IO, Pearson D, Elston CW, Nicholson RI, Blamey RW. Biological factors of prognostic significance in locally-advanced breast cancer. Breast Cancer Res Treat. 1994;29:259–64.
58. Houssami N, Ciatto S, Ellis IO, Ambrogetti D. Underestimation of malignancy in breast core-needle biopsy: concepts and precise overall and category-specific estimates. Cancer. 2007;109:487–95.
59. Houssami N, Ciatto S, Bilous M, Vezzosi V, Bianchi S. Borderline breast core needle histology: predictive values for malignancy in lesions of uncertain malignant potential. Br J Cancer. 2007;96:1253–7.
60. Ciatto S, Houssami N, Ambrogetti D, et al. Accuracy and underestimation of malignancy of breast core needle biopsy: the Florence experience of over 4000 consecutive biopsies. Breast Cancer Res Treat. 2007;101:291–7.
61. Lee AH, Denley HE, Pinder SE, et al. Excision biopsy findings of patients with breast needle core biopsies reported as suspicious of malignancy or lesion of uncertain malignant potential. Histopathology. 2003; 42:331–6.
62. Bonnett M, Wallis T, Rossmann M, et al. Histopathologic analysis of atypical lesions in image-guided core breast biopsies. Mod Pathol. 2003;16: 154–60.
63. Dillon MF, McDermott EW, Hill AD, O'Doherty A, O'Higgins N, Quinn CM. Predictive value of breast lesions of "uncertain malignant potential" and "suspicious for malignancy" determined by needle core biopsy. Ann Surg Oncol. 2007;14:704–11.
64. Margenthaler JA, Duke D, Monsees BS, Baraton PT, Clark C, Dietz JR. Correlation between core biopsy and excisional biopsy in breast high-risk lesions. Am J Surg. 2006;192:534–7.
65. Simpson JF, Page DL. Pathology of preinvasive and excellent-prognosis breast cancer. Curr Opin Oncol. 2001;13:426–30.
66. Page DL. Special types of invasive breast cancer, with clinical implications. Am J Surg Pathol. 2003;27: 832–5.
67. Pia-Foschini M, Reis-Filho JS, Eusebi V, Lakhani SR. Salivary gland-like tumours of the breast: surgical and molecular pathology. J Clin Pathol. 2003;56:497–506.
68. Weigel RJ, Ikeda DM, Nowels KW. Primary squamous cell carcinoma of the breast. South Med J. 1996;89:511–5.
69. Van Hoeven KH, Drudis T, Cranor ML, Erlandson RA, Rosen PP. Low-grade adenosquamous carcinoma of the breast. A clinicopathologic study of 32 cases with ultrastructural analysis. Am J Surg Pathol. 1993;17:248–58.
70. Toikkanen S. Primary squamous cell carcinoma of the breast. Cancer. 1981;48:1629–32.
71. Barnes PJ, Boutilier R, Chiasson D, Rayson D. Metaplastic breast carcinoma: clinical-pathologic characteristics and HER2/neu expression. Breast Cancer Res Treat. 2005;91:173–8.
72. Beatty JD, Atwood M, Tickman R, Reiner M. Metaplastic breast cancer: clinical significance. Am J Surg. 2006;191:657–64.
73. Foschini MP, Krausz T. Salivary gland-type tumors of the breast: a spectrum of benign and malignant tumors including "triple negative carcinomas" of low malignant potential. Semin Diagn Pathol. 2010;27: 77–90.
74. Ravdin PM. Should HER2 status be routinely measured for all breast cancer patients? Semin Oncol. 1999;26(4 Supp 12):117–23.
75. Yu JI, Choi DH, Park W, et al. Differences in prognostic factors and patterns of failure between invasive micropapillary carcinoma and invasive ductal carcinoma of the breast: matched case-control study. Breast. 2010;19:231–7.

76. Pettinato G, Manivel JC, Panico L, Sparano L, Petrella G. Invasive micropapillary carcinoma of the breast: clinicopathologic study of 62 cases of a poorly-recognized variant with highly-aggressive behavior. Am J Clin Pathol. 2004;121:857–66.
77. Wade PM Jr, Mills SE, Read M, Cloud W, Lambert MJ III, Smith RE: Small-cell neuroendocrine (oat-cell) carcinoma of the breast. Cancer. 1983;52:121–5; Shin SJ, DeLellis RA, Ying L, Rosen PP. Small-cell carcinoma of the breast: a clinicopathologic and immunohistochemical study of nine patients. Am J Surg Pathol. 2000;24:1231–8; Yamaguchi R, Tanaka M, Otsuka H, et al. Neuroendocrine small cell carcinoma of the breast: report of a case. Med Mol Morphol. 2009;42:58–61.
78. Richardson RL, Weiland LH. Undifferentiated small-cell carcinomas in extrapulmonary sites. Semin Oncol. 1982;9:484–96.
79. Moore JM. Undifferentiated adenocarcinoma of breast. Tex State J Med. 1953;49:603–4.
80. Kirsten F, Chi CH, Leary JA, Ng AB, Hedley DW, Tattersall MH. Metastatic adeno- or undifferentiated carcinoma from an unknown site – natural history and guidelines for identification of treatable subsets. Q J Med. 1987;62:143–61.
81. Soomro S, Shousha S, Taylor P, Shepard HJ, Feldmann M. c-erbB-2 expression in different histological types of invasive breast carcinoma. J Clin Pathol. 1991;44:211–4.
82. Martinazzi M, Crivelli F, Zampatti C, Martinazzi S. Epidermal growth factor receptor immunohistochemistry in different histological types of infiltrating breast carcinoma. J Clin Pathol. 1993;46:1009–10.
83. Miller WR, Ellis IO, Sainsbury J, Dixon JM. ABCs of breast diseases: prognostic factors. Br Med J. 1994;309:1573–6.
84. Mansour EG, Ravdin PM, Dressler L. Prognostic factors in early breast carcinoma. Cancer. 1994;74:381–400.
85. Seidman JD, Schnaper LA, Aisner SC. Relationship of the size of the invasive component of the primary breast carcinoma to axillary lymph node metastasis. Cancer. 1995;75:65–71.
86. Carter CL, Allen C, Henson DE. Relation of tumor size, lymph node status, and survival in 24, 740 breast cancer cases. Cancer. 1989;63:181–7.
87. Iwasa Y, Nowak MA, Michor F. Evolution of resistance during clonal expansion. Genetics. 2006;172:2557–66.
88. Garcia SB, Norelli M, Wright NA. The clonal origin and clonal evolution of epithelial tumors. Int J Exp Pathol. 2000;81:89–116.
89. Flanagan FL, McDermott MB, Barton PT, et al. Invasive breast cancer: mammographic measurement. Radiology. 1996;199:819–23.
90. Bloom HJ, Richardson WW. Histological grading and prognosis in breast cancer: a study of 1409 cases, of which 359 have been followed for 15 years. Br J Cancer. 1957;11:359–77.
91. Scarff RW, Torloni H. Histological typing of breast tumors. In: International histological classification of tumours, No. 2, Vol. 2. Geneva: World Health Organization; 1968. p. 13–20.
92. Le Doussal V, Tubiana-Hulin M, Friedman S, Hacene K, Spyratos F, Brunet M. Prognostic value of histologic grade nuclear components of Scarff-Bloom-Richardson (SBR): an improved score modification based on a multivariate analysis of 1262 invasive ductal breast carcinomas. Cancer. 1989;64:1914–21.
93. Simpson JF, Page DL. The role of pathology in premalignancy and as a guide for treatment and prognosis in breast cancer. Semin Oncol. 1996;23:428–35.
94. Simpson JF, Page DL. Status of breast cancer prognostication based on histopathologic data. Am J Clin Pathol. 1994;102(Suppl):S3–8.
95. Elston CW, Ellis IO. Pathological prognostic factors in breast cancer. I. The value of histological grade in breast cancer: experience from a large study with long-term followup. Histopathology. 1991;19:403–10.
96. Frierson Jr HF, Wolber RA, Berean KW, et al. Interobserver reproducibility of the Nottingham modification of the Bloom and Richardson histologic grading scheme for infiltrating ductal carcinoma. Am J Clin Pathol. 1995;103:195–8.
97. Contesso G, Jotti GS, Bonadonna G. Tumor grade as a prognostic factor in primary breast cancer. Eur J Cancer Clin Oncol. 1989;25:403–9.
98. Todd JH, Dowle C, Williams MR, et al. Confirmation of a prognostic index in primary breast cancer. Br J Cancer. 1987;56:489–92.
99. Imber G. Genius on the edge. New York: Kaplan; 2010.
100. Williams BC. The history of mastectomy. http://www.ehow.com/about_5505904_history-mastectomy.html. Accessed 19 June 2010.
101. Halsted WS. The results of radical operations for the cure of carcinoma of the breast performed at the Johns Hopkins Hospital from June 1889 to January 1894. Johns Hopkins Hosp Rep. 1894;4:297–327.
102. Bland CS. The Halsted mastectomy: present illness and past history. West J Med. 1981;134:549–55.
103. Wick MR. Principles of evidence-based medicine as applied to "sentinel" lymph node biopsies. Pathol Case Rev. 2008;13:102–8.
104. Fisher B, Wolmark N, Redmond C, et al. Findings from NSABP Protocol No. B-04: comparison of radical mastectomy with alternative treatments. II. The clinical and biologic significance of medial-central breast cancers. Cancer. 1981;48:1863–72.
105. Sanghani M, Balk EM, Cady B. Impact of axillary lymph node dissection on breast cancer outcome in clinically node negative patients: a systematic review and meta-analysis. Cancer. 2009;115:1613–20.
106. Collan YU, Eskelinen MJ, Nordling SA, et al. Prognostic studies in breast cancer – multivariate combination of nodal status, proliferation index, tumor size, and DNA ploidy. Acta Oncol. 1994;33:873–8.
107. Quiet CA, Ferguson DJ, Weichselbaum RR, Hellman S. Natural history of node-positive breast cancer: the curability of small cancers with a limited number of positive nodes. J Clin Oncol. 1996;14:3105–11.

108. Beal SH, Martinez SR, Canter RJ, Chen SL, Khatri VP, Bold RJ. Survival in 12, 653 breast cancer patients with extensive axillary lymph node metastasis in the anthracycline era. Med Oncol. 2010;27(4):1420–4.
109. Sahin AA, Guray M, Hunt KK. Identification and biologic significance of micrometastases in axillary lymph nodes in patients with invasive breast cancer. Arch Pathol Lab Med. 2009;133:869–78.
110. Hansen NM, Grube B, Ye X, Turner RR, Brenner RJ, Sim MS, et al. Impact of micrometastases in the sentinel node of patients with invasive breast cancer. J Clin Oncol. 2009;27:4679–84.
111. Viale G, Dell'Orto P, Biasi MO, et al. Comparative evaluation of an extensive histopathologic examination and a real-time reverse-transcription-polymerase chain reaction assay for mammaglobin and cytokeratin-19 on axillary sentinel lymph nodes of breast carcinoma patients. Ann Surg. 2008;247:136–42.
112. Douglas-Jones AG, Woods V. Molecular assessment of sentinel lymph nodes in breast cancer management. Histopathology. 2009;55:107–13.
113. Karam AK, Hsu M, Patil S, et al. Predictors of completion axillary lymph node dissection in patients with positive sentinel lymph nodes. Ann Surg Oncol. 2009;16:1952–8.
114. Pernas S, Gil M, Benítez A, et al. Avoiding axillary treatment in sentinel lymph node micrometastases of breast cancer: a prospective analysis of axillary or distant recurrence. Ann Surg Oncol. 2010;17:772–7.
115. Gurleyik G, Gurleyik E, Aker F, et al. Lymphovascular invasion, as a prognostic marker in patients with invasive breast cancer. Acta Chir Belg. 2007;107:284–7.
116. Nime FA, Rosen PP, Thaler HT, Ashikari R, Urban JA. Prognostic significance of tumor emboli in intramammary lymphatics in patients with mammary carcinoma. Am J Surg Pathol. 1977;1:25–30.
117. Rosen PP. Tumor emboli in intramammary lymphatics in breast carcinoma: pathologic criteria for diagnosis and clinical significance. Pathol Annu. 1983;18(Pt 2):215–32.
118. Lee AH, Pinder SE, Macmillan RD, Mitchell M, Ellis IO, Elston CW, et al. Prognostic value of lymphovascular invasion in women with lymph node negative invasive breast carcinoma. Eur J Cancer. 2006;42:357–62.
119. Trudeau ME, Pritchard KI, Chapman JA, et al. Prognostic factors affecting the natural history of node-negative breast cancer. Breast Cancer Res Treat. 2005;89:35–45.
120. de Mascarel I, MacGrogan G, Debled M, Sierankowski G, Brouste V, Mathoulin-Pélissier S, et al. D2-40 in breast cancer: should we detect more vascular emboli? Mod Pathol. 2009;22:216–22.
121. Kahn HJ, Marks A. A new monoclonal antibody, D2-40, for detection of lymphatic invasion in primary tumors. Lab Invest. 2002;82:1255–12557.
122. Arnaout-Alkarain A, Kahn HJ, Narod SA, Sun PA, Marks AN. Significance of lymph vessel invasion identified by the endothelial lymphatic marker D2-40 in node negative breast cancer. Mod Pathol. 2007;20:183–91.
123. Almholt K, Nielsen BS, Frandsen TL, et al. Metastasis of transgenic breast cancer in plasminogen activator inhibitor-1 gene-deficient mice. Oncogene. 2003;22:4389–97.
124. Kilinc N, Yaldiz M. p53, c-erbB-2 expression, and steroid hormone receptors in breast carcinoma: correlations with histopathological parameters. Eur J Gynaecol Oncol. 2004;25:606–10.
125. Reed W, Hannisdal E, Boehler PJ, Gundersen S, Host H, Marthin J. The prognostic value of p53 and c-erbB-2 immunostaining is overrated for patients with lymph node-negative breast carcinoma: a multivariate analysis of prognostic factors in 613 patients with a follow up of 14-30 years. Cancer. 2000;88:804–13.
126. Chiu CG, Masoudi H, Leung S, et al. HER-3 overexpression in prognostic of reduced breast cancer survival: a study of 4046 patients. Ann Surg. 2010;251:1107–16.
127. Blows FM, Driver KE, Schmidt MK, et al. Subtyping of breast cancer by immunohistochemistry to investigate a relationship between subtype and short and long term survival: a collaborative analysis of data for 10, 159 cases from 12 studies. PLoS Med. 2010;7(5):e1000279.
128. Putti TC, El-Rehim DM, Rakha EA, et al. Estrogen receptor-negative breast carcinomas: a review of morphology and immunophenotypical analysis. Mod Pathol. 2005;18:26–36.
129. Rakha EA, El-Sayed ME, Green AR, Lee AH, Robertson JF, Ellis IO. Prognostic markers in triple-negative breast cancer. Cancer. 2007;109:25–32.
130. Erdem O, Dursun A, Coskun U, Gunel N. The prognostic value of p53 and c-erbB-2 expression, proliferative activity, and angiogenesis in node-negative breast carcinoma. Tumori. 2005;91:46–52.
131. Horita K, Yamaguchi A, Hirose K, et al. Prognostic factors affecting disease-free survival rate following surgical resection of primary breast cancer. Eur J Histochem. 2001;45:73–84.
132. Lialiaris TS, Georgiou G, Sivridis E, et al. Prognostic and predictive factors of invasive ductal breast carcinomas. J BUON. 2010;15:79–88.
133. Lai P, Tan LK, Chen B. Correlation of HER-2 status with estrogen and progesterone receptors and histologic features in 3, 655 invasive breast carcinomas. Am J Clin Pathol. 2005;123:541–6.
134. Cao XX, Xu JD, Liu XL, et al. RACK1: a superior independent predictor for poor clinical outcome in breast cancer. Int J Cancer. 2009;127(5):1172–9.
135. Haupt B, Ro JY, Schwartz MR. Basal-like breast carcinoma: a phenotypically distinct entity. Arch Pathol Lab Med. 2010;134:130–3.
136. Mirza M, Shaughnessy E, Hurley JK, et al. Osteopontin-c is a selective marker of breast cancer. Int J Cancer. 2008;122:889–97.
137. Sigurdsson H, Baldetorp B, Borg A, et al. Indicators of prognosis in node-negative breast cancer. N Engl J Med. 2990;322:1045–53.
138. Sasano H. Histopathological prognostic factors in early breast carcinoma: an evaluation of cell

proliferation in carcinoma cells. Expert Opin Investig Drugs. 2010;19 Suppl 1:S5–11.
139. Reis-Filho JS, Lakhani SR. Breast cancer special types: why bother? J Pathol. 2008;216:394–8.
140. Weigelt B, Geyer FC, Natrajan R, et al. The molecular underpinning of lobular histological growth pattern: a genome-wide transcriptomic analysis of invasive lobular carcinomas and grade- and molecular subtype-matched invasive ductal carcinomas of no special type. J Pathol. 2010;220:45–57.
141. Schnitt SJ. Classification and prognosis of invasive breast cancer: from morphology to molecular taxonomy. Mod Pathol. 2010;23 Suppl 2:S60–4.
142. Schmidt C. Assays that predict outcomes make slow progress toward prime time. J Natl Cancer Inst. 2010;102:677–9.
143. Thuerigen O, Schneeweiss A, Toedt G, et al. Gene expression signature predicting pathologic complete response with gemcitabine, epirubicin, and docetaxel in primary breast cancer. J Clin Oncol. 2006;24: 1839–45.
144. Végran F, Boidot R, Coudert B, et al. Gene expression profile and response to trastuzumab-docetaxel-based treatment in breast carcinoma. Br J Cancer. 2009;101:1357–64.
145. Bohn OL, Nasir I, Brufsky A, et al. Biomarker profile in breast carcinomas presenting with bone metastasis. Int J Clin Exp Pathol. 2009;3:139–46.
146. Nuyten DS, Kreike B, Hart AA, et al. Predicting a local recurrence after breast-conserving therapy by gene expression profiling. Breast Cancer Res. 2006;8:R62.
147. Saal LH, Johansson P, Holm K, et al. Poor prognosis in carcinoma is associated with a gene expression signature of aberrant PTEN tumor suppressor pathway activity. Proc Natl Acad Sci USA. 2007;104:7564–9.
148. Karlsson E, Delle U, Danielsson A, et al. Gene expression variation to predict 10-year survival in lymph-node-negative breast cancer. BMC Cancer. 2008;8:254.
149. Konstantinovsky S, Smith Y, Zilber S, et al. Breast carcinoma cells in primary tumors and effusions have different gene array profiles. J Oncol. 2010;2010:969084.
150. Staaf J, Ringnér M, Vallon-Christersson J, et al. Identification of subtypes in human epidermal growth factor receptor 2–positive breast cancer reveals a gene signature prognostic of outcome. J Clin Oncol. 2010;28:1813–20.
151. Charpin C, Secq V, Giusiano S, et al. A signature predictive of disease outcome in breast carcinomas, identified by quantitative immunocytochemical assays. Int J Cancer. 2009;124:2124–34.
152. Kreipe HH, Ahrens P, Christgen M, Lehmann U, Langer F. Beyond staging, typing, and grading: new challenges in breast cancer pathology. Pathologe. 2010;31:54–9.
153. Giusiano S, Secq V, Carcopino X, et al. Immunohistochemical profiling of node negative breast carcinomas allows prediction of metastatic risk. Int J Oncol. 2010;36:889–98.
154. Cox G, Jones JL, Andi A, Waller DA, O'Byrne KJ. A biological staging model for operable non-small-cell lung cancer. Thorax. 2001;56:561–6.
155. Li AR, Chitale D, Riely GJ, et al. EGFR mutations in lung adenocarcinomas: clinical testing experience and relationship to EGFR gene copy number and immunohistochemical expression. J Mol Diagn. 2008;10:242–8.
156. Sholl LM, Xiao Y, Joshi V, et al. EGFR mutation is a better predictor of response to tyrosine kinase inhibitors in non-small cell lung carcinoma than FISH, CISH, and immunohistochemistry. Am J Clin Pathol. 2010;133:922–34.
157. Anonymous. Types of data. http://www.changingminds.org/explanations/research/measurements/types-data.htm. Accessed 19 June 2010.
158. Stroup RM, Pinkus GS. S100-immunoreactivity in primary and metastatic carcinoma of the breast: a potential source of error in immunodiagnosis. Hum Pathol. 1988;19:949–53.
159. Wick MR, Patterson JW. Multimodal pathologic diagnosis of malignant melanoma: integration of morphology, histochemistry, immunohistology, and electron microscopy. J Histotechnol. 2003;26:253–8.
160. Wick MR, Lillemoe TJ, Copland GT, Swanson PE, Manivel JC, Kiang DT. Gross cystic disease fluid protein-15 as a marker for breast cancer. Hum Pathol. 1989;20:281–7.
161. Miller RT, Swanson PE, Wick MR. Fixation and epitope retrieval in diagnostic immunohistochemistry: a concise review with practical considerations. Appl Immunohistochem Mol Morphol. 2000;8:228–35.
162. Idikio HA. Immunohistochemistry in diagnostic surgical pathology: contributions of protein life-cycle, use of evidence-based methods, and data normalization on interpretation of immunohistochemical stains. Int J Clin Exp Pathol. 2010;3:169–76.
163. Allred DC, Carlson RW, Berry DA, et al. NCCN Task Force Report: estrogen receptor and progesterone receptor testing in breast cancer by immunohistochemistry. J Natl Compr Cancer Netw. 2009;Suppl 6:S1–21.
164. Canadian Association of Pathologists-Association canadienne des pathologistes National Standards Committee, Torlakovic EE, Riddell R, Banerjee D, et al. Best practice recommendations for standardization of immunohistochemistry tests. Am J Clin Pathol. 2010;133:354–65.
165. Jacobs TW, Gown AM, Yaziji H, Barnes MJ, Schnitt SJ. Comparison of fluorescence in situ hybridization and immunohistochemistry for the evaluation of HER-2/neu in breast cancer. J Clin Oncol. 1999;17:1974–82.
166. Kakar S, Puangsuvan N, Stevens JM, et al. HER-2/neu assessment in breast cancer by immunohistochemistry and fluorescence in situ hybridization: comparison of results and correlation with survival. Mol Diagn. 2000;5:199–207.
167. Van de Vijver MJ. Assessment of the need and appropriate method for testing for the human epidermal

growth factor receptor-2 (HER2). Eur J Cancer. 2001;37 Suppl 1:11–7.
168. McCormick SR, Lillemoe TJ, Beneke J, Schrauth J, Reinartz J. HER2 assessment by immunohistochemical analysis and fluorescence in situ hybridization: comparison of HercepTest and PathVysion commercial assays. Am J Clin Pathol. 2002;117:935–43.
169. Lal P, Salazar PA, Hudis CA, Ladanyi M, Chen B. HER-2 testing in breast cancer using immunohistochemical analysis and fluorescence in-situ hybridization: a single-institution experience of 2, 279 cases and comparison of dual-color and single-color scoring. Am J Clin Pathol. 2004;121:631–6.
170. Ross JS, Fletcher JA, Bloom KJ, et al. HER-2/neu testing in breast cancer. Am J Clin Pathol. 2003;120(Suppl):S53–71.
171. Mrozkowiak A, Olszewski WP, Piascik A, Olszewski WT. HER2 status in breast cancer determined by IHC and FISH: comparison of the results. Pol J Pathol. 2004;55:165–71.
172. Ellis CM, Dyson MJ, Stephenson TJ, Maltby EL. HER2 amplification status in breast cancer: a comparison between immunohistochemical staining and fluorescence in situ hybridization using manual and automated quantitative image analysis scoring techniques. J Clin Pathol. 2005;58:710–4.
173. Dolan M, Snover DC. Comparison of immunohistochemical and fluorescence in situ hybridization assessment of HER-2 status in routine practice. Am J Clin Pathol. 2005;123:766–70.
174. Benohr P, Henkel V, Speer R, et al. HER-2/neu expression in breast cancer – a comparison of different diagnostic methods. Anticancer Res. 2005;25(3B): 1895–900.
175. Egervari K, Szollosi Z, Nemes Z, Kaczur V. Comparison of immunohistochemical and fluorescence in situ hybridization assessment of HER-2 status in routine practice. Am J Clin Pathol. 2006;125:155–6.
176. Sui W, Ou M, Chen J, et al. Comparison of immunohistochemistry (IHC) and fluorescence in situ hybridization (FISH) assessment for HER-2 status in breast cancer. World J Surg Oncol. 2009;7:83.
177. Mayr D, Heim S, Weyrauch K, et al. Chromogenic in situ hybridization for HER-2/neu-oncogene in breast cancer: comparison of a new dual-color chromogenic in situ hybridization with immunohistochemistry and fluorescence in situ hybridization. Histopathology. 2009;55:716–23.
178. Krug LM, Crapanzano JP, Azzoli CG, et al. Imatinib mesylate lacks activity in small cell lung carcinoma expression *c-kit* protein: a phase II clinical trial. Cancer. 2005;103:2128–31.
179. Koch CA, Gimm O, Vortmeyer AO, et al. Does the expression of *c-kit* (CD117) in neuroendocrine tumors represent a target for therapy? Ann NY Acad Sci. 2006;1073:517–26.
180. Sharma S. Applied multivariate techniques. Hoboken: Wiley; 1995.
181. Rasmussen BB, Thorpe SM, Norgaard T, Rasmussen J, Agdal N, Rose C. Immunohistochemical steroid receptor detection in frozen breast cancer tissue: a multicenter investigation. Acta Oncol. 1988;27:757–60.
182. Andersen J, Thorpe SM, King WJ, et al. The prognostic value of immunohistochemical estrogen receptor analysis in paraffin-embedded and frozen sections versus that of steroid-binding assays. Eur J Cancer. 1990;25:442–9.
183. Wilbur DC, Willis J, Mooney RA, Fallon MA, Moynes R, di Sant'Agnese PA. Estrogen and progesterone receptor detection in archival formalin-fixed, paraffin-embedded tissue from breast carcinoma: a comparison of immunohistochemistry with the dextran-coated charcoal assay. Mod Pathol. 1992;5:79–84.
184. Valgardsdottir R, Tryggvadottir L, Steinarsdottir M, et al. Genomic instability and poor prognosis associated with abnormal TP53 in breast carcinomas: molecular and immunohistochemical analysis. APMIS. 1997;105:121–30.
185. Sjogren S, Inganas M, Norberg T, et al. The p53 gene in breast cancer: prognostic value of complementary DNA sequencing versus immunohistochemistry. J Natl Cancer Inst. 1996;88:173–82.
186. Thorlacius S, Thorgilsson B, Bjornsson J, et al. TP53 mutations and abnormal p53 protein staining in breast carcinomas related to prognosis. Eur J Cancer. 1995;31A:1856–61.
187. Umekita Y, Kobayashi K, Saheki T, Yoshida H. Nuclear accumulation of p53 correlates with mutations in the p53 gene on archival paraffin-embedded tissues of human breast cancer. Jpn J Cancer Res. 1994;85:825–30.
188. MacGeoch C, Barnes DM, Newton JA, et al. p53 protein detected by immunohistochemical staining is not always mutant. Dis Markers. 1993;11:239–50.
189. Dunn JM, Hastrich DJ, Newcomb P, Webb JC. Maitland, Farndon JR: Correlation between p53 mutations and antibody staining in breast carcinoma. Br J Surg. 1993;80:1410–2.
190. Miles J: Getting the sample size right: a brief introduction to power analysis. http://www.jeremymiles.co.uk/misc/power/. Accessed 19 June 2010.
191. The Health Insurance Portability and Accountability Act. http://en.wikipedia.org/wiki/Health_Insurance_Portability_and_Accountability_Act/. Accessed 19 June 2010.
192. Anonymous. In-Memoriam: William L. McGuire. Breast Cancer Res Treat 1992;23:7–15.
193. McGuire WL. Breast cancer prognostic factors: evaluation guidelines. J Natl Cancer Inst. 1991;83:154–5.
194. Slamon DJ, Clark GM, Wong SG, Levin WJ, Ullrich A, McGuire WL. Human breast cancer: correlation of relapse and survival with amplification of the HER-2/neu oncogene. Science. 1987;235:177–82.
195. Trastuzumab. http://en.wikipedia.org/wiki/trastuzumab/. Accessed 19 June 2010.
196. Kute T, Lack CM, Willingham M, et al. Development of herceptin resistance in breast cancer cells. Cytometry. 2004;57A:86–93.
197. Tan AR, Swain SM. Ongoing adjuvant trials with trastuzumab in breast cancer. Semin Oncol. 2002;30 (5 Suppl 16):54–64.

198. Nahta R, Esteva FJ. HER-2-targeted therapy: lessons learned and future directions. Clin Cancer Res. 2003;9:5038–48.
199. Romond EH, Perez EA, Bryant J, et al. Trastuzumab plus adjuvant chemotherapy for operable HER-2-positive breast cancer. N Engl J Med. 2005;353:1673–84.
200. Piccart-Gebhart MJ, Procter M, Leyland-Jones B, et al. Trastuzumab after adjuvant chemotherapy in HER-2-positive breast cancer. N Engl J Med. 2005;353:1659–72.
201. Lewis R, Bagnall AM, Forbges C, et al. The clinical effectiveness of trastuzumab for breast cancer: a systematic review. Health Technol Assess. 2002;6:1–71.
202. http://www.bpac.org/nz/magazine/2007/april/herceptin.asp. Accessed 19 June 2010.
203. http://www.sws-pct.nhs.uk/PEC/2005/061205/Enc_08.pdf. Accessed 19 June 2010.
204. Anonymous: Herceptin or trastuzumab: efficacy and side effects. http://healthlifeandstuff.com/2009/12/herceptin-or-trastuzumab-efficacy-side-effects/. Accessed 19 June 2010.
205. Abelson J, Collins PA. Media hyping and the "herceptin access story:" an analysis of Canadian and UK newspaper coverage. Healthc Policy. 2009;4:e113–28.
206. Hedgecoe AM. It's money that matters: the financial context of ethical decision-making in modern biomedicine. Sociol Health Illn. 2006;28:768–84.
207. Williams C, Brunskill S, Altman D, et al. Cost-effectiveness of using prognostic information to select women with breast cancer for adjuvant systemic therapy. Health Technol Assess. 2006;10:1–204.
208. Nakhleh RE, Grimm EE, Idowu MO, Souers RJ, Fitzgibbons PL. Laboratory compliance with the American Society of Clinical Oncology/college of American Pathologists guidelines for human epidermal growth factor receptor 2 testing: a College of American Pathologists survey of 757 laboratories. Arch Pathol Lab Med. 2010;134:728–34.
209. Sauter G, Lee J, Bartlett JM, Slamon DJ, Press MF. Guidelines for human epidermal growth factor receptor-2 testing: biologic and methodologic considerations. J Clin Oncol. 2009;27:1323–33.
210. Turashvili G, Leung S, Turbin D, et al. Interobserver reproducibility of HER2 immunohistochemical assessment and concordance with fluorescent in situ hybridization (FISH): pathologist assessment compared to quantitative image analysis. BMC Cancer. 2009;9:165.
211. Jacobs TW, Prioleau JE, Stillman IE, Schnitt SJ. Loss of tumor marker-immunostaining intensity on stored paraffin slides of breast cancer. J Natl Cancer Inst. 1996;88:1054–9.
212. Mandrekar SJ, Sargent DJ. Predictive biomarker validation in practice: lessons from real trials. Clin Trials. 2010;7(5):567–73.
213. Richter-Ehrenstein C, Muller S, Noske A, Schneider A. Diagnostic accuracy and prognostic value of core biopsy in the management of breast cancer: a series of 542 patients. Int J Surg Pathol. 2009;17:323–6.
214. Nassar A, Radhakrishnan A, Cabrero IA, Cotsonis GA, Cohen C. Intratumoral heterogeneity of immunohistochemical marker expression in breast carcinoma: a tissue microarray-based study. Appl Immunohistochem Mol Morphol. 2010;18(5):433–41.
215. Powell WC, Hicks DG, Prescott N, et al. A new rabbit monoclonal antibody (4B5) for the immunohistochemical (IHC) determination of the HER2 status in breast cancer: comparison with CB11, fluorescence in situ hybridization (FISH), and interlaboratory reproducibility. Appl Immunohistochem Mol Morphol. 2007;15:94–102.
216. Wasielewski R, Hasselmann S, Ruschoff J, Fisseler-Eckhoff A, Kreipe H. Proficiency testing of immunohistochemical biomarker assays in breast cancer. Virchows Arch. 2008;453:537–43.
217. Terry J, Torlakovic EE, Garratt J, et al. Implementation of a Canadian external quality assurance program for breast cancer biomarkers: an initiative of Canadian Quality Control in immunohistochemistry (cIQc) and Canadian Association of Pathologists (CAP) National Standards Committee/Immunohistochemistry. Appl Immunohistochem Mol Morphol. 2009;17:375–82.
218. Hanley KZ, Birdsong GG, Cohen C, Siddiqui MT. Immunohistochemical detection of estrogen receptor, progesterone receptor, and human epidermal growth factor receptor 2 expression in breast carcinomas: comparison on cell block, needle-core, and tissue block preparations. Cancer Cytopathol. 2009;117:279–88.
219. Liu YH, Xu FP, Rao JY, et al. Justification of the change from 10% to 30% for the immunohistochemical HER2 scoring criterion in breast cancer. Am J Clin Pathol. 2009;132:74–9.
220. Davoli A, Hocevar BA, Brown TL. Progression and treatment of HER2-positive breast cancer. Cancer Chemother Pharmacol. 2010;65:611–23.
221. Walker JR, Singal PK, Jassal DS. The art of healing broken hearts in breast cancer patients: trastuzumab and heart failure. Exp Clin Cardiol. 2009;14:e62–7.
222. Köninki K, Barok M, Tanner M, et al. Multiple molecular mechanisms underlying trastuzumab and lapatinib resistance in JIMT-1 breast cancer cells. Cancer Lett. 2010;294:211–9.
223. Tagliabue E, Balsari A, Campiglio M, Pupa SM. HER2 as a target for breast cancer therapy. Expert Opin Biol Ther. 2010;10:711–24.
224. Geiger S, Lange V, Suhl P, Heinermann V, Stemmler HJ. Anticancer therapy-induced cardiotoxicity: review of the literature. Anticancer Drugs. 2010;21:578–90.
225. Baselga J. Herceptin alone or in combination with chemotherapy in the treatment of HER2-positive metastatic breast cancer: pivotal trials. Oncology. 2001;61 Suppl 2:14–21.
226. Dawood S, Broglio K, Buzdar AU, Hortobagyi GN, Giordano SH. Prognosis of women with metastatic breast cancer by HER2 status and trastuzumab treatment: an institutional-based review. J Clin Oncol. 2010;28:92–8.

227. Elkin EB, Weinstein MC, Winer EP, Kuntz KM, Schnitt SJ, Weeks JC. HER-2 testing and trastuzumab therapy for metastatic breast cancer: a cost-effectiveness analysis. J Clin Oncol. 2004;22:854–63.

228. Fitzgibbons PL, Page DL, Weaver D, et al. Prognostic factors in breast cancer. College of American Pathologists Consensus Statement 1999. Arch Pathol Lab Med. 2000;124:966–78.

Principles of Classification and Diagnosis in Anatomic Pathology and the Inevitability of Problem Cases

6

Michael Hendrickson

Keywords
Classification in anatomic pathology • Diagnostic principles in anatomic pathology • Problem cases in anatomic pathology • Complexity of individual neoplasms • Neoplastic kinds as family resemblance groups • Oncopathological reality

In this chapter, I set out a framework for thinking critically about oncopathological classification and diagnosis (C&D), organizing the discussion around the central elements of the classification process: (1) the individual cases being classified (e.g., the individual neoplasm, I_{Neop}), (2) the groups formed by aggregating individual cases similar in relevant respects (the neoplastic kind, K_{Neop}), and (3) the classifier-diagnostician whose essential contribution is evident at every stage of the process. Current research in molecular-genetic oncology suggests that I_{Neop}'s are best regarded as evolutionary processes, that the groups formed by aggregating them with respect to their histogenesis are extensionally indeterminate family resemblance groups and that our view of the world of neoplasms at any given time results both from the way the world is and, equally, how we chose to visualize and conceptualize it.

We and the world co-create oncological reality and problem cases – in-between cases, hybrid cases, and novel cases – are instructive in pointing to the inevitable failure of static classificatory grids to do justice to the complexity of the individual neoplasm. This perspective has fundamental consequences for the issues of concern to contemporary evidence based pathology (EBP).

Evidence-Based Pathology and Classification and Diagnostic Practices in Anatomic Pathology

Evidence-based medicine (EBM) is a contentious topic with, for some, a problematic name. It is presented by its advocates as the long-needed antidote to "clinical judgment" with what they take to be its subjective, anecdotal character and its privileging of uncodified clinical expertise over published population-based experience. The antidote to anecdote offered by EBM is the statistical analysis of populations. The fruits of this approach are the evidence provided by interventional studies (e.g., controlled clinical trials) and observational studies (e.g., techniques of clinical epidemiology). Integration of such studies yields, among other things, clinical guidelines of various sorts for

M. Hendrickson (✉)
Department of Pathology, Stanford University Medical Center, Stanford, CA 94305, USA
e-mail: hendrickson@stanford.edu

A.M. Marchevsky and M.R. Wick (eds.), *Evidence Based Pathology and Laboratory Medicine*,
DOI 10.1007/978-1-4419-1030-1_6,

medical conditions and a critical approach to biological markers used either for diagnosis or for hazarding a clinical prediction (i.e., risk, prognostic or predictive markers).

On the other hand, EBM's detractors draw attention to the fundamental problem of population-based studies – such studies tell us about populations, not individuals. Thus, while clinical judgment and case-based reasoning (CBR) self-consciously attend to the particularity and uniqueness of the individual under consideration, population-based studies scrupulously strip away all of that detail replacing it with a handful of observed features. This is in service of generating stable, statistically credible population averages. Paradoxically, the use of EBM techniques still requires clinical judgment to decide whether the findings of a population-based study really apply to an individual patient who is not an exact fit to mythical "average patient" in the population studied; a special case is the patient with more than one disease. Particularly annoying for some critics of EBM is the name itself: it is seen as ideological and suggests, rather pointedly, that whatever physicians had been using to make diagnoses and decisions prior to the advent of EBM methodologies was not evidence-based. They argue that elevating a particular way of thinking about clinical medicine – statistical reasoning as instantiated in EBM – to the exclusion of others is wrongheaded and unrealistic. The polemic continues to this day.

EBP, the recruitment of EBM principles in clinical and anatomic pathology, is in the process of defining itself. What part of this methodology has relevance to pathology? Certainly, much of the methodological focus of EBM is irrelevant to diagnostic and predictive pathology: professionally, we have little to do with making decisions about alternative therapies given a particular diagnosis. Ours is largely a noninterventional, nonexperimental descriptive literature that finds itself in last place in the EBM quality ranking of types of clinical research. In addition, anatomic pathology faces unique difficulties in defining its study groups; transforming what is basically a complex, primarily visual classificatory experience into language sufficiently precise to be followed by other pathologists and serve as the basis for reproducible assignments.

I prefer to think of both EBM and, by implication, EBP in less polemical terms. Statistical reasoning is one mode of thinking; CBR is another; and taxonomic reasoning, the style that dominates oncopathological classification, is yet another. Navigating through the complexities of an individual case – whether it be the clinical details of a patient or the histological particulars of that patient's tissue – requires the application of all three. There are no non-ideological reasons to privilege one mode over another; they all play a role.

The spirit of EBP is reformatory. Do our current C&D practices in anatomic pathology need fixing? Before I answer this question, I need to take an unvarnished look at oncopathological classifications, their construction and evolution, and the biological basis for the particular "messy" structure of their constituent elements: disease entities or neoplastic kinds (K_{Neop}'s). It is the purpose of this chapter to provide a twenty-first century sketch of the situation.

This is not an easy topic as the foundational problems we confront in oncopathological C&D are widespread in the natural sciences. Indeed, much thought has been given to these topics in a variety of disciplines. Our discussion draws upon sources in contemporary molecular-genetic oncology, biological systematics, the philosophy of biology (and more broadly, the philosophy of science), cognitive and judgmental psychology, and statistics. Taking our problems in oncopathology seriously requires this kind of intellectual outreach.

Problem Cases in Anatomic Pathology

Efficient day-to-day diagnosis is, for the well-trained surgical pathologist, usually straightforward. The majority of cases can be assigned without much difficulty, using the classification *de jour*, to established diagnostic categories. In this chapter, we will be concerned with the minority of problem cases that challenge us. Prominent examples include (1) in-between cases ("grey-zone" cases or borderline cases) that fall into the apparently seamless morphological multivariate continuum that bridges two kinds of neoplasms (K_{Neop}'s); (2) hybrid cases that present confusing combinations of distinct patterns from two or more distinguishable K_{Neop}'s; and

(3) novel cases that combine features in a way that have never before been encountered. Problem cases are analogous to the patients with rare genetic metabolic defects that played a crucial role in developing our understanding of normal metabolic pathways; their analysis helps us understand how all oncopathological classification works.

Some Preliminaries

Scientific and Managerial Classifications of Neoplasms

We currently have two general strategies for the classification of neoplasms in surgical pathology and cytopathology: scientific classifications (S-classifications) in service of explanation and managerial classifications (M-classifications) in service of clinical prediction. S-classifications answer questions like "why this particular shared neoplastic phenotype?" Histogenetic classifications (HG-classifications) are paradigmatic of (but do not exhaust) S-classifications. By contrast, M-classifications are responsive to the question "What does the future hold for a patient suffering from an individual neoplasm (I_{Neop}) with a particular phenotype?" M-classifications are fashioned to forecast future biological events based on clinical phenotype, $\Phi_{Clin}(t)$, such as the risk of developing an invasive carcinoma given a particular histomorphologic feature (risk); the future clinical course after no specific therapy – prognosis; and the likely response to a specific therapy – prediction. Grading systems for common adult malignancies are paradigmatic instances of M-Classifications.

The canonical classifications in oncopathology are hybrids of M-classification grids superimposed on HG-classifications. The image to have in mind is that of a topological survey map with one set of boundaries marking the distribution of physical features such as peaks (the HG-classification) superimposed upon which is a second set of pragmatic ("political") boundaries reflecting the various discrete classes of an M-classification. The spirit of these two classificatory activities is quite different and involves very different types of taxonomic models: histogenetic models and statistical (or probabilistic) models, respectively. Histogenetic investigations are pursued in the spirit of biological taxonomy (the Linnaean classification of plants, for example) and its associated mode of reasoning; managerial investigations are in the spirit of clinical epidemiology and its associated statistical and decision analytic mode of reasoning.

Diagnostic Problems Related to Lack of Expertise and Incomplete Information about an Individual Case

Many of the "problem" cases encountered in day-to-day pathology practice are resolved by gathering more information and/or by recruiting expert opinion. There is much to be said about these two strategies and when they should be employed; this is not my concern here. I am interested in the limiting case for which expertise and information are not at issue. Consider the relevant expert in possession of 'compete' information concerning a problematic case. A decision analytic device, the Clairvoyant, sharpens this idea. This is an imaginary figure with full knowledge, who can, and will, answer truthfully and completely any question put to her. [1] However, the Clairvoyant is temporally constrained in two ways: she won't tell you about the future state of the patient harboring the problematic I_{Neop} nor will she tell you about results that could be obtained employing technologies unavailable at the time of the expert's interrogation. For example, in 1950 it wouldn't do to ask her about the immunohistochemical findings for a particular problematic case. Why problem cases persist for the relevant expert with access to the Clairvoyant is the subject matter of this chapter.

Why Problem Cases Persist Even for the Relevant Expert with Access to a Clairvoyant?

I will use as an organizing framework for this discussion the principle players in C&D: (1) the complexity and uniqueness of individuals, the I_{Neop}'s, being classified; (2) the heterogeneity of groups (the K_{Neop}'s) formed by aggregating I_{Neop}'s similar in relevant respects; and (3) the classifier-diagnostician who puts it all together.

Complexity and Uniqueness of the Individual Neoplasm (I_{Neop})

Complexity

As illustrated in Fig. 6.1, it is convenient to discuss the complexity of the individual neoplasm (I_{Neop}) at three anatomic levels: the neoplastic *cell*, the neoplastic *tissue* (neoplastic cells embedded in the nonneoplastic cells that comprise their environment), and the clinically detectable neoplastic *mass* (Table 6.1). At the *cellular* level, the I_{Neop} inherits the functional and microanatomical complexity of its normal counterpart. The function of the normal cell is increasingly being framed in the language of biological systems and discussions of modules, pathways and global networks, nonlinear interactions, emergent properties, and "downward causation" fill the pages of molecular-genetics journals and textbooks [2]. Additionally, there has been a shift from an exclusive focus on the causal roles of genes to one that recognizes the importance of epigenetic modifications – DNA methylations and histone modifications. These conceptual shifts have been mirrored in cancer molecular genetics. Thus, in recent years exclusive focus on single cancer genes has given way to talk of the dysregulation of cancer cells at multiple levels of cellular control including epigenetic alterations, chromosome copy number changes, DNA point mutations, and inversions and translocations [3]. It is now clear that, in general, there is no gene or handful of genes that are the cause of cancer, or indeed, any particular kind of cancer [4–7]. As of 2009 at least 350 (1.6%) of the 22,000 protein-coding genes in the human genome have been reported to show recurrent somatic mutations in cancer with strong evidence that these contribute to cancer development [8]. Thus, the neoplastic cells of the common adult cancers are genetically highly complex. This is evident both from low-resolution cytogenetic studies and more recently in highly refined examinations cataloging sub-microscopic chromosomal abnormalities. The Circos diagrams of a group of breast cancers shown in Fig. 6.2 provide a striking graphical representation of this breathtaking complexity [9].

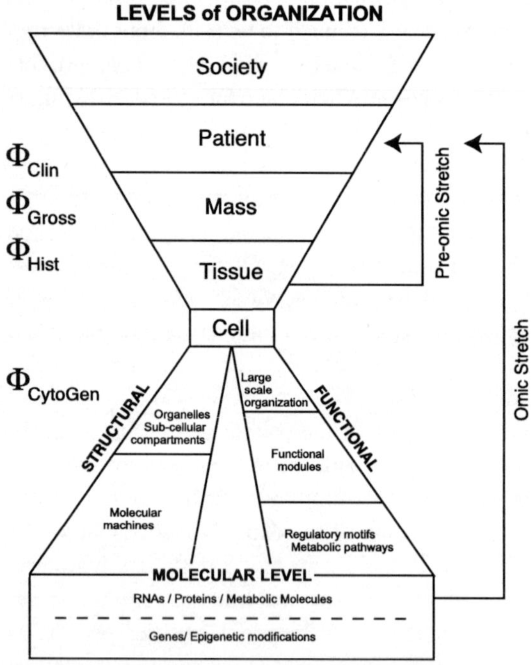

Fig. 6.1 Levels of organization. Cell and tissue levels are at the waist of the hourglass; they lie at the organizational midlevel. The molecular-to-cellular levels are split vertically between structural (*left*) and functional (*right*) levels; Oltvai and Barabási's complexity pyramid is represented by the functional branch on the *right* [66]. The phenotypes corresponding to various levels are indicated on the *left*: Φ_{Clin} = clinical phenotype (e.g., presenting signs and symptoms); $\Phi_{Clin}(t)$ = future clinical course (forecasts about risk, prognosis, prediction); Φ_{Gross} = naked eye phenotype whether seen by the pathologist in the gross room, by the surgeon intraoperatively or by the radiologist with imaging techniques; Φ_{Hist} = light microscopic phenotype; $\Phi_{CytoGen}$ = cytogenetic phenotype. "Level-hopping" is indicated on the *right* both -omic (gene expression arrays, proteomics, etc.) and pre-omic

Table 6.1 Characteristics of I_{Neop}'s

Complexity
Cellular level
Tissue level
Mass level
Context sensitivity
Uniqueness
Summarizing Metaphors
Malignant gestation
Viral quasi-species

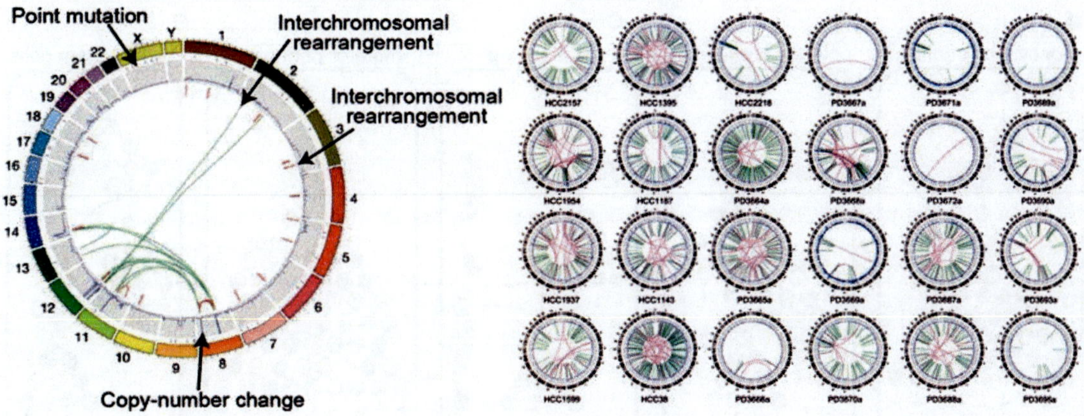

Fig. 6.2 The uniqueness of the I_{Neop}: Circos diagrams; molecular-genetic "train wrecks." Circos plots of the somatic rearrangements of 24 different invasive breast cancers make clear the molecular-genetic heterogeneity of this group of neoplasms. *Left*: The symbolic conventions of the circos plot [6]. Individual chromosomes are depicted on the outer circle followed by concentric tracks for point mutation, copy number, and rearrangement data relative to mapping position in the genome. *Arrows* indicate examples of the various types of somatic mutation present in this cancer genome. *Right*: The Circos plot of twenty four individual breast cancers. Note: each Circos diagram is really the superposition of the many diverse cytogenetic abnormalities of the different clones comprising I_{Neop} [9]

The I_{Neop} viewed as a *tissue* exhibits another layer of complexity. Neoplastic tissues have two constituents: neoplastic cells, typically arranged into parodies of structures normal to the anatomic site of origin, and nonneoplastic cells. The construction, evolution, and maintenance of a neoplastic tissue involve communication among the tumor cells and relevant nonneoplastic cell types. Well-studied examples include the vascularization of the I_{Neop} [10], the prominent role of the macrophage in cancer initiation and malignant progression [11], and participation of myoepithelial and various stromal cells in modulating the proliferation, survival, polarity, differentiation state, and invasive capacity of breast cancer cells [12–14]. In conclusion, while it is generally accepted that tumor initiation and progression are predominantly driven by acquired genetic alterations of neoplastic cells, the crucial importance of the microenvironment has become apparent in recent years. Taken together, neoplastic cells and their nonneoplastic interactants constitute a microecological system [15].

The I_{Neop} viewed as a clinically detectable *mass* reveals yet another level of complexity: evolutionary complexity. The earliest radiologically detectable solid malignancy has typically gone through at least 30 replications and consists of a billion or more cells. Histologically, this mass appears as a crazy quilt of dozens of genealogically related neoplastic clones each mingled with nonneoplastic constituents – cells and matrix – to form a complex of multiple microecologies. Moreover, the crazy quilt of patterns in a tumor evolves over time; the originally diagnosed I_{Neop} often has a different appearance than the recurrence.

What accounts for synchronic and diachronic *intratumor heterogeneity* [16–18]? There are two contributions: hereditary (inherited somatic mutations) and nonhereditary (phenotypic plasticity). Since the 1970s, I_{Neop}'s have been regarded as Darwinian evolutionary processes and the clinically detected cancer as a collection of genealogically related clones, themselves the product of a contingent, historical process [15, 18, 19]. Each I_{Neop} is the outcome of a process of Darwinian evolution occurring among cell populations within their microenvironments. The heritable variation is provided by the genetic instability of the cancer cell yielding a range of phenotypes and their associated microenvironments upon which selection can operate. Navin has recently reviewed various models – including stem cell variants – of somatic mutation generated heterogeneity, illustrated in Fig. 6.3 [16, 18]. The second reason for tumor heterogeneity, phenotypic plasticity, has two origins.

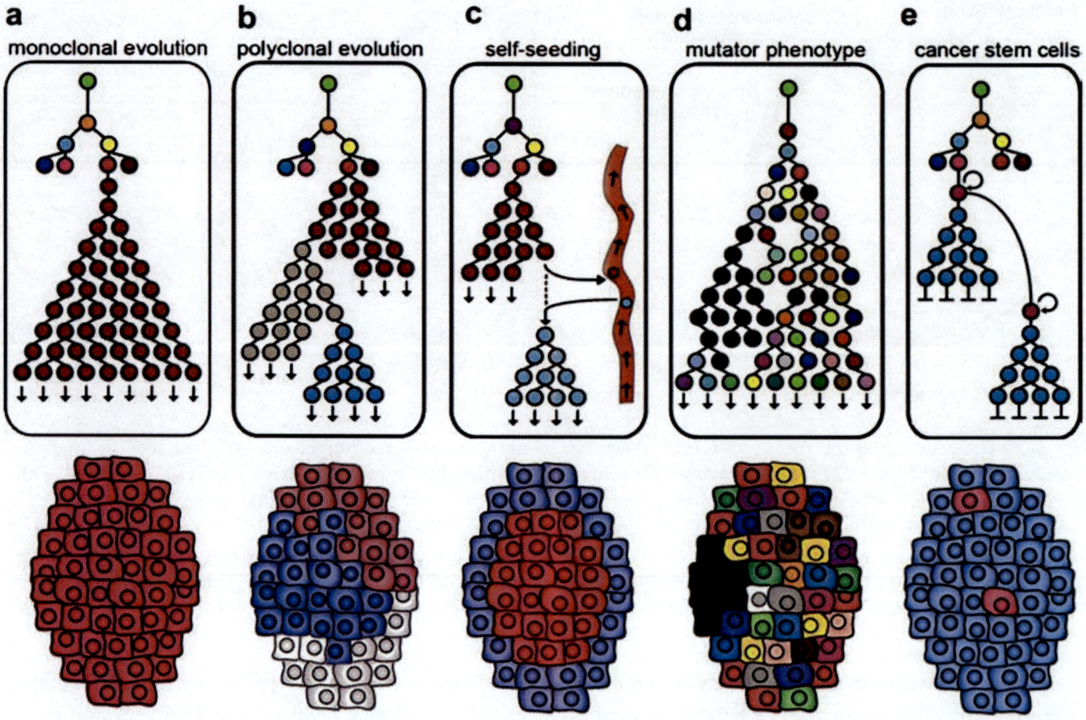

Fig. 6.3 Tumor progression models and lineages. Navin and Hicks have illustrated five models of tumor progression and their phenotypic consequences [18]. Green root nodes represent normal diploid cells, colored nodes are different tumor clones. (**a**) Monoclonal evolution forms a monogenomic tumor. (**b**) Polyclonal evolution forms a polygenomic tumor. (**c**) Self-seeding results in a tumor with a divergent peripheral subpopulation. (**d**) Mutator phenotype generates a tumor with many diverse clones. (**e**) Cancer stem cell progression results in a tumor with a minority of pink cancer stem cells

First, there is the heterogeneity that can be attributed to phenotypic variations on a single specified "cell of origin." This is exemplified for by the spectrum of grades within a single phenotype observed in the common adult cancer. The second source of heterogeneity implicates the developmental history of the TIC. For example, the normal uterine cervix is populated by glandular, squamous, and indifferent (or metaplastic) cells. The occurrence of confusing mixtures of these three phenotypes in an invasive cervical cancer can be understood as the TIC inscribing these developmental potentials in the clonal phenotypes of the I_{Neop} it gives rise to. Müllerian neoplasia offers a more dramatic example. Commonly, surface epithelial neoplasms of the ovary exhibit more than one phenotype. When this is striking, we call them "mixed." This amounts to the TIC retracing the possible developmental pathways open to the components of the müllerian ducts. Of course, germ cell neoplasms exhibit the greatest degree of phenotypic plasticity; this was dramatically demonstrated in the mouse teratocarcinoma studies by Mintz et al. [20]. It is as if the neoplastic cell can, in its confusion, take more than one developmental pathway; in other words, to follow Yogi Berra's advice: "when you come to a fork in the road, take it!"

There is one more layer of microecological complexity. There is growing evidence that there are important interactions among the distinct clones that make up an I_{Neop}. Here the clones play the role of species and the non-neoplastic cells, the role of the environment opening the way to an ecological analysis of neoplasia. This topic is reviewed by Marusyk and Polyak [17].

There are practical implications of this dynamic view of the I_{Neop}. The escape of an I_{Neop}

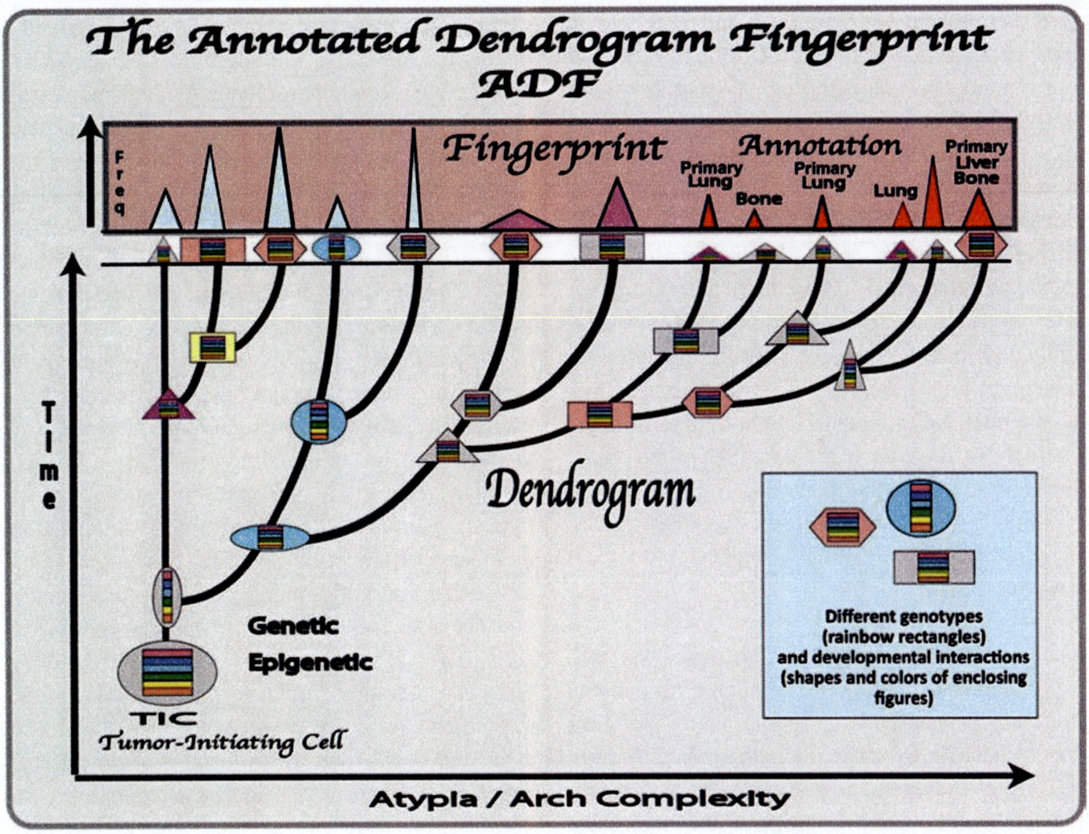

Fig. 6.4 The annotated dendrogram fingerprint (ADF). The Nowell's evolutionary trajectory is represented by the dendrogram with its root in the tumor initiating cell, the normal cell that has undergone malignant transformation. Time is represented vertically; an idealized summary of phenotype horizontally. Each node in the dendrogram represents a neoplastic clone; each node consists of a central multicolored rectangle set within a background figure. The *rectangle* symbolizes the multilevel genetic and epigenetic dysfunction of the constituent cells of the clone; different shaped rectangles represent different patterns of cellular dysfunction. The background figure represents the co-constructed microenvironment of that particular clone. The *top* panel depicts a snapshot of the I_{Neop} at a particular time. Here the horizontal axis again represents phenotype but now the vertical axis represents the percentage contribution of each clone (the nodes) to the composite tumor phenotype, or fingerprint. For example, the first seven peaks go into the make-up of the patient's primary tumor; the labeled peaks to metastatic deposits in various sites. This is just one possible snapshot; a slice across some other time would yield a different fingerprint. Thus, we have a representation of synchronic and diachronic tumor heterogeneity. To summarize, the ADF symbolizes the three levels of complexity of the I_{Neop}: the functional (epi)genetic complexity of the malignant cell by the rectangle; the micro-ecological complexity of the malignant tissue by its containing figure; and the evolutionary complexity of the clinically detectable mass by the dendrogram

from previously effective chemotherapy appears largely to have an evolutionary basis. Examples include the development of imatinib resistance in chronic myelogenous leukemia [21–23] and in gastrointestinal stromal tumors [24–26].

In Fig. 6.4 I introduce some symbolism, a modification of Nowell's 1976 diagram that serves to keep before us the multilevel complexity – cell, tissue, mass – of the I_{Neop}: what I will call the *annotated dendrogram fingerprint* (ADF).

Context Dependency

The clinical evolution (clinical phenotype) of a particular I_{Neop} is context dependent. For example, histomorphologically identical invasive squamous carcinomas exhibit very different clinical behaviors depending upon their precise location in the mouth and oropharynx. Similarly, the clinical presentation and the operability of a glioma of fixed grade depends crucially on anatomic location.

The complexity of neoplasms and their context dependency reminds us that the implicit reductive moves made in oncopathological classifications: first, the reduction of the patient to the patient's I_{Neop} second, the reduction of the I_{Neop} to a small set of gross, histological, immunological, and molecular-genetic characterizations and, third, the further reduction of these characterizations to a vector of categorical, ordered or interval values. The unique particularities of each patient are inevitably lost in this process. These considerations challenge any thoughts of strict, context-free histological, or molecular-genetic determinism. There will always be, in the language of the epidemiologist, confounding factors.

Uniqueness

It should be obvious from this discussion that each I_{Neop} is nontrivially unique. The altered normal cell from which it arises is as unique as the patient's fingerprints. Superimposed on this baseline individuality is the uniqueness imposed by the contingencies of the steps leading to the malignant transformation of the normal cell to produce a tumor initiating cell (e.g., the specific order in which cancer pathways are destabilized), the contingent interaction of those malignant cells with the patient's unique physiologic microenvironment, the contingency of the evolutionary pathways that constitute tumor progression, and finally, the contingencies of the tumor's precise location and time of clinical detection. All of these factors guarantee that the clinical behavior of groups of similar I_{Neop}'s will only admit a statistical formulation. The Circos diagrams remind us of this uniqueness (see Fig. 6.2).

The I_{Neop} Is a Dynamic Process, Not a Static Object

The foregoing discussion forces the conclusion that I_{Neop}'s are difficult to conceptualize and more usefully viewed as dynamic processes rather than static objects. It is, on the one hand, a single entity (certainly in the sense of the single disease of the patient who harbors it); on the other hand, it is a complex collection of interacting, evolving, physically distinguishable parts, the constituent clones. What are suitable metaphors for the individual neoplasm? One is the "malignant gestation"; a metaphor that emphasizes the maldevelopmental character of the process and its continuous spatiotemporal variation. Microbiology is the source of another metaphor: the viral quasispecies as exemplified by hepatitis C and HIV [27–30]. Both of these viral infections begin with an inoculum having one genetic composition but which then rapidly evolves into large numbers of derivative "species" under the selective pressure exerted by both the host's immune response and therapy. This metaphor comes closest to capturing the truth about the I_{Neop}. The distinguishable clones of an I_{Neop} are analogous to the species produced in the course of terrestrial organismic evolution. That is, each component of an I_{Neop}'s fingerprint is analogous to a species. In light of this discussion, we anticipate that the static classifications created by grouping relevantly similar I_{Neop}'s into kinds will be a problematic. It reminds us of the skepticism expressed by Darwin in his *Origins of the Species* about the reality of static Linnaean species.

Intrinsic Heterogeneity of Neoplastic Kinds (K_{Neop}'s)

Preliminaries

So far I have sketched out the multilevel complexity of the I_{Neop} and emphasized its uniqueness. How do we aggregate individually unique I_{Neop}'s into groups based on relevant similarities? It should be clear at the outset that the uniqueness of the I_{Neop}'s guarantees the intragroup heterogeneity of the classes that comprise *any* classification of I_{Neop}'s we can imagine.

Before we address the specifics of this process we need to lay some groundwork by setting out some preliminary definitions and make some observations about the classification process in general.

Classification Contrasted with Diagnosis

These two terms are used in inconsistent and confusing ways. In this chapter, I will use *classification* to denote either the process or the product of partitioning a particular domain (e.g., epithelial proliferations of the breast) into a set of mutually exclusive and collectively exhaustive kinds. *Diagnosis* denotes the process of assigning an as yet unexamined case to one (or more) of the kinds set out in the classification.

Classification Pluralism

It is a commonplace that there are many ways to classify objects in Nature depending upon one's interests. Consider the many classifications of plants: that of the curator of a botanical garden, that of the green grocer, the herbalist, or the landscape architect. No one botanical classification is privileged, they all serve different purposes. This homely example prepares us for the surprise that there is substantial, often acrimonious and heated, dispute over the scientific term "species." There are the phenetic species, the biological species, the ecospecies, and the evolutionary species [31]. Each species definition answers to the peculiarities of different domains (viruses, bacteria, vertebrates) and different research concerns (e.g., field identification, evolution, ecology) and their differing organizing principles. Thus, there is no sense to be made of "the one correct classification" independent of the research community's investigatory concerns.

Geometry of Classification: The Phenospace

In the following discussion I will employ some of the vocabulary of mathematical-statistical classification. The ideas are sketched out in the legend accompanying Fig. 6.5.

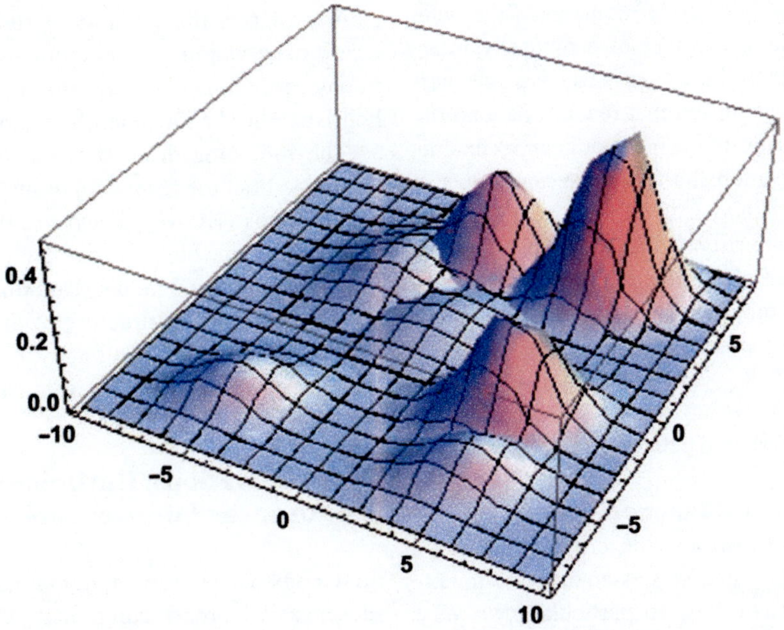

Fig. 6.5 An idealized tumor phenospace. Phenospaces for I_{Neop}'s are constructed by reducing the objects of study (I_{Neop}'s in our discussion) to some fixed number of ordered observations (say, tumor size, extent of necrosis, mitotic index, etc.) and then representing each analyzed case as a point in a suitably dimensioned space: a "feature space" or, synonymously, a "phenospace." It will meet our needs for this discussion to confine ourselves to two continuous features and use the third dimension, the height, to exhibit the number of cases taking on a particular pair of values. In general, this process yields peaks and valley and sparsely populated or unoccupied regions. Several questions are suggested by this plot. The existence of structure invites speculation about underlying generative mechanisms: does the presence of seven peaks suggest seven distinguishable generative mechanisms? If there are seven, where do the products of one leave off and the products of the other begin? That is, are there natural borders to these phenotypic clusters?

Relational Kinds and Structural Kinds

Kinds that occur in nature can be divided into two types: structural and relational (sometimes termed historical) depending upon whether the defining feature is a structural predicate or a relational one. That I have a mass of 79.5 kg is a structural property; that I am an uncle is a relational one. Structural kinds are those whose defining organizing principle is intrinsic to the objects being classified; it is to be found in each member of the kind. The paradigmatic structural kinds are atomic and molecular species (e.g., elemental gold, benzene, isoleucine); to determine whether two pure samples are of the same kind, one has only to examine the structure (physico-chemical properties etc.) of each sample. By contrast, relational kinds are those whose definition appeals to a relationship to something external to the objects being classified. Paradigmatic examples of relational kinds are biological species. One definition of the category species (of many possible definitions) is the biological species: to be members of the same species is to be a member of a naturally interbreeding group. To be a tiger is to have tiger parents. This is a definition that reaches beyond the intrinsic properties of the individual under examination to its relationship to an external object, a mother and a father. It is an empirical question whether there are structural features of each tiger (e.g., features of genomic organization) that pick out tigers (and only tigers) from their mimics. So far this does not appear to be the case. As I shall see, histogenetic K_{Neop}'s are relational kinds; what binds them into a group is not a shared structural "essence" but a shared cell of origin.

Oncopathological Taxonomic Models

I would like to re-frame the creation of oncopathological classifications as an exercise in taxonomic model building; in particular, two very different kinds of models – histogenetic models and statistical models.

Models play a major role in many scientific contexts. Examples include the billiard ball model of an ideal gas and its various elaborations, the Bohr model of the atom, the double helix model of DNA, and the general equilibrium model of financial markets [32, 33]. There are a number of advantages to talking in terms of models. First, it emphasizes that models are the constructs of the classifier. Second, it shifts the discussion from metaphysics (distinction between "real entities" and "pseudo-entities") to consideration of the empirical adequacy of competing explanatory models. Finally, discussions of models allow us to distinguish structurally different classes of models used in oncopathology: histogenetic and managerial.

Histogenetic Neoplastic Kinds (HG-K_{Neop}'s)

Histogenetic neoplastic kinds are collections of I_{Neop}'s presumed to share an origin from a particular normal cell or population of cells committed to a particular line of differentiation that have undergone malignant transformation. The plausibility of this theory is supported less by the direct observation of this temporal progression in any individual case but more by invoking the heuristic: "looks like, therefore came from."

The following discussion provides a way of thinking about the formation of histogenetic neoplastic kinds (HG-K_{Neop}) and has this sequential structure: (a) the observations that invite explanation; (b) a proposed model (Gouldian reruns); (c) a description of the structure of the groups predicted by the model; and finally, (d) the problem of conceptualizing and describing these groups.

The Observations: The Uninterpreted Phenospace of the Domain

First, consider a particular domain's phenospace, say invasive breast carcinoma. Choose 1,000 invasive breast carcinomas, each from a different patient. Characterize each I_{Neop}'s fingerprint. Plot the fingerprints for each of the 1,000 cases in a suitably dimensioned phenospace and structure emerges. Recall that in the phenospace, proximity reflects similarity with respect to the features that have been chosen by the investigator.

The resulting phenospace is occupied by clusters separated by thinly populated or unpopulated gaps. The phenospace has structure. So far, this is all description. How can we account for clustering? One guiding principle is: "Where there is structure, there is an underlying generative mechanism"; some mechanism that is responsible for the frequent covariation of the observed features in short, the clustering. Model building begins at this point.

The Model: Gouldian Reruns

Steven J. Gould in his book on the Cambrian Explosion, *Wonderful Life*, in making an argument about the plausibility of human intelligence arising a second time in the history of the planet, invites us to consider evolution run over and over again from a common temporal starting point [34]. I want to recruit this powerful image as a way to conceptualize HG-K_{Neop}'s. The discussion in the previous section left us with the remarkable image of the I_{Neop} as a *process*, an evolutionary trajectory resulting in the production of numerous genealogically related clones, each clone being analogous to an individual species. The Gouldian rerun idea is simply this: a HG-K_{Neop} is the superposition of the ADFs of all I_{Neop} sharing a common generative mechanism. This common mechanism is usually identified with the "cell of origin." Figures 6.6 and 6.7 and the accompanying legends elaborate this theme.

The Model's Consequences: Extensionally Indeterminate Core-Penumbra-Tierra Incognita Structure (Extnl-CoPeTI)

More generally, this process yields clusters separated by gaps in a suitably dimensioned phenospace. Each cluster has an internal substructure consisting of one or more concentrations of typical (core) cases, a fringe of looser concentrations

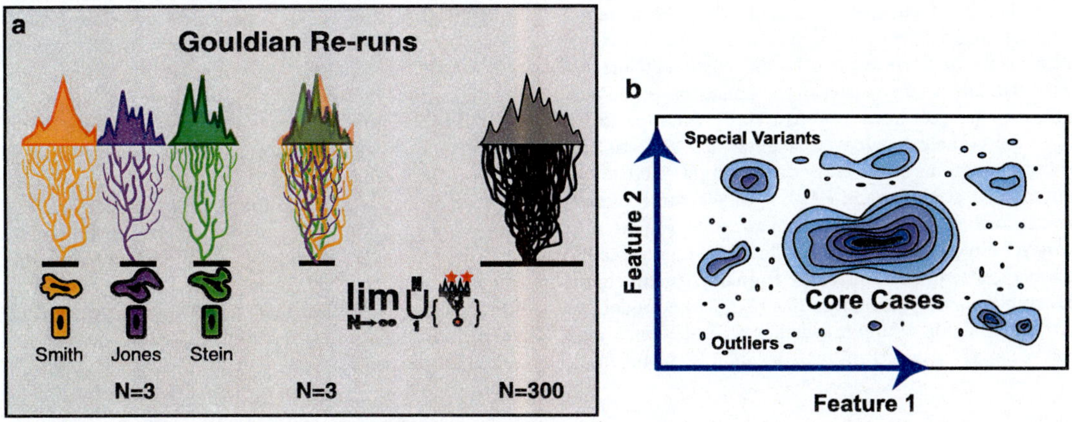

Fig. 6.6 Histogenetic neoplastic kinds: Gouldian reruns. Each patient (Smith, Jones, and Stein) harbors an invasive breast cancer, each with its unique ADF. Each one would fill in patches in a suitably dimensioned breast carcinoma phenospace. Each is thought to arise from a normal differentiated cell, counterparts of which are present in the breasts of all three. Fix that intersubjectively normal phenotype and now imagine each individual's ADF "starting off" from a malignant version of that common normal cell type. Malignant transformation of that normal cell leads to the corresponding tumor initiating cell (TIC). Think of all three neoplasms arising from that common root and then superimpose the three trajectories. This leads to the filling out of our breast cancer phenospace with contributions from all three I_{Neop}'s. Now increase the number to 300 and we get something like what is pictured at the extreme *right*. Panel B shows a contour diagram that might be produced by this experiment. In more abstract terms, we can think of a HG-K_{Neop} arising from a specified normal cell type "A" (HG-K_{Neop} [A]) as the set theoretical union (what we have been calling a superposition) of a large number of ADFs ("*n*") and then let *n* increase indefinitely. The increase in *n* amounts to gathering more experience about the range of variation of HG-K_{Neop} [A]

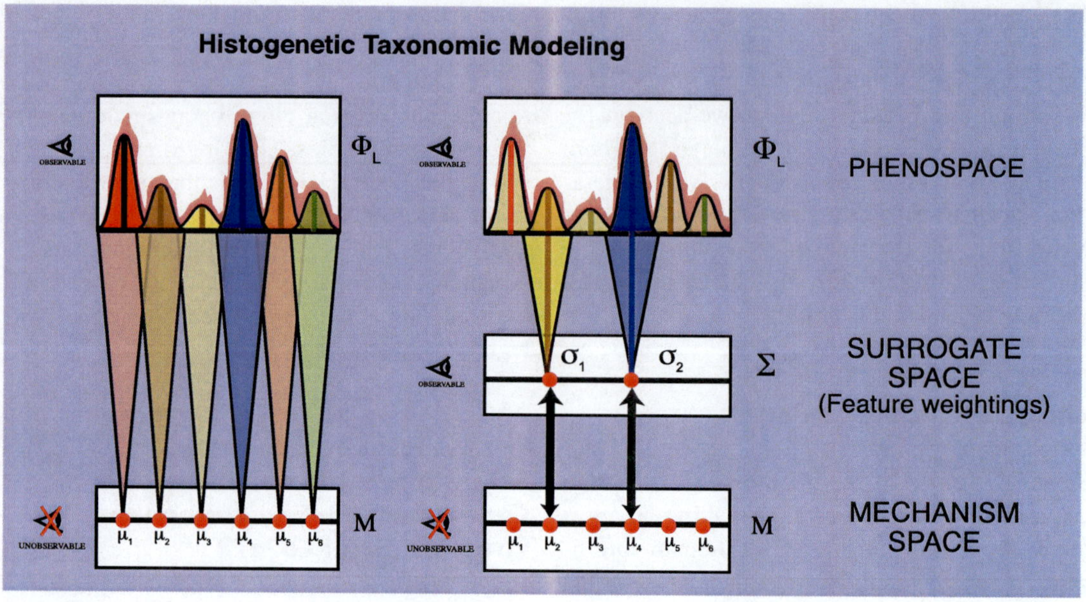

Fig. 6.7 The histogenetic taxonomic model schema. Making sense of "Gold Standards" involves analyzing a little more closely the relationship between the phenospace and the taxonomic model we use to make sense of the phenospace. *Left-hand side*: The Phenospace: this silhouette represents the observed phenospace (the result of studying a large number of cases in the particular domain) featuring six more or less ill defined but overlapping peaks. The Mechanism space: we decided that there are six generating histogenetic mechanisms. These individual mechanisms (μ's) correspond to the postulated mechanisms that lead to the cluster in the phenospace; the passage, for example, from a normal cell phenotype to the K_{Neop}; the complex maldevelopmental and evolutionary process that produces the crazy quilt of light microscopic patterns that comprise the HG-I_{Neop}'s. We can represent these in another space, the mechanism space. Importantly, we never directly observe the mechanisms represented in this space; we infer their presence from the structure in the observable phenospace. Given this taxonomic model, we can then ask, for example, whether an in-between case represents an instance of one or another histogenetic mechanism instantiated by the peaks on either side of the problematic case. *Right hand panel*: The Surrogate space: sometimes we decide on empirical grounds that some observable feature can be a stand-in for the, in principle, unobservable mechanism. The interposed surrogate space, Σ, is populated by the observable stand-ins for the corresponding set of postulated but nonobservable mechanisms. An example would be the SYT-SSX gene fusion for synovial sarcoma. Sometimes these are referred to as "Gold Standards" but this is misleading. If the requirement for a "Gold Standard" feature is that it is both necessary and sufficient for the diagnosis of a particular K_{Neop}, then the fusion product is not one; the usual claim in the case of synovial sarcoma is that 90% of cases show this feature. Moreover, currently, the relationship between the presence of a surrogate and the generative mechanism is completely mysterious; the most that can be said is that the "Gold Standard" feature and the mechanism are strongly correlated. Surrogates of this sort are more usefully regarded as features that are heavily weighted in an overall assessment of all the clinicopathological features used in diagnosis.

of atypical cases (penumbra) and cases that fade off in a diagnostically problematic way into "neighboring" entities ("terra incognita"), for short, *CoPeTI clusters*. Figures 6.8 and 6.9 illustrate this general concept. There is another consequence of the model: since the number of possible trajectories produced by a particular generative mechanism is, in principle, unlimited, we will always encounter new fingerprints. Thus, these phenospace clusters have the additional property of being "open" or, more precisely, extensionally indeterminate; the boundaries delimiting a parti-cular K_{Neop} are, according to this model, essentially undefined. In summary, the Gouldian rerun model predicts relational kinds that have an extensionally indeterminate CoPeTI structure (or *ExtnI-CoPeTI*, for short). The structure of K_{Neop}'s is reminiscent of that of

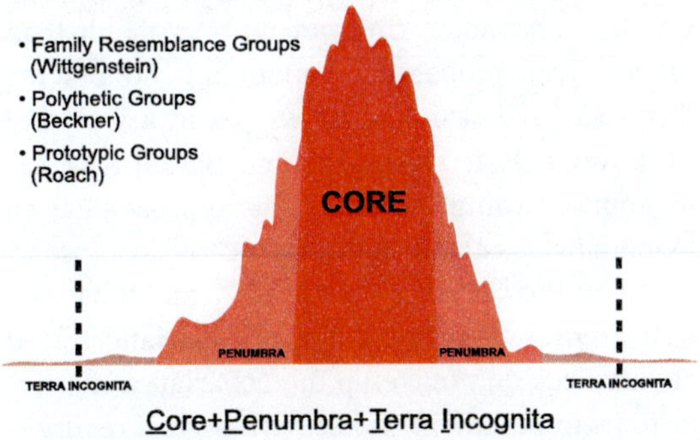

Fig. 6.8 The CoPeTI group. Biological variability in whatever domain tends to produce uni-modal or multi-modal "bell-shaped" like curves; K_{Neop}'s are no exception. If, from our phenospace, I extract a peak and take a cross-section through it and its immediate environment, I usually obtain something like this figure. Clustered around the mean are typical cases (the core) and as I move away from the mean I encounter less typical cases (the penumbra) and finally move into no-man's land (the terra incognita). For the sake of brevity and for us to keep this structure in mind I will use the acronym: CoPeTI

disease kinds in rheumatology, for example, systemic lupus or rheumatic fever a K_{Neop} is, in this sense, a morphologic syndrome.

Phenospace structure, then, is a reflection of a variety of factors that more or less constraint the population of I_{Neop}'s – each one of which is a contingent, unique evolutionary trajectory — originating from a particular TIC. These constraints include (1) phenotypic plasticity, the regenerative and developmental potential of the TIC, and (2) the contexts (anatomic, microanatomic, humoral, etc.) of the I_{Neop}. At this point, three questions arise: First, how many scientifically credible mechanisms are suggested by the structure? (How many K_{Neop}'s are there in the particular domain?) Second, how are the projections of these mechanisms into the phenospace to be delimited? That is, what are the boundaries separating K_{Neop}'s? Third, what attitude should I

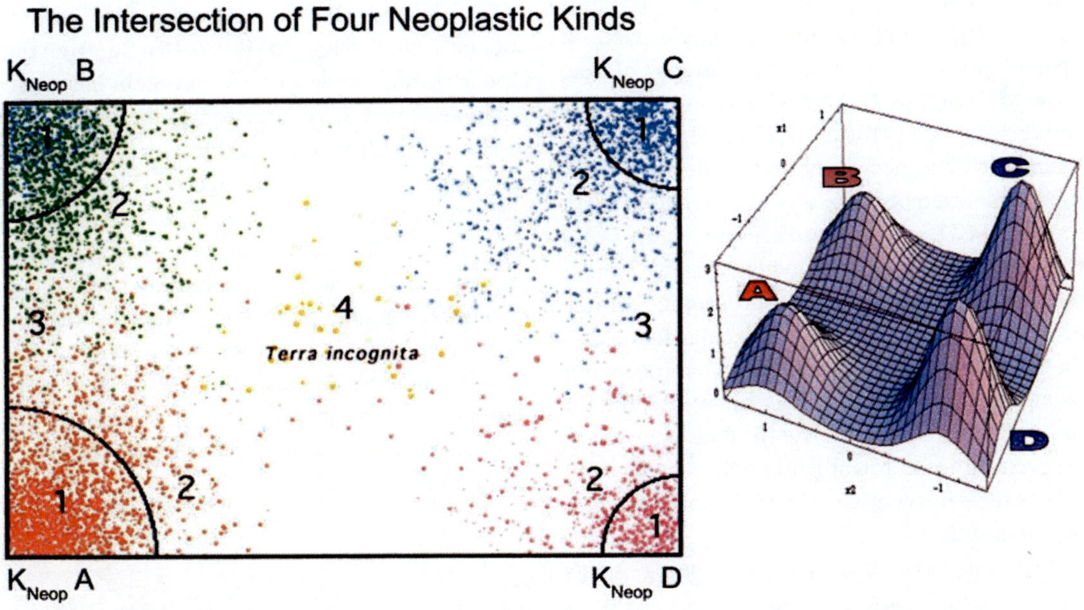

Fig. 6.9 Two representations of a typical patch of a domain's phenospace. The valley formed by four peaks in a two dimensional phenospace is shown. On the right is a three-dimensional depiction – the frequency of cases is indicated on the *z*-axis. On the *left* is a depiction of the same phenospace but this time each case is represented by a point; the density of points corresponds with the frequency of cases in a particular region of the phenospace. The histogenetic taxonomic model assumes four mechanism; the colors indicate the theoretical results of Gouldian reruns starting off from four types of transformed normal cell types. The CoPeTI naming is employed here: 1 = core cases; 2 = penumbral cases; 3 = in-between cases; and 4 = terra incognita ("there dragons be")

have toward problem cases viewed from this new perspective?

How many distinguishable histogenetic mechanism can be supported by our data?
This can be thought of as a model parameter to be specified by the investigator in much the same way that in cluster analysis one has to specify a range of values for the anticipated number of clusters to be "discovered" in unsupervised classification. "Lumpers" prefer a low number for this parameter; "splitters" prefer a higher number.

How, if at all, are the K_{Neop}'s to be delimited? To grid or not to grid
A grid imposed on a phenospace is the geometric equivalent of a crisply defined classificatory partition – the division of the phenospace into a set of high-dimensional volumes that are non-overlapping mutually exclusive regions that collectively exhaust the phenospace. The extensional indeterminacy of the Gouldian rerun model guarantees that any gridding will be problematic. Any partitioning of the phenospace in unambiguous, crisp characterizations of the observed features (the grid) will fail at a fine enough level of partitioning. Indeed, both crisp boundaries and necessary and sufficient conditions for membership are incompatible with ExtnI-CoPeTI groups. Furthermore, there is no refinement of a partition – whether using a more nuanced treatment of light microscopic features or employing thousands of molecular features – that will escape this problem. That does not mean that the current grid is not sufficient for most diagnostic work. But it does suggest a different attitude toward problem cases; *problem cases are symptomatic of this fundamental incompatibility.*

One approach that avoids gridding treats K_{Neop}'s as multivariate probability distributions with ranges that include all possible values that the features can assume in the phenospace. For any region of the phenospace, there is a nonzero probability that any of the posited generative mechanisms (the HG-K_{Neop}'s) could take on values in that region. Anything is possible for the HG-K_{Neop}, but some kinds are more probable than others. This probabilistic modeling honors the ExtnI-CoPeTI structure of K_{Neop}'s in a way that grids do not. It should be mentioned that the machine-learning version of this approach has an essentialist cast: the multivariate mean is interpreted as the "essence" of the K_{Neop} and the variation (represented by values of variances and covariances that make up the covariance matrix) as reflecting random "noise." Biological reality is sacrificed in this model; much of the "noise," far from being random, may well be biologically relevant signal [35, 36].

How Are Problem Cases to be Handled?

At this point, the reader may say: "All of this is well and good but the practice of oncopathology requires some manageable partition of the phenospace." The response is, of course, this is true and the existing systems perform surprisingly well. What our analysis suggests is that grids are pragmatic solutions and not to be taken too seriously, theoretically, as reflecting our current understanding of K_{Neop}'s (Fig. 6.10). So, from the Gouldian reruns perspective, problem cases are guaranteed and draw attention to the limitations of gridding. What to do? From a practical point of view, if there is *no* managerial distinction at issue, then forcing a problem case into one category or another seems at best, of academic importance only, at worst, pointless. If there *is* a managerial gradient involved, then the discussion must shift into a totally different mode: decision analytic and, as will be discussed, indeterminacy of histogenetic assignment, by no means, paralyzes clinical decision making (see Chap. 10).

Representing ExtnI-CoPeTI Structure in Concepts and Language:

How do should we conceptualize and talk about the continuous, multidimensional, spatio-temporal variation characteristic of I_{Neop}'s on the one hand and the ExtnI-CoPeTI groups (K_{Neop}'s) into which

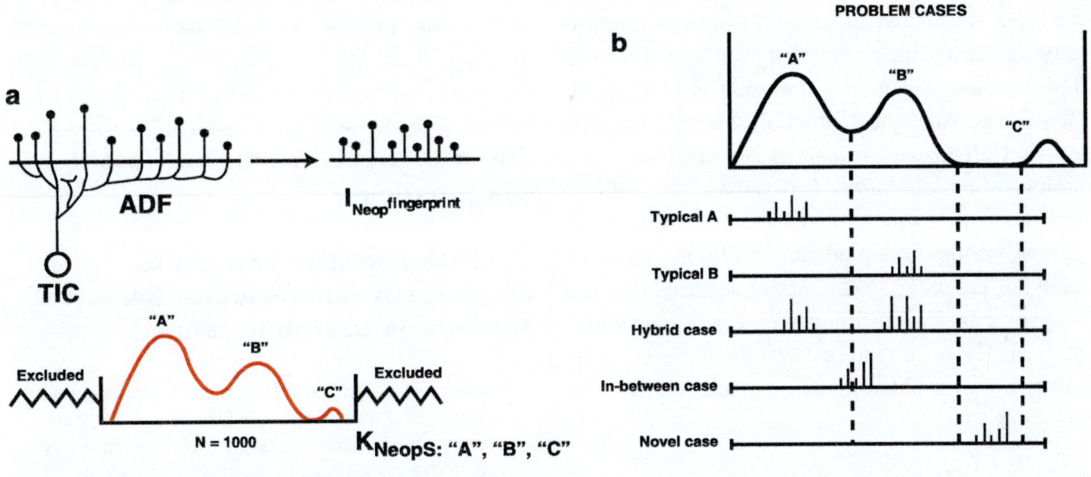

Fig. 6.10 Problem cases. (**a**) A stylized ADF is simplified into its associated fingerprint, a snapshot of the I_{Neop}'s heterogeneity at the moment of biopsy. (**b**) The relevant domain is represented by a silhouette with labels "A," "B," and "C"; for example, I call things in this region "K_{Neop}(A)." The silhouette represents the results of plotting 1,000 I_{Neop}'s from this domain. (C) The fingerprints of both typical cases and problem cases are depicted

they cluster? We have recourse to vague concepts and vague language. It is important to emphasize that vagueness is a property of concepts and predicates. The world is not vague; the world is, well, what it is [37].

As an illustrative example, let us take synovial sarcoma. Our Gouldian rerun model tells us that I should expect that this neoplastic kind should have an ExtnI-CoPeTI structure. Consider a set of instruction for diagnosing the HG-K_{Neop}, synovial sarcoma and separating it from its mimics. Many of the phenotypic features that we are advised to evaluate are imprecise. We have "synovial sarcomas are large" instead of providing a numeric size range; We have terms like "most" (50%?, 95%?) and "cellular." This vagueness of feature specification extends to integer-valued, countable features of the I_{Neop}. For example, the difficulty with providing a mitotic count frequency (say, maximum number of mitotic figures/ten high power fields) for a uterine smooth muscle neoplasm is *not* in the counting part (statistical and sampling issues, though there are) but in deciding whether something is or is not a mitotic figure. In other words, the feature itself is an extensionally indeterminant CoPeTI category. Not only are individual criterial features vague, criteria for membership in synovial sarcoma are also vague. How many of these features are required? Should some be weighted more heavily than others?

What Sort of Concept Is a K_{Neop}?

Cognitive psychologists and linguists studying concepts have written extensively on classes with this structure beginning in the 1970s with the work of Eleanor Rosch and George Lakoff. Terms used for these groups include "family resemblance groups," "cluster concepts," "prototype groups," and "polythetic groups [38–43]." Common features include a high level of intragroup heterogeneity; a graded architecture (there are better and worse examples in the class); prototypic examples; and, most importantly, an *absence* of a defining set of individually necessary and jointly sufficient (INJS conditions) for membership. The last amounts to the assertion that the groups have no essences. It became clear in the 1970s that most nontechnical concepts and their linguistic representation do not have a classical (i.e., satisfying INJS conditions) structure; many have a prototype structure. Traditionally, the kinds that occur in nature have been thought to have a classical, essentialist structure. This is a tradition that began with Aristotle in Hellenistic Greece and was taken up wholesale by Linnaeus in the 18th C. and informed his structuring of biological classification. It is only in the 20th C. that the grip of essentialism has been relaxed. It is now widely accepted that biological species have no 'essences.' What about features that are said to be "Gold Standard" for a particular K_{Neop}'s? These are more usefully thought of as surrogates for histogenetic mechanisms (see Fig. 6.7).

Managerial Neoplastic Kinds ($M\text{-}K_{Neop}$'s)

If histogenetic classifications have the flavor of biological systematics, managerial classifications are more in the spirit of commercial risk analysis, say, fashioning risk categories for credit card applicants (good risk, intermediate risk, bad risk) using applicant characteristics (age, credit history, income, etc.). Managerial classifications are formed by playing off a wide variety of descriptors (features) against a clinical outcome of interest; in machine-learning terms, they are exercises in *supervised classification* (see Chap. 7 and 10.) The basic ideas are illustrated in Fig. 6.11. Paradigmatic examples are grading systems for common adult malignancies; these are managerial classifications that discretize a multivariate continuum into statistically credible, distinct $\Phi_{Clin}(t)$ groups or lotteries (Fig. 6.12). The "benign-malignant" dichotomous classification and its expansions can be regarded as "extended grading systems" (Fig. 6.13).

Managerial classifications are engrafted on underlying histogenetic classifications; managerial classifications both inherit the diagnostic problems of the underlying histogenetic classification and lead to diagnostic difficulties of their own. Managerial grey zones are quite different and dealing with them involves a change in conceptual register from histogenetic considerations to decision-analytic ones. Please see discussion in Chap. 7 and 10.

The Human Element: The Classifier/ Diagnostician

The Pathologist and the World Co-create Oncopathological Reality: The Conceptual Fabric Defined

> The true, insightful, and fundamental statement that science, as a quintessentially human activity, must reflect a surrounding social context does not imply either that no accessible external reality exists, or that science, as a socially constructed institution, cannot achieve progressively more adequate understanding of nature's facts and mechanisms.
>
> Stephen Jay Gould [44]

We co-construct our view of oncopathological reality. I mean this, not is some spooky extreme postmodernist way but in the noncontroversial sense that classifications issue from our attempts conceptualize and describe an undifferentiated world, a world that doesn't come presorted into 'natural kinds.' Construed most broadly, classifications embody our attempts to structure a world initially experienced, in William James phrase, "as one great blooming, buzzing confusion." We bring our current conceptual scheme and the methodologies (*conceptual fabric*) available to us at a particular time to bear on a particular domain (Table 6.2). The parsings (or classifications) of individuals in that domain have changed and will continue to change as we acquire new experience and our conceptual fabric changes. In other words, our classifications and their constituent kinds, the things we count as "real," change with the times (Table 6.2).

Coarse Grained Taxonomic Instability (Macro-Revisions)

Both nonmanagerial and managerial classifications evolve under the pressure of both additional experience and changes in the conceptual fabric. In the process, old K_{Neop}'s either disappear (or are radically transformed) or new ones take their place. Theory change is, of course, a standard topic in the

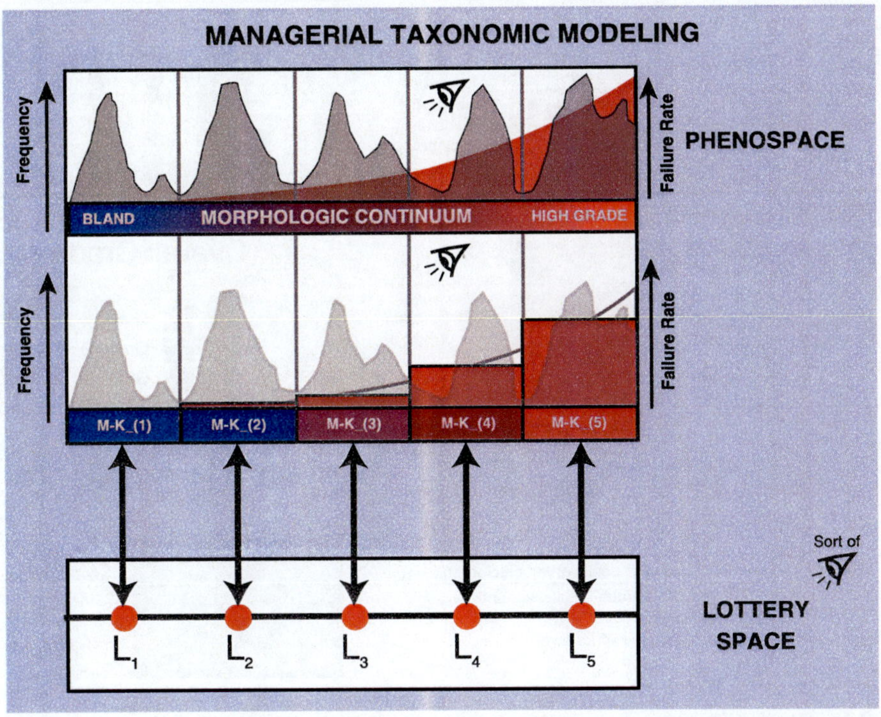

Fig. 6.11 The basic ideas behind managerial lotteries. *Upper panel*: the phenospace depicting both a continuous risk funtion and its discretized version. The x-axis represents some continuous composite measure of cytological atypia and architectural complexity. The y-axis represents two features: on the *left*, the frequency of cases having a particular morphologic index value and, on the *right*, the failure rate associated with a given morphologic index value. The *top half* of the panel depicts, in *grey*, a silhouette of the phenospace against which is plotted a continuous, monotonically increasing risk level. In the *bottom half* panel, the phenospace has been discretized into risk categories; the step function represents the average risk for each of the newly formed categories. These managerial neoplastic kinds are indicated in the bottom strip. For example, managerial K_{Neop} 1 or M-K-(1) etc. The lottery space (*bottom panel*) makes explicit the distinct lotteries associated with each managerial K_{Neop}. The 'eye' reminds us that we observe the morphology and associate the case with a specific lottery. The 'sort of' reminds us that our observations of the lottery characteristics for any given partition evolve over time with the acquisition of more clinicopathological experience. This evolution is one of the forces (among others) that drives the managerial classification macro-revisionary cycle (see discussion). Case assignment is problematic at the boundaries of categories; different assignments yield different predictions. This is an artifact of the discretizing procedure; a more realistic prediction would be that such a boundary case would have a behavior intermediate between the two straddled lotteries. Until recently, it was conventional to employ the dichotomous classification – "benign-malignant"; clinically more useful is the refined classification that recognizes additional distinct interpolated between 'benign' and 'malignant,' for example 'low malignant potential' tumors

philosophy of science; its most famous expounder in recent years was Thomas Kuhn [45, 46].

Recall the lymphoma histogenetic classification wars that roiled the world of hematopathology in the 1970s [47]. Discussions surrounding managerial revisions can be equally energetic. The debate over the existence of a "low malignant potential tumor" in the ovarian serous neoplasia spectrum is an example. Should the morphologic continuum be partitioned into "benign-malignant" versus "benign-LMP-malignant [48–52]?"

The dynamics of classification change can be represented as two evolutionary processes, one for M-classifications (the clinicopathologic spiral) and the other for S-classifications (the scientific spiral); the two trajectories mutually inform one another as they coevolve. Importantly, there is traffic between the two sides; some landscape features begin as

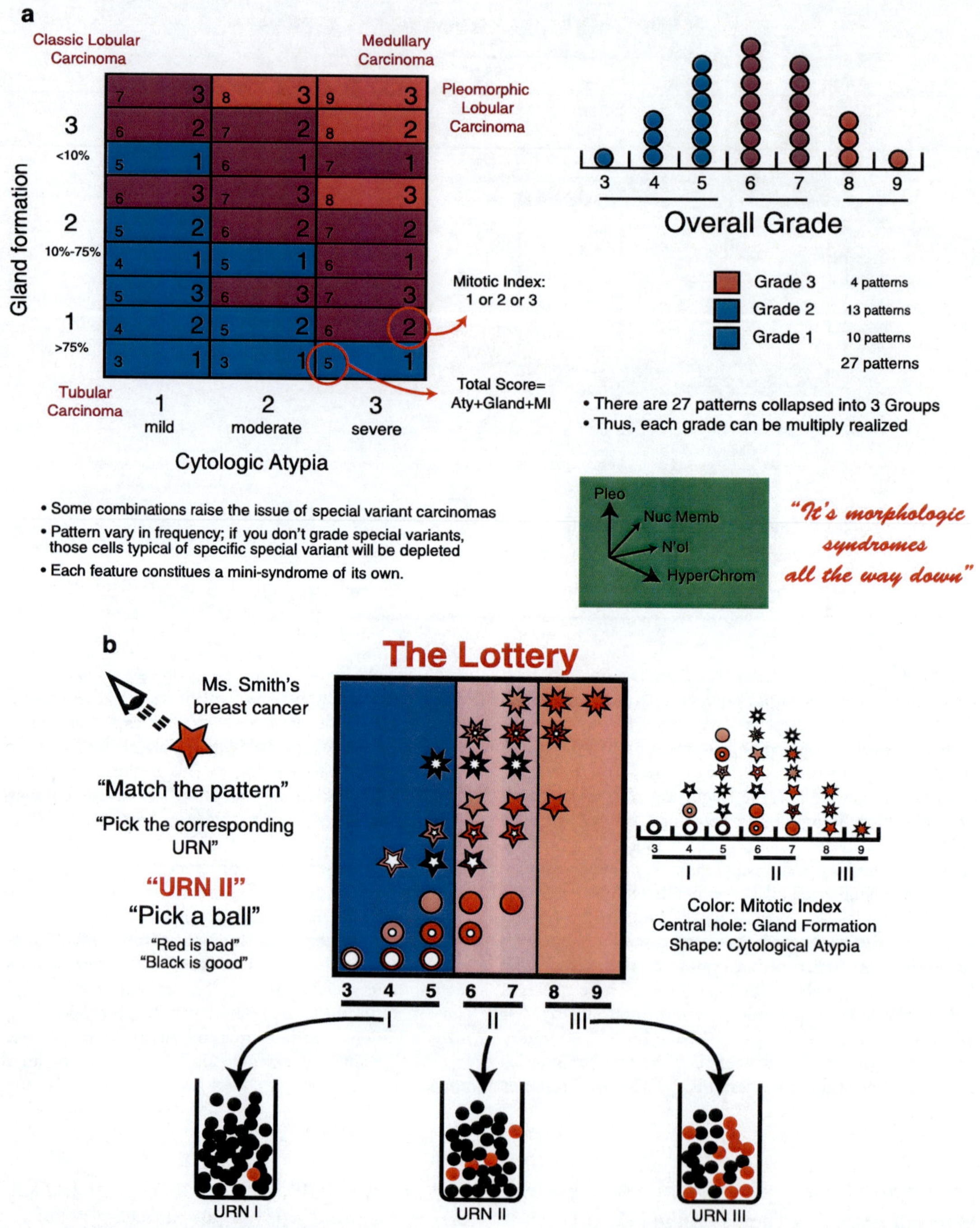

Fig. 6.12 Grading infiltrating ductal carcinoma of the breast – Nottingham Scarff-Bloom-Richardson (NSBR). Grading systems are paradigmatic examples of managerial classifications. The NSBR grading of invasive ductal carcinoma (IDC) serves as an example [67, 68]. (**a**) A representation of the IDC phenospace. Given a case of IDC one makes three observations: percentage gland formation, degree of cytological atypia, and mitotic index. Each of these three features can take on one of three values (1, 2, or 3). Add up the scores for the case being examined (ranges from 3 to 9) and assign the case a composite Grade using the scheme illustrated on the *right*. (**b**) The IDC Lottery: an interpretation of the IDC taxonomic model

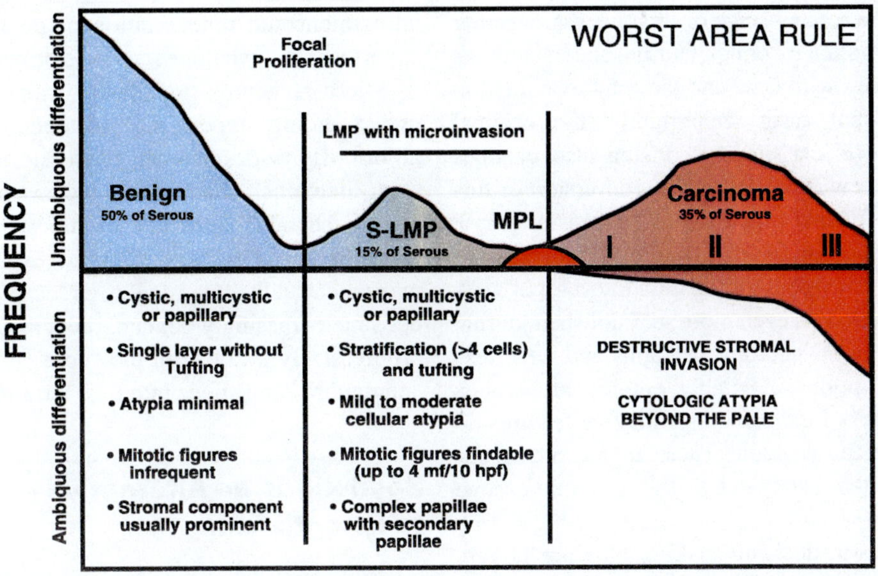

Fig. 6.13 The scheme applied to the ovarian serous neoplasia spectrum. In this figure the *y*-axis serves two purposes: the total width, for any fixed value of *x*, represents frequency; location below the *x*-axis indicate the extent to which serous differentiation is easily recognized. For example, the serous phenotype becomes increasingly attenuated as one moves into the Grade III carcinoma range. *S-LMP* serous low malignant potential neoplasm; *MPL* micropapillary lesion

Table 6.2 The oncopathological conceptual fabric

Methodologies available at a particular time
Global theories in the supporting sciences
Domain-specific theories (for example, theories about the etiology and pathogenesis of neoplasia)
Domain-specific knowledge accumulated to date
Styles of scientific reasoning (for example, statistical reasoning, case-based reasoning [65], taxonomic reasoning, and experimental reasoning) [69–71]

S-distinctions and evolve into M-distinction. This passage, for example, is the investigative focus for researchers validating proffered cancer markers (see Chap. 7 for a discussion of validation).

Transmission and Translation of a Classification

One session over a multiheaded microscope with an expert pathologist reviewing her cases is sufficient to disabuse one of the idea that experts diagnose using explicit criteria. Recognition comes first, criteria to justify the diagnosis, later. It is also clear that substantial nonhistopathologic knowledge is recruited in arriving at a diagnosis. Bartels sees this as an instance of "sensor fusion – the combining of sensory data with data from other sources such that the resulting information is in some sense better than would be possible when these sources are used individually [53]." Both of these observations prompt my use of the term "classificatory vision" to denote the pathologist's complex interior sense of "the map of the terrain"; the term reminds us that whatever makes up the expert's sense of some oncopathological domain, it is largely nonlinguistic and draws widely on many elements of the conceptual fabric. The later informs the way the expert navigates around a slide; chooses which microscopic fields to examine, which to ignore; in short, to decide what is "signal" and what is "noise."

Under ideal circumstances, the *transmission* of a classificatory vision from the investigator to a potential user involves the back and forth communication of the two over a mutiheaded microscope. It is an exercise in iterative ostensive teaching: pointing, naming, and correcting. Even under these ideal circumstances, there is an ineliminable indeterminacy of transmission. We never know, at any stage of this process, whether we have "gotten it" or not. Our misunderstandings emerge only with time and the joint examination of additional cases. Importantly, the original investigator's classificatory vision also changes with this new experience. The conversion of this "sensory fusion" process into spoken language, the translation problem, is itself challenging; summarizing that verbal formulation into a set of written instructions is even more so. Published journal articles rely on photomicrographs and terse textual descriptions inevitably employ ambiguous language. As I indicated, quantitative features do not escape this problem. These are anemic substitutes for the back and forth of a microscope session.

Diagnostic decision making aids are largely dedicated to facilitating this communicative task. They attempt to recapture the originary scene of ostensive classification transmission by making available extravagant numbers of images and modeling the "expert's" intuitions with rule based or probabilistic computer models. This topic is expanded upon in Chaps. 7 and 10.

Fine-Grained Taxonomic Instability (Micro-Revisions)

I discussed public large-scale revisions above; there is another kind of classificatory revision, "micro-revisions." By this I mean the ongoing, daily adjustments in the classificatory vision of the pathologist, the expert in particular, that is occasioned by her confronting a novel case and assimilating it to one or another K_{Neop}'s by, for example, using criteria that go beyond those extracted from the literature. If memory serves, the next time she sees another case like this one, she will make the same diagnosis. In these situations, the expert is *both classifying and diagnosing at the same time*. The way to understand the expert reporting: "I communed privately with the case for a long time and decided it was K_{Neop}(A) rather than K_{Neop}(B) or K_{Neop}(C)" is as a classificatory act. Returning to the map metaphor, we can think of this as the ongoing adjustment and renegotiation of details of the expert's grid – whether scientific or managerial.

Micro-revisions provide a framework for understanding expert disagreement, which is notoriously widespread in anatomic pathology. Over time, micro-revisionary cycles lead inevitably to the noncongruence of the private maps (classificatory visions) of different experts. Their maps are usually congruent over "core" cases but become increasingly noncongruent as one moves progressively away from the "core" through the "penumbra" and slides into the "terra incognita."

Boyd Kinds, an Alternative to Essentialism

Here is a puzzle that raises important issues: Is the K_{Neop}, synovial sarcoma of 1950, the same or different from the K_{Neop} synovial sarcoma of 2010? If not how are they related? Synovial sarcoma was first described about 90 years ago. The extension (the I_{Neop}'s included under the term) of the K_{Neop} synovial sarcoma has changed over the years with, for example, the acceptance of a monophasic variant. In the late 1980s, a consistent, specific translocation involving chromosomes X and 18 was discovered to be widely distributed in synovial sarcomas as then defined [54]. The fusion product of this translocation, SYT-SSX chimeric RNA, can be detected by reverse-transcriptase polymerase chain reaction and this procedure is now used in routine diagnostic test. It now has become customary to talk of the presence of the fusion product SYT-SSX as the "Gold Standard" for the diagnosis of synovial sarcoma, despite the fact that not all "classic" synovial sarcomas exhibit this feature. In recent years, the extension of synovial sarcoma has been expanded, using the SYT-SSX criterion, to include a variety of sarcomas that, on light microscopy examination, either possess a distinctive phenotype more characteristic of another type of sarcoma or are undifferentiated [55, 56].

The history of synovial sarcoma and, in particular, after the acceptance of SYT-SSX as the "Gold Standard" traces a general pattern. First, there is an early impression of distinctive H&E

histomorphological similarities justifying a grouping; I dub it "K_{Neop}(A)." Then, I posit some underlying generative mechanism. Next, I refine the initial characterization in light of new observations or reconceptualization under the pressure of changes in theory. Throughout this process, the K_{Neop} (A) retains the same name and I have the sense that I am approaching asymptotically the "true" K_{Neop}(A) with each cycle. This is the historical and contingent process of classificatory evolution. What happens to the K_{Neop}(A) during this process? Clearly its extension changes. What remains constant? It cannot be anything like a classical "essence," (i.e., "Gold Standard," set of INJS conditions) as I have seen. These are subtle and difficult issues and space only permits hints at a solution.

The traditional conception of "natural kinds" (i.e., groupings that occur in nature independent of our interest) has involved INJS conditions. It turns out that almost none of the categories investigated in biology, nor in most of the other special sciences – such as psychology, meteorology, astronomy, economics, or linguistics – involve shared intrinsic characteristics that are necessary and sufficient for membership [57–59].

The philosopher, Richard Boyd, has proposed an alternative understanding of natural kinds that does not involve necessary and sufficient membership conditions; he calls these "homeostatic property clusters natural kinds [60–62]." They feature Wittgensteinian families of properties that tend to be nonaccidentally coinstantiated, in that something that possesses some of the properties in the cluster makes it more likely that it will also possess the other properties in the cluster. Boyd has argued that biological species, higher taxa and many of the categories studied in economics and geology, have this character. Thus, categories can occur in nature prior to our classificatory schemes without any intrinsic characteristics or "essences" that all members of the category have in common. I think K_{Neop}'s with their ExtnI-CoPeTI structure are instances of Boyd kinds. The model also effectively deals with both what has been termed macro-revisions and micro-revisions. Chiong provides a medically oriented summary in the context of defining "brain death" [63].

Conclusions: The Mythology of Classificatory and Diagnostic Pathology (Table 6.3)

We can summarize the arguments of this chapter by setting out the major conclusions as a collection of myths. I have already discussed the myths of the homogeneous, static I_{Neop}'s and of histopathologic or molecular-genetic determinism.

Naïve Realism

> My guess is that I have a folk theory of categorization itself. It says that things come in well-defined kinds, that the kinds are characterized by shared properties, and that there is one right taxonomy of the kinds [64].
>
> It is easier to show what is wrong with a scientific theory than with a folk theory. A folk theory defines common sense itself. When the folk theory and the technical theory converge, it gets even tougher to see where that theory gets in the way – or even that it is a theory at all [39], p. 33.

Naïve realism in oncopathology takes roughly this form: There are the histogenetic neoplastic kinds "out there" waiting to be discovered. The attuned investigator by careful examination can identify these kinds in an unmediated way. The oncopathological taxonomist is like the field biologist venturing forth into the rainforest to identify and describe all the species of orchids encountered.

Essentialism

Naive realism is essentialist in that it asserts that while the individual neoplasms comprising a neoplastic kind show great variation, behind that variation there is an essence that is shared by all of the members of the kind. This essence amounts to a set of necessary and sufficient conditions for membership in the kind; I have referred to these as criterial features. Furthermore, this "essence" can be approximated by the averages of all the criterial features of the examined members of the group; in telecommunication jargon, the average is the "signal"; the variation is the "noise."

Table 6.3 Some myths of oncopathology

The myth	Opposed to the myth
The myth of the homogeneous, static neoplasm	The ADF and the histomorphologic crazy quilt; the individual neoplasm as a multiplicity of evolving clones
The myth of histological determinism	Anatomic context dependency
The myth of molecular-genetic determinism ("smallism", i.e., privileging the causal role of lower levels of the organizational pyramid over higher levels)	Levels of organization and complexity; emergent properties of integrated systems; context dependency
The myths of naïve realism about K_{Neop}'s	
• Realism (we have unmediated direct access to the way the World is structured)	We have no direct access to the 'real'; our interactions with the World are mediated by a 'conceptual fabric'; we co-create oncological reality
• Essentialism (all members of a K_{Neop}'s share a set of properties that are both necessary and sufficient for membership; i.e., they share an 'essence.')	K_{Neop}'s possess no essences; K_{Neop}'s are ExtnI CoPeTI groups; histo-morphologic syndromes
• Classification monism (there is one correct and true way to classify natural individuals into natural kinds)	Classification pluralism; the form and structure of a classification depends upon the background questions being asked. The coexistence of S-classifications and M-classifications instantiate this principle in oncopathology Classificatory macro-revisions
• Experts in the relevant domain have access to the 'true' diagnosis	The problem of expert disagreement For the expert when confronting problem cases (in possession of 'complete' information) the normally separate acts of diagnosis and classification collapse into a single activity Pathology experts are the 'language police' of the oncopathological community
The myth of the disappearance of problem cases in the fullness of time	Each I_{Neop} is non-controversially unique There are fundamental limitations to imposing a static essentialist grid onto an evolutionary process. This is true whether one is dealing with biological organisms or I_{Neop}'s. Aristotle meets Darwin

This metaphysical outlook pervades our oncopathological literature; it is our folk theory of classification and is encouraged by daily contact with case material that is easily and nonproblematically diagnosed using the vague guidelines available. Using any half-way functional classification, the ADF of most cases, of course, will be located near the center of some CoPeTI group. This pragmatic fact about an evolved classification is insufficient to warrant a belief in oncopathological essentialism.

Classification Monism

The myth of classification monism suggests that in the "Recording Angel's Book" is inscribed the one true classification of neoplasms. Our terrestrial efforts, over time, gradually converge on this true order.

The Role of the Expert

This myth amounts to the belief that the expert, examining a problematic case, can see through the troublesome variation of the individual neoplasm to its essence and, in possession of this insight, make the 'correct' assignment.

Conclusions

The analysis of clinically vivid defects of metabolism (e.g., alkaptonuria) led, historically, to an understanding of normal metabolic pathways. Similarly, an analysis of problem cases led us to reflections on how classification and diagnosis usually proceeds in oncopathology and, ultimately, the sketch of C&D presented in this chapter. This perspective has it that these "naïve realist" positions are wrong in just about every respect. Noncontroversially, there is nothing more real than the individual cancer afflicting a patient. The realist stance has it that the neoplastic kind to which the individual cancer belongs is as real as Ms. M's cancer. There are the neoplastic types out there to be discovered; decades of accumulated 'field' experience has produced the current canonical list of the named neoplastic kinds discovered to date. When talking about them we use locutions like: "most cases of X" or "sometimes X's can be confused with Y's because..." or "it can be very difficult to tell an X from a Y" or "X's never have feature a..." Other realist discourse includes: "It used to be thought that X was a real entity, but now we know it not to be, it is only a phenotype" or "We report 59 cases of a previously unrecognized vulvar soft tissue neoplasm.." or "Undifferentiated sarcoma: does it exit?" Opposed to *naïve realism* is the idea that a classification reflects not only what the world has to offer but also the conceptual fabric in which the investigator is embedded. In other words, oncopathological classifications are a coconstruction of investigator and the world. K_{Neop}'s do not have *essences* any more than biological species or medical genetic disorders have essences. I have argued that K_{Neop}'s have an ExtnI-CoPeTI structure; they are open-ended and not defined by any set of necessary and sufficient conditions. "Gold Standard" for the diagnosis of a K_{Neop} is always talk about privileged surrogates. I have suggested that Boyd's perspective is a promising alternative to essentialism. First, it frees us of a conceptual structure that has not worked in, for example, biological systematics. It realistically reflects what actually goes on in biological classification by accommodating: (1) groups that are faithful to the continuous spatial and temporal variation of K_{Neop}'s; and (2) the dynamics of both public macro-revisions and private micro-revisions so characteristic of oncopathological classification and diagnosis.

Opposed to *classification monism* is classification pluralism; the commonplace that, even in biological systematics, we parse a particular domain in many different ways depending upon our interests. The managerial and nonmanagerial classifications instantiate this principle in oncopathology.

Against this background, what is the role of the expert pathologist in a particular oncological domain? To answer this question we need to move beyond the naïve realist view of the expert as a trained but neutral observer reading off the structure of the world in a theory neutral way. This is all wrong. Oncological classification and diagnosis is a community activity and the expert plays an essential regulatory role in that community. Experts determine the correct usage of neoplastic kind terms; they are the arbiters of the taxonomic boundary disputes I alluded to above. Thus, the only Gold Standard is Expert Consensus and in the absence of that consensus, the 'right' answer is undefined. The *expert* is accomplished in many ways, but one of them is not the impossible task of identifying essences. When the expert says: "I have never seen an case of 'A' that had feature 'x'..." this is not to be construed as a claim about his special access to essences; it is to be taken as an convoluted expression of his taxonomic conventions. A more realistic claim is that the expert has refashioned the 'boundaries' of the entity (in some principled way, it is hoped) to accommodate the problematic case. The expert's classificatory vision has changed; he is both classifying and diagnosing at the same time.

Eventual Disappearance of Problem Cases

Naïve realism encourages the belief that with further work problem cases will eventually disappear. The perspective that this analysis provides, on the contrary, insures the persistence of hybrid, in-between, and unique cases; indeed, at a fine enough level of examination, all cases are problem cases. We can think of each type of problem case as an exaggeration of features central to typical I_{Neop}'s. *Hybrid cases* are, taxonomically speaking, *embarrassingly* heterogeneous either because they have reached back into their developmental history or, in their neoplastic maldevelopment, have taken all the forks in the road; *novel cases* are *embarrassingly* unique; *in-between cases* have tapped more shallowly into their developmental history in a way that has them phenotypically bridge two or more developmentally related standard trajectories for tissues in that anatomic site. Think of the neoplastic counterparts of the uterine cervical cells that have both glandular and squamous features. There is little hope that the flood of molecular-genetic data generated by the rapidly proliferating high-throughput technologies will change these facts of diagnostic and classificatory life. The central obstacle to this project is summarized by the historian Forrester: "*The ideal of science as certain knowledge is of course Aristotle's ideal. One version of how Aristotle's vision was finally contested and overthrown focuses on Darwinian evolution. The pre-Darwinian Aristotelian theory of the natural world is founded, it is argued, on the category or species, arranged hierarchically in order of generality. Darwin's fundamental break with the Aristotelian tradition was to see classes or species as constituted by populations of individuals which vary along an indefinite number of axes. ... the claim is that it is populations of independently varying individuals that constitute the base matter of the natural and human worlds. All categories or species are artificial, imprecise and ultimately misleading attempts to portray in the outmoded Aristotelian language of predication [that is, in crisp, unambiguous criteria] a fundamental dynamic reality which can be represented only statistically.*" [65]

What Does Our Analysis Mean for Evidence-Based Pathology?

EBP, whatever it turns out to be, must address the issues raised in this essay: the complexity of I_{Neop}'s; the ExtnI-CoPeTI structure of K_{Neop}'s and the creative role of the classifier-diagnostician. To the extent that EBP is chiefly concerned with managerial distinctions, EBM has much to teach us. While there are certainly no essences and extensional indeterminacy is a reality, continua can be discretized, for managerial purposes, in an arbitrary but principled ways. This theme is further elaborated in Chaps. 7 and 10 discussing validation and decision analysis.

Acknowledgment This chapter represents a precis of a book-length work in preparation expanding on these topics. I am indebted to Prof Charitini Douvaldzi (Stanford University) for invaluable discussions of this material.

References

1. Howard RA. Foundations of professional decision analysis: a Manuscript in process. Stanford Course Notes; 1998.
2. Klipp E, Liebermeister W, Wierling C, Kowald A, Lehrach H, Herwig R. Systems biology: a textbook. Wiley-VCH; 2009.
3. Wang E, editor. Cancer systems biology. Boca Raton: CRC Press; 2010.
4. Hanahan D, Iinberg RA. The hallmarks of cancer. Cell. 2000;100(1):57–70.
5. Vogelstein B, Kinzler KW. Cancer genes and the pathways they control. Nat Med. 2004;10(8):789–99.
6. Ledford H. Big science: the cancer genome challenge. Nature. 2010;464(7291):972–4.
7. Iinberg RA. Biology of cancer. New York: Garland Science; 2006.
8. Stratton MR, Campbell PJ, Futreal PA. The cancer genome. Nature. 2009;458(7239):719–24.
9. Stephens PJ, McBride DJ, Lin ML, et al. Complex landscapes of somatic rearrangement in human breast cancer genomes. Nature. 2009;462(7276):1005–10.
10. Folkman J. Role of angiogenesis in tumor growth and metastasis. Semin Oncol. 2002;29(6 Suppl 16):15–8.
11. Qian BZ, Pollard JW. Macrophage diversity enhances tumor progression and metastasis. Cell. 2010;141(1):39–51.
12. Polyak K. Breast cancer: origins and evolution. J Clin Invest. 2007;117(11):3155–63.
13. Polyak K, Kalluri R. The role of the microenvironment in mammary gland development and cancer. Cold Spring Harb Perspect Biol. 2010;2(11):a003244. Epub 2010 Jun 30.
14. Iigelt B, Bissell MJ. Unraveling the microenvironmental influences on the normal mammary gland and breast cancer. Semin Cancer Biol. 2008;18(5):311–21.
15. Merlo LM, Pepper JW, Reid BJ, Maley CC. Cancer as an evolutionary and ecological process. Nat Rev Cancer. 2006;6(12):924–35.
16. Navin N, Krasnitz A, Rodgers L, et al. Inferring tumor progression from genomic heterogeneity. Genome Res. 2010;20(1):68–80.
17. Marusyk A, Polyak K. Tumor heterogeneity: causes and consequences. Biochim Biophys Acta. 2010;1805(1):105–17.

18. Navin NE, Hicks J. Tracing the tumor lineage. Mol Oncol. 2010;4(3):267–83.
19. Nowel PC. The clonal evolution of tumor cell populations. Science. 1976;194(4260):23–8.
20. Mintz B, Welmensee K. Normal genetically mosaic mice produced from malignant teratocarcinoma cells. Proc Natl Acad Sci U S A. 1975;72(9):3585–9.
21. Hofmann WK, Komor M, Wassmann B, et al. Presence of the BCR-ABL mutation Glu255Lys prior to STI571 (imatinib) treatment in patients with Ph+ acute lymphoblastic leukemia. Blood. 2003;102(2):659–61.
22. Roche-Lestienne C, Soenen-Cornu V, Grardel-Duflos N, et al. Several types of mutations of the Abl gene can be found in chronic myeloid leukemia patients resistant to STI571, and they can pre-exist to the onset of treatment. Blood. 2002;100(3):1014–8.
23. Shah NP, Nicoll JM, Nagar B, et al. Multiple BCR-ABL kinase domain mutations confer polyclonal resistance to the tyrosine kinase inhibitor imatinib (STI571) in chronic phase and blast crisis chronic myeloid leukemia. Cancer Cell. 2002;2(2):117–25.
24. Corless CL, Heinrich MC. Molecular pathobiology of gastrointestinal stromal sarcomas. Annu Rev Pathol. 2008;3:557–86.
25. Gramza AW, Corless CL, Heinrich MC. Resistance to tyrosine kinase inhibitors in gastrointestinal stromal tumors. Clin Cancer Res. 2009;15(24):7510–8.
26. Liegl B, Kepten I, Le C, et al. Heterogeneity of kinase inhibitor resistance mechanisms in GIST. J Pathol. 2008;216(1):64–74.
27. Solé RV, Deisboeck TS. An error catastrophe in cancer? J Theor Biol. 2004;228(1):47–54.
28. Solé R, Goodwin B. Signs of life: how complexity pervades biology. New York: HarperCollins Publishers; 2002.
29. Nowak MA. Evolutionary dynamics. Exploring the equations of life. Cambridge: The Belknap Press of Harvard University Press; 2006.
30. Mas A, Lopez-Galindez C, Cacho I, Gomez J, Martinez MA. Unfinished stories on viral quasispecies and Darwinian views of evolution. J Mol Biol. 2010;397(4):865–77.
31. Ereshefsky M. Species. Stanford: Stanford Encyclopedia of Philosophy; 2010.
32. Frigg R, Hartmann S. Models in science. Stanford: Stanford Encyclopedia of Philosophy; 2006.
33. Giere RN. Scientific perspectivism. Chicago: University Of Chicago Press; 2006.
34. Gould SJ. Wonderful Life: the Burgess Shale and the nature of history. New York: W. W. Norton; 1989.
35. Bartels PH. Future directions in quantitative pathology: digital knowledge in diagnostic pathology. J Clin Pathol. 2000;53(1):31–7.
36. Mehta T, Tanik M, Allison DB. Towards sound epistemological foundations of statistical methods for high-dimensional biology. Nat Genet. 2004;36(9):943–7.
37. Russell B. Vagueness. In: Keefe R, Smith P, editors. Vagueness: a reader Cambridge. MA: The MIT Press; 1999.
38. Beckner M. The biological way of thought. New York: Columbia Univ Press; 1959.
39. Lakoff G. Women, fire, and dangerous things. Chicago: University of Chicago Press; 1987.
40. Margolis E, Laurence S. Concepts and cognitive science. Concepts: core readings. Cambridge: The MIT Press; 1999. p. 3–81.
41. Rosch E. Principles of categorization. Cognition and categorization. Hillsdale: Lawrence Erlbaum Associates; 1978. p. 312–22.
42. Vineis P. Definition and classification of cancer: monothetic or polythetic? Theor Med. 1993;14(3):249–56.
43. Wittgenstein L. Philosophical investigations. New York: Macmillan; 1953.
44. Gould SJ. The Hedgehog, the Fox, and the Magister's Pox: Mending the Gap Between Science and the Humanities: Harmony; 2003.
45. Kuhn TS. The structure of scientific revolutions. Chicago: The University of Chicago Press; 1962.
46. Kuhn TS. The Copernican revolution: planetary astronomy in the development of western thought. Cambridge, Massachusetts: Harvard University Press; 1976.
47. Dorfman RF. Classifications of the malignant lymphomas. Am J Surg Pathol. 1977;1(2):167–70.
48. Hendrickson MR, Kempson RL. Reply: the citadel defended-The counterattack. Hum Pathol. 2000; 31(11):1440–2.
49. Kempson RL, Hendrickson MR. Ovarian serous borderline tumors: the citadel defended [editorial; comment]. Hum Pathol. 2000;31(5):525–6.
50. Seidman JD, Kurman RJ. Ovarian serous borderline tumors: a critical review of the literature with emphasis on prognostic indicators [see comments]. Hum Pathol. 2000;31(5):539–57.
51. Seidman JD, Soslow RA, Vang R, et al. Borderline ovarian tumors: diverse contemporary viewpoints on terminology and diagnostic criteria with illustrative images. Hum Pathol. 2004;35(8):918–33.
52. Kurman RJ, Seidman JD. Ovarian serous borderline tumors: the citadel defended. Hum Pathol. 2000; 31(11):1439–42.
53. Bartels PH, Montironi R. Quantitative histopathology: the evolution of a scientific field. Anal Quant Cytol Histol. 2009;31(1):1–4.
54. Fisher C. Synovial sarcoma. Ann Diagn Pathol. 1998;2(6):401–21.
55. van de Rijn M, Barr FG, Xiong QB, Hedges M, Shipley J, Fisher C. Poorly differentiated synovial sarcoma: an analysis of clinical, pathologic, and molecular genetic features. Am J Surg Pathol. 1999;23(1): 106–12.
56. Krane JF, Bertoni F, Fletcher CD. Myxoid synovial sarcoma: an underappreciated morphologic subset. Mod Pathol. 1999;12(5):456–62.
57. Hull DL. The effect of essentialism on taxonomy – two thousand years of stasis (I). Br J Philos Sci. 1964;61:314–26.
58. Hull DL. The effect of essentialism on taxonomy – two thousand years of stasis (II). Br J Philos Sci. 1965;16(61):1–18.

59. Hull D, Ruse M. The philosophy of biology. Oxford: Oxford University Press; 1998.
60. Boyd R. Homeostasis, species, and higher taxa. Species: new interdisciplinary essays. Cambridge: The MIT Press; 1999. p. 141–86.
61. Boyd R. Scientific realism. Stanford: Stanford Encyclopedia of Philosophy; 2002.
62. Keller RA, Boyd R, Wheeler QD. The illogical basis of phylogenetic nomenclature. Bot Rev. 2003;69(1): 93–111.
63. Chiong W. Brain death without definitions. Hastings Cent Rep. 2005;35(6):20–30.
64. Wilson RA. Genes and the agents of life. The individual in the fragile sciences – biology. Cambridge: Cambridge University Press; 2005.
65. Forrester J. If p, then what? Thinking in cases. Hist Human Sci. 1996;9(3):1–25.
66. Oltvai ZN, Barabási AL. Systems biology. Life's complexity pyramid. Science. 2002;298(5594):763–4.
67. Dalton LW, Pinder SE, Elston CE, et al. Histologic grading of breast cancer: linkage of patient outcome with level of pathologist agreement. Mod Pathol. 2000;13(7):730–5.
68. Elston CW, Ellis IO. Pathological prognostic factors in breast cancer. I. The value of histological grade in breast cancer: experience from a large study with long-term follow-up. Histopathology. 1991;19(5):403–10.
69. Crombie AC. Styles of Scientific Thinking in the European Tradition. The history of argument and explanation especially in the mathematical and biomedical sciences and arts. London: Duckworth; 1994.
70. Hacking I. Style for historians and philosophers. Historical ontology. Cambridge: Harvard University Press; 2002. p. 159–77.
71. Hendrickson M. Exorcizing Schrödinger's ghost: reflections on what is life? And its surprising relevance to cancer biology. In: Gumbrecht HU, Harrison R, editors. Schrodinger. Palo Alto: Stanford University Press; 2010.

Evaluating Oncopathological Studies: The Need to Evaluate the Internal and External Validity of Study Results

7

Michael Hendrickson and Bonnie Balzer

Keywords
Evaluation of oncopathological studies • Prognostic classification rules • Evidence-based pathology • Validity of study results • Gene expression arrays

Published oncopathological studies purport to tell us not only how the world appears to the investigator but makes the stronger additional claim that the world will look the same way to us. What guarantees are there that the data presented by the investigator justifies his view of the world? The term *'internal validity'* captures this worry. Threats to internal validity can be grouped into problems related to either chance or bias. *Chance issues*: did the investigators look at a large enough sample to develop an accurate picture of the domain they are describing? This is the statistician's problem of Type I/II error, study power and sample size calculations. Worries of this sort are allayed by maximizing the sample size. Another question: is their picture of the world more nuanced and detailed than their data warrants? This is the problem of 'over-fitting' and has at its heart the 'curse of dimensionality.' This problem is particularly acute for the high dimensional data produced by –omics research. The simple, but sometimes unrealistic, cure for this worry is the validation of the study's conclusions using a completely different set of cases drawn from the relevant domain. In the absence of such an independent sample, there are a number of cross-validation techniques that can partially address this problem. *Bias* refers to the systematic erroneous association of some characteristic with a group in a way that distorts a comparison with another group. Bias is directly addressed through the appropriate design of experimental studies and by randomization in clinical interventional trials; there are no such safeguards in non-experimental observational research. *Investigator intra-observer and inter-observer agreement*: No two pathologists have (in the language of Chap. 6) an identical classificatory vision. Are there important differences among the investigators in their agreement on the morphologic evaluations presented in the study?

External validity: What guarantees are there that the investigator's view of the world will be ours? The study may pass internal validity tests but the vision it provides may have little to do with the world as we will perceive it. This is a question about generalizability, or 'external validity.' For example, one may question whether valid conclusions drawn from a study of cases extracted from the expert pathologist's files have much to do with community pathology practice.

M. Hendrickson (✉)
Department of Pathology, Stanford University Medical Center, Stanford, CA 94305, USA
e-mail: hendrickson@stanford.edu

A.M. Marchevsky and M.R. Wick (eds.), *Evidence Based Pathology and Laboratory Medicine*,
DOI 10.1007/978-1-4419-1030-1_7, © Springer Science+Business Media, LLC 2011

Table 7.1 Evaluation of an oncopathological study

Overall study design	
	Managerial claim study?
	Scientific claim study?
	Unsupervised or supervised classification
Internal validity	
	Chance
	Is sample size adequate?
	Is the data overfitted?
	Biases
	Missing data bias
	Short follow-up bias
	Referral (selection) bias
	Spectrum bias
	Confounding factor bias
	Verification bias
External validity	
	Can the results of this study be generalized to other cases?
Communicability	
	Observer agreement among the authors
	Communication of classificatory vision to potential users
	Were the morphologic distinctions described in the study communicated successfully?
Relevance to the reader	
	Are the study results of practical significance to my practice?

Another problem central to oncopathological studies is the *communication* of the investigator's 'classificatory vision'. As discussed in *Chapter 6*, surgical pathology C&D is, obviously, a highly visual, impressionistic activity and passing from the visual to the conceptual and verbal poses challenges not faced by other clinical disciplines. Failure to communicate the relevant morphological criteria can occur at several levels and may undermine the impact of an otherwise valid study.

In this chapter we will survey these topics (Table 7.1). For narrative convenience we depart from the strict outline of the table at various points. We will draw upon several Stanford gynecologic pathology studies to make these points. We do this, not to slight other workers, but because these are the problems with which we have most hands on experience. We finish with a brief overview of the substantial informatics problems faced by genomic studies.

The Overall Design of an Oncopathological Study

What Is the Goal of the Study? Managerial Classification or Something Else?

As discussed in Chap. 6, it is important in oncopathology to distinguish between those studies whose purpose is to make serious risk/prognostic/predictive (RPP) claims – future clinical course or clinical phenotype, $\Phi_{Clin}(t)$ for short – and those that do not. Histogenetic classifications, an example of a scientific classification and managerial classifications, are quite different on a number of counts. Histogenetic modeling involves postulating a number of plausible mechanism that produce the observed phenotypes of the neoplasms in a given domain (see Fig. 6.7 and related discussion). For managerial classifications the taxonomic modeling exercise now takes the form of fashioning statistically credible, distinct lotteries by dividing, in a suitable way, a multivariate continuum (Figs. 6.12–6.14).

The first step in analyzing a oncopathological report is to have a clear idea of the investigator's intent and the type of classification modeling in which the authors are engaged. Is the study presenting an interesting new neoplastic type or kind (K_{Neop}) ("stroll through the phenospace") or perhaps a new K_{Neop} with some comments on clinical outcome but, with no serious managerial claim? Or, is the study making a serious managerial claim? These usually conclude with something like: "It's essential that you make this distinction or patients will be disadvantaged!"

Supervised and Unsupervised Classification Models

The managerial/nonmanagerial distinction can be sharpened by turning to the machine learning contrast between *supervised* and *unsupervised* classification. Supervised learning is the task of inferring a classification rule from a "supervising" *training set*. That is, the observed features are partitioned into "predictors" (typically, individual gross or histomorphologic features) and "outcomes" (some aspect of $\Phi_{Clin}(t)$). The training set consists of a set of cases with known outcomes. A supervised learning algorithm analyzes the training data and, with one eye on the outcome, uses the predictors to group cases that concentrate, for example, "good actors" and "bad actors"; that is, it produces a classification rule, almost invariably with some misclassification rate. The hope is that the classification rule will predict the correct outcome for any collection of unexamined cases *test sets* in the domain. Realization of this hope requires the learning algorithm to accurately generalize from the training data to unseen situations encountered in the test set. Again, there is always a misclassification rate, and almost always the misclassification rate is higher for the test set than for the training set.

In unsupervised classification, on the other hand, all observed features are taken as an unpartitioned ensemble and a search is undertaken for "natural" grouping or clustering in the data. Despite its apparent objectivity ('letting the observations speak for themselves') this is not, by any means, a theory-free process. These techniques require substantial input from the investigator: among other things, the selection of the individuals to be studied, the features to be examined (or not), the scales used to evaluate those features, statistical pre-processing of those measurements, to normalize them or not, a choice of similarity metric (e.g., Eulidean, Mahalanobis), a choice of clustering techniques, a specification of the number of clusters the investigator thinks is present in the data, a specification of a threshold for forming groups, the kind of intracluster structure one is looking for (e.g., Gaussian), etc. Cluster analysis in its various forms is the tool employed in unsupervised classification [1–3].

Recasting in these terms, our original question about the oncopathological study under examination, then, is: "Is this study, structurally, some version of supervised or unsupervised classification and, if supervised, is the supervising feature some $\Phi_{Clin}(t)$?"

Exploratory and confirmatory statistics and computers

The advent of high-speed computation, made exploratory data analysis possible. Exploratory data analysis (EDA) is an approach to analyzing data for the purpose of suggesting hypotheses worth testing. EDA complements the tools of classical statistics designed to test hypotheses. No longer were statisticians' analyses confined to hypothesis testing using mathematically tractable parametric techniques (e.g., normal distribution theory), but they could examine high-dimensional data using nonparametric computer intensive techniques. Exploratory data analysis of high dimensional data sets brought with it the need for directly visualizing this data in a perspicuous and convenient way [4]. Through the use of rotating scatter plots, color coding, the use of a variety of symbols, high-dimensional data could be examined and manipulated. These capabilities are now standard in laptop statistical programs like JMP or StatView and plots of this sort appear routinely in the -omic literature.

We have employed these techniques in several Stanford studies since the 1980s. The graphics used in our study of problematic uterine smooth muscle neoplasms (Fig. 7.1) and our study of serous low malignant potential tumors (Fig. 7.2) illustrate this point.

Diagnostic and Predictive Components of Oncopathological Studies

Oncopathological observational studies inherit all the methodological complications of clinical observational studies [5, 6] but have the added special problems of reproducibly making and communicating histopathological distinctions.

For the purposes of this discussion, we can distinguish the predictive components of the study (internal and external validity) and the diagnostic component (investigator observer agreement and the translation and transmission problems peculiar to oncopathological communications).

The Predictive Component: Internal and External Validity

Anatomic surgical pathology is a largely regulation-free discipline; we do our own policing. There is no FDA oversight of conventional light microscopic distinctions that are employed routinely in

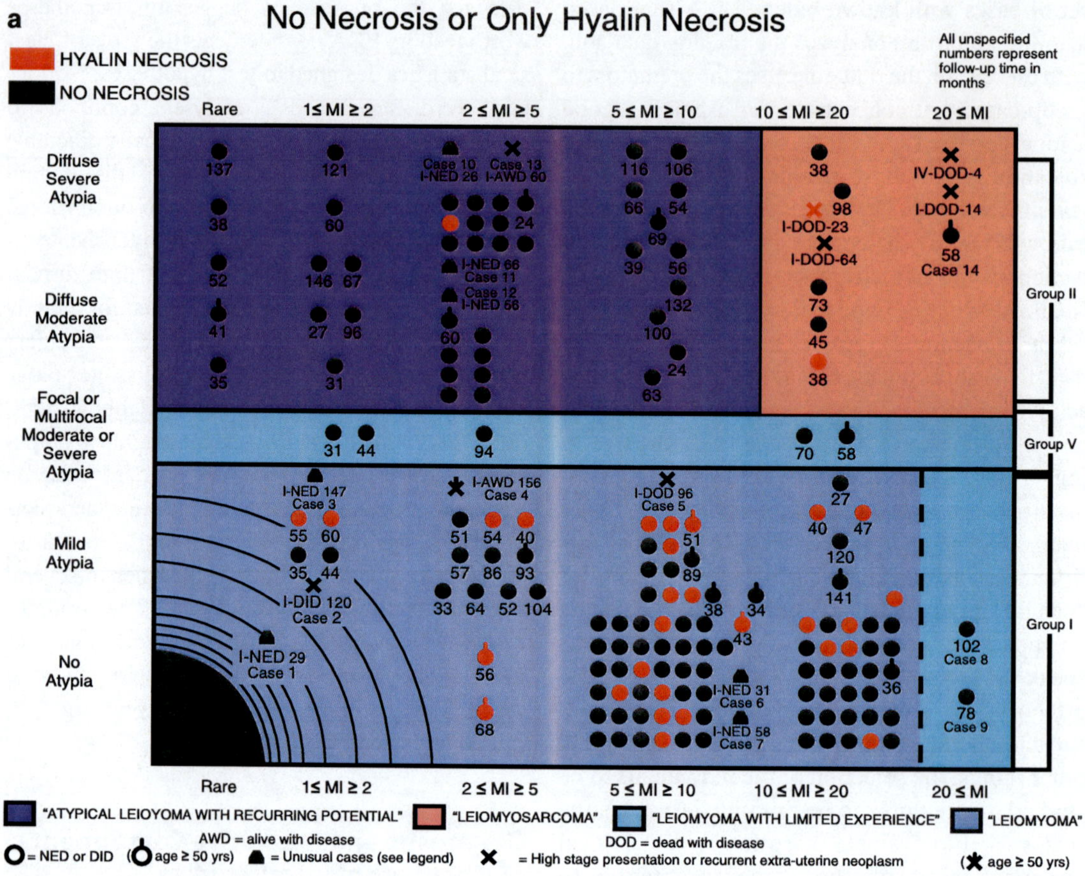

Fig. 7.1 Uterine smooth muscle charts. Taking the two plots together, six dimensions of data are depicted; our assignments (color coding of regions of the phenospace) are a seventh. Graphical displays preserving the covariance structure of the data set and are easier to assimilate than entries in a complex table [71]. We employed *contour lines* to make clear important exclusion from this study. In the no-necrosis/hyaline-necrosis plot the *bottom left contour lines* remind us of the Mt. Everest of mitotically inactive leiomyomas not included in the study that serve to put "benign metastasizing leiomyoma" in its proper context. In the coagulative tumor cell necrosis plot, the *bottom left* reminds the reader of the large number of acutely infarcted leiomyomas not included in the study and the *top right contour lines*, the larger number of diagnostically nonproblematic leiomyosarcomas that were not part of the study group

patient care decision-making or, for that matter (as the disclaimer on all our surgical pathology reports makes explicit), immunohistochemical tests. Treatment recommendations are often made on the basis of what, in the cancer marker world, would be Level 4–5 (Level 1, being the best) evidence. By contrast, prognostic and predictive gene expression array (GEA) markers have received intense scrutiny. In the service of evidence-based reasoning in pathology, it is useful to start thinking of proffered $\Phi_{\text{Clin}}(t)$ claims within the framework of cancer marker studies and clinical prediction rules.

The evidentiary rules for *cancer marker studies* have been extensively discussed in the recent literature by Hayes and his group and others [7–11]. Table 7.2 provides a list designed for GEA markers. How would these apply to oncopathological classification using conventional light microscopic features? A variant of breast cancer is reported: "A distinctive clinicopathological entity … with a particularly good (or bad) prognosis: report of 54 cases." This can be framed as a prognostic cancer marker claim. Questions to ask: (1) really? – validity issues; and (2) am I better off with this marker than the -existing ones? What is the incremental

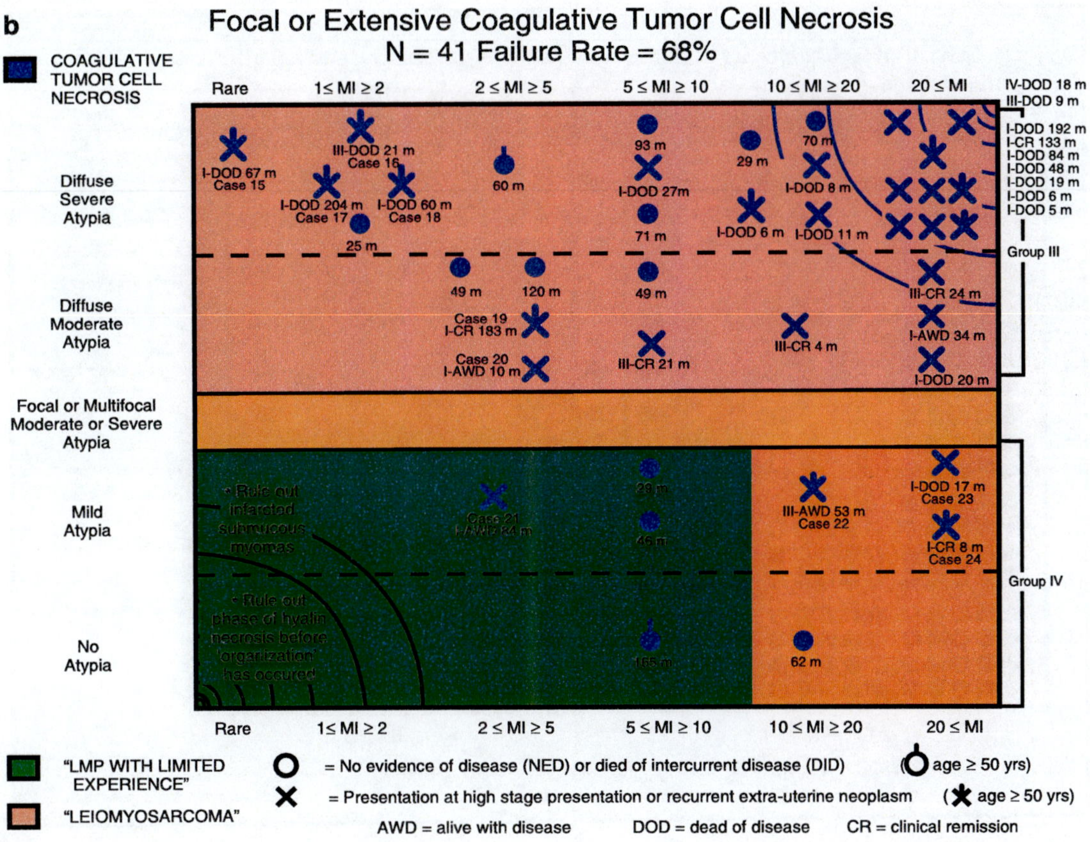

Fig. 7.1 (continued)

Φ_{Clin}(t) insight from this classification over and above the classifications I usually employ? Would the usual grading scheme have picked up this difference? These are the basic questions addressed in the cancer marker analytic literature.

Clinical prognostic models use a variety of patient descriptors to fashion a multivariate classification rule that assigns the patient to an outcome category, for example, low, intermediate, and high risk. Examples include the Nottingham prognostic index to estimate the long-term risk of cancer recurrence or death in breast cancer patients [12]. The notions of training set/test set, overfitting, validation, curse of dimensionality, etc. permeate the analytic literature in this area. Several brief, accessible introductions to prognostic models have appeared recently [13–18]. An introduction to multivariate statistics is provided by Katz [19, 20].

The histopathologic version of this takes as predictors a variety of gross and histological features and plays them off against a specified Φ_{Clin}(t). For example, the Stanford study attempting to fashion a clinically relevant morphologic definition of well-differentiated endometrial adenocarcinoma was cast in the format of a prognostic model using myoinvasion as a surrogate for clinically relevant disease [21]. All promising H&E features were recorded and, with the aid of CART feature selection and validation, a subset was selected that optimally concentrated myoinvasive positive/negative cases. Other examples are provided by various multivariate classification rules using gross and histological features to separate adrenal cortical neoplasms into clinically benign and malignant groups [22] and sorting thymomas into prognostically relevant histopathological groups [23–26].

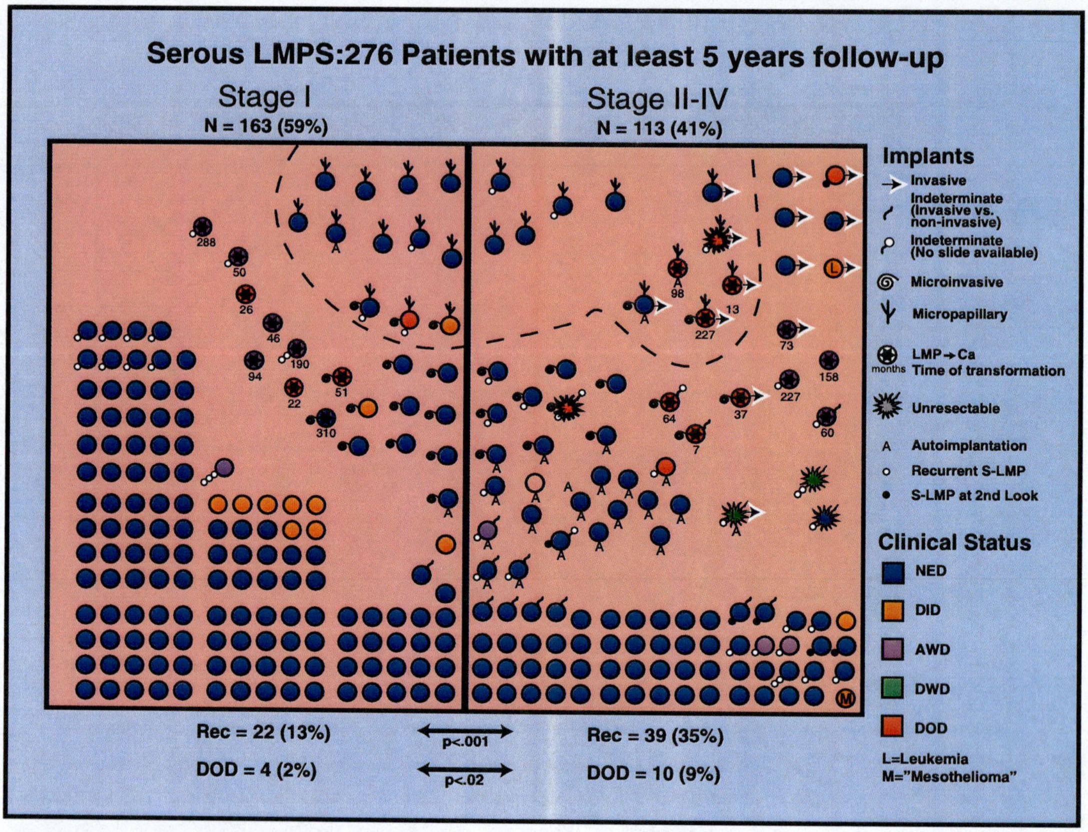

Fig. 7.2 Ovarian serous low malignant potential tumors (S-LMPs). In this figure, the abscissa and ordinate serve nonnumeric functions: low stage vs. high stage and, roughly, "interesting" and "uninteresting case." All of the cases in the study are represented; most of the cases are, from the perspective of our study goals, relevant only in making clear important denominators. The *top part* of the plot is used to spread out cases of interest: those exhibiting microinvasion, micropapillary features, those that transitioned to well-differentiated carcinoma, the character of the implants, etc. These are represented by symbols; color codes for clinical outcome. Again, we have preserved the covariance structure of the data; for example, the covariation of micropapillary features and microinvasion. An additional advantage of this sort of representation is that the reader can query our database. A glance provides the reader with the distribution of our cases and an idea of the confidence one can have in statistics relating to specific subgroups of cases. A picture is, it turns out, worth more than a thousand words [72]

Critical Evaluation of the Validity of Oncopathological Studies

The critical evaluation of an oncopathological study involves answering five questions: (1) What was the role of chance in producing the claimed results (issues of sample size and overfitting)? (2) Are biases implicated in producing the results (e.g., selection bias, spectrum bias, confounding factors)? (3) Can the results of this study be generalized to other cases? (4) Were the morphologic distinctions described in the study communicated successfully? (5) Are the study results of practical significance?

Sampling Issue: What Has Been Included in the Study? Carving Out the Study Group from the Larger Domain

Using the metaphor of the phenospace developed in Chap. 6, we can think of the investigator's study group as being formed by carving a (high dimensional) patch out of the phenospace. This patch will include cases exhibiting features over a certain multivariate range and will exclude cases falling outside those ranges. Fig. 6.12 of invasive ducal carcinomas conveys this image.

Table 7.2 Study design

What is the goal of the study?	Descriptive ("stroll through the phenospace")? Correlated feature? Managerial claim?
Type of data collection	Retrospective Prospective
Sample size	Is the sample sufficiently large to detect in a statistically credible way the difference claimed (or, alternatively) not found?
Sampling method	Sample of convenience Stratified sampling Random sampling
Study material	What has been included? What is the spectrum of cases? What has been excluded?

Evaluation of the phenospace being evaluated in the study raises the following general questions: What is the spectrum of cases included in the study? What did the investigators' cases look like? What features were regarded as criterial? Were some features more important than others? What were salient but noncriterial features? What is required is a multivariate representation that preserves the covariance structure of the case data and, in particular, links the clinical outcome with each case.

Another Sampling Issue: What Was Excluded from the Study?

As discussed above, the entity the investigator is reporting is embedded in a study is typically only part of a larger phenospace. The question of what was left out is particularly important when the investigators are making a managerial claim. How was the cut made along the boundaries delimiting "good actors" and "bad actors" within this sample? These distinctions are usually found in the differential diagnosis section in the discussion section of the paper. That discussion should go beyond reporting the typical features of the contrasted entity; rather, it is more helpful to discuss the resolution of problem cases at that boundary and how the authors resolved them. The uterine smooth muscle scatter plot makes these cuts explicit in Fig. 7.1. *Venn diagrams* provide another tool for depicting high-dimensional data in two dimensions and seldom represent more than three dichotomous variates. The British mathematician A. W. F. Edwards developed a simple method of generalizing Venn diagrams to higher dimensions [27, 28]. Fig. 7.3 illustrates one use.

Yet Another Sampling Issue: Is the Sample Large Enough to Support the Study's Conclusions?

More experience is better than less experience. This simple thought elaborated in the hypothesis testing framework yields the mathematically sophisticated apparatus of sample size calculations; the number of cases required to detect a specified difference between two groups [29–31]. The statistical hypothesis model is set out in Fig. 7.4. The behavioral psychologist have identified inattention to the importance of sample size as the belief in the "law of small numbers"; that, for example, the averages calculated from small samples are as good as those derived from large samples [32]. The essentialism discussed in Chap. 6 appears to ground this belief. After all, says the confirmed essentialist, you don't need many cases to identify the clinicopathologic essence of a particular K_{Neop}. Symptomatic of small sample size problems are the outcome statistics of series with small number of cases – rare diseases especially – yield unstable measures of clinical outcome; "survival ranges from 20 to 80%": translation, "you almost certainly will be cured of this disease," or "you almost certainly will die of this disease." For example, the large and conflicting literature about the prognostic relevance of heterologous elements in malignant mixed tumors of the uterus is based on studies with few subjects. Prognoses, from these underpowered studies, for tumors with various types of heterologous elements studies ranged from "very bad" to "irrelevant" to "good." It took a large GOG study of clinical stage I cases to begin to sort this out [33].

The lesson: if a serious claim is made about differences in prognosis between two tumor types, it should be against the background of sample size calculations. How many cases would need to be studied to establish, in a statistically credible way, the claimed RPP difference? A related issue is the problem of testing *multiple hypotheses*; this is particularly a problem for high-dimensional data.

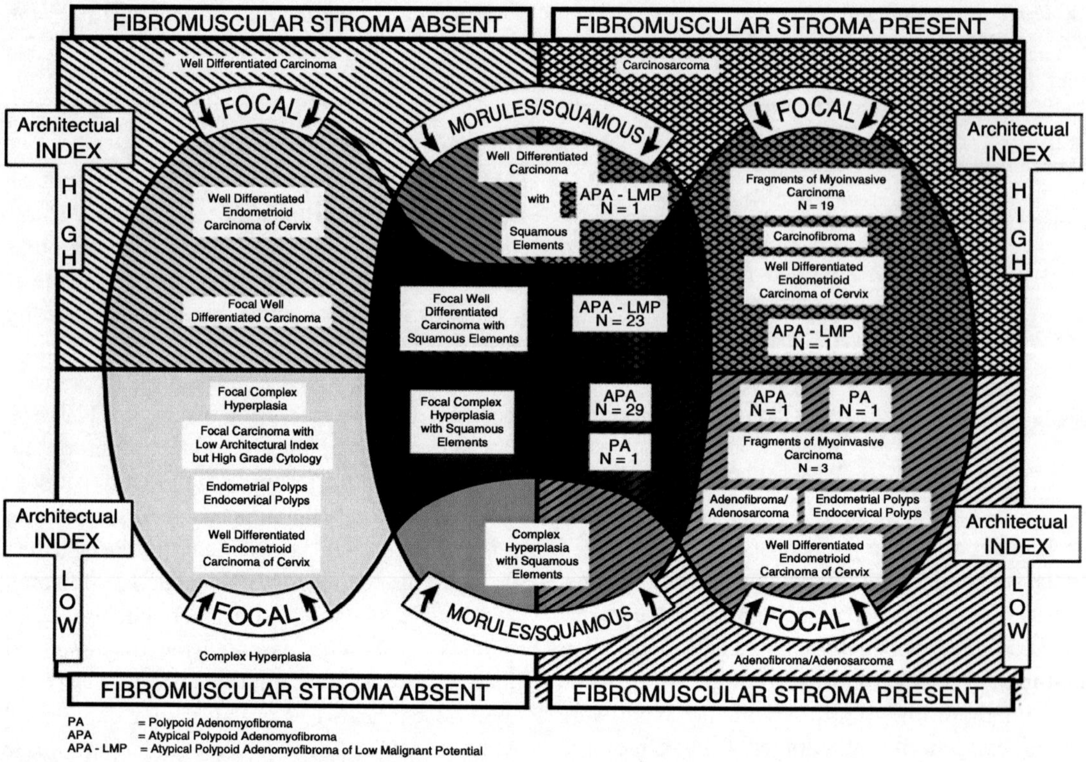

Fig. 7.3 The atypical polypoid adenomyofibroma study: differential diagnosis Venn diagram. We used a four variates Venn diagram to depict the differential diagnosis of atypical polypoid adenomyofibroma. In each of the cells defined by this partition, we list the differential diagnostic possibilities. Four morphologic features are depicted: (**a**) architectural index (*top half*, high; *bottom half*, low); (**b**) the presence of a prominent fibromuscular stroma (*right half of rectangle*) or its absence (*left half of rectangle*); (**c**) the focality of the process (*inside dumbbell*, focal; *outside dumbbell*, diffuse) manifest in the hysterectomy specimen as focality and in a sampling as dimorphism; and (**d**) the presence of squamous or morular differentiation (*inside central oval*) or its absence (*outside central oval*). The presence or absence of each of these four features defines 16 different morphological combinations. The diagnostic possibilities that correspond to these patterns are set out in the appropriate overlap regions. In summary, this diagram both indicates differential diagnostic possibilities and the 'carving out' process that resulted in our study group [73]

Is the Level of Detail of the Conclusions Unrealistic Given the Sample Size?

Less well appreciated than underpowered studies is the problem of *overfitting*. More information about a fixed number of cases may not be better when it comes to forecasting a $\Phi_{Clin}(t)$. That is, the addition of refinements (new features) to a classification rule recorded from a fixed number of cases may be unhelpful. Recall the discussion of training and test sets above. The problem is with "overfitting" the training set; that is, providing too elaborate a characterization of the study group used in training the classification rule. This would be fine if the world was exactly like the sample, sadly, it is not [34]. This is a serious problem for high dimensional biology (HDB) (see below) but also a problem for the lower dimensional biology of histopathological prediction rules.

The simple (but often unrealistic) remedy for overfitting is the *validation* of the classifier using a completely different set of cases. Some protection against overfitting is provided by *cross-validation*. The method involves sequentially leaving out parts of the original sample ("split-sample") and conducting a classifier; the process is repeated until the entire sample has been assessed. The results are combined into a final

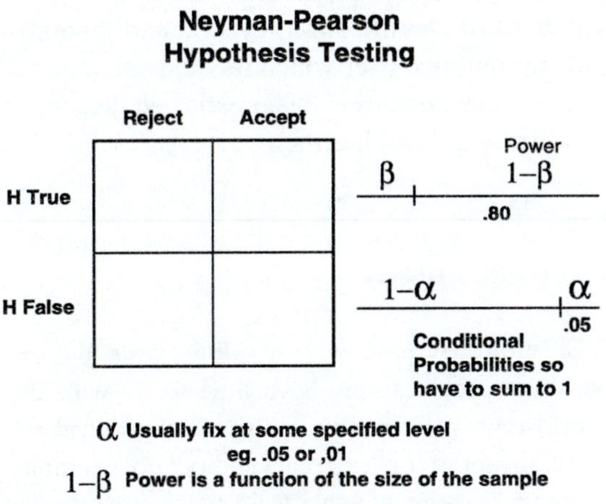

Fig. 7.4 Type I and Type II errors in α 2×2 table. The hypothesis is that a difference exists between two groups. Type I α error amounts to the erroneous conclusion that there is a difference between compared groups when no difference exists. We can think of it as the false discovery rate. Similarly, type II error (β error) is the false-negative conclusion that there is no difference when, in fact, a difference does exist. Power is defined as (1−β); the probability of correctly identifying a difference. The probabilities of these two kinds of error are parameters that are set by the investigator. Typical choices are: $\alpha=0.05$ and $(1-\beta)=0.80$. While neither error can ever entirely be avoided, a simple method to decrease their probability is to increase the sample size. Interestingly (and controversially), Ioannidis by analyzing the logic behind hypothesis testing and the usual choices for the size of type I and II errors (controversially) concluded that most published studies produced false conclusions [36]

model that is the product of the training step [34]. CART (classification and regression tree analysis) incorporates cross-validation as it constructs an optimal decision tree [35]. We used CART in our study of endometrial carcinoma [21]. The exploratory tree (constructed using all of the data in the training set in all its particularity) was very elaborate and contains dozens of nodes; cross-validation typically prunes the tree down to three or four nodes.

Effect of Missing Data

Missing data can be fatal to the conclusions of the study, or not. Certainly, studies that make serious $\Phi_{Clin}(t)$ claims and are missing much of the follow-up information are suspect. This also applies to important potentially confounding factors that would bear on $\Phi_{Clin}(t)$: size of tumor, location, resectability, etc.

Bias

Bias refers to the systematic erroneous association of some characteristic with a group in a way that distorts a comparison with another group. Ioannidis defines bias as "the combination of various design, data, analysis, and presentation factors that tend to produce research findings when they should not be produced [36]." Vineis defines bias as "results that are the consequence of an erroneous study design [37]." There is a substantial epidemiology literature on dozens of forms of bias; most of these are not directly relevant to biases in the oncopathological literature [38].

Bias is directly addressed through the appropriate design of experimental studies and by randomization in clinical interventional trials, but there are no such safeguards in nonexperimental observational research.

Short Follow-up Bias: This is a particularly important source of bias, obviously, for studies of neoplasms that have a long clinical course. Examples from gynecologic pathology include serous borderline surface epithelial neoplasms, endometrial stromal neoplasms, and granulosa cell tumors. For example, the initial impression of granulosa tumors was that they were clinically benign, but longer follow-up studies from Britain and Scandinavia disabused us of this notion. So, short follow-up of such neoplasms yields misleadingly high relapse-free survival estimates.

Referral (Selection) Bias and Spectrum Bias: It is a commonplace that university practice differs substantially from community practice. It follows that emptying the consultants' files at a university center will yield a different set of cases than a comparable emptying of the community pathologist's files. The bias reflects that fact that consultants tend not to get straightforward cases (so atypical cases are overrepresented) and university oncology units tend to get therapeutically challenging cases (so bad actors tend to be overrepresented)

In general, there is an overrepresentation of difficult cases and clinically malignant cases. For example, the natural history of leiomyosarcoma as depicted in the Stanford study is completely atypical; the number of young women is way out of proportion to national age distributions for this disease. Reason: pathologists send in cases from young women for verification. In summary, the spectrum of cases reported reflects the accrual practices of the institution (either the clinical services or the consultation practice of the pathologist) both in terms of recruitment into the study and the spectrum of clinical outcomes in the study group.

Confounding Factors: We discussed in Chap. 6 the myth of histopathologic determinism. Another way of thinking about this is in terms of confounding factors. One has the impression from some of our morphological literature that the only phenotypic feature that matters for a patient is the histopathologic phenotype of her I_{Neop}. The huge success of the TNM staging system reminds us of the importance of nonhistopathological features in determining $\Phi_{Clin}(t)$.

Verification Bias: There is a straightforward question to be asked of a study: Were the cases all diagnosed in the same way? Did the reviewing pathologist see all the cases? If immunohistochemistry played a role in case assignment, was this performed on all cases?

However, there are deeper issues at play here that we can illustrate with the example of marker studies. We need to distinguish two different scenarios. First, studies that promote a marker for distinguishing two, in principle, separable but phenotypically overlapping clusters (say, distinguishing primary from metastatic mucinous carcinomas of the ovary). There is a fact of the matter determined in a methodologically independent way; there is, or is not, a primary in the place predicted by the marker. Here, talk of test characteristics: sensitivity, specificity, etc. make sense. The second situation, concerns markers, claimed to clear up some muddled region of a phenospace, for example, poorly (or undifferentiated) mesenchymal neoplasms of the uterus. Here we find ourselves dealing with issues (discussed in Chap. 6) of classification revision and theoretical stipulations, over which the relevant experts may or may not agree. Diagnostic test discourse is weirdly out of place here.

External Validity

The study may pass internal validity tests, but the vision it provides may have little to do with the world as we will perceive it. This is a question about generalizability, or "external validity." For example, one may question whether valid conclusions drawn from a study of cases extracted from the expert pathologist's files have much to do with community pathology practice.

Relevance

Assume that the chance and bias hurdles have been satisfactorily addressed. We are left with the question of the relevance of the study to general practice. Would my patient's tumor have been included in this study and do the summary statistics reported in the study apply to my patient? Oncopathological studies should, and usually do, include relevant nonhistopathological features: age, gender, comorbidity, symptoms, gross features, details of treatment, etc.

Clinicopathology is a work in progress

Typically, in the course of delineating the feature of a K_{Neop} over time, initial studies have had limited generalizability. In time a fuller picture of the K_{Neop}'s neighborhood in the phenospace emerges, and the morphologic spectrum of the K_{Neop} becomes clearer. It may be that the clinical aggressiveness of a K_{Neop} is overestimated (e.g., aggressive angiomyxoma), or the diagnostic significance of a particular pattern is overestimated (the myxoid pattern for uterine myxoid leiomyosarcoma) by a failure to attend to K_{Neop}s in the neighborhood. Thus, external validity is incremental; later studies typically review earlier studies and modify their conclusions accordingly. Explorations of the phenospace are always works in progress. This is very reminiscent of the decay of marker test characteristics over time [7–11].

Other Diagnostic Issues in Oncopathological Studies: The Communicative Component

Reproducibility of the assessment of features or classifications employed in the study

How do we know that the investigators agreed on the morphological evaluations detailed in the study? Intraobserver and interobserver disagreement is common in daily diagnostic life – the great scandal of diagnostic anatomic pathology – and well documented in our literature. The assessment of cytological atypia in endometrial hyperplasia, an important managerial distinction, is a notorious example [39].

Translation and Transmission of the Investigator's Classificatory Vision

Another important question is how effectively did the paper communicate the classificatory vision of the authors? What compromises my ability to imitate the investigators in my diagnostic work when confronted with a case that would fall in the domain of the study group? Published journal articles rely on photomicrographs and terse textual descriptions inevitably employing imprecise language. Quantitative features do not escape the problem of vagueness as discussed in Chap. 6.

Both these concerns have their roots in issues discussed in Chap. 6: (1) the extensionally indeterminant CoPeTI structure of the classes being considered; (2) the inevitable linguistic imprecision that attaches to both the characterization of the features used to define these unruly groups and the characterization of the groups themselves; (3) the observer's ongoing classificatory, private, micro-revisions prompted by the examination of problem cases; and (4) the difficulties of translating and transmitting a classificatory vision.

This last problem lies at the heart of our oncopathological enterprise; it is the gorilla sitting in the middle of the drawing room; we can put a negligee of statistics on it but the gown does not conceal the fact that it is a gorilla. The question is how effectively did the study under consideration study deal with the gorilla? A diagram of the study's phenospace is one way of partially addressing this problem. Gleason pioneered this technique with his ubiquitous grading chart and, following his example, we employed diagrams to convey architectural patterns in our endometrial cancer study (Fig. 7.5) [40]. Additional assurances

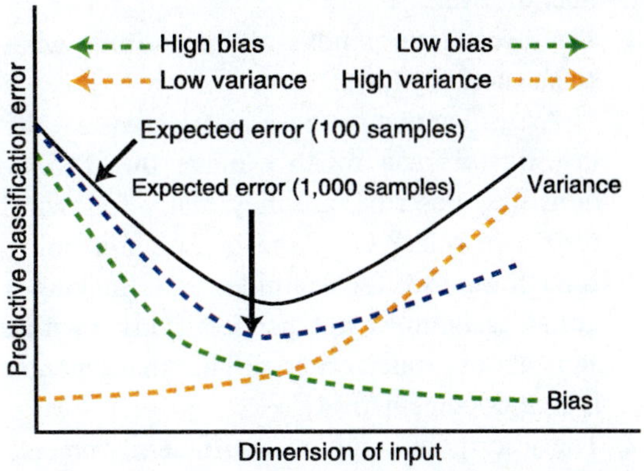

Fig. 7.5 The bias-variance dilemma. What makes for a good classifier? Much has been written about this by researchers in the machine-learning and pattern recognition fields. The performance of a classifier, as measured by its misclassification rate, depends on the interrelationship among (1) sample size, (2) the dimensionality of the data (how many features are evaluated), and (3) the complexity of the model – how many parameters have to be estimated within tolerable error limits. Imagine that we have several different, but equally good, training data sets. A classification rule is *biased* for a particular set of training sets if, when trained on each of these data sets, it is systematically incorrect when predicting the correct outcome. This, for example, occurs when the classification rule is too simple; univariate rules typically have this character; they "under-fit" the data. A classification rule has high *variance* if it predicts different outcomes when trained on different training sets. This occurs when the classification rule is too complex; complex multivariate rules typically have this character; they "overfit" the data. The *misclassification rate* of a classifier is related to the sum of the bias and the variance of the classification rule. In the diagram, the expected error curve is the sum of the bias cure and the variance curve. Generally, the rule designer must negotiate a trade-off between bias and variance as a function of the dimensionality of the data; thus, the error curves have a minimum. Two expected error curves are shown: the larger the number of cases the lower the expected error. A classifier with low bias must be "flexible" so that it can fit the data well. But if the classifier is too flexible, it will fit each training data set differently, and hence have high variance [3]

that the translation-transmission problem was addressed by the investigators are provided by an assessment of the level of agreement among the investigators [21].

Sources of Communication Failures

Effective transmission of information can fail at a number of levels:

1. The investigator is not really describing what he/she actually does:

   Assuming that we have assurances that the investigators can reliably make the distinctions they describe, are they really following their own rules? Or is the investigator doing something else; for example, is he making a gestalt assignment and then justifying it with a story about explicit criteria? This phenomenon is well documented [41].
2. The descriptions employ insufficiently precise language:

   Ambiguous language travels with the vague predicates and vague categories required to conceptualize and verbalize continuously varying features and extensionally indeterminant CoPeTI groups. "Confluent growth," "papillary growth"; "large" vs. "small" cells; "mitotic figure." In our study of endometrial carcinoma, we spent many hours trying to understand what Kurman and Norris, in their excellent and thorough study, meant by "confluent growth" and "fibrous stroma" [21, 42].
3. The descriptions are incomplete:

   Common omissions include: unstated criteria or feature-weighting strategies; failure to address unanticipated combinations of criterial features; and a failure to address the ubiquitous problem of tumor heterogenity
4. The authors have not provided instructions for dealing with the expected problem cases in the domain they are describing:

   What help is provided for problem cases – hybrids, in-between cases, and novel cases? As Chap. 6 suggests, completely anticipating such cases is impossible. That said, typical problem cases in the investigator's experience should be presented.

Genomic Studies

Genomics, GEA particularly, currently dominate our literature. Our journals are filled with articles promoting expression array patterns as cancer markers, as the basis for revising conventional light microscopic classifications of neoplasms, as prognostic and predictive markers or – more in the basic science literature – as ways elucidate cell signaling pathways. The mood has been upbeat. In 2005, Ioannidis ironically summed up the prevailing optimistic perspective of GEAs in a 2005 Lancet editorial entitled, "Microarrays and molecular research: noise discovery?"

> The promise of microarrays has been of apocalyptic dimensions. As put forth by one of their inventors, "all human illness can be studied by microarray analysis, and the ultimate goal of this work is to develop effective treatments or cures for every human disease by 2050 [43]." All diseases are to be redefined, all human suffering reduced to gene-expression profiles. Cancer has been the most common early target of this revolution and publications in the most prestigious journals have heralded the discovery of molecular signatures conferring different outcomes and requiring different treatments [44].

This editorial was occasioned by a pessimistic "forensic statistics" analysis of several published prognostic GEA signatures for a variety of cancers in the same issue. These authors concluded:

> …the list of genes included in a molecular signature … depends greatly on the selection of the patients in training sets. Five of the seven largest published studies addressing cancer prognosis did not classify patients better than chance. This result suggests that these publications were overoptimistic. [-----] Studies with larger sample sizes are needed before gene expression profiling can be used in the clinic [45].

In the same vein, Dupuy and Simon reported a detailed account of 42 peer-reviewed studies published in 2004. Fifty percent of them contained at least one of the following three basic flaws:

> 1) in outcome-related gene finding, an unstated, unclear, or inadequate control for multiple testing; 2) in class discovery, a spurious claim of correlation between clusters and clinical outcome, made after clustering samples using a selection of outcome-related differentially expressed genes; or 3) in

supervised prediction, a biased estimation of the prediction accuracy through an incorrect cross-validation procedure [46].

These are more than just quibbles; these failures fatally compromise the usefulness of such results [46]. Why is this not working? What are the problems? Some of them – multiple testing and validation – are familiar from the discussion above. Others are more complicated. First, what is *not* addressed by the majority of GEA studies?

The Biological Perspective

Let us locate these worries within the context that was sketched out in Chap. 6. The material for most expression array studies is a convenience sample – banked tissue of some sort (frozen, paraffin blocks, etc.) from which mRNA is extracted and from which cDNA is prepared. Studies of such material do not directly address several essential aspects of the I_{Neop}.

1. *I_{Neop} heterogeneity and evolution*: The sampled I_{Neop} is caught in a moment of time, a snapshot; the "signal" represents the average of the genetically and epigenetically heterogeneous cells and populations in the sample. For example, in Chap. 6, the Circos plots of "individual" breast cancers are really graphical summaries of all of the cytogenetic abnormalities of individual cells present in the sample.
2. *Context dependency of the neoplastic cell*: it is a commonplace that cells behave differen-tly in different micro-environments. Deciding whether a gene or the elements of a genetic pathway are inappropriately upregulated or downregulated requires knowledge of the context; precisely the thing that is lost in the homogenization required for GEA studies.
3. *I_{Neop} microenvironment*: there is the problem of separating the signal from the nonneoplastic elements in the sample from the signal of the neoplastic elements. In recent years, microdissection techniques and single cell GEA have begun to address this problem [47, 48].
4. I_{Neop} cellular complexity – functional and micro-anatomic – and the context dependency of cellular function. Clarke et al. refer to these issues as the "confound of multimodality" (COMM):

> problems that are associated with extracting truth [read, an empirically adequate model] from complex systems. ... COMM refers to the potential that the presence of multiple interrelated biological processes will obscure the true relationships between a gene or gene subset and a specific process or outcome, and/or create spurious relationships that may appear statistically or intuitively correct and yet may be false [3].

Clarke et al. provide a number of illuminating examples: the multiple functions of transforming growth factor β1 and the transcription factors tumor necrosis factor α and estrogen receptor α (ERα) [3]. Whether these are up or downregulated depends upon a context, again, precisely what is lost in GEA studies.

Methodological Problems

What are the issues peculiar to GEA publications? There are four basic problems: (1) The confusion between an observational study and an experimental study; (2) High dimensional biology (HDB) and the "small sample scenario"; (3) Fishing expeditions and the role of modeling in biology; (4) Noisy experimental data.

1. *Observation studies vs. experimental studies*: One recurrent theme is the failure of many genomic researchers to distinguish between an observational and experimental design. We can frame our discussion in terms of *"level-hopping."* Sotiriou and Pusztai distinguish between "top-down" and "bottom-up" studies [49]. In the *"top-down"* approach, gene-expression data from cohorts of patients with known clinical outcomes are compared to identify genes that are associated with prognosis without any a priori biologic assumption. In short, the jump is from a molecular profile to a $\Phi_{Clin}(t)$. Genomic techniques inherit all the problems of correlating conventional light microscopic features with $\Phi_{Clin}(t)$ and another substantial set of problems involved in moving the starting point back to the molecular level. Bypassed in this additional trajectory are, respectively, molecular motifs, signaling pathways, and cell-wide networks. This structure

of such a correlative, level-hopping study is observational and, the fact that genes are the predictors notwithstanding, not experimental. In the *"bottom-up"* approach, gene-expression patterns that are associated with a specific biologic phenotype or a deregulated molecular pathway are first identified and then subsequently correlated with the clinical outcome. In the *candidate-gene approach*, selected genes of interest on the basis of existing biologic knowledge are combined into a multivariate predictive model. Both of these designs discipline the study with certain a priori modeling assumptions and, as we shall see, the results are crucially dependent on the truth of those assumptions [49].

Potter describes the consequences of this shift from an experimental to an observational perspective:

> When a cancer sample is compared with normal tissue, attributing differences in gene expression to differences in disease state is entirely inappropriate in the absence of data regarding the age, sex, genetic profile, histology and treatment of the person from whom the sample came. This involves, not the failure to control confounding, but often the failure even to measure any of the other relevant exposures. If unaffected tissue from the same patient is used as a comparison, there are still the problems of the existence of field effects and of selection bias [50].

Potter suggests education as the culprit for this common misapprehension:

> The reason for this failure to distinguish between observational and experimental designs might be that, although observational scientists are trained in experimental methods, the reverse is seldom true. Furthermore, making the observations with new and powerful technology seems to induce amnesia as to the original nature of the study design. It is as though astronomers were to ignore everything they knew both about how to classify stars and about sampling methods, and instead were to point spectroscopes haphazardly at stars and note how different and interesting the pattern of spectral absorption lines were [50].

This theme is also picked up on by Ransohoff

> The culture of laboratory medicine does not appreciate that, when the tools of molecular biology are applied to heterogeneous groups of people, it is not experimental research anymore but rather is observational epidemiology, with its own rules of evidence, in which molecular biology simply provides a measuring tool [51].

I think there is a deeper issue of ideology involved here. Recall my discussion of histological determinism, the unstated background belief that what drives prognosis are the histological features of the I_{Neop}. This, as I discussed, encourages an inattention to other known determinants of prognosis. I believe something similar – molecular determinism – is responsible for the failure to appropriately frame GEA studies as observational studies vulnerable to all the biases well known to epidemiologists.

2. *Mathematical-statistical problems in HDB*:

> *Toto,* I've a feeling *we're not in Kansas anymore*
>
> – Wizard of Oz

The mathematical-statistical issues involved in high-dimensional spaces are formidable. Passing from the mathematics of *t*-tests, chi-squared test and linear regression – the conventional, and very important, biostatistical topics – to the mathematics and statistics of high-dimensional spaces is like moving from reading a bestselling detective novel to tackling James Joyce's *Finnegans Wake*. Thus, a critical reading of gene expression literature is challenging, even for the statistician; indeed, a cottage industry of "forensic statisticians" has been prompted by the mathematical-statistical difficulties presented by what has come to be known by many workers as "genomic signal processing." [52] The lesson for anatomic pathologists: the first thing to check on any paper that employs genomic techniques is whether a statistician is among the authors.

The "tall, skinny matrix" or "small sample scenario" problem: The problems arise because of the peculiar topology of high-dimensional spaces and the relative paucity of data points in those spaces. Clarke et al. summarizes the basic problem [3, 53]:

> Most univariate and multivariate probability theories were derived for data space where N (number of samples) > D (number of dimensions). Expression data are usually very different (D>>>N). A study of 100 mRNA populations

(one from each of 100 tumors) arrayed against 10,000 genes can be viewed as each of the 100 tumors existing in 10,000-D space. This data structure is the inverse of an epidemiological study of 10,000 subjects (samples) for which there are data from 100 measurements (dimensions), yet both data sets contain 100 data points.

By way of contrast, a widely used rule of thumb in the pattern recognition field is to have at least ten training samples per feature dimension [54]. In microarray studies, this ratio is often closer to 0.01 samples per dimension [55].

Curse of dimensionality: The performance of a statistical model (classifier) depends upon the interrelationship of three things: (1) sample size, (2) data dimensionality, and (3) model (classification rule) complexity. The "curse of dimensionality" refers to the breakdown of optimal model fitting using statistical learning techniques in high dimensions. The ability of an algorithm to converge to a "true" model degrades rapidly as the data dimensionality increases. The number of training cases required to maintain optimality goes up exponentially with the dimensionality (the number of features examined per case) of the feature space [2, 3, 53, 56]. Fig. 7.6 and the accompanying legend have more details.

These observations can be reframed in terms of the "bias/variance dilemma [54]." Simple models may be biased but will have low variance. More complex models have greater representation power (low bias) but overfit to the particular training set (high variance). Thus, the large variance associated with using many features (including those with modest discrimination power) defeats any possible classification benefit derived from these features. With severe limits on available samples in microarray studies, complex models using high-feature dimensions will severely overfit, greatly compromising classification performance [53].

Some form of the curse's reach, manifest as overfitting, extends to a wide variety of applications: classifiers using conventional light microscopic features, multivariate regression techniques, and artificial neural networks (ANN).

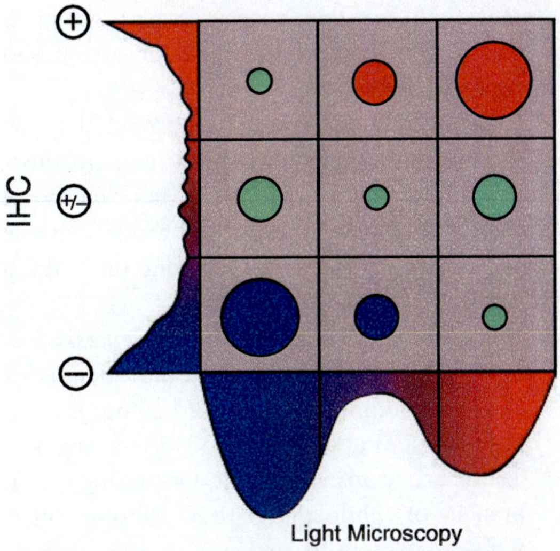

Fig. 7.6 A simple example of the "curse of dimensionality." The *x*-axis depicts a typical conventional light microscopic (H&E) morphological continuum ranging from "core" cases of Blues through in-between cases (*shades of purple*) to "core" cases of Red. In the language of Chap. 6 we have two overlapping ExtnI CoPeTI clusters. An immunohistochemical test is performed that can result in a negative, a positive or an inconclusive, result. The possible results are displayed in a 3×3 matrix. The size of the *circles* corresponds to the proportion of cases in each category. Most "core" cases of Blue are negative; most core cases of Red are positive. Some of the light microscopically in-between cases travel with the Blues, some with the Reds, and some remain indeterminate. The usual diagnostic interpretation is that the IHC test has disambiguated the purple region into true Blues and true Reds. What about the other cells? Some typical Blue cases are positive; some typical Red cases are negative. It is a *classificatory* decision to continue to call B/+ cases "B" and R/− cases "R"; similar decisions are required for the other possibilities. There are 3^3 possible diagnostic/classificatory decisions to make choices. It is easy to see that with the addition of new features, each of which can take on three values, the possibilities will go up exponentially with the number of features; 3^n for n features. It is also clear that, if the number of investigated cases remains constant, the possible combinations outstrip the number of cases. This is another version of the "curse of dimensionality." Immunohistochemical panels present us with this alarming vista

A related counterintuitive property of high-dimensional space is the following: the investigator is often in the position of finding a data point's nearest neighbor in the feature space. Here is the awkward fact: the distance to a point's farthest neighbor approaches that of its nearest neighbor when the dimensionality of the space increases to as few as 15 [3]. This has implications for case-based reasoning (CBR) (see Chap. 10).

Richard Simon's group has provided many accessible introductions to these mathematical-statistical problems [57–59]. The "curse of dimensionality" can be glimpsed using a simple example that pathologists confront on a daily basis (Fig. 7.7).

3. *Epistemological concerns – is hypothesis-free data mining really science at all?* Genomics and data mining have raised a number of deeper issues about what constitutes science. These are worries about epistemology, that branch of philosophy that, among other things, attempts to understand what constitutes the scientific method. A good place to begin is with the critique of Sydney Brenner, the 2004 Nobel Laureate for, among many other things, his *C. elegans* work. Sydney Brenner, with his characteristic talent for getting to the heart of the matter, frames the data mining problem in broad mathematical terms, as an ill-posed inverse problem. The generic forward problem involves positing a model, deriving predictions from that model, and then comparing predictions with the data. The generic inverse problem involves deducing a model from the data without any a priori assumptions about the model. Data mining amounts to an ill-posed (theory-poor) inverse problem. His argument is worth quoting in its entirety:

> I want to show here that this approach is bound to fail, because even though the proponents seem to be unconscious of it, this claim of systems biology is that it can solve the inverse problem of physiology by deriving models of how systems work from observations of their behavior. It is known that inverse problems can only be solved under very specific conditions. A good example of an inverse problem is the derivation of the structure of a molecule from the X-ray diffraction pattern of a crystal. This cannot be achieved because information has been lost in making the measurements. What is measured is the intensity of the reflection, which is the square of the amplitude, and since the square of a negative number is the same as that of its positive counterpart, phase information has been lost. There are three ways to deal with this. The obvious way is to measure the phase; the question then becomes well-posed and can be answered. The other is to try all combinations of phases. There are 2n possible combinations, where n is the number of reflections; this approach might be feasible where n is small but is not possible where n is in the hundreds or thousands, when we will exceed numbers like the total number of elementary particles in the Universe. The third method is to inject new a priori knowledge; this is what Watson and Crick did to find the right model. That a model is correct can be shown by solving the forward problem, that is, by calculating the diffraction pattern from the molecular structure. The universe of potential models for any complex system like the function of a cell has very large dimensions and, in the absence of any theory of the system, there is no guide to constrain the choice of model. In addition, most of the observations made by systems biologists are static snapshots and their measurements are inaccurate; it will be impossible to generate nontrivial models of the dynamic processes within cells, especially as these occur over an enormous range of time scales—from milliseconds to years. Any nonlinearity in the system will guarantee that many models will become unstable and will not match the observations. Thus, as Tarantola [60] has pointed out in a perceptive article on inverse problems in geology, which every systems biologist should read, the best that can be done is to invalidate models (in the Popperian sense) by the observations and not use the observations to deduce models since that cannot be successfully carried out [61].

An engaging expansion of this argument is available online: Sydney Brenner's lecture: "Much ado about nothing: systems biology and the inverse problem [61]."

Brenner is concerned with hypothesis-free data exploration. A more detailed argument along these same lines has been made by systems biologist Dougherty and coworkers in a series of publications (See Dougherty, 2008 for references [62]). After an extensive review of the history of the scientific method, they conclude that studies that depart from the model-data interaction schema (i.e., hypothesis-driven research) shouldn't count as science at all. They summarize their dismissal of data mining by citing Immanuel Kant's famous dictum: "A concept without a percept [observation] is empty; a percept without a concept is blind."

So, there are fatal downsides to sifting through massive amounts of data in a theory-free way. There are also downsides, in this data rich environment, of having partial theories. Clarke

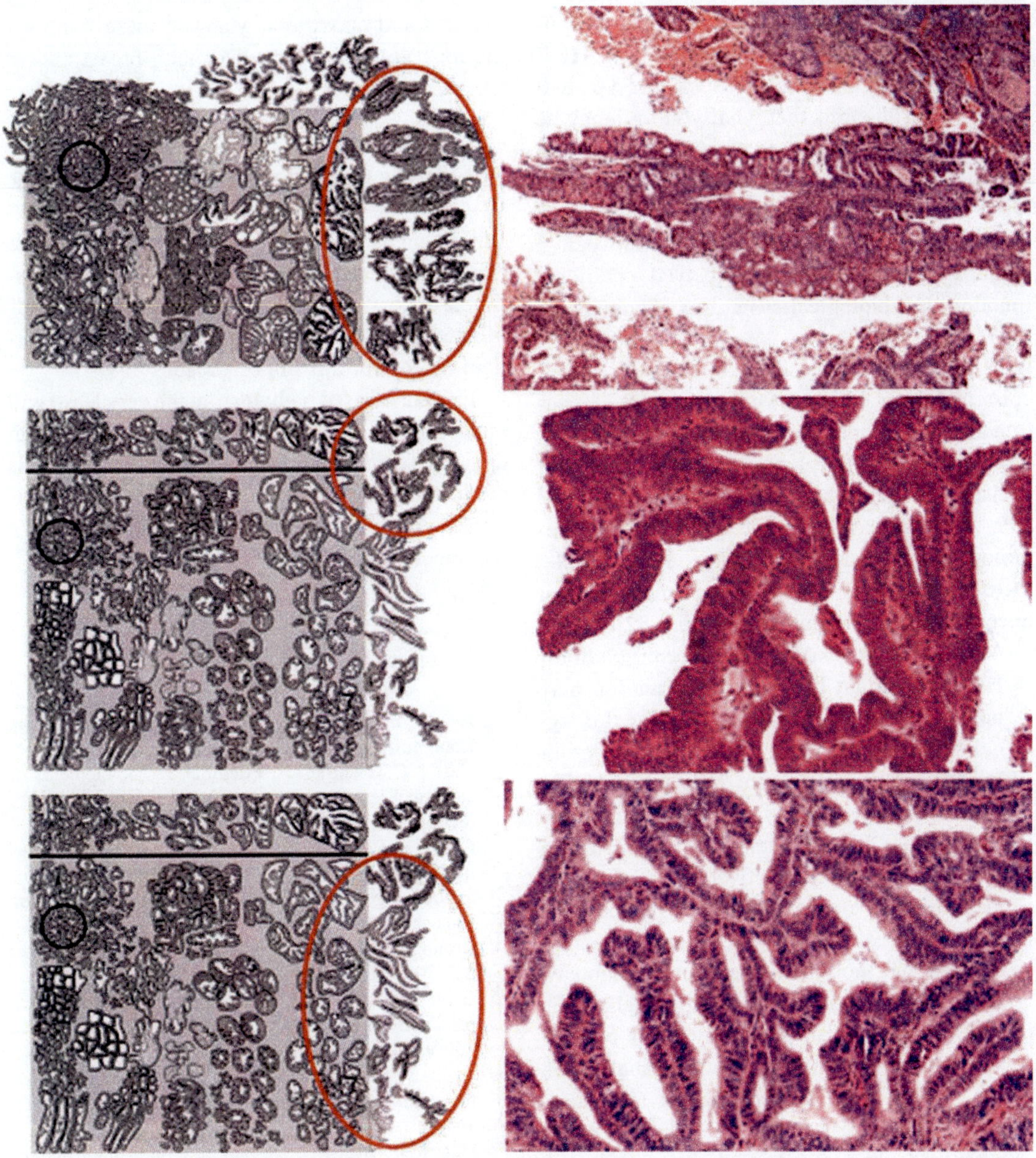

Fig. 7.7 Endometrial cancer chart [40]. Schematic of endometrial glandular proliferations with small budding glands, macroglands, and exophytic papillae. The *lower one-half* of the chart represents proliferations with very low risk for myometrial invasion in the hysterectomy specimen (<0.05%) and are designated as "complex endometrial hyperplasia" (with or without atypia), whereas the *upper one-half* of the chart represents proliferations with a sufficiently high risk for myometrial invasion in the hysterectomy specimen to warrant diagnosis as "well-differentiated endometrial adenocarcinoma." Proliferations with intermediate degrees of complexity are depicted immediately above the *solid horizontal line* on the *lower one-half* of the chart and are designated as "borderline, cannot exclude well-differentiated endometrial adenocarcinoma." These latter lesions have an intermediate risk for myoinvasion in the hysterectomy specimen (approximately 5%). For example, the *circles* denote low, intermediate, and high-risk exophytic papillary patterns. Similar circles can be drawn for the macroglandular and small budding glandular patterns. They are correlated with photomicrographs of corresponding cases

et al. warn us against the *self-fulfilling prophesy*. If you are committed to a model, in HDB you can usually confirm it; "seek and ye shall find." The problem is that what you find may be erroneous. "With thousands of measurements and the concurrent presence of multiple sub-phenotypes, intuitively logical but functionally incorrect associations may be implied between a signal's (gene or protein) perceived or known function in a biological system or phenotype of interest [3]."

Finally, at a more technical, statistical level, epistemological issues intrude. Mehta et al. caution that many papers aimed at the HDB community describe the development or application of statistical techniques whose validity is questionable, and betray a misunderstanding of the epistemological foundations of statistics. For example, there is sometimes a confusion of measurement uncertainty with biological variation [52].

4. *Noisy data*: Noisy data is a major problem for HDB. Important biological information may have a very low signal, and separating this signal from measurement noise is highly problematic. GEA data are typically highly correlated: this correlation could either represent "signal" (true correlations of, for example, elements of an activated pathway) or measurement "noise" in the data. Indeed, spurious correlations are a property of high-dimensional, noisy data sets and, obviously, are a problem for statistical approaches that seek to define a data set solely by its correlation structures. Although data normalization can remove spurious correlation (and also, unfortunately, real correlations) the results are sensitive to the particular technique employed; in other words, the same data set can yield different models using different techniques.

The Marker Study Perspective

GEA studies designed to make M-Class distinction (risk, prognosis, prediction) are properly evaluated within the cancer marker framework. There are many excellent surveys of this evaluation process as applied to proffered GEA markers and classifiers. Many of these focus on the most intensively studied field, breast cancer [9, 34, 49, 63–70].

Relevance to Evidence-Based Pathology

In this chapter, we have suggested applying the framework of tumor marker studies and prognostic classification rules to histopathologic claims of managerial relevance and emphasized the particular need for this in GEA results.

Evidence-based pathology, at the very least, will involve acquiring the conceptual tools to deal with the issues discussed in the Genomics section. This is a formidable task; remember the forensic statisticians. What anatomic pathologists can provide is a measure of morphologic "common sense."

References

1. Everitt B, Landau S, Leese M. Cluster analysis. London: Arnold; 2001.
2. Hastie T, Tibshirani R, Friedman J. The elements of statistical learning. Data mining, inference, and prediction. New York: Springer; 2001.
3. Clarke R, Ressom HW, Wang A, et al. The properties of high-dimensional data spaces: implications for exploring gene and protein expression data. Nat Rev Cancer. 2008;8(1):37–49.
4. Breiman L. Statistical modeling: two cultures. Stat Sci. 2001;16(3):199–231.
5. Grimes DA, Schulz KF. An overview of clinical research: the lay of the land. Lancet. 2002; 359(9300):57–61.
6. Grimes DA, Schulz KF. Descriptive studies: what they can and cannot do. Lancet. 2002;359(9301): 145–9.
7. Hayes DF, Bast RC, Desch CE, et al. Tumor marker utility grading system: a framework to evaluate clinical utility of tumor markers. J Natl Cancer Inst. 1996;88(20):1456–66.
8. Hayes DF. Do we need prognostic factors in nodal-negative breast cancer? Arbiter. Eur J Cancer. 2000;36(3):302–6.
9. Henry NL, Hayes DF. Uses and abuses of tumor markers in the diagnosis, monitoring, and treatment of primary and metastatic breast cancer. Oncologist. 2006;11(6):541–52.
10. Harris L, Fritsche H, Mennel R, et al. American Society of Clinical Oncology 2007 update of recommendations for the use of tumor markers in breast cancer. J Clin Oncol. 2007;25(33):5287–312.

11. Weigelt B, Horlings HM, Kreike B, et al. Refinement of breast cancer classification by molecular characterization of histological special types. J Pathol. 2008;216(2):141–50.
12. Galea MH, Blamey RW, Elston CE, Ellis IO. The Nottingham Prognostic Index in primary breast cancer. Breast Cancer Res Treat. 1992;22(3):207–19.
13. Altman DG, Vergouwe Y, Royston P, Moons KG. Prognosis and prognostic research: validating a prognostic model. BMJ. 2009;338:b605.
14. Moons KG, Altman DG, Vergouwe Y, Royston P. Prognosis and prognostic research: application and impact of prognostic models in clinical practice. BMJ. 2009;338:b606.
15. Moons KG, Royston P, Vergouwe Y, Grobbee DE, Altman DG. Prognosis and prognostic research: what, why, and how? BMJ. 2009;338:b375.
16. Royston P, Moons KG, Altman DG, Vergouwe Y. Prognosis and prognostic research: Developing a prognostic model. BMJ. 2009;338:b604.
17. Justice AC, Covinsky KE, Berlin JA. Assessing the generalizability of prognostic information. Ann Intern Med. 1999;130(6):515–24.
18. Mallett S, Royston P, Waters R, Dutton S, Altman DG. Reporting performance of prognostic models in cancer: a review. BMC Med. 2010;8:21.
19. Katz MH. Multivariable analysis: a primer for readers of medical research. Ann Intern Med. 2003;138(8):644–50.
20. Concato J, Feinstein AR, Holford TR. The risk of determining risk with multivariable models. Ann Intern Med. 1993;118(3):201–10.
21. Longacre TA, Chung MH, Jensen DN, Hendrickson MR. Proposed criteria for the diagnosis of well-differentiated endometrial carcinoma. A diagnostic test for myoinvasion. Am J Surg Pathol. 1995;19(4):371–406.
22. Lau SK, Weiss LM. The Weiss system for evaluating adrenocortical neoplasms: 25 years later. Hum Pathol. 2009;40(6):757–68.
23. Gupta R, Marchevsky AM, McKenna RJ, et al. Evidence-based pathology and the pathologic evaluation of thymomas: transcapsular invasion is not a significant prognostic feature. Arch Pathol Lab Med. 2008;132(6):926–30.
24. Marchevsky AM, Gupta R, McKenna RJ, et al. Evidence-based pathology and the pathologic evaluation of thymomas: the World Health Organization classification can be simplified into only 3 categories other than thymic carcinoma. Cancer. 2008;112(12):2780–8.
25. Marchevsky AM, McKenna Jr RJ, Gupta R. Thymic epithelial neoplasms: a review of current concepts using an evidence-based pathology approach. Hematol Oncol Clin North Am. 2008;22(3):543–62.
26. Begg CB, Cramer LD, Venkatraman ES, Rosai J. Comparing tumour staging and grading systems: a case study and a review of the issues, using thymoma as a model. Stat Med. 2000;19(15):1997–2014.
27. Edwards AWF. Cogwheels of the mind. The story of Venn Diagrams. Baltimore: Johns Hopkins University Press; 2004.
28. Stewart I. Another fine math you've got me into. New York: W.H. Freeman and Company; 1992.
29. Hennekens CH, Buring JE. Epidemiology in medicine. Boston: Little, Brown and Company; 1987.
30. Matthews DE, Farewell VT. Using and understanding medical statistics. 4 Rev Enl edition ed. Switzerland: S. Karger AG; 2007.
31. Florey CD. Sample size for beginners. BMJ. 1993;306(6886):1181–4.
32. Tversky A, Kahneman D. Belief in the law of small numbers. Judgment under uncertainty: heuristics and biases. Cambridge: Cambridge University Press; 1982. p. 23–31.
33. Silverberg S, Major F, Blessing J, et al. Carcinosarcoma (malignant mixed mesodermal tumor) of the uterus. A Gynecologic Oncology Group pathologic study of 203 cases. Int J Gynecol Pathol. 1990;9(1):1–19.
34. Ransohoff DF. Rules of evidence for cancer molecular-marker discovery and validation. Nat Rev Cancer. 2004;4(4):309–14.
35. Breiman L, Friedman JH, Olshen RA. Classification and regression trees. Belmont: Wadsworth International Group; 1984.
36. Ioannidis JP. Why most published research findings are false. PLoS Med. 2005;2(8):e124.
37. Vineis P. History of bias. Soz Praventivmed. 2002;47(3):156–61.
38. Chavalarias D, Ioannidis JP. Science mapping analysis characterizes 235 biases in biomedical research. J Clin Epidemiol 2010;63:1205–15.
39. Kendall BS, Ronnett BM, Isacson C, et al. Reproducibility of the diagnosis of endometrial hyperplasia, atypical hyperplasia, and well-differentiated carcinoma. Am J Surg Pathol. 1998;22(8):1012–9.
40. McKenney JK, Longacre TA. Low-grade endometrial adenocarcinoma: a diagnostic algorithm for distinguishing atypical endometrial hyperplasia and other benign (and malignant) mimics. Adv Anat Pathol. 2009;16(1):1–22.
41. Einhorn HJ. Expert judgment: some necessary conditions and an example. Judgment and decision making: an interdisciplinary reader. Vol 2. Cambridge: Cambridge University Press; 2000. p. 336–47.
42. Kurman R, Norris H. Evaluation of criteria for distinguishing atypical endometrial hyperplasia from well-differentiated carcinoma. Cancer. 1982;49(12):2547–59.
43. Schena M. Microarray analysis. New York: Wiley-Liss; 2003.
44. Ioannidis JP. Microarrays and molecular research: noise discovery? Lancet. 2005;365(9458):454–5.
45. Michiels S, Koscielny S, Hill C. Prediction of cancer outcome with microarrays: a multiple random validation strategy. Lancet. 2005;365(9458):488–92.
46. Dupuy A, Simon RM. Critical review of published microarray studies for cancer outcome and guidelines on statistical analysis and reporting. J Natl Cancer Inst. 2007;99(2):147–57.

47. Navin N, Krasnitz A, Rodgers L, et al. Inferring tumor progression from genomic heterogeneity. Genome Res. 2010;20(1):68–80.
48. Marusyk A, Polyak K. Tumor heterogeneity: causes and consequences. Biochim Biophys Acta. 2010; 1805(1):105–17.
49. Sotiriou C, Pusztai L. Gene-expression signatures in breast cancer. N Engl J Med. 2009;360(8):790–800.
50. Potter JD. At the interfaces of epidemiology, genetics and genomics. Nat Rev Genet. 2001;2(2):142–7.
51. Ransohoff DF. Discovery-based research and fishing. Gastroenterology. 2003;125(2):290.
52. Mehta T, Tanik M, Allison DB. Towards sound epistemological foundations of statistical methods for high-dimensional biology. Nat Genet. 2004;36(9):943–7.
53. Wang Y, Miller DJ, Clarke R. Approaches to working in high-dimensional data spaces: gene expression microarrays. Br J Cancer. 2008;98(6):1023–8.
54. Jain AK, Duin RPW, Mao J. Statistical pattern recognition: a review. IEEE Trans Pattern Anal Mach Intell. 2000;22:4–37.
55. Allison DB, Cui X, Page GP, Sabripour M. Microarray data analysis: from disarray to consolidation and consensus. Nat Rev Genet. 2006;7(1):55–65.
56. Duda RO, Hart PE, Stork DG. Pattern classification. New York: Wiley; 2001.
57. McShane LM, Radmacher MD, Freidlin B, Yu R, Li MC, Simon R. Methods for assessing reproducibility of clustering patterns observed in analyses of microarray data. Bioinformatics. 2002;18(11):1462–9.
58. Simon R. Interpretation of genomic data: questions and answers. Semin Hematol. 2008;45(3):196–204.
59. Simon RM, Korn EL, McShane L, Radmacher M, Wright GW, Zhao Y. Design and analysis of DNA microarray investigations. New York: Springer; 2003.
60. Tarantola A. Popper, Bayes and the inverse problem. Nat Phys. 2006;2:492–4.
61. Brenner S. Much ado about nothing: systems biology and the inverse problem. Reading the human genome with Sydney Brenner. 2009. http://thesciencenetwork.org/programs/reading-the-human-genome-with-sydney-brenner/much-ado-about-nothing-systems-biology-and-inverse-problems. Accessed on April 5, 2011.
62. Dougherty ER. On the epistemological crisis in genomics. Curr Genomics. 2008;9(2):69–79.
63. Ioannidis JP. Is molecular profiling ready for use in clinical decision making? Oncologist. 2007; 12(3):301–11.
64. Pusztai L. Lost in translation – prognostic signatures for breast cancer. Nat Clin Pract Oncol. 2008; 5(7):363.
65. Pusztai L. Current status of prognostic profiling in breast cancer. Oncologist. 2008;13(4):350–60.
66. Pusztai L, Iwamoto T. Breast cancer prognostic markers in the post-genomic era. Breast Cancer Res Treat. 2011;125:647–50.
67. Pusztai L, Mazouni C, Anderson K, Wu Y, Symmans WF. Molecular classification of breast cancer: limitations and potential. Oncologist. 2006;11(8): 868–77.
68. Ransohoff DF. Bias as a threat to the validity of cancer molecular-marker research. Nat Rev Cancer. 2005; 5(2):142–9.
69. Ross JS, Hatzis C, Symmans WF, Pusztai L, Hortobagyi GN. Commercialized multigene predictors of clinical outcome for breast cancer. Oncologist. 2008;13(5):477–93.
70. Sotiriou C, Wirapati P, Loi S, et al. Gene expression profiling in breast cancer: understanding the molecular basis of histologic grade to improve prognosis. J Natl Cancer Inst. 2006;98(4):262–72.
71. Bell SW, Kempson RL, Hendrickson MR. Problematic uterine smooth muscle neoplasms. A clinicopathologic study of 213 cases. Am J Surg Pathol. 1994;18(6):535–58.
72. Longacre TA, McKenney JK, Tazelaar HD, Kempson RL, Hendrickson MR. Ovarian serous tumors of low malignant potential (borderline tumors): outcome-based study of 276 patients with long-term (> or = 5-year) follow-up. Am J Surg Pathol. 2005;29(6): 707–23.
73. Longacre TA, Chung MH, Rouse RV, Hendrickson MR. Atypical polypoid adenomyofibromas (atypical polypoid adenomyomas) of the uterus. A clinicopathologic study of 55 cases. Am J Surg Pathol. 1996;20(1):1–20.

Power Analysis and Sample Sizes in Pathology Research

8

Robin T. Vollmer

Keywords
Power analysis • Sample size in pathology research • Pathology research • Experimental design in pathology research • Statistical power in pathology research

For decades research in pathology has occurred with little attention paid to the formalities of experimental design and issues of sample size and statistical power, and it still happens this way. Pathology research often begins with an intuition or a question arising from cumulative observations made on tissue specimens, followed by the more formal step of collecting exploratory data for study and analysis. However, this process is now evolving as a result of changes in the research environment. In most academic institutions, research in pathology is increasingly being controlled by institutional review boards (IRBs) and their statisticians. Plans for pathology research are now expected to follow known experimental designs and include analyses of sample size and statistical power. Nevertheless, in spite of the foregoing there will always be a role for exploratory studies, which require minimal attention to the details of formal experimental design. In fact, analysis of sample size and statistical power cannot be done until preliminary exploratory studies are completed.

R.T. Vollmer (✉)
Department of Laboratory Medicine, VA Medical Center, 508 Fulton Street, Durham, NC 27705, USA
e-mail: Robin.Vollmer@va.gov

Effect of Sample Size on Testing of Hypothesis

Most of us know that studies of few patients do not produce statistically significant results. Less intuitive are the occasional observations that studies with large numbers of patients can yield low *p* values on effects that eventually prove of limited importance [1]. Consider a hypothetical example. Let *T* symbolize a laboratory test, which is positive in 25% of patients. In preliminary observations, 35% of patients negative for *T* had the disease, *D*, and 45% of those with positive *T* had *D*. The change in prevalence of *D* from 35 to 45% is known as the size of the effect, or simply the effect size. How many patients are required to demonstrate that *T* and *D* are significantly associated? The following plot shows the relationship between the *p* value for a chi-square test of independence between *T* and *D* vs. the number of study patients.

Figure 8.1 shows that using fewer than 200 patients yields high *p* values, that over 400 patients produce *p* values less than 0.05 and that large numbers of study patients can yield very low *p* values even when the size of the test effect is modest. Scrutiny of this plot leads to two alternative conclusions. First, for the test *T* any study with less than

A.M. Marchevsky and M.R. Wick (eds.), *Evidence Based Pathology and Laboratory Medicine*,
DOI 10.1007/978-1-4419-1030-1_8, © Springer Science+Business Media, LLC 2011

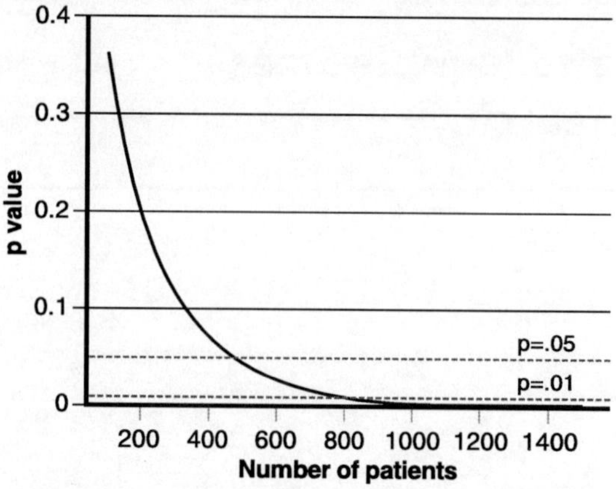

Fig. 8.1 Plot of p value obtained from a chi-square test of independence vs. the number of patients studied. The results come from the binomial model to be discussed in subsequent sections. All plots and results in this chapter were generated from S-PLUS software or programs written in C language by the author using the algorithms listed in the chapter and in the references

400 patients is of insufficient size to reach a statistically significant result, that is, it is "underpowered." Now, alternatively, consider a preliminary study of just 100 patients for this test. Clearly, such a study should result in a high p value but in doing so will tell us that the effect size of T for D is small and perhaps too small to be of practical interest.

Statistical Errors Types I and II: Definition of Power

In classical statistical analysis, the investigator formulates what is called the null hypothesis. This is the hypothesis that there are no significant effects between two or more populations of interest and that all observed results are due to randomness. In this setting, one can make two errors. The first is the type I error, which is the rejection of the null hypothesis, when in fact the null hypothesis is true. For a given experiment, the probability of making a type I error is the same as the p value for the statistical test. The second error, a type II, develops when we accept the null hypothesis although it is false. The probability of a type II error is commonly symbolized as β, and power equals $1-\beta$. Thus, the lower the probability of type II error, the higher is the statistical power for the study and its statistical test.

Table 8.1 Information necessary to calculate sample sizes: the general case

α	The p value one wants to meet, or probability of type I error
β	The probability of type II error (power is $1-\beta$)
Effect size	The magnitude of result one wants to find

Estimating Sample Sizes and Power: The General Case

Fortunately, statistical software packages in common use readily calculate both sample sizes and power for most common experimental designs. These include S-PLUS (www.spotfire.tibco.com), SAS (www.sas.com), SPSS (www.spss.com), and NCSS (www.ncss.com). All one need do is to select three key pieces of information: the p value one hopes to meet, the power level for the test, and the minimal size of the experimental effect (Table 8.1).

Common choices for α are 0.05 or 0.01. Common choices for β are 0.2 and 0.1. Because power equals $1-\beta$, the choosing 0.2 for β is equivalent to a choosing 0.8 for the power (sometimes expressed as 80%). Choice of the minimal effect size to be detected depends on the nature of the random variables used. For example, in survival analysis one might want to detect a difference in survival of as little as 2 months in a disease that is rapidly fatal. For other studies, the choice of 2 months would be too small to matter. Regardless, the choices of α, β, effect size, and sample size are made by the investigator and the values used by the software to estimate β and the power. What follows are several examples for common types of studies.

Estimating Sample Sizes and Power: Two Binary Random Variables

For this type of study, the motivation is to discover an association between a binary outcome and a binary explanatory variable. A common example in pathology is the study of how a specific diagnosis relates to an immunohistochemical stain (IHC). The outcome is the diagnosis,

Table 8.2 Information necessary to calculate sample sizes: the binomial case

α	The p value one wants to meet
β	The probability of type II error (power is $1-\beta$)
Effect size	The change in frequency of outcome one wants to detect
fp	The frequency of a positive result for the explanatory variable

and the explanatory variable is the IHC result. In this situation, the binomial model provides estimates of either sample size or power. The model requires one to select values for α and β as well as at least two additional variables (Table 8.2).

Finding a value for fp, the fraction of patients whose tissue will stain positive, requires preliminary studies or a search of prior literature. Then one must select the size of the effect to be detected. For example, if we expect that the frequency of the diagnosis to be 0.25 of patients and want to see if a positive IHC stain increases the frequency of diagnosis to 0.45, then the effect size would be an increase from 0.25 to 0.45. If preliminary studies indicated that fp was approximately 0.25, then the binomial model with $\alpha=0.05$ and $\beta=0.2$ would estimate that the sample size should be 295 patients. Now suppose that for the above study the investigator has just 125 patients. What would be the power of his study be to detect the same effect with $\alpha=0.05$? The binomial model indicates that the power would be 0.4 (in percentages 40%). In other words with just 125 patients, the probability of making a type II error would be 0.6.

Figure 8.2 summarizes the strong, positive relationship between power (expressed as a fraction) and the number of patients studied and was designed for the above study and its choices of α, β, and effect size.

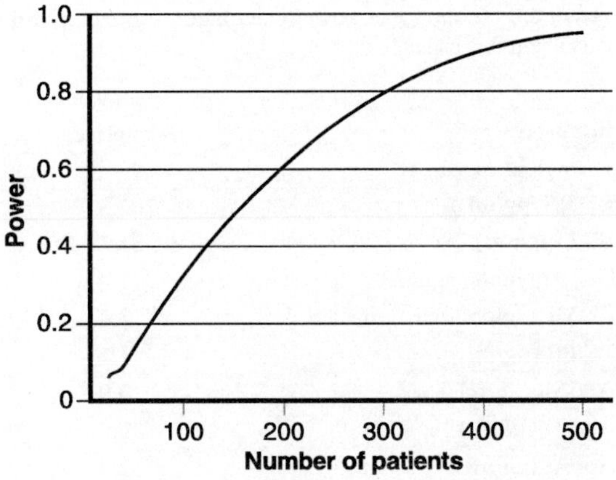

Fig. 8.2 Plot of calculated power vs. number of patients studied for associating a IHC stain with a diagnosis, when $\alpha=0.05$ and the size of effect is a change in frequency of diagnosis from 0.25 to 0.45

Table 8.3 Information necessary to calculate sample sizes: the case for means

α	The p value one wants to meet
β	The probability of type II error (power is $1-\beta$)
Effect size	The change in mean value one wants to detect
sd's	The standard deviations of the dependent continuous variable for the populations studied

Estimating Sample Sizes and Power: Means of Continuous Random Variables

If the random variable of interest is continuous, like a clinical chemistry test result, and the outcome variable is binary like the presence of a disease, then a common research question is whether the mean value of the result differs for those with and without the disease. For example, in 2008 Zhang et al. published mean values of several biomarkers measured in cerebral spinal fluid (CSF) in patients with either Alzheimer or Parkinson disease [2]. Although the authors' primary motivation was not to test for differences in means of biomarkers between these two diseases, their data provide a useful example of sample size and power applied to chemical tests. As before, one must select values for α and β. However, for such a study selecting the size of the effect implies selecting differences in mean values of the biomarkers for the two diseases (Table 8.3).

Finally, one must know approximate values for the standard deviations of each continuous variable to be tested, and this information must come from

Table 8.4 Example of power calculation for testing differences in mean values of CSF biomarkers in Alzheimer and Parkinson diseases

Biomarker	Mean values Alzheimer	Parkinson	Power	β
τ Amyloid (pg/mL)	1,425	387.8	1.0	0
BDNF (pg/mL)	202.3	184	0.7	0.3
IL-8 (pg/mL)	37.4	36.3	0.05	0.95
β42 Amyloid (pg/mL)	371.8	510.6	1.0	0
β2-Microglobulin (μg/mL)	1.4	1.6	0.3	0.7
VDPB (μg/mL)	1.1	1.2	0.1	0.9
ApoAll (μg/mL)	0.9	0.8	0.07	0.93
ApoE (μg/mL)	2.5	2.3	0.1	0.9
ApoAl (μg/mL)	2.3	2.4	0.06	0.94
Haptoglobin (μg/mL)	2.3	3.8	0.2	0.8

BDNF stands for brain-derived neurotrophic factor. IL-8 stands for interleukin 8. β Amyloid stands for amyloid [A] β 42. VDPB stands for vitamin D binding protein. Apo stands for apolipoprotein. Sample size was fixed at 48 patients in the Alzheimer group and 40 in the Parkinson group, and for this analysis α was fixed at 0.05. Mean values come from Table 2 of Zhang et al. [2]

preliminary studies. With these choices made, one can then estimate sample sizes. Alternatively, if one knows the sample sizes, then the software can estimate the power (and β) for detecting the effect.

For example, let us examine the power available to detect the differences in mean values reported by Zhang et al. (Table 8.4). The authors had a total of 88 patients, and they found that the means for both τ amyloid and β42 amyloid were significantly different between the two diseases. By contrast, they did not find significant differences in mean values for BDNF, IL-8, β2-microglobulin, VDBP, ApoAll, ApoE, ApoAl, and haptoglobin. Table 8.4 also shows the power available for detecting significant differences in means for the ten biomarkers. For each of the eight non-significant biomarkers, the power for detecting the observed difference in means was less than 0.8, also implying that the probability of type II errors was relatively high (range from 0.3 to 0.95). By contrast, the power for finding significant differences in means for τ amyloid and β42 amyloid between the two diseases was essentially 1.

Estimating Sample Sizes for the Logistic Model

The logistic regression model allows us to examine the relationship between a single, binary outcome random variable and one or more explanatory random variables. For example, the logistic regression model is ideal when we want to see if a combination of explanatory variables can predict the presence or absence of a disease. The binary outcome could alternatively be the presence of absence of a response to treatment or the presence or absence of failure after treatment. The greatest strength of the logistic model comes when there are multiple or continuous explanatory variables. In this circumstance of multiple explanatory variables, estimating sample sizes and power for the logistic model requires the information listed in Table 8.5.

For example, consider the situation for just one continuous, explanatory variable, $x1$. First, some preliminary data are necessary. From this data, one calculates the mean, $mx1$, and standard deviation, $s1$, of $x1$ as well as the overall probability of a positive outcome, Po. Po also approximates the conditional probability of a positive outcome when the $x1$ variable equals $mx1$, so that Po can be written as $P(y=1 \mid x1=mx1)$. Next, we use either the preliminary data to estimate the probability of a positive outcome when $x1=mx1+s1$ or we select some threshold probability we wish to detect. This second probability is the conditional probability $P(y=1 \mid x1=mx1+s1)$, which for simplicity we will symbolize as $P1$.

Table 8.5 Information necessary to calculate sample sizes: the logistic regression model

α	The p value one wants to meet
β	The probability of type II error (power is $1-\beta$)
Po	The baseline probability of positive outcome
Effect size	The odds ratio one wants to detect
nx	The number of explanatory x variables to be used
x details	Details about the x variables such as mean and standard deviations

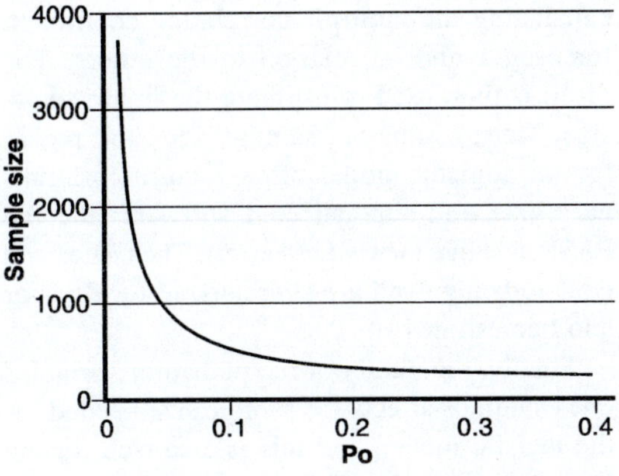

Fig. 8.3 Plot of required sample size vs. Po, the underlying probability of a positive outcome for a logistic regression analysis at a fixed OR of 1.5. The relationship between sample size and Po comes from equations given by Hosmer and Lemshow and is determined for a single continuous x variable with α=0.05 and β=0.2

Finally, we must consider the odds ratio, OR, defined as:

$$\text{OR} = \frac{P1/(1-P1)}{\text{Po}/(1-\text{Po})}.$$

If higher levels of $x1$ increase the chance of a positive outcome, then the OR will exceed 1.0. If higher levels of $x1$ decrease the chance of a positive outcome, then the OR will be less than 1.0. Thus, by estimating or selecting a value of $P1$ that we want to detect, we also select an OR. With values chosen for α and β as before, then one can use the tables published by Hsieh or available software packages to estimate the sample size [3].

Common sense tells us that if we are trying to study uncommon outcomes, then we need larger sample sizes. This is true for the logistic model, where the value of Po can dramatically affect the size of the sample needed to detect a particular OR effect. The following figure demonstrates this relationship with a plot of sample size vs. the value of Po.

Figure 8.3 shows that when a positive outcome is uncommon, over 1,000 patients are needed to detect an OR of 1.5. By contrast, when the outcome is as common as 0.2 (i.e., 20% of patients), then just 274 patients are needed.

Similarly, the value of the OR to be detected dramatically affects the size of the sample. Figure 8.4 demonstrates this affect for fixed values of Po=0.2, α=0.05, and β=0.2.

The plot demonstrates that for fixed values of Po, α and β, the closer the projected value of OR is to 1.0, the larger will be the required sample size. By contrast when the projected OR is as low as 0.7, just 350 patients are needed, and when the OR is as high as 1.5, just 274 patients are needed.

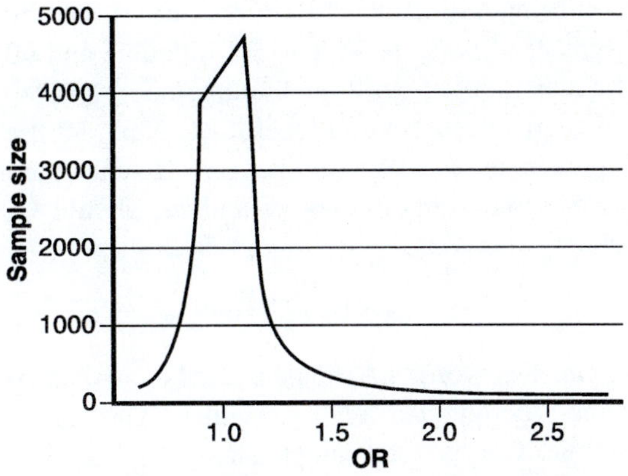

Fig. 8.4 Plot of sample size vs. OR, the odds ratio of a positive outcome for an x variable at a value one standard deviation above its mean and for a fixed Po of 0.2. The relationship between sample size and OR comes from equations given by Hosmer and Lemshow and is determined for a single continuous x variable with α=0.05 and β=0.2 (values of OR between 0.9 and 1.05 were excluded)

If there is more than one x variable, then an additional step is necessary and consists of calculating the multiple correlation coefficient for each x and its relation to the others. The result is then used to estimate the final sample size. Thus, estimating sample sizes and power for the logistic model often requires preliminary data and sophisticated software like the PASS package (www.ncss.com). The issues and equations involved are summarized by Hosmer and Lemeshow [4].

Finally, the number of explanatory variables one examines affects the sample size needed for the logistic model, and this is also true for the Cox survival model. If the number of x variables is large and the number of patients with observed positive outcomes is small, multivariate logistic regression analyses can yield unreliable results due to overestimated and underestimated variances. Logistic models in this situation may overfit the data and then not validate well with new data. Hosmer and Lemeshow suggest the following guidelines [4]. First, let $n1$ be the number of patients with a $y=1$ outcome and $n0$ be the number with $y=0$ outcome. Pick the lower of these two and label it nL. Next, let the number of x variables be nx. Hosmer and Lemeshow suggest that nx and nL should be chosen such that:

$$nx+1 \leqslant nL/10.$$

In other words, nL should exceed more than 10 times the number of x variables. This result implies that the total sample size should be even larger. In the author's experience, it is most often the number of patients with a positive outcome that will be smaller and therefore of greatest importance for comparing with the number of x variables.

Consider an example. Suppose we plan a study with five explanatory x variables ($nx=5$) and suppose that the fraction of patients with a positive outcome is 0.2. Then nL must be such that

$$nL \geqslant 10 \times (5+1) = 60$$

and the total number of patients needed (n) will be at least

$$n \geqslant 60/0.2 = 300.$$

Hosmer and Lemeshow also caution that contingency tables of outcome by values of the x variables should contain at least ten patients per cell. Because current studies of either nucleic acid microarrays or serum proteonomics often include thousands of x variables and just several hundreds of total patients, the above considerations suggest that it is possible such studies may not validate well with new patients.

Estimating Sample Sizes for Survival Analysis

Estimating sample size and power for survival analysis is more complex than for other analyses, because the outcome in survival analysis is a composite of two random variables: time and status at the last time. To understand the process, let us consider the survival times of two groups of patients, A and B. Groups A and B might be defined by the presence or absence of a molecular marker or stain. Alternatively, groups A and B might be defined by values of a continuous variable x below or above a cutpoint. For this kind of study, the information needed to estimate sample sizes is given in Table 8.6.

The effect size to be detected is the hazard ratio, which in turn relates directly to the change in survival one wants to detect. For the two groups

Table 8.6 Information necessary to calculate sample sizes: survival analysis

α	The p value one wants to meet
β	The probability of type II error (power is $1-\beta$)
PA	Proportion of patients in group A
PB	Proportion of patients in group B
Td	Planned duration in time for the study patients
Pd	The overall probability of death at Td
Effect size	The hazard ratio, hr, one wants to detect
nx	The number of explanatory x variables to be used
x details	Details about the x variables such as mean and standard deviations

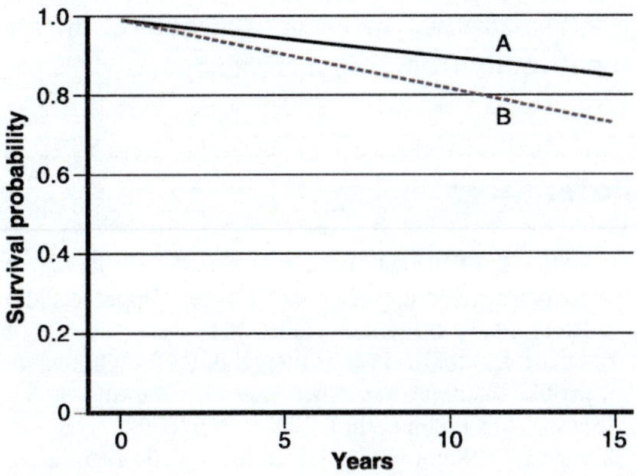

Fig. 8.5 Plot of survival probability for two simulated patient groups, A and B

of patients, A and B, the ratio of their hazard functions would be hr=hA/hB, and the relationship between their survival functions, SA and SB, relates to this ratio as follows:

$$SA = SB^{(hr)}.$$

Now consider the following plot of survival probabilities for patient groups A and B (Fig. 8.5).

The survival probabilities at 10 years for groups A and B are respectively 0.90 and 0.78. Suppose, we plan a study with a control group whose survival is equal to group A and we want to detect a drop in survival equivalent to that of group B. The proportional hazard model implies that the hazard ratio, hr, for group B relative to group A is:

$$hr = hB / hA = \ln(SB) / \ln(SA) = \ln(0.78) / \ln(0.90) = 2.4.$$

(Here, ln stands for the natural logarithm.) Thus, the hr to be detected would be approximately 2.4. To put this in perspective, Therneau and Grambsch suggest that many clinical studies are designed to detect much more modest values of hr – for example, values ranging from 1.15 to 2.00. On the other hand, detecting lower hr requires more study patients. Having selected values for the variables in Table 8.6, we use the software to determine sample sizes needed for survival studies (see, e.g, Therneau and Grambsch and Scheoenfeld).

Consider a specific example. Recently Marotti et al. reported the results of estrogen receptor-β (ER-β) expression in invasive breast cancer [5]. They found that in ER-α positive tumors, the presence of ER-β implied an improvement in proportion surviving at 30 years from approximately 0.64–0.74. This difference in survival corresponds to a hazard ratio of approximately 0.68. In their study, the *p* value for this result was 0.10, so that they concluded that the difference in survival was not significant. For this subset of their data, the authors had 470 patients with ER-α positive tumors. Now consider how many would be required to show that the effect of ER-β on survival was significant at a *p* value of 0.05 and with a power of 0.8? The answer is 222 patients with observed times of death. Because most of the study patients were living at the last time of observation, the authors had fewer than 150 with observed times of death. Thus, their study did not have sufficient power to detect this small change in survival.

Issues Relevant to Follicular Variant of Papillary Carcinoma of the Thyroid

One of the more controversial topics in anatomic pathology concerns the definition of the follicular variant of papillary carcinoma of the thyroid (PTC) [6–10]. This tumor has come to be recognized as a variant of PTC even when encapsulated and when papillary structures are absent. In fact, the defining morphological features of PTC have come to comprise several nuclear phenomena, about which there is much debate and documented disagreements. If an encapsulated follicular tumor is not a follicular variant of PTC, then what would it be? The answer is a follicular adenoma. Thus, for encapsulated follicular tumors the major distinction to be made is between follicular variant of PTC and follicular adenoma. Clearly, the prognosis for follicular adenoma should be excellent. By contrast, there are well-documented cases of follicular variant of PTC with recurrence and metastases after sufficiently long follow-up. Thus, some experts now suggest that to resolve the dilemmas about definition of PTC and its distinction from follicular adenoma what are needed are studies with long-term follow-up. Let us consider this issue in further detail.

Experts agree that the long-term prognosis for most patients with PTC is good. The AJCC lists the 5-year survival of stage I PTC as 0.971 and the 5-year relative survival as 0.998 [11]. This implies that the baseline 5-year survival for a group without PTC should be approximately 0.9729. Now let us suppose that the 5-year survival for an encapsulated follicular adenoma should approximate the baseline for the population (i.e., 0.9729). Next, let us suppose that the 5-year survival for encapsulated PTC should approximate that for stage I PTC (i.e., 0.971). How many patients would it take to detect a significant difference in survival for encapsulated PTC vs. follicular adenoma? If the total follow-up were to be 10 years with $\alpha=0.05$ and $\beta=0.2$, then the answer is approximately 120,000 patients, or 1,200,000 patient-years of follow-up. These numbers suggest that it will be unlikely that studies of survival in these tumors will ever answer the question of whether survival in encapsulated PTC differs significantly from follicular adenoma.

References

1. Miller I, Miller M, John E. Freund's mathematical statistics with applications. 7th ed. Upper Saddle River: Pearson Prentice Hall; 2004.
2. Zhang J, Sokal I, Peskin ER, et al. CSF multianalyte profile distinguishes Alzheimer and Parkinson diseases. Am J Clin Pathol. 2008;129:526–9.
3. Hsieh FY. Sample size tables for logistic regression. Stat Med. 1989;8:795–802.
4. Hosmer DW, Lemeshow S. Applied logistic regression. 2nd ed. New York: Wiley; 2000.
5. Marotti JD, Collins LC, Hu R, Tamimi RM. Estrogen receptor-β expression in invasive breast cancer in relation to molecular phenotype: results from the Nurses' Health Study. Mod Pathol. 2010;23:197–204.
6. Rosai J. Papillary thyroid carcinoma: a root-and-branch rethink. Am J Clin Pathol. 2008;130:683–6.
7. Baloch ZW, LiVolsi VA. Follicular-patterned lesions of the thyroid. The bane of the pathologist. Am J Clin Pathol. 2002;117:143–50.
8. Hunt JL, Dacic S, Barnes EL, Bures JC. Encapsulated follicular variant of papillary thyroid carcinoma. Am J Clin Pathol. 2002;118:602–3.
9. Baloch Z, LiVolsi VA, Henricks WH, Sebak BA. Encapsulated follicular variant of papillary thyroid carcinoma. Am J Clin Pathol. 2002;118:603–4.
10. Chan JKC. Encapsulated follicular variant of papillary thyroid carcinoma. Am J Clin Pathol. 2002; 118:605.
11. Edge SB, Byrd DR, Compton CC, Fritz AG, Greene FL, Trotti III A, editors. AJCC cancer staging manual. 7th ed. New York: Springer; 2010. p. 87–96.

Meta-Analysis: A Statistical Method to Integrate Information Provided by Different Studies

9

Eleftherios C. Vamvakas

Keywords

Meta-analysis for evaluation of therapies • Statistical methodology for medical literature review • Epidemiology of study results • Evidence-based pathology • Diagnostic test accuracy

Meta-analysis or statistical overview is the structured and systematic integration of information from different studies of a given problem [1]. It refers to the disciplined synthesis of previous research findings where the results of multiple reports on the effect of an exposure or treatment are compared, contrasted, and reanalyzed. When the results are discrepant, the purpose of the meta-analysis is to investigate reasons for disagreements among the studies. When the results are concordant, the goal of an overview is to derive, through the application of a number of quantitative methods, a measure of the effect of the exposure or treatment across the combined investigations. This measure is referred to as the "average" or "summary" effect of the exposure or treatment under study [1–5].

Meta-analysis differs from the traditional narrative reviews of the literature in that: (1) all completed investigations on the effect of an exposure or treatment that meet specific eligibility criteria are retrieved and considered for inclusion in the overview; (2) the quality of the retrieved studies is assessed systematically; (3) the degree of agreement among the studies is evaluated – both conceptually and based on statistical criteria – and the synthesis of the findings proceeds if the variation in reported results is sufficiently modest to be attributed to chance; and (4) quantitative methods are used to calculate the "average" effect of the intervention across the available studies, and to test that effect for statistical significance [1–5]. If a meta-analysis is conducted in accordance with these principles, it can provide the reader with "an objective view of the research literature, unaffected by the sometimes distorting lens of individual experience and personal preference that can affect a less structured review" [6].

Meta-analysis has two generally accepted applications and one controversial use. It can serve to integrate the findings of studies which report a treatment effect operating in the same direction, but varying substantially in size between reports. The purpose of the synthesis is to provide a more precise estimate of the most likely magnitude of the treatment effect, so that a definitive randomized controlled trial (RCT) can be designed, enrolling as many patients as are needed

E.C. Vamvakas (✉)
Department of Pathology and Laboratory Medicine, Cedars-Sinai Medical Center, 8700 Beverly Blvd., Los Angeles, CA 90048, USA
e-mail: vamvakase@cshs.org

DOI 10.1007/978-1-4419-1030-1_9, © Springer Science+Business Media, LLC 2011

to establish the existence of that effect. Alternatively, meta-analysis can be used to investigate reasons for disagreements among studies which report treatment effects operating in opposite directions or differing markedly in size when they all point in the same direction. The aim of the analysis is to explain discrepancies among published results, based on relevant characteristics of the patients who were included in the available studies, the treatments that were administered, or the quality of study design and analysis.

The third, and controversial, application of meta-analysis is to integrate the findings of studies that report a treatment effect operating in the same direction, but not attaining statistical significance in any study, perhaps because of the small sample size and inadequate statistical power of each report. Here, the purpose of the synthesis is to establish the existence of a treatment effect by combining the patient populations enrolled in separate studies. This proposed use of statistical overviews makes meta-analysis appear as a possible alternative to an RCT undertaken to establish the efficacy of a therapeutic intervention. Overviews, however, best serve as a supplement (as opposed to an alternative) to RCTs.

This is because – even when a definitive RCT for establishing the efficacy of a therapeutic intervention is, eventually, conducted – its findings may not necessarily apply to all patients. Trialists use highly restrictive inclusion/exclusion criteria for patient enrollment, because they strive to include a patient population as homogeneous as possible, to make it easier to detect a treatment effect untainted by confounding factors. The results of an RCT may therefore not apply to patients who do not meet the eligibility criteria of the study. Thus, RCTs constitute the gold standard for evaluating the efficacy of therapeutic interventions, but need to be supplemented by meta-analyses in order to broaden the applicability of their findings [1–7].

A meta-analysis integrates the findings of separate studies, which usually differ in many aspects of their design. This variation in the design attributes of reports included in a meta-analysis results in greater generalizability of the findings of a statistical overview, compared to the results of an RCT, because – by combining studies with disparate design characteristics – a meta-analysis permits examination of the effect of an intervention in many different situations. If the treatment effect is consistent in all the studies, this consistency favors a true treatment effect, rather than one due to chance, or some systematic error, or uncontrolled factor that may have compromised the results of all completed investigations.

To appreciate the contribution of meta-analyses in the medical literature, it is appropriate to think of an overview as an original report consisting of two parts: a qualitative component and a quantitative one [1, 6, 7]. According to Jenicek [1], the first phase of a statistical overview should be a "qualitative" meta-analysis, which must precede the "quantitative" phase of the report. An assessment of the quality of all retrieved studies should be made, and studies of unacceptable quality should be excluded from the overview. In Goodman's opinion, a meta-analysis should "raise research and editorial standards, by calling attention to the strengths and weaknesses of the body of research in an area" [6]. O'Rourke and Detsky assert that the major contribution of a meta-analysis lies in the attention that it draws to flaws in the design and conduct of previous studies [7]. When all published studies are subjected to a detailed review of the methods – with a focus on the impact of the methods on the validity of the results – inadequacies can be identified and their resolution encouraged. Recognized shortcomings can be thus avoided in future individual research efforts, so that more valid results are produced.

For their initially-intended purpose (i.e., for the investigation of the effects of therapeutic interventions), meta-analyses were limited to RTCs [8–10]. The rationale and tools for conducting a meta-analysis were thus developed for RCTs, that is, the controlled clinical experiments undertaken to establish that a new treatment achieves a better clinical outcome than standard therapy; and which can be presumed to be free of the effects of selection bias and confounding factors, as well as free of the effect of observation bias when they are double-blind [11]. Meta-analysis was used in pathology (i.e., for the study of diagnostic-test accuracy) several years after the method had been widely used in clinical medicine.

Studies of diagnostic-test accuracy conducted at different centers often produce estimates of the sensitivity and specificity of a test that vary widely. Such variation may be due to random sampling variation, differences in study quality, differences in the characteristics of the test and the enrolled patients, and/or differences in the cutoff points used to calculate the published estimates of sensitivity and specificity [12–17]. The wide variation across studies in the reported accuracy of a laboratory test limits the value of the information provided by traditional reviews of the literature presenting the range of available estimates. What is often needed, instead of this range, is insight into the reasons for the differences in the reported estimates of accuracy, and – if possible – a summary estimate of the sensitivity and specificity of the test based on all available data.

Meta-analysis has thus been used to: (1) produce valid summary estimates of the diagnostic accuracy of laboratory tests; (2) explain the variation in the results of published reports; and (3) improve the quality of the primary studies by identifying their methodologic shortcomings. However, there are differences between RCTs and studies of diagnostic-test accuracy, as well as methodologic obstacles to the use of meta-analysis in diagnostic pathology [16], which must be carefully addressed by meta-analysts of studies of diagnostic-test accuracy.

The purpose of this chapter is to provide practicing pathologists with the necessary background for reading and evaluating published reports of meta-analyses of RCTs as well as overviews of studies of diagnostic-test accuracy. The first part of the chapter describes the applications of meta-analysis in the domain of RCTs. The second part discusses how these same concepts and (appropriately modified) methods can be used to integrate results of studies of diagnostic-test accuracy. The rationale for quantitative research synthesis is presented and the component parts of a meta-analysis are described. A recommended approach to the medical interpretation of overviews is then presented. All concepts are illustrated using as an example the meta-analysis [18] of the RCTs of white-blood-cell (WBC) reduction of red-blood-cell (RBC) components, by means of prestorage or poststorage filtration, to prevent the purportedly deleterious immunomodulatory effects of WBC-containing allogeneic blood transfusion (ABT) [19]. Transfusion-related immunomodulation may predispose patients to an increased risk of bacterial infection, and perhaps also mortality, during or shortly after a hospitalization [20].

The Unit of Observation in Meta-Analysis

Meta-analysis is the epidemiology of study results. Clinical studies use the individual patient as the unit of observation. In contrast, the unit of observation in meta-analysis is either the adverse effect of an exposure or the beneficial effect of an intervention, as calculated from each individual original report. For example, published RCTs of the deleterious effect of exposure to WBC-containing ABT or, alternatively, of the efficacy of the intervention of WBC reduction of RBC components to prevent this purported ABT adverse effect, used the individual patient as the unit of observation [21–34]. On the contrary, the meta-analyses of these reports [18, 35, 36] used as the unit of observation one or more measures of the adverse ABT effect as calculated from within each reported study. More specifically, the odds ratio (OR) of either bacterial infection [21–32] or all-cause mortality [21, 23–29, 31, 33, 34] represented the clinical effect of the deleterious immunomodulatory or pro-inflammatory effects of ABT [19, 20] as calculated from within each RCT [21–34].

Each study [21–34] thus contributed to the meta-analysis [18] one or more estimates of the effect of WBC-containing ABT in increasing the risk of either infection or mortality. Figures 9.1 and 9.2 show the results of these individual RCTs [21–34] as calculated from intension-to-treat-analyses. The OR of bacterial infection or short-term (up to 3-month posttransfusion) mortality (Figs. 9.1 and 9.2, respectively) was calculated from each RCT if the authors had reported the four counts of a 2×2 contingency table (Table 9.1). Two RCTs [30, 32] had presented only "as-treated" analyses of patients transfused with non-WBC-reduced vs. WBC-reduced RBCs, vs. subjects randomly allocated preoperatively to receive either non-WBC-reduced or WBC-reduced

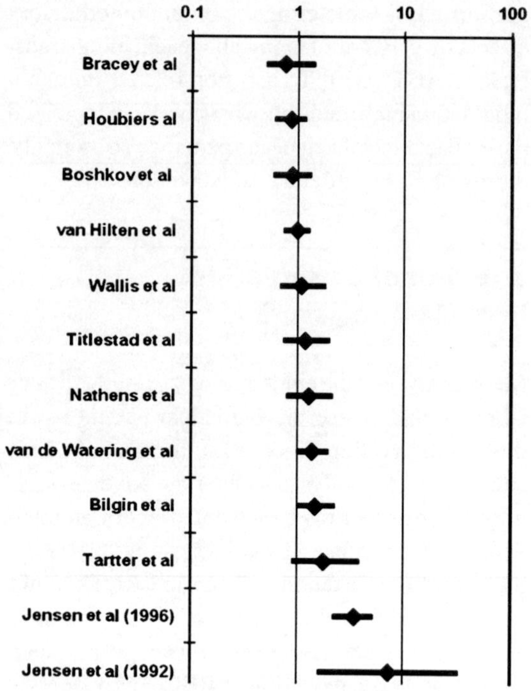

Fig. 9.1 RCTs investigating the association of WBC-containing ABT with bacterial infection ranked in the order of magnitude of the ABT effect that they reported [21–32]. For each RCT, the figure shows the OR of bacterial infection in subjects randomized to receive non-WBC-reduced vs. WBC-reduced allogeneic RBCs or whole blood, as calculated from an intention-to-treat analysis (Table 9.2). Each OR is surrounded by its 95% CI. If the 95% CI of the OR includes the null value of 1, the ABT effect is not statistically significant ($p>0.05$). A deleterious ABT effect is indicated by an OR > 1, provided that the associated 95% CI does not include the null value of 1

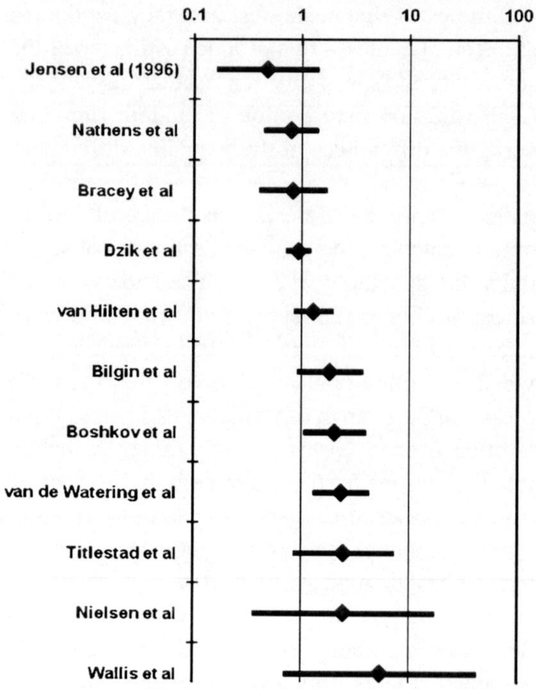

Fig. 9.2 RCTs investigating the association of WBC-containing ABT with short-term (up to 3-month posttransfusion), all-cause mortality ranked in the order of magnitude of the ABT effect that they reported [21, 23–29, 31, 33, 34]. For each RCT, the figure shows the OR of mortality in subjects randomized to receive non-WBC-reduced vs. WBC-reduced allogeneic RBCs, as calculated from an intention-to-treat analysis

RBCs who had not needed ABT perioperatively. For these two studies, which reported only on bacterial infection as an outcome (Fig. 9.1 and Table 9.2), the minimal number of infections recorded in the third comparison group of patients not needing perioperative transfusion was allocated [18] to the two randomization arms to produce approximate 2×2 contingency tables for an intention-to-treat analysis. One RCT [23] followed-up postrandomization (recording the adverse events of infection and/or death) only the transfused patients. Figures 9.1 and 9.2 show the results of these RCTs [21–34] ranked in the order of magnitude of the ABT effect on bacterial infection or mortality calculated from within each study.

A meta-analysis integrates exposure or intervention (treatment) effects calculated from separate studies, such as the deleterious effects of WBC-containing ABT shown in Figs. 9.1 and 9.2. It is important to appreciate that a meta-analysis integrates the exposure or treatment effects calculated from individual studies, as opposed to "pooling" the data on the individual patients enrolled in each RCT. Thus, the ABT effect from each RCT, as incorporated into the analysis of an overview [18, 35, 36], is based exclusively on the outcomes of the recipients of non-WBC-reduced vs. WBC-reduced ABT within each individual study. In Table 9.1, patients preoperatively randomized to receive WBC-containing ABT (in the event that they need perioperative transfusion) constitute the treatment arm, because – by receiving non-WBC-reduced RBCs – they are exposed to the immunomodulatory

Table 9.1 2×2 Contingency table counts for the randomized controlled trials investigating the relationship between WBC-containing ABT and bacterial infection or short-term (up to 3-month posttransfusion) all-cause mortality

	Treatment arm (subjects randomized to receive non-WBC-reduced ABT[a])	Control arm (subjects randomized to receive WBC-reduced ABT[a])
Subjects developing infection[b]	*a*	*b*
Subjects remaining free of infection[c]	*c*	*d*

Odds of infection or mortality in treated patients $= \dfrac{a/(a+c)}{c/(a+c)} = \dfrac{a}{c}$

Odds of infection or mortality in controls $= \dfrac{b/(b+d)}{d/(b+d)} = \dfrac{b}{d}$

odds ratio (OR) $= \dfrac{\text{odds of infection or mortality in treated patients}}{\text{odds of infection or mortality in controls}} = \dfrac{a/c}{b/d} = \dfrac{ad}{bc}$

a = count of patients randomized to receive non-WBC-reduced ABT developing infection[b]
b = count of patients randomized to receive WBC-reduced ABT developing infection[b]
c = count of patients randomized to receive non-WBC-reduced ABT not developing infection[c]
d = count of patients randomized to receive non-WBC-reduced ABT not developing infection[c]
[a] In the event that they needed perioperative transfusion
[b] Or dying within 3 months posttransfusion
[c] Or surviving up to 3 months posttransfusion (to the completion of each study's follow-up period)

or pro-inflammatory effects of allogeneic WBCs [19, 20]. Patients preoperatively randomized to receive non-WBC-reduced ABT constitute the control arm, that is, the unexposed subjects.

Controls from one RCT cannot serve as controls for patients being exposed to allogeneic WBCs in another RCT. Such a comparison would be invalid, because the various studies included in a meta-analysis differ from one another in various characteristics of the enrolled patients, the exposure(s) received, as well as attributes relating to study design and analysis (Table 9.2). These differences among the studies are often likely to affect the outcome of interest (e.g., the odds of infection (Fig. 9.1) or all-cause mortality (Fig. 9.2)). Thus, because of multiple differences among the available studies, it is invalid to compare directly the experience of individual patients from one study to that of subjects from another RCT. An overview compares the *effect* of an exposure or intervention in one study with the effect of that exposure or intervention in other RCTs.

For example, Table 9.2 lists some of the differences between the RCTs [21–34] investigating the association of WBC-containing ABT with bacterial infection or all-cause mortality recorded up to 3 months posttransfusion. Among other differences between the studies, these RCTs differed in the RBC product transfused to the non-WBC-reduced arm, the RBC product transfused to the WBC-reduced arm, and/or the clinical setting. All but four RCTs, including all RCTs published after 1998, transfused to the WBC-reduced arm allogeneic RBCs filtered *before* storage (Table 9.2). Thus, for patients in the WBC-reduced arm, these RCTs abrogated both any ABT effects mediated by immunologically-competent allogeneic mononuclear cells [37–39] and any ABT effects mediated by WBC-derived soluble mediators that progressively accumulate in the supernatant fluid of RBCs during storage [40–43]. In contrast, three RCTs published between 1992 and 1998 [30–32], as well as one of three randomization arms employed in the RCT of van de Watering et al. [28], transfused to the WBC-reduced arm allogeneic RBCs or whole blood filtered *after* storage. For patients in the WBC-reduced arm, these RCTs [28, 30–32] prevented effects mediated by immunologically-competent allogeneic mononuclear cells [37–39], but not effects mediated by WBC-derived soluble mediators that accumulate during storage [40–43].

Five RCTs [21, 23, 25, 28, 29] were conducted in cardiac surgery and five [22, 26, 30–32] in gastrointestinal surgery. The ABT effect may be

Table 9.2 Design of RCTs investigating the association of WBC-containing allogeneic blood transfusion with bacterial infection and/or short-term, all-cause mortality

References	Year of publication	Clinical setting	Sample size	Non-WBC-reduced allogeneic RBC component given to the treatment arm	WBC-reduced allogeneic RBC component given to the control arm	Country in which the study was conducted
Bracey et al. [21]	2002	Cardiac surgery	443	Unmodified RBCs	Prestorage-filtered RBCs	US
Houbiers et al. [22][a]	1994	Colorectal cancer resection	697	Buffy-coat-reduced RBCs	Prestorage-filtered RBCs	The Netherlands
Boshkov et al. [23]	2004	Cardiac surgery	562[b]	Unmodified RBCs	Prestorage-filtered RBCs	US
van Hilten et al. [24]	2004	Acute ($n=79$) or elective ($n=413$) aortic aneurysm repair; resection of gastrointestinal malignancy	1,052	Buffy-coat-reduced RBCs	Prestorage-filtered RBCs	The Netherlands
Wallis et al. [25]	2002	Cardiac surgery	597	Buffy-coat-reduced ($n=204$) or plasma-reduced[c] ($n=198$) RBCs	Prestorage-filtered RBCs	United Kingdom
Titlestad et al. [26]	2001	Colorectal surgery	279	Buffy-coat-reduced RBCs	Prestorage-filtered RBCs	Denmark
Nathens et al. [27]	2006	Trauma patients	324[d]	Unmodified RBCs stored for <25 days	Prestorage-filtered RBCs	US
van de Watering et al. [28]	1998	Cardiac surgery	914	Buffy-coat-reduced RBCs	Prestorage ($n=305$) or poststorage ($n=303$) filtered RBCs	The Netherlands
Bilgin et al. [29]	2004	Cardiac surgery	474	Buffy-coat-reduced RBCs	Prestorage-filtered RBCs	The Netherlands
Tartter et al. [30][a]	1998	Gastrointestinal surgery	221	Unmodified RBCs	Poststorage-filtered RBCs	US
Jensen et al. [31]	1996	Colorectal surgery	586	Buffy-coat-reduced allogeneic RBCs	Poststorage-filtered RBCs	Denmark
Jensen et al. [32][a]	1992	Colorectal surgery	197	Unmodified whole blood	Poststorage-filtered whole blood	Denmark
Dzik et al. [33][e]	2002	All hospitalized patients	2,780	Unmodified RBCs	Prestorage-filtered RBCs	US
Nielsen et al. [34][e]	1999	Burn trauma patients	24	Buffy-coat-reduced RBCs	Prestorage-filtered RBCs	Denmark

[a] RCTs reporting data on bacterial infection (but not mortality)
[b] Transfused patients only (as opposed to all randomized patients)
[c] In terms of its WBC content, this component is equivalent to nonbuffy-coat-reduced (i.e., unmodified) RBCs
[d] All randomized patients ($n=324$) were used in the analysis of mortality; patients who did not refuse consent ($n=268$) were used in the analysis of infection
[e] RCTs reporting data on mortality (but not infection)

enhanced in the setting of cardiac surgery, because WBC-derived soluble mediators and/or allogeneic mononuclear cells may act as a second inflammatory insult, compounding the diffuse inflammatory response to the extracorporeal circuit and predisposing to postoperative complications [44]. Alternatively, the ABT effect may be enhanced in the "unclean" setting of gastrointestinal surgery. Either way, it is possible for a deleterious ABT effect to become manifest only in the presence of cofactors, such as the special conditions that exist in cardiac or gastrointestinal surgery.

In addition, there was great variation among the RCTs in the amount of blood transfused and the frequency of a diagnosis of postoperative infection. As few as 26.7% of randomized subjects needed perioperative transfusion in some gastrointestinal surgery studies [26]; in contrast, as many as 94.7% of randomized subjects needed perioperative transfusion in some cardiac-surgery studies [28]. In gastrointestinal surgery, the frequency of postoperative infection ranged from 8.1% [32] to 33.4% [22]. The differences in the proportion of transfused patients reflected patient-related selection factors (severity of underlying illness) as well as setting- and surgeon-related selection factors (subjective application of liberal or conservative transfusion criteria during an operation – when objective laboratory indicators of the need for transfusion are unavailable). The differences in the frequency of postoperative infection reflected differences in the patients' severity of illness and the employed diagnostic criteria for infection, differences in the types of infections evaluated in each study, and perhaps also the effects of observation and/or selection bias (since not all RCTs were double-blind and, in most cases, the details of the randomization procedure[s] were not reported).

Thus, it is most unlikely that all RCTs targeted an increase in the risk of postoperative infection or all-cause mortality mediated by a deleterious ABT effect that was *biologically* the same in all the cases. Instead, these RCTs [21–34] most likely targeted effects of non-WBC-reduced ABT that differed both in magnitude and/or nature – being mediated by either allogeneic mononuclear cells [37–39] or WBC-derived soluble mediators accumulating during storage [40–43] or both; and being compounded (or not) by other cofactors (such as a diffuse inflammatory response to the extracorporeal circuit used in cardiac surgery [44]). Accordingly, a meta-analysis integrating the results of all available studies would not establish an effect attributed to a specific biologic mediator or mechanism. Stated in other words, the medical heterogeneity of the available RCTs made it inappropriate to combine the results of all available RCTs in a meta-analysis [45].

Assessment of the Eligibility of Original Reports for Inclusion in a Meta-Analysis

Meta-analysis is based on the assumption that all studies evaluating the effect of an exposure or intervention are retrieved. Some of these reports are then selected for inclusion in the analysis, based on eligibility criteria specified in advance. Exclusions are initially determined by the medical scope of the overview. If the medical question asked is a general one, broad selection criteria may be used; if it is a more specific one, the criteria are stricter. The hypothesis under investigation must be defined in precise terms, so that the selection of studies for analysis can be made in an objective and reproducible manner. Additional criteria for exclusion may include the date of publication (because a study may no longer be clinically relevant), the language of publication (if reports not published in English cannot be properly evaluated), the length of follow-up (if this is considered too short for a meaningful assessment of the outcome under study), and the completeness of the presented information (if the four counts of a contingency table (Table 9.1) cannot be extracted from an abstract, letter to the editor, or other summary report of a study). Excluded studies should be listed in the report of the meta-analysis, and the reasons for their exclusion should be explicitly stated.

When subjects are randomly allocated preoperatively to receive non-WBC-reduced vs. WBC-reduced ABT in the event that they need perioperative transfusion (Table 9.2), patients from either arm of the RCT should have the same baseline probability of developing bacterial infection, of dying within 3 months of the transfusion, and of needing perioperative ABT. Provided that the number of the enrolled subjects is *very* large, the play of chance will distribute equally between the treatment and control arms all prognostic factors for mortality or development of bacterial infection other than the receipt of non-WBC-reduced (as opposed to WBC-reduced) ABT. Therefore, in the absence of any intervention (such as WBC reduction of the administered RBCs), the same proportion of patients from either randomization arm should be expected to develop infection or die within 3 months of the transfusion from any cause. For this reason, any difference in the odds of infection or mortality between the two randomization arms can be ascribed to the receipt of non-WBC-reduced (vs. WBC-reduced) ABT.

The intent to investigate the existence of a causal relationship is the reason why – when meta-analyses were initially introduced in medicine – only RCTs used to be eligible for inclusion in an overview. When results from observational studies are also available, the findings of observational studies are either not considered at all or integrated separately from the results of RCTs. As it will be discussed later, however, investigations of diagnostic-test accuracy are, in their vast majority, observational studies.

Assessment of the Quality of Randomized Controlled Trials Included in a Meta-Analysis

The assessment of the quality of studies meeting the eligibility criteria for inclusion in a meta-analysis was listed as a necessary part of any statistical overview in the early guidelines for meta-analysis in clinical research [1, 2, 6–8]. Formal instruments for assessing the quality of RCTs have been (and continue to be) developed [46–50]. Chalmers et al. [46] developed a detailed list of items to be used for scoring the quality of published RCTs on a scale from 0 to 1. Guidelines for evaluating observational studies were initially presented by Lichtenstein et al. [51] and Feinstein [52] and several more scales followed.

A simple instrument was developed by Jadad et al. [53] for use by all readers of RCTs. The maximum quality score that can be given to a study based on this instrument is 5. Two points are given to a report for random assignment of subjects to treatment and control groups; 2 points are granted for blinding both investigators and patients; and 1 point is added if the number of patients excluded from the analysis, along with the reasons for all dropouts and withdrawals, are presented in the report of the RCT. With regard to the randomization procedure, 1 point is given if a study is designated as "randomized," but the randomization procedure is not described; 0 point is given if the randomization procedure is described, but is judged to be inappropriate; and 2 points are given if the randomization procedure is described, and is appropriate. In regard to the blinding technique, 1 point is given if a study is designated as "double-blind," but the procedure for blinding investigators and patients is not described; 0 point is given if the blinding procedure is described, but is judged to be inappropriate; and 2 points are given if the blinding procedure is described, and is appropriate.

Moher et al. [54] used the instrument of Jadad et al. [53] to measure the quality of 127 RCTs from the medical literature. Few RCTs had reported either the method used to generate the randomization sequence (15%), or the method used to conceal this sequence until the point of randomization occurred (14%). RCTs that had not adequately described the measures taken to conceal the treatment allocations, exaggerated the effect of the intervention under study by 37% ($p<0.01$), compared to RCTs that had adequately reported the method(s) used for concealment. Furthermore, RCTs receiving a low total quality score (≤ 2) exaggerated the estimate of the effect of the intervention by 34%, compared with high-quality trials (>2) ($p<0.001$). Moher et al. [54] concluded that the pooling of the findings of low-quality RCTs results in a clinically important and statistically significant exaggeration of the efficacy of an intervention under study.

Therefore, after a quality score has been assigned to each study that is eligible for inclusion in a meta-analysis, meta-analysts must confront the contentious issue whether studies of inferior quality are to be included in the calculation of the "average" treatment effect. The main argument for including studies that are not of the best quality is that a larger number of studies permits examination of the effect of the intervention in more situations. However, this advantage must be balanced against the disadvantage of including questionable results. There is a general consensus that, if studies of poor quality are to be included, the differences in quality must be taken into account in the analysis [55, 56]. Computational methods used in meta-analysis assign weights to each study that are proportional to a study's sample size [57, 58]. In theory, the quality scores could also be incorporated into the weights assigned to each report, so that the calculated "average" treatment effect can depend more heavily on the findings of investigations of superior quality [55]. Alternatively, the studies could be stratified by quality score, so that an "average" treatment effect can be calculated separately for each stratum of quality. If the effects differ across strata, the "average" effect calculated from studies of superior quality can be considered to be the valid one.

Overviews in the health field have sometimes adjusted for the quality of the combined studies by statistical techniques [59]. Some experts have recommended that minimal quality standards be set in advance, in the form of criteria for inclusion, and that studies that do not meet them be excluded. Others have proposed that only the "best" of the available studies be used [60, 61]. Quality scores have been criticized, however, as being based on the report of a study, which is not necessarily an accurate measure of the truth about some elements of quality. The standards for reporting details of the methods used have become more stringent over the last decade [62, 63], and studies published more recently tend to attain higher quality scores for that reason.

Rationale for Quantitative Research Synthesis

An overview compares the effect of an exposure or treatment in one study with the effect of that exposure or treatment in other studies. A meta-analysis by the *fixed-effects* method [57, 58] combines a series of 2×2 contingency table counts (Table 9.1), as though the tables were strata of patients enrolled in the same study (and stratified according to the level of a confounding factor in an epidemiologic investigation or by admitting hospital in a multicenter RCT). The findings from these individual strata are integrated, according each stratum a weight commensurate with its sample size. An assumption is made that there is a uniform or "fixed" treatment effect in all of the strata (or in all of the studies included in the meta-analysis). Studies are thought to have generated different estimates of this fixed effect solely because of random sampling variation. The results of a meta-analysis by the fixed-effects method are thus valid only if this is a reasonable assumption to make.

This assumption cannot be reasonably made if the combined studies differ with respect to important design attributes (Table 9.2). If current medical knowledge suggests that the effect of an intervention should differ in various situations (such as those shown in Table 9.2), it is probably *unreasonable* to assume that the exposure or treatment under study has had the same effect in all the reported studies. A meta-analysis by the *random-effects* method [66] is advocated for these circumstances. The assumption of a random-effects analysis is that the effect of the exposure or treatment varies from study to study, being randomly positioned about some central value. This value is the summary or "average" effect of the exposure or treatment across the combined studies.

In a fixed-effects analysis, only *within-studies* variation influences the uncertainty of the summary effect across the combined studies that are calculated by the overview. "Within-studies" variation refers simply to random sampling variation from study to study, that is, the variation that results each time that a study sample is drawn, at random, from the target population of all eligible patients. This sampling variation is inversely proportional to the sample size of each report. No *between-studies* variation is presumed to exist when a fixed-effects analysis is conducted, as all included studies are assumed to measure the same (fixed) effect of the exposure or treatment. Therefore, the differences among the studies in the magnitude and direction of the reported treatment effect do not influence the uncertainty that surrounds the summary effect calculated by the meta-analysis.

On the contrary, in a random-effects analysis, both within-studies and between-studies variation influence the uncertainty surrounding the calculated summary effect. The uncertainty associated with the measured estimate of the effect increases if the sample size of the combined studies is small, because small sample sizes result in large within-studies variation. The uncertainty increases further if the combined studies differ in important design characteristics (such as those shown in Table 9.2), because such differences among the reports imply that the individual studies should be expected to measure different exposure or treatment effects. The more the combined studies differ in important design characteristics, the greater the expected differences in the estimates of the effect(s) calculated by these studies; therefore, the greater also the between-studies variation, and the greater the uncertainty surrounding the summary effect calculated by the meta-analysis.

The 95% confidence interval (CI) of the summary effect measures this uncertainty which surrounds the "average" treatment effect calculated by the meta-analysis. The 95% CI calculated from a fixed-effects analysis is an estimate of the within-studies variation in the combined studies. In contrast, the 95% CI calculated from a random-effects analysis is an estimate of *both* the within- and between-studies variation, thus being, wider than the 95% CI calculated from a fixed-effects analysis. The difference between these two 95% CIs is proportional to the between-studies variation, or the magnitude of the differences in study-design attributes as well as in reported results.

Small studies have more of an impact on the calculated "average" effect when a random- (as opposed to fixed-) effects analysis is undertaken. When the literature eligible for analysis consists of one (or a few) large investigations and many small studies, a single large report may dominate the findings of an overview conducted by a fixed-effects method. This analysis would take only the within-studies variation into account, and would thus weigh studies with large sample sizes (and small within-studies variation) more favorably than small reports. Therefore, the conclusions of the overview could, for the most part, reflect the results of these few large studies, as opposed to the composite evidence from all completed studies. In contrast, the findings of a meta-analysis by the random-effects method would reflect the combination of within- and between-studies variation. The more the combined studies differ in important design attributes, the more important the between-studies variation becomes, as compared to the within-studies variation. As a result, the more the influence of a single large study diminishes, and the more the stated conclusions of the overview accomplish the purpose of the meta-analysis, which is to examine the effect of an exposure or treatment in many, different situations.

If there are no important design differences between the combined studies, random- and fixed-effects analyses will produce similar results. On the contrary, if there are substantive differences among the studies, the two methods of analysis will produce disparate results [64]. Fixed- and random-effects analyses are based on different conceptions of the proper role, scope, and meaning of meta-analysis. Despite the differences in assumptions delineated above, there are strong opinions about the appropriateness of both lines of analysis [65–68].

Assessment of the Combinability of the Reports Included in the Meta-Analysis

Results of separate studies should be combined by the methods of meta-analysis only when the estimates of effect size that they have reported are sufficiently close to one another. This prerequisite is referred to as *homogeneity* of effects.

The opposite situation – that is, when sizable differences exist between investigations in study attributes and the reported estimates of effect – is known as *heterogeneity* of effects. A discussion of the homogeneity (or heterogeneity) of the studies must precede any integration of studies in a meta-analysis. Study results should not be integrated in the presence of unexplained heterogeneity, although this principle is very often not adhered to in published meta-analyses. Statistical reviewers of the U.S. Food and Drug Administration have denigrated as mere computational exercises all overviews that had combined heterogeneous reports [69–71].

Homogeneity is assessed statistically by the *Q* test statistic, which examines whether the variation in the findings of the studies is sufficiently modest to have arisen by chance [1–7]. If $p<0.05$ for the *Q* test statistic, there is a smaller than 5% probability that the variation in the results of the available studies might have arisen by chance. In this situation, the hypothesis of homogeneity is rejected, and the results of the studies should not be combined. Such statistical heterogeneity generally reflects the *medical* heterogeneity of the studies. For example, in Fig. 9.1, the effect of WBC-containing ABT varies from a 20% reduction to a 7.3-fold increase in the risk of infection. This extreme statistical heterogeneity ($p<0.001$ for the *Q* test statistic, that is, a smaller than 1/1,000 probability that the variation in the findings of the studies [21–32] might have arisen by chance) reflects the considerable medical heterogeneity of the studies (Table 9.2).

The Q test statistic is a chi-square test with $n-1$ degrees of freedom (where n = number of studies included in the overview). Because the *Q* test statistic depends on the number of studies – being less sensitive to heterogeneity when the number of studies available for meta-analysis is small – an alternative test (I^2) has been proposed to assess the extent of heterogeneity among studies [72, 73]. I^2 does not inherently depend on the number of studies included in the analysis, and it is expressed as a percentage (i.e., the percentage of total variation across studies attributed to heterogeneity). For this reason, it has intuitive meaning to the reader, and it can be directly compared between meta-analyses. Low heterogeneity corresponds to I^2 values of <25%, while high heterogeneity is reflected in I^2 values of >75% [72]. However, Higgins et al. [72] did not indicate any specific cutoff value (e.g., >75%) past which it is inappropriate to integrate studies owing to heterogeneity. Instead, they suggested that quantification of heterogeneity is only one component of a wider investigation of variability across studies; and that the interpretation of a given degree of heterogeneity will differ according to whether the estimates of effect from the various studies show the same direction of effect.

When studies are heterogeneous, instead of integrating results, meta-analysts should present an analysis of the possible reasons for variation in the findings of the available studies [74–78]. The simplest method for explaining heterogeneity is a stratification of the eligible studies based on design, quality, and/or characteristics of enrolled patients and/or administered interventions or exposures. Providing that the hypothesis of homogeneity is not rejected within each stratum following such stratification of the available studies, the calculated stratum-specific "average" treatment effects may help explain the disagreements among the available reports.

In the case of the RCTs of WBC-containing ABT and infection (Fig. 9.1 and Table 9.2), meta-analyses of clinically-homogeneous subsets of RCTs by a random-effects method [79] produced results diametrically opposed to the findings expected from the theory that attributes the effect of non-WBC-reduced ABT to WBC-derived soluble mediators [40–43]: there was a reduction in the risk of postoperative infection in association with *poststorage* (as opposed to *prestorage*) WBC reduction [18]. More specifically, across nine relatively homogeneous RCTs [21–29] that transfused allogeneic RBCs filtered before storage to the WBC-reduced arm, no increase in the risk of postoperative infection was detected in association with non-WBC-reduced ABT (summary OR = 1.06, 95% CI, 0.91–1.24; $p>0.05$ – middle panel in Fig. 9.3). If the ABT effect were mediated by WBC-derived soluble mediators, prestorage filtration should have abrogated an

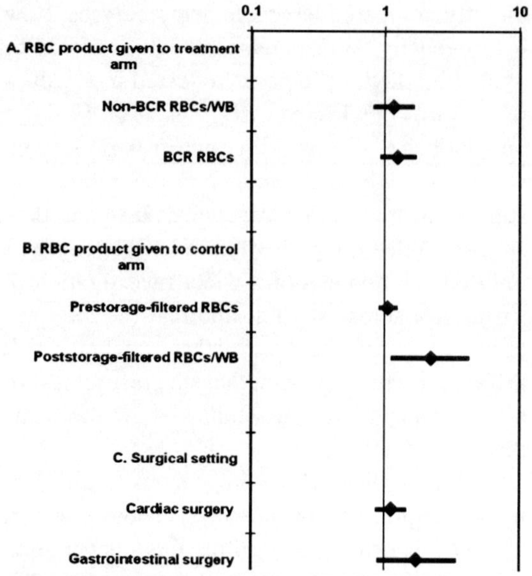

Fig. 9.3 Possible sources of variation in the findings of RCTs investigating the association between WBC-containing ABT and bacterial infection. Stratified meta-analyses are presented of studies that administered the same RBC product to their treatment or control arm or were conducted in the same clinical setting. The summary ORs calculated across the studies that transfused buffy-coat-reduced allogeneic RBCs to the treatment arm (seven studies; see Table 9.2) or were conducted in gastrointestinal surgery (five studies) are shown solely for the purpose of illustration, because these study subgroups were heterogeneous ($p<0.01$ and <0.001, respectively, for the Q test statistic), precluding a medically-meaningful integration of their findings. Only the subgroup analysis of the studies that administered *poststorage-filtered* allogeneic RBCs or whole blood to the control arm produced a statistically significant ($p<0.05$) ABT effect (summary OR=2.25; 95% CI, 1.12–4.25). Thus, the purported deleterious effect of WBC-containing ABT appeared to be prevented by the transfusion of WBC-reduced RBCs filtered after – but not before – storage. The subgroup of four studies [28, 30–32] transfusing poststorage-filtered allogeneic RBCs [28, 30, 31] or whole blood [32] to the control arm was the smallest ($n=1{,}616$) of all subgroups shown in the figure and consisted of early studies published before 1999 (Table 9.2). Transfusion of poststorage-filtered allogeneic RBCs or whole blood is now rarely (if ever) used in the US. *BCR* buffy-coat-reduced; *WB* whole blood

increased infection risk associated with non-WBC-reduced ABT, because it would have removed the allogeneic WBCs from the components given to the WBC-reduced arm of each study before the WBCs could release any significant amounts of mediators into the supernatant fluid of the components.

In contrast, across four RCTs [28, 30–32] that transfused RBCs filtered after storage to the WBC-reduced arm, there was a more than two-fold increase in the risk of infection in association with non-WBC-reduced ABT (middle panel in Fig. 9.3). If the ABT effect were mediated by WBC-derived soluble mediators, poststorage filtration should not have abrogated an increased infection risk associated with non-WBC-reduced ABT, because it would not have removed such mediators from the supernatant fluid of the stored RBCs given to the WBC-reduced arm of the studies. Yet, this was the only clinically-homogeneous subset of studies in which an adverse effect of WBC-containing ABT was detected (Fig. 9.3).

Investigation of the sources of variation in the results of RCTs of WBC-containing ABT and all-cause mortality did generate a clinically-meaningful result, however (Fig. 9.4). Across the (also statistically-homogeneous) cardiac-surgery studies, there was a 72% increase in mortality in association with non-WBC-reduced (compared with WBC-reduced) ABT. This result conforms to what would have been expected from the immunomodulation theory [44] (that there would be more of an immunomodulatory ABT in cardiac surgery where the pro-inflammatory effect of the extracorporeal circuit acts as a cofactor than in other settings), and it is also calculated in adherence to the rule of integrating only medically- and statistically-homogeneous studies.

Regression techniques offer a more elegant method for explaining heterogeneity among studies [80]. If ten or more original reports on the effect of WBC-containing ABT on increasing the risk of bacterial infection or all-cause mortality were available per explanatory variable included in the model, the variation in the results of those RCTs might be explained by the following regression model:

$$\ln(\text{odds of infection or mortality}) = \alpha + \beta_1 X_1 + \beta_2 X_2 + \beta_3 X_3 + \beta_T T,$$

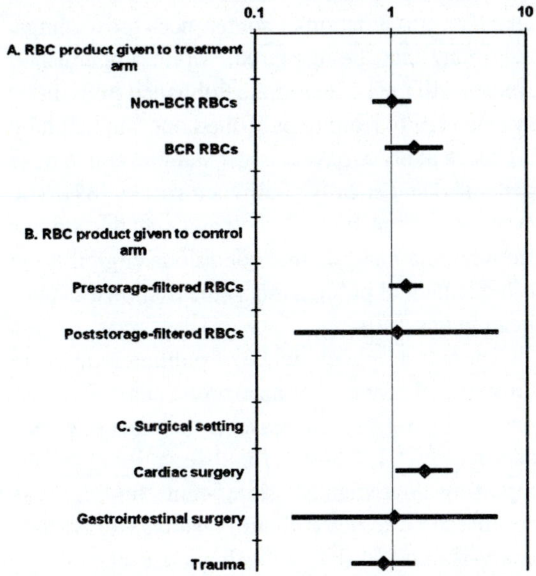

Fig. 9.4 Possible sources of variation in the findings of RCTs investigating the association between WBC-containing ABT and short-term (up to 3-month posttransfusion), all-cause mortality. Stratified meta-analyses are presented of studies that administered the same RBC product to their treatment arm or control arm or were conducted in the same clinical setting. The summary ORs calculated across the studies that transfused poststorage-filtered allogeneic RBCs (two studies [28, 31]) or were conducted in gastrointestinal surgery (two studies [26, 31]) are shown solely for the purpose of illustration, because these study subgroups were heterogeneous ($p=0.02$ for the Q test statistic in both cases). Only the subgroup analysis of studies conducted in cardiac surgery [21, 23, 25, 28, 29] produced a statistically significant ($p<0.05$) ABT effect (summary OR=1.72; 95% CI, 1.05–2.81). Across the six remaining studies conducted at other settings [24, 26, 27, 31, 33, 34], the summary OR was 0.99 (95% CI, 0.73–1.33). Both the cardiac-surgery and the noncardiac-surgery studies were homogeneous ($p>0.10$ and $p=0.20$, respectively, for the Q test statistic). Cardiac-surgery studies enrolled a total of 2,990 patients; noncardiac-surgery studies a total of 5,045. *BCR* buffy-coat-reduced

where

ln = natural logarithm

a = intercept (i.e., a constant)

X_1 = RBC component given to the treatment arm (nonbuffy-coat-reduced or buffy-coat-reduced RBCs or whole blood)

X_2 = RBC component given to the control arm (WBC-reduced RBCs or whole blood filtered before or after storage)

X_3 = clinical setting (cardiac surgery, gastrointestinal surgery, or other)

$\beta_1, \beta_2, \beta_3$ = partial regression coefficients for the variables thought to represent possible sources of variation in the results of available studies (i.e., partial regression coefficients for the study descriptors [or explanatory variables] X_1, X_2, X_3 above)

β_T = partial regression coefficient for being randomly allocated to the WBC-containing arm of an RCT, that is, corresponding to the exposure or treatment under study

If some of the calculated estimates of the partial regression coefficients for the predictor variables in this model (b_1, b_2, b_3) differed from zero to a statistically significant extent, the heterogeneity among studies might be explained by the corresponding study descriptor(s). For example, if b_1, b_2, and b_3 all differed significantly from zero, the conclusion of the analysis would be that the RBC product given to the treatment and control arm, as well as the cardiac-surgery (vs. noncardiac surgery) clinical setting, could be responsible for the extreme variation in the results of the reported studies. With the sources of heterogeneity thus explained, the effect of random assignment to the receipt of non-WBC-reduced (vs. WBC-reduced) ABT (b_T) could then be calculated, as well as tested for statistical significance.

The Medical Interpretation of Overviews

In overviews addressing medical issues, research questions must be stated with no less thorough a biologic discussion than would appear in a traditional review, and the findings must be discussed in the context of a review of pathophysiologic principles and results of basic laboratory research and individual RCTs [78]. Most importantly, the relevance of the findings to patient care must be explained to the reader. In addition, readers of overviews must be reminded that meta-analyses use historical material from studies published over a considerable period, because this historical nature of the material may influence the applicability of the findings to contemporary clinical practice.

For example, the only adverse effect detected with WBC-containing ABT vis-à-vis the development of bacterial infection derived from RBC components (middle panel in Fig. 9.3) no longer used in the US. Regardless of any methodologic reasons that may have produced this finding across four studies [28, 30–32], the only analysis that is clinically relevant today is the comparison between prestorage-filtered WBC-reduced and non-WBC-reduced RBCs. In this latter comparison, no adverse effect of WBC-containing ABT on bacterial infection was detected.

The finding that WBC-containing ABT may be related to increased all-cause mortality in cardiac-surgery (lower panel in Fig. 9.4) is most relevant today, however, because not all blood transfusion services in the US administer WBC-reduced components to patients undergoing open-heart surgery.

The value of meta-analysis in combining patient populations enrolled in separate studies for the purpose of documenting the existence of an exposure or treatment effect is not universally accepted [80–82]. The reason is that meta-analyses and large RCTs disagree 10–35% of the time, that is, more often than would be expected by chance [83–86]. This is probably because the findings of meta-analyses are susceptible to the effects of selection and observation bias, in a manner similar to the results of traditional observational original reports.

An observational study conducted at a single institution and investigating the effect of an exposure or treatment on a disease must enroll all patients who are sequentially admitted to that hospital or service with a specific diagnosis. If subjects are missed or excluded, selection bias could result. Similarly, the validity of a meta-analysis depends on the complete sampling of all the studies performed on a particular topic. Validity can be preserved if a representative sample is obtained, but any incomplete sample is a potentially biased one [87]. Unfortunately, meta-analysts may not be able to locate all published studies, because computerized data bases do not cover all periodicals, search algorithms often fail to identify relevant articles, and the indexing of studies is imperfect [88]. Even if the literature is optimally searched, studies published as government reports, book chapters, dissertations, conference proceedings, etc., may not be captured, while unpublished studies will not be identified. Published trials differ systematically from unpublished ones, in that they are more likely to have a larger sample, and to have generated statistically significant results [89]. The systematic exclusion of small and negative studies from a meta-analysis that conditions eligibility on achievement of publication status is known as publication bias [90].

There is ample evidence of publication bias in the medical literature. Easterbrook et al. [91] documented a 3.8-fold increase in the odds of publication (95% CI, 1.5–9.8) for observational studies reporting statistically significant findings, as compared to studies with null results. Multivariate analysis showed that the better odds of publication could not be explained by the quality of study design. On the contrary, there was a trend towards a greater number of statistically significant results with poorer quality studies [91].

Selection bias can arise not only during retrieval of studies from the literature, but also during assessment of the eligibility of the retrieved reports. In evaluating the quality of investigations, analysts may be influenced by knowledge of the study results or journal of publication. They may even be inclined to modify eligibility criteria, so as to include in the overview reports from prestigious journals. According to Felson [87], selection bias is the principal reason for discrepant results in meta-analyses. Different teams of analysts may base their conclusions on alternate sets of original reports, generating either statistically significant or null (i.e., statistically insignificant) findings. This was also the explanation for the discrepant results between the meta-analysis [18] whose results are depicted in Figs. 9.3 and 9.4 and the earlier overviews [35, 36] that had included a smaller number of RCTs whose findings had been made available through 2002 [92].

Meta-Analyses of Studies of Diagnostic-Test Accuracy

Development of new fields often requires the development of new methods [93]. The cardinal difference between RCTs and studies of the

Table 9.3 Diagnostic accuracy of a laboratory test

	Disease status		
	Present	Absent	Totals
Positive test results	True-positives (TP)	False-positives (FP)	TP+FP
Negative test results	False-negatives (FN)	True-negatives (TN)	FN+TN
Totals	TP+FN	FP+TN	All individuals tested

$$\text{Accuracy} = \frac{\text{Number of correct test results}}{\text{Number of people tested}}$$

$$\text{Sensitivity} = \frac{\text{Number of true - positive test results}}{\text{Number of people with disease tested}} = \frac{\text{TP}}{\text{TP} + \text{FN}}$$

$$\text{Specificity} = \frac{\text{Number of true - negative test results}}{\text{Number of people without disease tested}} = \frac{\text{TN}}{\text{TN} + \text{FP}}$$

$$\text{Positive predictive value} = \frac{\text{Number of true - positive test results}}{\text{Number of all positive test results}} = \frac{\text{TP}}{\text{TP} + \text{FP}}$$

$$\text{Negative predictive value} = \frac{\text{Number of true - negative test results}}{\text{Number of all negative test results}} = \frac{\text{TN}}{\text{TN} + \text{FN}}$$

accuracy of diagnostic tests is that *all* patients enrolled in RCTs have the disease of interest; whereas studies of diagnostic-test accuracy include a *mixed* population of subjects with and without disease. Moreover, RCTs measure one quantity, that is, the effect of a therapeutic intervention in treated patients vs. controls; whereas studies of diagnostic-test accuracy measure *two* quantities, that is, the sensitivity and specificity of a test. These two quantities are interdependent, and they also depend on the cutoff point used in each study for judging the results of the test to be positive; sensitivity can be increased by decreasing the cutoff point and decreasing the specificity, or vice versa. Sensitivity and specificity are thus negatively correlated.

In combining the findings (Table 9.3) of studies of diagnostic-test accuracy, an assumption is made that the published estimates of the sensitivity and specificity of a test are likely to vary among studies, because of differences between the studies in the cutoff point used for judging the results of the test to be positive. Accordingly, methods for integrating the findings of these reports must address the interdependence between sensitivity and specificity, and the influence of the cutoff point used in each study on the corresponding estimate of accuracy. To meet the former objective, the estimates of sensitivity are not combined independently of the estimates of specificity, but the two components of accuracy obtained from each study are considered jointly. To remove the effect that the variation of the cutoff point has on accuracy, the diagnostic accuracy of a laboratory test across the available studies is summarized in the form of a summary receiver-operating characteristic (ROC) curve that plots the "average" true-positive (TP) proportion calculated for the test against the "average" false-positive (FP) proportion (Table 9.4) [12–17]. If this initial analysis shows that the accuracy of the laboratory test is constant within a range of

Table 9.4 Interrelationships between the sensitivity and specificity of a diagnostic test

True-positive proportion (TPP) = Sensitivity
True-negative proportion (TNP) = Specificity
False-positive proportion (FPP) = 1 − Specificity
False-negative proportion (FNP) = 1 − Sensitivity
TPP + FNP = (Sensitivity) + (1 − Sensitivity) = 1
TNP + FPP = (Specificity) + (1 − Specificity) = 1
Sensitivity = $P\ (T+/D+)^a$ = TPP
Specificity = $P\ (T-/D-)^b$ = TNP
1 − Specificity = $P\ (T+/D-)^c$ = FPP
1 − Sensitivity = $P\ (T-/D+)^d$ = FNP

[a] Probability of the test's being positive given the presence of disease

[b] Probability of the test's being negative given the absence of disease

[c] Probability of the test's being positive given the absence of disease

[d] Probability of the test's being negative given the presence of disease

clinically relevant cutoffs, a point estimate of the summary accuracy of the test – the summary OR – is also calculated, in lieu of (or in addition to) the summary OR curve. Statistical methods for integrating data on laboratory test accuracy have both been developed and are under development [94, 95].

To control for the interdependence between the estimates of sensitivity and specificity derived from each primary study, meta-analyses combine these two quantities into an OR, and they then use the OR as the overall measure of the accuracy of the laboratory test as calculated from each study (Table 9.5). The OR is defined as the odds of a TP test result, divided by the odds of a FP test result, that is, the odds of obtaining a positive test result as calculated from a person with disease, divided by the odds of obtaining a positive test result in a person without disease. The natural logarithm of the odds of a TP test result (i.e., ln[TPP ÷ (1 − TPP)]) is designated as logit (TPP). The natural logarithm of the odds of a FP test result (i.e., ln[FPP ÷ (1 − FPP)]) is designated as logit (FPP). The natural logarithm of the OR, designated as *D*, equals the difference between these logits (i.e., *D* = logit [TPP] − logit [FPP]). *D* is a logodds ratio that measures how well the test discriminates between subjects with and without the disease. *S* is a measure of the threshold for classifying a test result to be positive, and it equals the sum of the logits (i.e., *S* = logit [TPP] + logit [FPP]); it is large and positive if both the TPP and the FPP are large, and it is negative when they are small [95, 96].

The calculations involved in estimating the position of a summary ROC curve across studies included in a meta-analysis are summarized in Table 9.6. From each primary study, the meta-analysts extract

Table 9.5 Overall diagnostic accuracy of a laboratory test, as determined by the odds ratio

$$\text{Odds ratio} = \frac{\text{odds of a true - positive test result}}{\text{odds of a false - positive test result}}$$

or

$$\text{Odds ratio} = \frac{\text{odds of obtaining a positive test result in a person with disease}}{\text{odds of obtaining a positive test result in a person without disease}}$$

or

$$\text{Odds ratio} = \frac{(\text{true - positive proportion})/1-(\text{true - positive proportion})}{(\text{false - positive proportion})/1-(\text{false - positive proportion})}$$

or

$$\text{Odds ratio} = \frac{(\text{sensitivity})/1-(\text{sensitivity})}{1-(\text{specificity})/(\text{specificity})}$$

Sensitivity (%)	Specificity (%)	Odds ratio	Natural logarithm of odds ratio[a]
99.9	99.9	999,000.00	13.8
99.8	99.8	249,500.00	12.4
99.5	99.5	39,800.00	10.6
99.0	99.0	9,802.00	9.2
98.0	98.0	2,402.00	7.8
95.0	95.0	361.00	5.9
90.0	90.0	81.00	4.4
80.0	80.0	16.00	2.8
70.0	70.0	5.44	1.7
60.0	60.0	2.25	0.8
50.0	50.0	1.00	0.0

[a]Measure of the overall accuracy of a laboratory test used in the meta-analyses of studies of the diagnostic accuracy of laboratory tests

Table 9.6 Calculation of a summary receiver-operating characteristic (ROC) curve[a]

A. Calculate the quantities D_i and S_i for each study included in the analysis

1. Extract 2×2 contingency table counts from the report of each study:

	Disease status	
Test results	Present	Absent
Positive	True-positives (TP)	False-positives (FP)
Negative	False-negatives (FN)	True-negatives (TN)

2. Calculate the TPP, FPP, and OR_i for each study:

$$\text{True - positive proportion (TPP)} = \frac{\text{TP}}{\text{TP} + \text{FN}}$$

$$\text{False - positive proportion (FPP)} = \frac{\text{FP}}{\text{FP} + \text{TN}}$$

$$\text{Odds ratio } (\text{OR}_i) = \frac{\text{TPP} \div (1 - \text{TPP})}{\text{FPP} \div (1 - \text{FPP})}$$

3. Calculate the quantities D_i and S_i for each study:

$$\text{D}_i = \ln(\text{OR}_i) = \text{logit (TPP)} - \text{logit (FPP)}$$

$$\text{S}_i = \text{logit (TPP)} + \text{logit (FPP)}$$

where ln is the natural logarithm, logit (TPP) is the natural logarithm of the odds of a true-positive test result; and logit (FPP) is the natural logarithm of the odds of a false-positive test result

B. Fit a simple linear regression model using the quantities D_i and S_i from each study

$D = \alpha + \beta S$

C. Transform this model back to the conventional axes of TPP vs. FPP, and draw a summary ROC curve over the range of the data

[a]See Littenberg and Moses [95] and Moses et al. [96]

data for a 2×2 contingency table showing the reported TP, FP, true-negative (TN), and false-negative (FN) results of the laboratory test under evaluation. They then compute a true-positive proportion (TPP=TP÷[TP+FN]) and a false-positive proportion (FPP=FP÷[FP+TN]) for each contingency table, and calculate the logit (TPP) and the logit (FPP), as well as the difference between the logits (*D*) and the sum of the logits (*S*). Having summarized the data from each primary study with these two quantities (e.g., D_i and S_i for the *i*th study), they fit a simple linear regression model using *D* as the dependent variable and *S* as the predictor variable: [95, 96]

$$D = \alpha + \beta S.$$

By employing this logarithmic transformation, it is possible to use a line to represent a curvilinear relationship. The fitted regression line can then be transformed back to the conventional axes of an ROC curve (i.e., a plot of the TPP vs. the FPP), and depict a summary ROC curve across the combined studies [95, 96].

The intercept of the model (*a*) is the estimated logodds ratio when the accuracy of the test remains constant as the cutoff point varies from study to study. The regression coefficient or slope (*β*) provides an estimate of the extent to which the logodds ratio depends on the cutoff used. When *β* is near zero (or, at least, if $-0.5 < \beta < +0.5$), the shape of the curve calculated by the transformed model approximates that of a traditional ROC curve. Also if *b* does not differ significantly from zero, the accuracy of the test does not depend on the particular cutoff point used in each study, and the accuracy of the test across the combined studies can be summarized by the logodds ratio given by the intercept *a*. The larger this intercept is, the closer the curve is positioned to the upper left corner in the ROC space, which indicates a greater diagnostic accuracy for the test [95, 96].

Obstacles to the Use of Meta-Analysis for the Integration of Findings of Studies of Diagnostic-Test Accuracy

As discussed previously in the context of RCTs: (1) low-quality studies should be either excluded from a meta-analysis or weighed in proportion to their quality; and (2) available studies should be combined only if the variation in reported results is sufficiently modest to be attributed to chance. In the case of RCTs, the Q test statistic quantifies the probability that the variation in the results of the available studies is sufficiently modest to permit their integration by the methods of a meta-analysis. The meta-analytic methods are still being refined, however, for use with studies of diagnostic-test accuracy, and the lack of as fully developed methods can be somewhat of an impediment to the use of meta-analysis in pathology. The calculations presented in Table 9.6 are sometimes deemed to be too complicated, and many investigators succumb to the temptation of integrating estimates of sensitivity independently of the corresponding estimates of specificity; as well as estimates of specificity independently of the corresponding estimates of sensitivity. Although it is easy to do so with the meta-analysis software made widely available for RCTs, such a simplistic approach to the analysis is valid only when the meta-analysts have demonstrated a lack of dependence of the diagnostic-test accuracy on the cutoff employed in each retrieved study.

The most important obstacle, however, to the use of meta-analysis for integrating results of studies of diagnostic-test accuracy are the suboptimal technical or scientific merits of the studies available for analysis. Several aspects of study design and analysis [97–99] need thus be considered by analysts in judging the quality of studies of diagnostic-test accuracy (Table 9.7). These issues have been discussed in detail by Sackett et al. [100].

When the accuracy of an index laboratory test is investigated, an assumption is made that the employed "gold standard" can *definitively* discriminate between individuals with and without disease. If the available "gold standard" is imperfect, there will be an error in the initial estimation of the accuracy of the laboratory test [101–103]. Available tests with established diagnostic accuracy rarely meet the definition of a "gold standard"; however, those evaluating the diagnostic accuracy of new laboratory tests must strive to use the best available method for ascertaining the presence of disease in their study population.

Table 9.7 Questions to be considered in assessing the quality of studies of the diagnostic accuracy of laboratory tests

Was the "gold standard" used definitive?
Was the "gold standard" used independent of the test under evaluation?
Were *all* individuals included in the study – or a *random* subset of individuals – tested by the "gold standard?"
Did the individuals included in the study represent a consecutive series or a randomly selected study population?
Were any individuals withdrawn from the analysis following their inclusion in the study, because of equivocal test results or any other reason?
Did the performance of the test under evaluation and the "gold standard" conform to the standard of practice?
Was the uncertainty surrounding the calculated estimates of sensitivity and specificity of the test quantified?
Was the cutoff point used for interpreting the results of the test as positive clinically appropriate, and/or was it varied within a clinically relevant range?
Was the clinical setting in which the test was evaluated adequately described?

Ideally, all enrolled patients should undergo complete diagnostic work-ups without knowledge of the results of the laboratory test under evaluation. However, if the "gold standard" requires an invasive procedure, it may be desirable to restrict its use to a subset of the study population. This approach is acceptable only if the selection of patients for verification by the "gold standard" is random. If the patients who undergo the invasive procedure are selected based on abnormal results from other tests, or because they have risk factors for disease, etc., verification bias is introduced which can seriously distort the results of the study. The effects of this systematic error on the diagnostic accuracy of the test are unpredictable, and they cannot be corrected statistically [103–105].

The accuracy of a laboratory test should be assessed in consecutive patients, or patients selected randomly for inclusion in the study, and all enrolled patients should be included in the analysis. No withdrawals of patients can be permitted following their inclusion in the study, because of equivocal test results or any other reason. The methods for carrying out the test under evaluation and the *gold standard* should be described in sufficient detail, and the cutoff point used for judging either test to be positive should be specified. Moreover, the uncertainty surrounding the calculated estimates of sensitivity and specificity should be communicated to the reader, by reporting 95% CIs for these proportions. To remove the influence of an arbitrary cutoff point on the reported estimates of sensitivity and specificity, the cutoff for the test should be varied within a clinically relevant range, and the diagnostic accuracy of the test should be reported in the form of an ROC curve. Alternatively, if a single cutoff point is used, the clinical appropriateness of the chosen cutoff point should be discussed. The clinical setting in which the test is evaluated should be stated explicitly, and a description of the characteristics of the enrolled patients (e.g., age, gender, symptoms, results of other diagnostic tests, etc.) should be provided.

Once all studies of diagnostic-test accuracy conform to the STARD guidelines [106], perhaps the most important obstacle to the use of meta-analysis for integrating the results of studies of diagnostic-test accuracy will have been overcome. Further guidelines (for both the conduct and the reporting of studies) are provided in the STROBE statement [107], which applies to observational studies in general.

When the available studies of the accuracy of a laboratory test differ in important study characteristics (such as the employed cutoff point or the disease prevalence in the included population), the diagnostic accuracy of the test should be assumed to differ from study to study, according to the varying characteristics of each study. Therefore, in such a situation, a random-effects method should be used to integrate the findings of the available studies. Random-effects methods that take into account the dependence of sensitivity and specificity on the cutoff point used in each study continue to be developed. The fixed-effects method delineated in Table 9.6 for the calculation of a summary ROC curve [95, 96] can be modified to conform to the assumptions of a random-effects analysis.

Another impediment to the use of meta-analysis in pathology is that individuals included in studies of diagnostic-test accuracy are not allocated randomly by the investigators to have (or to not have) the disease of interest. The validity of statistical tests is guaranteed only if the allocation of subjects to comparison arms is random. In RCTs, randomization makes it possible to ascribe a probability distribution to the difference in outcome between two arms that receive equally effective treatments under the null hypothesis. Knowledge of this distribution is a prerequisite for assigning significance levels to any observed differences. If the allocation of subjects to groups is not random, the validity of tests of significance depends on additional assumptions about the comparability of the groups and the appropriateness of the statistical models. The veracity of these latter assumptions is difficult to establish.

Finally, in the case of RCTs, there is ample evidence of publication bias in the medical literature, and meta-analyses of RCTs consider the possible effect(s) of this bias on the stated conclusions. The effect of publication bias on studies of diagnostic-test accuracy is not as well researched, but many investigators suspect that the published studies of diagnostic-test accuracy are a biased subset that tends to overestimate the diagnostic accuracy of the test under evaluation. Since the studies of diagnostic-test accuracy are – in their vast majority – observational, it is likely that publication bias may have an even larger impact on meta-analyses of studies of diagnostic-test accuracy than on meta-analyses of RCTs.

Conclusions

Meta-analyses are a supplement to RCTs, which remain the gold standard for evaluating the efficacy of therapeutic interventions, but need to be supplemented by meta-analyses in order to broaden the applicability of the findings. Furthermore, meta-analyses can be an important research tool for the systematic evaluation of the quality of published studies and for the disciplined investigation of reasons for disagreements among reports. Overviews can identify errors and shortcomings in completed studies and may be able to explain why trial results differ. In the past, narrative reviews of the literature served these functions in a less formal manner. Meta-analyses are much better suited for these purposes, because of their objective and quantitative nature.

Since meta-analysis is a technical statistical method, many clinicians find themselves unable to appreciate its nuances and limitations in the same way that they can appreciate those of a traditional original report. However, readers of the medical literature need to be familiar with the definitions and assumptions of fixed- vs. random-effects analyses, as well as with the meaning of the results of the Q test statistic or other tests for homogeneity [108]. This is because health-policy guidelines – as well as recommendations for patient management – are already being based, and are likely to be increasingly based in the future, on input from statistical overviews.

Meta-analysis has several potential uses when the diagnostic accuracy of laboratory tests is investigated, but it is a rather new field of study that needs to refine its tools and establish its credibility. Validated instruments for assessing the quality of studies, statistical tests for judging the combinability of studies, and random-effects methods for integrating the findings of studies are well-developed for RCTs, and continue to be developed for studies of diagnostic-test accuracy. In the future, meta-analysis should become as powerful a tool for technology assessment in pathology as it is for clinical medicine.

References

1. Jenicek M. Meta-analysis in medicine: where we are and where we want to go. J Clin Epidemiol. 1989; 42:35–44.
2. L'Abbé KA, Detsky AS, O'Rourke K. Meta-analysis in clinical research. Ann Intern Med. 1987;107: 224–33.
3. Cooper H, Hedges LV, editors. The handbook of research synthesis. New York: Russell Sage Foundation; 1994.
4. Cook TD, Cooper H, Gordray DS, et al. Meta-analysis for explanation: a casebook. New York: Russell Sage Foundation; 1992.
5. Glasziou P, Irwig L, Bain C, Colditz G. Systematic reviews in health care: a practical guide. Cambridge: Cambridge University Press; 2001.
6. Goodman SN. Have you ever met a meta-analysis you didn't like? Ann Intern Med. 1991;114:244–6.
7. O'Rourke K, Detsky AS. Meta-analysis in medical research: strong encouragement for higher quality in individual research efforts. J Clin Epidemiol. 1989;42: 1021–4.
8. Chalmers TC, Levin H, Sacks HS, Reitman D, Berrier J, Nagalingam R. Meta-analysis of clinical trials as a scientific discipline. I. Control of bias and comparison with large co-operative trials. Stat Med. 1987; 6:315–25.
9. Peto R. Why do we need systematic overviews of randomized trials? Stat Med. 1987;6:233–40.
10. Yusuf S. Obtaining medically meaningful answers from an overview of randomized clinical trials. Stat Med. 1987;6:281–6.
11. Vamvakas EC. Statistical associations and cause-and-effect relationships. In: Vamvakas EC. Evidence-based practice of transfusion medicine. Bethesda: AABB Press; 2001. p. 21–64.
12. Irwing L, Tosteson AN, Gatsonis C, et al. Guidelines for meta-analyses evaluating diagnostic tests. Ann Intern Med. 1994;120:667–76.
13. Irwig L, Macaskill P, Glasziore P, Fahey M. Meta-analytic methods for diagnostic test accuracy. J Clin Epidemiol. 1995;48:119–30.
14. Vamvakas EC. Meta-analyses of studies of the diagnostic accuracy of laboratory tests: a review of the concepts and methods. Arch Pathol Lab Med. 1998;122:675–86.
15. Boissel JP, Cucherat M. The meta-analysis of diagnostic test studies. Eur Radiol. 1998;8:484–7.
16. Vamvakas E. Applications of meta-analysis in pathology practice. Am J Clin Pathol. 2001;116 Suppl 1:S47–64.
17. Glasziou P, Irwing L, Bain C, Colditz G. Diagnostic tests. In: Systematic reviews in health care: a practical guide. Cambridge: Cambridge University Press; 2001. p. 74–89.
18. Vamvakas E. White-blood-cell containing allogeneic blood transfusion and postoperative infection or

mortality: an updated meta-analysis. Vox Sang. 2007; 92: 224–32.
19. Blajchman MA, Bordin JO. Mechanisms of transfusion-associated immunosuppression. Curr Opin Hematol. 1994;1:457–61.
20. Vamvakas E, Blajchman MA. Transfusion-related immunomodulation: an update. Blood Rev. 2007;21: 327–48.
21. Bracey AW, Radovancevick R, Nussimeier NA, LaRocco M, Vaughn WK, Cooper JR. Leukocyte-reduced blood in open-heart surgery patients: effects on outcome. Transfusion. 2002;42(Suppl):5S.
22. Houbiers JGA, Brand A, van de Watering LMG, et al. Randomized controlled trial comparing transfusion of leucocyte-depleted or buffy-coat-depleted blood in surgery for colorectal cancer. Lancet. 1994;344: 573–8.
23. Boshkov LK, Furnary A, Morris C, Chien G, van Winkle D, Reik R. Prestorage leukoreduction of red cells in elective cardiac surgery: results of a double-blind randomized controlled trial. Blood. 2004;104: 112a.
24. van Hilten JA, van de Watering LMG, van Bockel JH, et al. Effects of transfusion with red cells filtered to remove leukocytes: randomized controlled trial in patients undergoing major surgery. BMJ. 2004;328: 1281–4.
25. Wallis JP, Chapman CE, Orr KE, Clark SC, Forty JR. Effect of WBC reduction of transfused RBCs on postoperative infection rates in cardiac surgery. Transfusion. 2002;42:1127–34.
26. Titlestad IL, Ebbesen LS, Ainsworth AP, Lillevang ST, Quist N, Georgsen J. Leukocyte-depletion of blood components does not significantly reduce the risk of infectious complications: results of a double-blind, randomized study. Int J Colorectal Dis. 2001;16: 147–53.
27. Nathens AB, Nester TA, Rubenfeld GD, Nirula R, Gernsheimer TB. The effects of leukoreduced blood transfusion on infection risk following injury: a randomized controlled trial. Shock. 2006;26:342–7.
28. van de Watering LMG, Hermans J, Houbiers JGA, et al. Beneficial effect of leukocyte depletion of transfused blood on post-operative complications in patients undergoing cardiac surgery: a randomized clinical trial. Circulation. 1998;97:562–8.
29. Bilgin YM, van de Watering LMG, Eijsman L, et al. Double-blind, randomized controlled trial on the effect of leukocyte-depleted erythrocyte transfusions in cardiac valve surgery. Circulation. 2004;109:2755–60.
30. Tartter PI, Mohandas K, Azar P, Endres J, Kaplan J, Spivack M. Randomized trial comparing packed red cell blood transfusion with and without leukocyte depletion for gastrointestinal surgery. Am J Surg. 1998;176:462–6.
31. Jensen LS, Kissmeyer-Nielsen P, Wolff B, Quist N. Randomized comparison of leukocyte-depleted versus buffy-coat-poor blood transfusion and complications after colorectal surgery. Lancet. 1996;348:841–5.
32. Jensen LS, Andersen AJ, Christiansen PM, et al. Postoperative infection and natural killer cell function following blood transfusion in patients undergoing elective colorectal surgery. Br J Surg. 1992;79: 513–6.
33. Dzik WH, Anderson JK, O'Neill EM, Assman SF, Kalish LA, Stowell CP. A prospective, randomized clinical trial of universal WBC reduction. Transfusion. 2002;42:1114–22.
34. Nielsen HJ, Hammer J, Kraup AL, et al. Prestorage leukocyte filtration may reduce leukocyte-derived bioactive substance accumulation in patients operated for burn trauma. Burns. 1999;25:162–70.
35. Fergusson D, Khanna MP, Tinmouth A, Hébert PC. Transfusion of leukoreduced red blood cells may decrease postoperative infections: two meta-analyses of randomized controlled trials. Can J Anaesth. 2004;51:417–24.
36. Blumberg N, Zhao H, Wang H, Messing S, Heal JM, Lyman GH. The intention-to-treat principle in clinical trials and meta-analyses of leukoreduced blood transfusions in surgical patients. Transfusion. 2007;47: 573–81.
37. Blajchman MA, Bardossy I, Carmen R, Sastry A, Singal DP. Allogeneic blood transfusion-induced enhancement of tumor growth: two animal models showing amelioration by leukodepletion and passive transfer using spleen cells. Blood. 1993;81:1880–2.
38. Mincheff MS, Meryman HT, Kapoor V, Alsop P, Wotzel M. Blood transfusion and immunomodulation: a possible mechanism. Vox Sang. 1993;65: 18–24.
39. Kao KJ. Induction of humoral immune tolerance to major histocompatibility complex antigens by transfusions of UV-B irradiated leukocytes. Blood. 1996;88:4375–82.
40. Ghio M, Contini P, Mazzei C, Brenci S, Barbaris G, Filaci G, et al. Soluble HLA Class I, HLA Class II, and Fas ligand in blood components: a possible key to explain the immunomodulatory effects of allogeneic blood transfusion. Blood. 1999;93:1770–7.
41. Bordin JO, Bardossy L, Blajchman MA. Growth enhancement of established tumors by allogeneic blood transfusion in experimental animals and its amelioration by leukodepletion: the importance of timing of the leukodepletion. Blood. 1994;84: 344–8.
42. Nielsen HJ, Reimert CM, Pedersen AN, Brunner N, Edvarsen L, Dybkjaer E, et al. Time-dependent spontaneous release of white cell- and platelet-derived bioactive substances from stored human blood. Transfusion. 1996;36:960–5.
43. Innerhofer P, Luz G, Spotl L, Hobish-Hagen P, Schobersberger W, Fischer M, et al. Immunologic changes following transfusion of autologous or allogeneic buffy-coated-poor versus leukocyte-depleted blood in patients undergoing arthroplasty. I. Proliferative T-cell responses and T-helper/T-suppressor cell balance. Transfusion. 1999;39:1089–96.

44. Fransen E, Maessen J, Denterner M, Senden N, Buurman W. Impact of blood transfusion on inflammatory mediator release in patients undergoing cardiac surgery. Chest. 1999;116:1233–9.
45. Diversity and heterogeneity [monograph on the Internet]. Oxford: The Cochrane Collaboration. 2002. http://www.cochrane-net.org/openlearning/HTML/mod13-5.htm.
46. Chalmers TC, Smith Jr H, Blackburn B, et al. A method for assessing the quality of a randomized controlled trial. Control Clin Trials. 1981;2:31–49.
47. Detsky AS, Naylor CD, O'Rourke K, McGeer AJ, L'Abbe KA. Incorporating variations in the quality of individual randomized trials into meta-analysis. J Clin Epidemiol. 1992;45:255–65.
48. Zelen M. Guidelines for publishing papers on cancer clinical trials: responsibilities of editors and authors. J Clin Oncol. 1983;1:164–9.
49. Moher D, Jadad AR, Nichol G, Penman M, Tugwell P, Walsh S. Assessing the quality of randomized controlled trials: an annotated bibliography of scales and checklists. Control Clin Trials. 1995;16:62–73.
50. Moher D, Jadad AR, Tugwell P. Assessing the quality of reports of randomized trials. Int J Technol Assess Health Care. 1996;12:195–208.
51. Lichtenstein MJ, Mulrow CD, Elwood PC. Guidelines for reading case-control studies. J Chronic Dis. 1987;40:893–903.
52. Feinstein AR. Twenty scientific principles for trohoc research. In: Feinstein AR, editor. Clinical epidemiology: The architecture of clinical research. Philadelphia: Saunders; 1985. p. 543–7.
53. Jadad AR, Moore RA, Carroll D, et al. Assessing the quality of reports of randomized trials: is blinding necessary? Control Clin Trials. 1996;17:1–12.
54. Moher D, Jones BA, Cook DJ, et al. Does quality of reports of randomized trials affect estimates of intervention efficacy reported in meta-analyses? Lancet. 1998;352:609–13.
55. Steinberg KK, Thacker SB, Smith SJ, et al. A meta-analysis of the effect of estrogen replacement therapy on the risk of breast cancer. JAMA. 1991;265:1985–90.
56. Berlin JA, Colditz GA. A meta-analysis of physical activity in the prevention of coronary heart disease. Am J Epidemiol. 1990;142:612–28.
57. Mantel N, Haenszel W. Statistical aspects of the analysis of data from retrospective studies of disease. J Natl Cancer Inst. 1959;22:719–48.
58. Yusuf S, Peto R, Lewis J, Collins R, Sleight P. Beta blockade during and after myocardial infarction: an overview of the randomized trials. Prog Cardiovasc Dis. 1985;27:335–71.
59. Klein S, Simes J, Blackburn GL. Total parenteral nutrition and cancer clinical trials. Cancer. 1986;58: 1378–86.
60. Slavin RE. Best-evidence synthesis: an alternative approach to traditional and meta-analytic reviews. Educ Res. 1986;15(9):5–11.
61. Slavin RE. Best-evidence synthesis: why less is more. Educ Res. 1987;16(5):15–6.
62. Begg C, Cho M, Eastwood S, et al. Improving the quality of reporting of randomized controlled trials: the CONSORT statement. JAMA. 1996;276:637–9.
63. Mahoer D, Schulz KF, Altman DG. The CONSORT statement: revised recommendations for improving the quality of reports of parallel-group randomized trials. J Am Podiatr Med Assoc. 2001;91:437–42.
64. Berlin JA, Laird NM, Sacks HS, Chalmers RC. A comparison of statistical methods for combining event rates from clinical trials. Stat Med. 1989;8: 141–51.
65. Thompson SG, Pocock SJ. Can meta-analysis be trusted? Lancet. 1991;338:1127–30.
66. Demets DL. Methods for combining randomized clinical trials: strengths and limitations. Stat Med. 1987;6:341–8.
67. Meier P. Commentary on "Why do we need systematic overviews of randomized trials?". Stat Med. 1987;6:329–31.
68. Bailey KR. Inter-study differences: how should they influence the interpretation and analysis of results? Stat Med. 1987;6:351–8.
69. Huque MF. Experiences with meta-analysis in FDA submissions. Proc Biopharm Sect Am Stat Assoc. 1988;2:28–33.
70. Dubey S. Regulatory considerations on meta-analysis and multicenter trials. Proc Biopharm Sect Am Stat Assoc. 1988;2:18–27.
71. Stein RA. Meta-analysis from one FDA reviewer's perspective. Proc Biopharm Sect Am Stat Assoc. 1988;2:34–8.
72. Higgins JPT, Thompson SG, Deeks JJ, Altman DG. Measuring inconsistency in meta-analyses. BMJ. 2003;327:557–60.
73. Altman DG, Bland MJ. Interaction revisited: the difference between two estimates. BMJ. 2003;326:219.
74. Abramson JH. Meta-analysis: a review of pros and cons. Public Health Rev. 1990/91;18:1–47.
75. Greenland S, Longnecker MP. Methods for trend estimation from summarized dose-response data, with applications to meta-analysis. Am J Epidemiol. 1992;135:1301–9.
76. Greenland S, Salvan A. Bias in the one-step method for pooling study results. Stat Med. 1990;9:247–52.
77. Cook TD, Cooper H, Cordray DS, et al. Meta-analysis for explanation: a casebook. New York: Russell Sage Foundation; 1992.
78. Ellenberg SS. Meta-analysis: the quantitative approach to research review. Semin Oncol. 1988;15:472–81.
79. DerSimonian R, Laird N. Meta-analysis in clinical trials. Control Clin Trials. 1986;7:177–88.
80. Greenland S. Quantitative methods in the review of epidemiologic literature. Epidemiol Rev. 1987; 9:1–30.
81. Bailar III JC. The promise and problems of meta-analysis. N Engl J Med. 1997;337:559–61.
82. Meta-analysis under scrutiny. Lancet. 1997;350:675.
83. Villar J, Carrolli G, Belizan JM. Predictive ability of meta-analyses of randomized controlled trials. Lancet. 1995;345:772–6.

84. Cappelleri JC, Ioannidis JPA, Schmid CH, et al. Large trials versus meta-analyses of small trials: how do their results compare? JAMA. 1996;276:1332–8.
85. LeLorier J, Grégoire B, Benhaddad A, et al. Discrepancies between meta-analyses and subsequent large randomized, controlled trials. N Engl J Med. 1997;337:536–42.
86. Ioannidis JPA, Cappelleri JC, Lau J. Issues in comparisons between meta-analyses and large trials. JAMA. 1998;279:1089–93.
87. Felson DT. Bias in meta-analytic research. J Clin Epidemiol. 1992;45:885–92.
88. Haynes RB, McKibbon KA, Walker CJ, et al. Computer searching of the medical literature: an evaluation of MEDLINE search systems. Ann Intern Med. 1985;103:812–6.
89. Begg CB, Berlin JA. Publication bias and dissemination of clinical research. J Natl Cancer Inst. 1989;81:107–14.
90. Dickersin K, Chan S, Chalmers TC, et al. Publication bias and clinical trials. Control Clin Trials. 1987;8: 343–53.
91. Easterbrook PJ, Berlin JA, Copalan R, Matthews DR. Publication bias in clinical research. Lancet. 1991;337:867–72.
92. Vamvakas EC. Why have meta-analyses of the randomized controlled trials of the association between non-white-blood-cell reduced allogeneic blood transfusion and postoperative infection produced discordant results? Vox Sang. 2007;93:196–207.
93. Sackett DL. Discussion of the paper "Meta-analytic methods for diagnostic test accuracy" presented at the Potsdam International Consultation on Meta-analysis (Potsdam, Germany; March 1994). J Clin Epidemiol. 1995;48:131–2.
94. Midgette AS, Stukel TA, Littenberg B. A meta-analytic method for summarizing diagnostic test performances: receiver-operating-characteristic summary point estimates. Med Decis Making. 1993;13: 253–7.
95. Littenberg B, Moses LE. Estimating diagnostic accuracy from multiple conflicting reports: a new meta-analytic method. Med Decis Making. 1993;13: 313–21.
96. Moses LE, Shapiro D, Littenberg B. Combining independent studies of a diagnostic test into a summary ROC curve: data-analytic approaches and some additional considerations. Stat Med. 1993;12: 1293–316.
97. Arroll B, Schechter MT, Sheps SB. The assessment of diagnostic tests; a comparison of the recent medical literature – 1982 versus 1985. J Gen Intern Med. 1988;3:443–7.
98. Cooper LS, Chalmers TC, McCally M, et al. The poor quality of early evaluations of magnetic resonance imaging. JAMA. 1988;259:3277–80.
99. Bean CA, Sostman HD, Zheng JY. Status of clinical MR evaluations, 1985–1988: baseline and design for further assessments. Radiology. 1991;180:265–9.
100. Sackett DL, Straus SE, Richardson WS, Rosenberg W, Haynes RB. Evidence-based medicine. Edinburgh: Churchill Livingstone; 2000.
101. Valenstein PN. Evaluating diagnostic tests with imperfect standards. Am J Clin Pathol. 1990;93: 252–8.
102. Phelps CE, Hutson A. Estimating diagnostic test accuracy using a "fuzzy gold standard". Med Decis Making. 1995;15:44–57.
103. Begg CB. Biases in the assessment of diagnostic tests. Stat Med. 1987;6:411–23.
104. Begg CB, Greenes RA. Assessment of diagnostic tests when disease verification is subject to selection bias. Biometrics. 1983;39:207–15.
105. Gray R, Begg CB, Greenes RA. Construction of receiver operating characteristic curves when disease verification is subject to selection bias. Med Decis Making. 1984;4:151–64.
106. Bossuyt PM, Reitsma JB, Burns DE, et al. Towards complete and accurate reporting of studies of diagnostic accuracy: the STARD explanation and elaboration. Ann Intern Med. 2003;138:W1–12.
107. Vandenbroucke JP, von Elm E, Altman DG, et al. Strengthening the Reporting of Observational Studies in Epidemiology (STROBE): explanation and elaboration. Ann Intern Med. 2007;147: W163–94.
108. Moher D, Liberati A, Tetzlaff J, Altman DG, and the PRISMA Group. Preferred reporting items for systematic reviews and meta-analyses: the PRISMA statement. PLoS Med. 2009;6:e1000097, p. 1–6. Available at: www.plosmedicine.org.

Decision Analysis and Decision Support Systems in Anatomic Pathology

10

Michael Hendrickson and Bonnie Balzer

Keywords
Decision analysis • Anatomic pathology decision support systems • Evidence-based pathology

In this chapter, we discuss two aspects of decision-making in anatomic pathology: decision analysis (DA) and decision support systems (DSS). As background information for our discussion of DA, we will distinguish two kinds of ignorance: vagueness and probabilistic uncertainty and then discuss the two dominant interpretations of probability – stable relative frequencies (frequentist) and degrees of belief (Bayesian).

Subjective Probability and Decision Analysis

Subjective probability is the language of DA. DA provides the conceptual machinery to integrate a suitable characterization of the basic elements of the decision – actions, information, and preferences – to produce the best alternative. In considering ways in which these concepts can be usefully deployed in day-to-day anatomic diagnostics, we can ask several questions. We start by asking the question: is there a clinically relevant decision to be made? Other questions involve the important decision analytic concepts of the value of information, Bayesian updating, sensitivity analysis, and cost functions. Finally, we will discuss strategies for dealing with diagnostic assignment uncertainty that persists after information gathering strategies have been exhausted.

Decision Support Systems

DSS are computer-based classifiers that evaluate evidence and classify a situation either in service of morphological diagnosis or the prediction of some aspect of a patient's future, such as the risk for developing invasive cancer, prognosis or prediction. Diagnostic systems are basically imitative. *Rule-based expert systems* attempt to model the diagnostic performance of expert pathologists. They have limitations that will be discussed against the background of topics discussed in Chap. 6. Prognostic systems employ what is termed "case-based reasoning (CBR)," matching a set of patient predictors with those of a large number of database patients for whom predictors and clinical outcomes are known. The use of this term has little to do with *clinical* CBR and, in mathematical-statistical

M. Hendrickson (✉)
Department of Pathology, Stanford University Medical Center, Stanford, CA 94305, USA
e-mail: hendrickson@stanford.edu

A.M. Marchevsky and M.R. Wick (eds.), *Evidence Based Pathology and Laboratory Medicine*,
DOI 10.1007/978-1-4419-1030-1_10, © Springer Science+Business Media, LLC 2011

terms, amounts to a nearest-neighbor search. The "curse of dimensionality" discussed in Chap. 7 again intrudes.

DSS are basically classifiers; they evaluate evidence and classify a situation either in service of diagnosis or prediction of some aspect of a patient's future clinical phenotype, $\Phi_{Clin}(t)$. In this discussion, we are interested less in the specifics of DSSs and more in locating them within the classificatory and diagnostic framework explained in Chap. 6. From that perspective, we ask what can we expect from diagnostic DSSs given the problems presented to expert systems by the translation-transmission problem and the private, microrevisionary changes that constantly shift the individual expert's landscape and boundaries. In short, that an expert's opinion is a moving target and that experts' mental "maps" of the classificatory terrain are almost always, particularly in the neighborhood of boundaries. noncongruent.

Scope-Side Decision Analysis

DA and modern mathematical probability were born at the same time in France in the seventeenth century [1, 2]. These ideas have been elaborated and systematized over the ensuing 300 years and, in the twenty-first century, subjective expected utility (SEU) theory informs the way we think about everything from economics to public health policy to personal decision-making. Its principles have become today's common sense and they form the core of EBM. In the past 50 years, DA has become a discipline in its own right with its own journals and academic departments. The current mathematical formulations of DA are daunting, but the core ideas are easily stated and quite intuitive. Sox provides a detailed account, with worked examples, of DA in a medical setting [3].

We are interested here in setting out the basic ideas of DA and believe that the quality of both the teaching and practice of diagnostic surgical pathology would be improved by informing day-to-day decision-making with these principles.

The Basic Ideas of Decision Analysis: The Decision Basis

Decisions involve choosing among alternatives that will yield uncertain futures, for which we have preferences. There are three elements of any decision: (1) what you can *do* or the alternative actions that can be taken; (2) what you *know*, the information you have; and (3) what you *want*, your preferences. Collectively, these three represent the *decision basis*, the specification of the decision. DA provides the logic that operates on the decision basis – actions, information, preferences – to produce the best alternative. Crucial to this process is a clear description by the decision maker of precisely what decision is under consideration at the time – the *framing* of the decision. This frame will inform all elements of the decision basis [4].

Vagueness vs. Probabilistic Uncertainty

DA deals with uncertainty of a very specific type and not with other types; it is crucial to understand the difference. There are two kinds of uncertainty: vagueness and probabilistic uncertainty [5]. As discussed in Chap. 6, *vagueness* is a characteristic of verbal descriptions of both the features that figure in the morphologic definition of an entity and the delimitation of a neoplastic kind (K_{Neop}'s) from its neighbors in the phenospace; vagueness gives rise to assignment uncertainty. *Probabilistic uncertainty* is predicated of either unexamined features of members of a particular precisely defined class or their future behavior. We may be in doubt about whether a particular individual neoplasm (I_{Neop}) is A or B (an in-between case) after our exhaustive examination – that's vagueness. On the other hand, we may be certain that the I_{Neop} is an "A," but uncertain whether that patient will experience a recurrence or not – that's probabilistic uncertainty. This is what motivated my use of the lottery metaphor to model managerial K_{Neop}'s. Vagueness is uncertainty about which lottery the patient is in; probabilistic uncertainty is intrinsic to the lottery.

DA banishes vagueness – assignment uncertainty – from the modeling process by insisting that predicates (feature descriptors, like "large," "crowded," "atypical") and category designations ("complex atypical endometrial hyperplasia") pass, what the decision analyst, Ron Howard, calls a "clarity test."

"Consider a clairvoyant who knew the future, who had access to all future newspapers, readings of physical devices, or any other determinable quantity. The clarity test asks whether the clairvoyant [literal at the level of Asperger's syndrome] would be able to say whether or not the event in question occurred or, in the case of a variable, the value of the variable." *He exemplifies this with the term* "technical success" "[this] would have to be defined in such terms as 'able to operate x hours under conditions y without failure' [...]" [6]. *This insistence is* appropriate for decision analytic modeling: probabilistic reasoning is predicated on crisp, unambiguously defined categories; the foundation of mathematical probability is classical set theory. Something is either "A" or "not A," there is nothing in-between; this is Aristotle's law of the excluded middle.

For most situations involving vagueness (Chap. 6), this requirement seems forced and arbitrary and has led to the development of alternative, more flexible logics. Fuzzy theory (fuzzy set theory, fuzzy logic, fuzzy categories) was developed in the 1960s in by a U.C. Berkeley engineer, Lotfi Zadeh, in response to these problems [7]. There are several accessible introductions [8–10]. The medical applications have been explored in a series of publications by Sadegh-Zadeh [11]. Some of these techniques have been incorporated in DSS [12].

Interpretations of Mathematical Probability

Mathematical probability refers to an axiomatic branch of mathematics and is used, noncontroversially, to model games of chance (classical probability). Controversy arises in extending the model to real-world situations outside the casino. There are two main schools of thought (and many variants): frequentist and subjectivist (or personalist). The *frequency* interpretation holds that probability should model long-run stable empirical frequencies. For example, repeated tosses of a coin yields a relative frequency of 0.5 for a "fair" coin. In many real-world applications, long-run frequencies are commonly never achieved. For example, we talk about the probability of it raining on a particular day or the probability of a successful space craft launching (e.g., the *Challenger* space shuttle). A different notion of probability is required to handle these situations. One general response to these situations is to view probability as a measure of belief. People who interpret probability in this way are called *subjectivists or personalists*. Formally, for them, a probability is cashed out for a willingness to bet on one possibility over another; DA is committed to this view of probability. The probabilist Spiegelhalter describes an experiment that helps to fix these concepts. He is addressing a lay audience.

> I hold a coin and ask, "What is the chance this will come up heads?" They cheerfully say something like "50%" or "half-and-half." I then toss the coin, catch it, flip it onto the back of my hand without revealing it, and ask, "What is the probability this is heads?" Pause. Then someone, less confidently, mumbles "50%." I reveal the coin to myself, but not to them, and ask, "What is your probability that this is heads?" Very grudgingly they might eventually admit "50%." In this experiment I have gone from pure aleatory [games of chance, or frequentist interpretation] uncertainty to pure epistemological [subjectivist] uncertainty, showing (1) epistemological uncertainty is "in the eye of the beholder" (my probability was eventually 0% or 100%, whereas theirs was still 50%), (2) that the language of probability applied to both forms, and (3) that these different types of uncertainty may be perceived differently [13].

Much has been written in the statistical and machine learning literature on these often contentious issues of interpretation; Hacking and Hájek are good places to start [2, 14, 15].

The Clinician's Lament

Equipped with these distinctions, we can now examine a common complaint about pathologists. The disgruntled clinician points out: "I have to have a certain diagnosis in order to proceed with my clinical work." There is, of course, no question of eliminating probabilistic uncertainty; most of us discover this shortly after emerging from the womb. Voltaire observed: "Doubt is not a pleasant condition, but certainty is absurd." What are we to make of the clinician's insistence on certainty from pathologists? When clinicians insist on certainty, it is usually *assignment* uncertainty they are worrying about. Their therapies are indexed by our assignments; clinicians are usually completely comfortable with probabilistic uncertainty *given a fixed assignment*; in other words, as long as they know what lottery they are dealing with. Again, the macho surgical pathologist's response – "May be wrong, but never in doubt" – is about assignment uncertainty.

Applying the Basic Intuitions of Decision Analysis to Diagnostic Pathology

How does DA help in oncopathological diagnosis? The underlying strategy here is to locate a particular diagnostic problem in the patient's specific clinical context and ask: "What information does the clinician require to move the patient's clinical management along to the next step?" In this first section, we discuss some generalizations and guiding principles useful in day-to-day diagnosis in surgical pathology.

Our heritage from the legendary surgical pathologists of the mid-twentieth century was admission to the clinical decision-making process. Pathologists throughout the world emerged from their hospital basements and became full participants in patient care management. This activist tradition emphasized the importance of locating anatomic diagnoses within a clinical decision-making framework. Exhilarating, though this was, it came with a price; the exposure of an elaborate nineteenth and early twentieth century tumor taxonomy to the minimalism of pragmatic oncopathology. For example, there is the taxonomically unglamorous truth that the status of the excision margins and tumor size are more important than which of five different subspecies of tumor "A" (all, currently, calling for the same therapy) might be afflicting the patient. There was a growing appreciation of the distinction one of us (MH) made in Chap. 6 between S-classifications (I used histogenetic classifications as a example) and M-classifications. I commented there that S-classifications are fine-grained and mark all the myriad salient phenotypic distinctions that can be made; M-classifications are coarse-grained and codify the much fewer clinically relevant distinctions. The public working out of this sentiment is seen in the several attempts to group HG-K_{Neop}'s into managerially relevant categories. Examples include the soft tissue neoplasms and gynecologic mesenchymal proliferations [16, 17]. We are now confronted with a new challenge – both practical and pedagogical; the mapping of the many HG-K_{Neop}'s into a handful of managerial classes. In other words, there has been a gradual move toward the diagnosis that is "good enough to get on with clinical management" and away from the "histogenetically right diagnosis."

The "Future Utility of the Distinction" Argument

Elaborate histological, cytogenetic, and molecular-genetic workups are often justified on the grounds that something useful will turn up that will be of use in the future. "How are we ever going to know if a distinction is important if we don't record it?" The problem with unsponsored research efforts of this sort is that they will ultimately have to be repeated in a disciplined way (see internal validity discussion in Chap. 7) and it may well interfere with cost-effective, efficient, patient management. So, the liberal use in our literature of locutions like "It is important to distinguish 'A' from 'B,' 'C' and 'D' have to be critically examined; the obligatory follow-up questions: 'Why?' 'Important for whom?' It may well be that the distinction is one that can, in principle, be made, but should a clinical manager be willing to pay for this distinction? What is the evidence that something different should be done in light of this new information? The problem is compounded when the clinician, innocent of our classificatory ways, assumes that because we have a name for something, it is a distinction he should worry about. Of course, this problem can run the other way. In the absence of any convincing evidence, clinicians, in their role of the final decision maker, coerce the pathologist to engage in many empty rituals. Searching for keratin positive cells in sentinel lymph node biopsies and performing CD117 examinations on random malignancies come to mind [18].

To date, discussions of histopathology employing EBM principles have concentrated exclusively on managerial distinctions. Let's take a look at some guiding principles and how they play out in day-to-day diagnostics.

Background Principles to be Considered in Decision Analysis

Good Decisions and Good Outcomes

It is important to distinguish between good/bad decisions and good/bad outcomes. Uncertainty in medicine is ineliminable; good decision-making consists in "taming chance," in employing a coherent decision-making strategy that uses one's best guess about uncertain quantities in light of current information. Good decision analytic technique doesn't guarantee a favorable outcome; the well thought-out model of a particular situation doesn't guarantee, obviously, that the outcome will be the one you want. It is also true that faulty decision-making may be followed by a favorable outcome. What DA promises is that if you follow its precepts, you will maximize your chances of the outcome you favor.

Uncertainty is Inescapable But Shouldn't Paralyze Decision-Making

If diagnostic assignments are crisp, there are no problems; the business of DA is uncertainty management. How might DA handle assignment uncertainty? One way to finesse this problem is to settle upon a taxonomic model; for example, that the region between peaks in the phenospace is populated by atypical cases from one or the other population and assign a probability to the two possibilities [5]. Other models are possible, for example, including a third population of "in-between" cases, a separate and distinct lottery (in the language of Chapter 6), and assigning probabilities to three possibilities.

Some Crucial Questions and Other Issues Related to Decisions in Pathology (Table 10.1)

Is There a Clinically Relevant Decision To Be Made?

The Stanford professor, Ron Howard, who first coined the term "decision analysis" in the 1960s, has often said that the most difficult part of consulting work in DA is discovering whether or not the client really does have a decision to make?

"If you have only one alternative, then you have no choice in what you do. If you do not have any information linking what you do to what will happen in the future, then all alternatives serve equally well because you do not see how your actions will have any effect. If you have no preferences regarding what will happen as a result of choosing any alternative, then you will be equally happy choosing any one" [4].

Howard was referring to the difficulty in exposing this structure in the typically complex details of the client's specific situation. Often what is required is someone to take a bird's eye view of the situation and point out the obvious. Another correlative point: DA has nothing to tell us about nonmanagerial distinctions; there is no clinical decision to be made. Scientific classification disputes are discussed in an entirely different framework. Histogenetic classification issues, for example, involve the scientific plausibility of competing embryological theories in a particular domain, issues quite remote from clinical decision making.

Table 10.1 Important questions to ask about a problematic case

Question 1: Is there a clinically relevant decision to be made?
Question 2: Do I need more information to make this clinically relevant decision? The value of information
Question 3: What have I learned from my new information? Bayesian updating
Question 4: Would I make a different clinically relevant decision if my probabilities were slightly adjusted? Sensitivity analysis
Question 5: What's at stake for this particular patient? Cost functions
Question 6: What do I do in the face of assignment uncertainty when it makes a clinical difference?

The Problem of the Burgeoning Oncopathological Zoo

Anatomic pathologists face a situation similar to that of Howard's client. The complexity of our diagnostic task stems from the hybrid character of oncopathological classification – a managerial overlay on a much more complicated histogenetic classification. We have hundreds of named entities but, in any particular domain, these entities fall into only a few managerial categories. Many of the named categories are associated with vague $\Phi_{Clin}(t)$ claims that probably would not stand up under the kind of scrutiny given to cancer markers (Chap. 7). These claimed distinctions, nevertheless, persist in the primary literature and the reviews of that literature. It is a major challenge keeping track of the exponentially proliferating neoplastic kinds and critically evaluating whether or not they should figure in patient care decisions. Molecular kinds will soon be making their contribution to this burden. It is at this point that the principles set out below become important as a way of effectively focusing on one's clinically relevant diagnostic efforts.

Guiding Principles in Clinical Decision-Making: What Are We Trying to Accomplish for a Particular Patient?

The guiding principle is to doggedly pursue the question: What's the clinical context? What does the clinician need to know about the specimen submitted to get on with the next stage of clinical decision-making? Let's look at this more carefully. Clinically relevant differential diagnostic sets are generated during the course of diagnosis. For example, we might initially sort the relevant possibilities into a differential diagnosis organized around phenotype. We then might sort the members of these phenotype sets into three groups: those associated with a benign clinical course ("good actors"), those with a clinically malignant course ("bad actors"), and those with an intermediate clinical behavior. Further diagnostic testing should have as a goal establishing to which broad category the case belongs. For example, when confronted with a high-grade malignancy in the soft tissues and having ruled out mimics (e.g., metastasis, local extension from another site, melanoma, hematolymphoid malignancy) and established that the tumor is descriptively a pleomorphic, high-grade primary soft tissue sarcoma, it can be argued that one's clinically relevant work is done. It remains an open question whether fine-tuning this diagnosis (Is it dedifferentiated liposarcoma, leiomyosarcoma, poorly differentiated synovial sarcoma, etc.?) is clinically useful. Once a case can be assigned unequivocally to one or the other category, from the point of view of clinical action, nothing more need be done. If all of the "benign" K_{Neop}'s in a particular location will be treated the same way and likewise for all the malignant K_{Neop}'s, further diagnostic efforts may be in service of nonmanagerial goals, but have nothing to do with clinical decision-making.

The Value of Information: Do I Need More Information to Make this Clinically Relevant Decision?

The question that should probably drive the elaborateness of the histopathological workup in a cost-effective environment should be: What does the clinician need to get on with clinical workup, treatment? The analysis may be different for different stages of the clinical workup. The answers to this question will differ for a needle biopsy of a mammographically suspicious lesion or a needle biopsy of a retroperitoneal soft tissue mass than for the respective resection specimens. The conventional lavish immunohistochemical (IHC) workup of a soft tissue neoplasm doesn't need to be performed on the limited sample provided by a needle biopsy; it can await the resection specimen. For a resection specimen, a more elaborate workup is conventional. When should we stop? Do diminishing returns set in when working up, for example, what is noncontroversially a high-grade pleomorphic soft tissue sarcoma? EBP has a role here in scrutinizing the claimed distinctions between the dozen denizens in this particular zoo.

We are painfully aware that standard of care consideration often does not reflect this practical approach to diagnosis. We may, for various compelling local reasons, respond to these pressures, but, even so, it is valuable to maintain a clear-eyed view of the evidentiary warrant (or lack) for these decisions. There are some requirements: (1) We need to start off with a focused question. For example, distinguishing "A" or "B" and what are the most discriminating tests to order?; (2) We need to know what we will do with possible results. For an IHC study, we need to know what we would do with a positive or negative or an inconclusive result. In short, don't order the test unless you know what you would do with the possible answers you might obtain. If you would make the same diagnosis given any possible test result, the test has a "value of information" of zero; you should not have ordered the test. When multiple tests are ordered, the "curse of dimensionality" rears its ugly head. It is not at all uncommon to receive a consult case with twenty or more IHC studies. It reminds us that "more information is not necessarily better." See the discussion in Chap. 7.

Often, of more value than additional IHC testing is clinical or radiological information. It makes no sense to try to leverage the location of a uterine cancer (from cervix or fundus) using an IHC panel when a call to the clinician might settle the issue. That's not to say that there are not cases of cancer centered on the uterine isthmus which are problematic; it's to argue against the reflex ordering of a panel to sort out what might well be a perfectly obvious clinical situation. It's like using the degree of actinic elastosis in a skin biopsy to ascertain the age of a patient as an alternative to looking at the age box in the pathology requisition. Again, whether a well-differentiated cartilaginous neoplasm of bone is "enchondroma" or "chondrosarcoma" is a distinction that the radiologist makes, not the pathologist on her own; the radiologic findings are constitutive elements of the final "pathologic" diagnosis.

What Have I Learned from My New Information? Bayesian Updating

Bayes Theorem is a trivial algebraic consequence of the axioms of mathematical probability. It becomes interesting when it is interpreted as a formula for learning from experience [2]. Bayesian thinking lies at the heart of DA. It tells us how to combine what we knew with what we found out to discover what we should now believe.

The odds formulation of Bayes Theorem is a particularly transparent way of visualizing this principle (Fig. 10.1). Diagnostic IHC studies can be understood only within this framework. IHC yields, in general, a set of likelihood ratios on diagnostic possibilities. Learning from some combination of test results requires a set of "input" prior odds on those possibilities [19].

Independence of Informational Evaluations

There are two attitudes assessing a patient's histology. The first, the integrative view, insists on having all the relevant background information (clinical history, imaging findings, etc.) before evaluating the histology of a case. Opposed to this is the attitude, the independent assessment view, that the independence of the histologic input should be preserved by examining the slides without any of that background information. There is truth in both approaches. "Independent assessment" is most consistent with Bayesian principles. To incorporate the radiological information in one's assessment of histology and in updating using *both* histology and radiology, treated as independently evaluated inputs, may lead to "double counting" of the radiologic evidence. It is also true that no histological assessment should be reported without a careful integration of the informational inputs provided by clinical and radiological features. Ideally, independent assessment should be followed by clinicopathological integration using Bayesian updating.

Would I Make a Different (Clinically Relevant) Decision if My Probabilities were Slightly Adjusted? Sensitivity Analysis

The question how robust is my diagnosis to "wiggling" my input probabilities? leads to the concept of sensitivity analysis: How sensitive is my

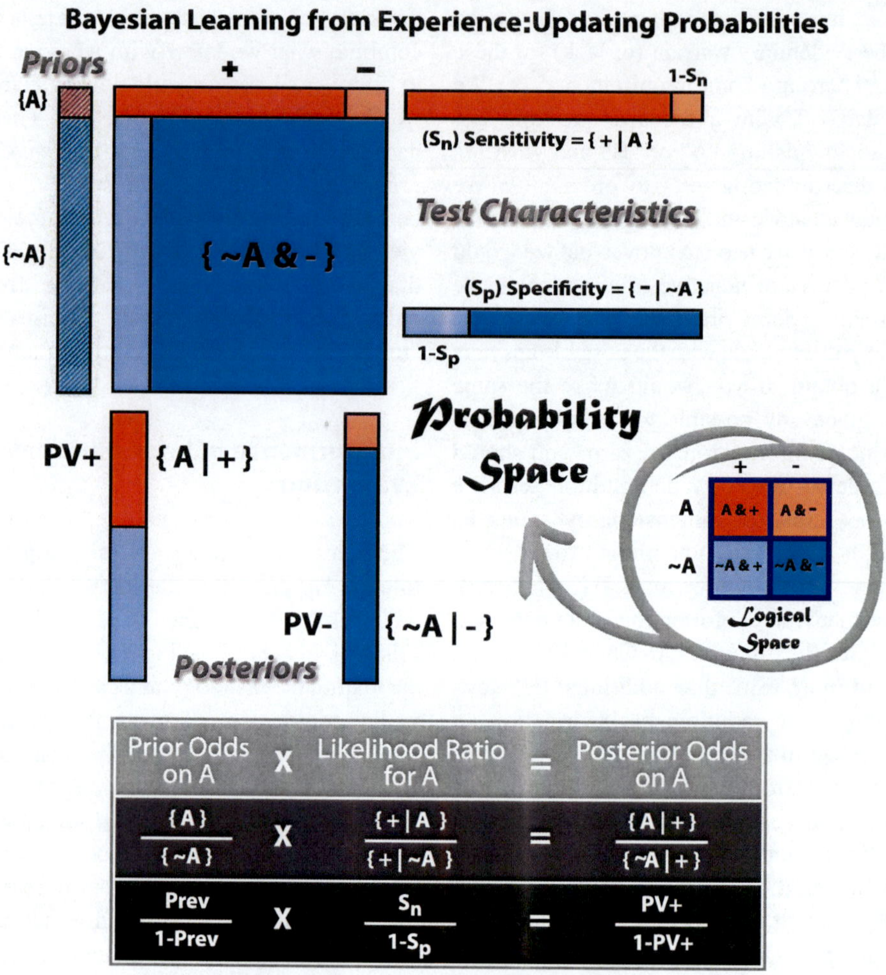

Fig. 10.1 The diagnostic test matrix and Bayes' odds. The unit area probability square provides a particularly intuitive representation of Bayes' theorem. The logical possibilities are color coded in the 'Logical Space' on the right. Red for true positives, light blue for false positives etc. The logical *possibility* squares are distorted to reflect the *probabilities* of each of these logical possibilities to produce the large probability square on the right. The 'Priors' rectangle depicts the total probability of true positives/negatives and has unit area; the other rectangles ('Test Characteristics' and 'Posteriors') represent conditional probabilities; each, of course, have unit area. This is a particularly intuitive formulation; it tells how we pass from what we knew prior to the test (the prior odds) and what we found out by doing the test (the likelihood ratio) to what we should now believe in light of that new evidence (the posterior odds). The rule is simple: multiply the prior odds by the likelihood ratio. The odds form of Bayes theorem can be evaluated visually by forming the ratios of the appropriate rectangles depicted in the probability space. For example, it is clear that with the situation depicted the posterior odds on disease given a positive test is roughly 0.5 (the ratio of the red patch over the light blue patch in the large probability square. Forming each of the ratios (visually) in the product makes this geometrically plausible. Bayesian updating of beliefs is an iterative process: the posterior odds can become the prior odds of another round of diagnostic tests. Applying this rule sequentially by multiplying the likelihood ratios makes the simplifying assumption that the tests are conditionally independent; this is usually an unrealistic assumption in most practical situations [39]. Bayesian networks can accommodate a feature dependency structure [27]

diagnosis under slight changes in my prior odds or my likelihood ratios? Would a change in diagnosis lead to a different action? Does sensitivity to one particular input suggest that I need more information to narrow that uncertainty? Do I need to perform more tests? These are the basic questions involved in the decision analyst's sensitivity analysis.

What's at Stake for this Particular Patient? Cost Functions

Decision analytic methodology insists on a separation of patient utilities from the action and information inputs into the process. Pathologists sometime engage in scope-side group DA. "How can I make a diagnosis of Grade I endometrial carcinoma in this 30 year old woman infertility patient when I know that the risk to life with such a lesion is minimal and that there are treatments short of hysterectomy that are sometimes curative?" One's natural impulse is to downshift one's diagnosis to "complex atypical hyperplasia." Given the same pattern in a postmenopausal woman with dysfunctional bleeding, one might have no hesitation in making a diagnosis of Grade I adenocarcinoma. Locating a process along a graded morphologic continuum is one thing; deciding what clinical action to take for a particular patient (or class of patients) with that histology is another. For example, what clinical action is warranted given a particular morphological patterns depends upon whether one is dealing with a "high penalty hysterectomy" situation (reproductive conservation important or the patient is a high-risk surgical candidate) or a "low penalty hysterectomy" situation (reproductive conservation not an issue and patient is a good surgical candidate). There is nothing paradoxical or mysterious about this; it is a straightforward issue of there being different "action threshold" along a morphological continuum for different classes of patients.

The basic idea behind managerial threshold setting is the cost function. Consider two overlapping bell-shaped curves; we want to determine the optimal threshold in the overlap area for shifting from calling cases "A" to calling cases "B." The optimal threshold is one that minimizes the total cost of misclassification. The inputs for this calculation are (1) the prior probabilities encountering an "A" or a "B" and (2) the costs that attach to errors of the two types: miscalling an "A" for a "B" and miscalling a "B" for an "A." Debate in histopathologic diagnosis is often erroneously focused on the details of morphology when it really is about utilities – anticipating the impact of a diagnosis.

This discussion raises a number of lessons: First, diagnoses are often not simply a report of objective findings, they may be value-laden. Second, there is sometimes confusion about who should be integrating clinicopathologic information to come up with treatment recommendations for the patient? A pathologist's diagnosis may amount to a recommendation for treatment rather than being a report of an objective finding, an informational input. Third, it is sometimes not clear whose utilities are being reflected in decision-making: the patient's, the pathologist's, the clinician's, or the insurance carrier's. These are difficult issues beyond the scope of this discussion.

What Do I Do in the Face of Irresolvable Uncertainty in Diagnosis when it Makes a Clinical Difference?

In Chap. 6, in discussing problem cases, one of us unhelpfully pointed out that it is in the nature of I_{Neop}'s that problem cases never disappear. I urged a philosophical attitude that these cases pointed to the inevitable failure of static, discretizing classification systems to do justice to evolving processes distinguished by their continuous spatio-temporal variation. I also pointed out that as one moves from "core" cases to cases occupying the "PeTI" region (or encounters taxonomically embarrassing heterogeneity), several things happen with great regularity: (1) for experts, diagnosis and classification collapse into a single activity; (2) experts' appeal to published criteria gives way to arbitrary (but often principled) stipulation using noncriterial features and (3) interexpert agreement degrades. It is further argued in Chap. 6 that, in the absence of expert consensus (when in possession of "complete" information), there is no fact of the matter about the correct assignment.

That is all well and good, the reader might say, but we are still left with the practical issue of diagnosing such cases. Here we are only concerned with assignments that make a managerial difference. The relevant experts will assign nonmanagerial problem cases by appeal to one or another oncogenetic or histogenetic theory. What about managerially relevant diagnostic decisions? Here the basic strategy is to "look up" from the microscope and ask if the clinician should care about the distinction you are trying to make. First, consider the K_{Neop}'s on either side of the in-between case. What is the claimed difference in behavior? The next question to ask is: "Are the claimed differences supported by credible evidence?" For example, low-grade serous carcinomas, psammocarcinomas, and serous borderline tumors of peritoneal origin are all part of a morphologic continuum. They are rare and there is limited information about their long-term behavior, although they all are, relative to the usual serous carcinoma of the ovary, clinically low grade. In this case, it is not at all clear from the literature that there are substantial differences in the long-term behavior of the three (nor, in fact, that mere mortals can follow the experts in distinguishing among them) [20]. What is one to do with an in-between case in this spectrum?

The next question to ask: "What's at stake?" Even if there are differences in behavior, are they sufficient to warrant different therapeutic approaches? Debulking is recommended for all three; there is no good evidence that chemotherapy is effective with these low-grade neoplasms. The issue, then, is whether to undertake radical debulking of disease (with removal of the internal genitalia) or conservative debulking, involving preservation of ovarian tissue and the uterus. Next question: "How old is the patient?" If reproductive conservation is relevant, then debulking with preservation of the uninvolved ovary and the uterus is indicated; if not, radical debulking is the appropriate choice. This would be the choice for all three. Thus, in the face of assignment uncertainty, attention turns to the pros and cons of various clinical options given that all three have more or less the same behavior, despite the fact that two are labeled "cancer" and the other is not.

The Rubber Band Paradox

The in-between case raises another curious diagnostic practice. A case lies between "A" and "B" along a multivariate morphologic continuum. After a good bit of extensive testing and hand-wringing, we decide that the balance of the evidence is for "A." A standard argument for this practice is that the behavior of "A" is substantially different from "B."

There are a number of ways of making sense of this. Here is a pragmatic argument: it may be the case that the chemotherapy for A is different from the chemotherapy for B or A is treated with surgery and B is not. This is all well and good and makes decision analytic sense particularly when the diagnostic dilemma is expressed probabilistically. That is: "I put 0.80 probability on A and the 0.20 on B." A cost function can be developed and an expected utility calculation done that issues in a decision.

What *doesn't* make sense is to conclude that, because you have – after long agonizing and in possession of "complete" information – decided that it's an "A" it will behave like the *average* "A." The rubber band image come to mind because the in-between cases "snap" to one or the other measure of central tendency in the neighborhood, A or B in this case. In fact, it is probably more important that the case was difficult to classify than that it was finally assigned to the "A" category. This rubber band move is a covert form of essentialism; cases either have an "A" essence or a "B" essence and that essence is captured by the measure of central tendency (the mean or the median); the variation (that the case has strayed into the in-between region) is confusing random "noise" that the pathologist has now, with his testing, seen through to the "signal." This view conflates random *measurement* variation with potentially important *biological* variation. As the late S.J. Gould put it: "The median is *not* the message!" [21]. It's important to look at the entire distribution, the Full House, in making clinical predictions.

The Novel Case and the "Closest Fit" Strategy

Just as the "hybrid case" can be thought of as the embarrassingly heterogeneous case, the "novel case" can be thought of as the embarrassingly unique case. These, as might be expected, are relatively common in a consultation practice. The basic strategy here is to roam the relevant phenospace in search of the "closest fit" and invoke the heuristic "Looks like therefore most likely will behave as." Examples include: "Histologically low-grade mesenchymal proliferation with potential for local recurrence (see learned comment wherein all of the relevant differential diagnostic possibilities are considered and serially discarded)."

The Fallible Reasoner: Judgmental Psychology

There are pitfalls in intuitive probabilistic reasoning; these errors in judgment have been an active area of research since the 1970s and a Nobel prize in economics was awarded to one of the founders of the field, Daniel Kahneman. Space does not permit a discussion of this topic, but an important element of the EBP program should be a study of the relevance of judgmental psychology to oncopathological decision-making. There are several accessible introductions to the important topic [3, 22–24].

Decision Support Systems

Space does not permit a review of DSS and we will only examine these efforts from the perspective set out in Chap. 6. DSS are basically classifiers that evaluate evidence and classify a situation either in service of morphological diagnosis or prediction. Diagnostic systems aim to simulate the diagnostic performance of experts in the domain; they are imitative and attempt to solve the "translation-transmission" problem set out in Chap. 6. The goal of predictive systems is to generate a clinical prediction using, what's been termed in the (DSS) literature, "case-based reasoning (CBR)." CBR amounts to matching the phenotype of the current patient (clinical features, histological features, etc.) with those contained in a database of thousands of patients about whom both phenotype and clinical outcome are known. The patient is assigned the prognosis of those database patients with the closest phenotype match.

Diagnostic Systems

One of the earliest applications of expert systems was to the task of medical diagnosis. In the 1980s, a very active area of research was the construction of expert systems – computer-based systems that replace or assist an expert in performing a complex task. The construction of a diagnostic program typically involves "downloading" the classificatory vision of an expert in the particular domain. This is exemplified by the Pathfinder expert system which was designed by David Heckerman, then a Stanford Medical student, and colleagues to simulate the diagnostic performance of expert hematopathologists in diagnosing lymph node pathology [25, 26]. I participated in some stages of this work. In its last versions, the model contained more than sixty different diseases and around a hundred different features. An extensive library of images accompanies this program. The basic idea was to capture the expertise of a group of academic hematopathologists as a Bayesian network. A Bayesian network, or belief network, is a graphical model that represents a set of random variables (nodes) and their conditional dependences (by lines connecting the nodes). Roughly, this can be thought of as a high-dimensional joint probability distribution relating observed features (both morphological and clinical) to diagnostic categories. Its diagnostic capabilities were evaluated using actual cases and comparing Pathfinder's performance with that of the experts who originally provided the expertise for the system. Knowledge-based expert systems of this sort have not caught on; there is very little about them in the literature after 2000. There are a number of reasons for this including legal liability issues for misdiagnoses and compatibility with the physicians' workflow [27]. Very few pathologists are willing to spend an hour entering data on a problem case; it is a lot easier to send the case off to an expert.

Attempts of this sort are, however, of theoretical interest. In the language of Chap. 6, Pathfinder and the like diagnostic systems are an attempt to solve the "translation-transmission" problem; the translation of the expert's classificatory vision into language and images and its transmission to a nonexpert user. We can make a number of preliminary observations, again, using Pathfinder as an example: (1) the system reflects a composite of several experts' expertise; realistically, we would anticipate that these experts would not always be in agreement on a particular case assignment; (2) the system is limited by the experts' knowledge; in particular, the experts' current location along the macrorevisionary cycle. This is a real problem for hematopathology; classifications change with some regularity; (3) the system can be anticipated to have difficulties with problem cases. The discussion of Chap. 6 of the expert's private microrevisionary cycles emphasized that when confronting problem cases, classification and diagnosis collapse into a single act. In diagnosing problem cases, the expert may depart from a prior rules to make his assignment; it appears, on the face of it, unlikely that the expert's diagnostic-classificatory moves would be anticipated by a set of conditional probabilities downloaded in a few interview during the construction of the program. In short, the expert doesn't know what his criteria will be until he encounters the problem case. Again, using the language of Chap. 6, we would expect excellent performance on "core" cases, but, for peripheral terra incognita (PeTI) cases, performance would degrade.

Advantages and Disadvantages of Predictive Systems and Case-Based Reasoning

There is a fundamental problem with population-based studies – such studies tell us about the characteristics of groups, not individuals. Thus, while clinical judgment and CBR self-consciously attend to the particularity and uniqueness of the individual under consideration, population-based studies scrupulously strip away all of that detail replacing it with a handful of observed features. This reductionist move is in service of generating stable, statistically credible population averages. Thus, evidence-based medicine has ideologically (and rhetorically) positioned itself against anecdotal CBR. The pendulum, however, swings!

CBR has become a popular approach to realize the goal "personal prognosis." CBR involves, in the language of Bartels et al., identification rather than classification [28]. *Classification*, the partitioning of a domain into classes, involves the selection of a relatively small, manageable number of features and representing each case in a feature space spanned by those dimensions. Limiting the number of features is forced by the "curse of dimensionality." (See Chap. 7 for discussion) They characterize this as a closed feature space. Clinical and morphologic prediction rules have this character. *Identification*, in contrast, uses as many dimensions as are available to establish the identity (or closest fit) to other cases in the database. The prediction for that case is that of the group of nearest neighbors. This is an open feature space.

Montironi et al. describe the role of CBR in prognostic support systems:

> CBR establishes a prognosis for a particular patient, and thus differs significantly from statistical classification, in which the patient is assigned to a group, all of whose members were given the same diagnosis. Statistical classification allows a prognosis on the basis of what is known for the group, for example, a probability to progress or survive for a certain period of time. However, statistical procedures are neither usually intended nor designed to characterize individuals. For example, for a given patient it is not possible to say whether the prognostic outlook is poor or better within the bounds given for the group. CBR, conversely, is designed to provide individual patient prognosis. Case based reasoning compares the new case with cases from a large database of cases for which the clinical outcome is known. From such a database, only the most similar cases are retrieved and used to predict the outcome. The data may include qualitative and quantitative histopathological feature values, patient anamnestic data, treatment, and observed response to treatment, thus providing a very detailed characterization of the patient's situation [29].

Except in the most general sense of searching for similar cases, the use of CBR is problematic. For Montironi et al., it is simply an application of the heuristic: "Looks like, therefore will act like." It is certainly a long way off from Osler sitting at the bedside puzzling over a singular patient, Sigmund Freud probing the psyche of Anna O., Sherlock Holmes in his Baker Suite rooms, or the other Holmes, Oliver Wendell Jr., mulling over issue of precedence in the Supreme Court [30].

In the DSS literature, CBR has two features: the patient's phenotype can be characterized using an open-ended number of features and the classification rule is: associate this patient's point in the feature space with the nearest (i.e., most similar) case(s) in the high-dimensional neighborhood. In mathematical-statistical terms, this is a *k*-nearest-neighbor (kNN) search.

It's worth recording the differences between the folksy examples I provided and a kNN search. A few example suffice: (1) the patient's particularity has to be reduced to a set of observed features and some subset of those features recorded. There are problems in including too much (what turns out, in the fullness of time, to be "noise") and too little (missed "signal"). Recall the years of our examining peptic ulcer surgery specimens and ignoring the Helicobacter organisms; (2) the observations have to be preprocessed into a computer digestible form, usually nonfuzzy; (3) a similarity measure must be selected from a large number of workable metrics (e.g., Euclidean, Mahalanobis). We discovered in Chap. 6 that high-dimensional biology is plagued by the "curse of dimensionality"; kNN searches are no exception. The "nearest neighbor" looses meaning with a modest increase in the dimensionality of the data. That is, as the dimensionality of the phenospace increases the ratio of the distance to the nearest neighbor and the distance to the most distant neighbor asymptotically approaches unity. See Chap. 7 for discussion.

Who Should Be Making the Decisions in Oncopathology?

Unguided statistical intuitions are notoriously flawed and keeping track, without assistance, of the large number of conditional probabilities involved in a practical decision-making problem is impossible. The evaluation of the tsunami of evidence from clinical trials, from genomic studies, requires, as we have seen, highly specialized knowledge from a variety of disciplines for which pathologists have little training. The futuristic vision of the unaided community (or academic) pathologist as integrator of information from multiple levels of organization – from cancer gene to histopathologic findings to $\Phi_{\text{Clin}}(t)$ – is a fantasy. We'll need some sort of help. There is much debate about who should be integrating this growing, complex quantity of patient information. Not surprisingly, some pathologists argue that it should be the pathologist [31, 32].

However, this issue may be settled, there is no question that light microscopy is an essential organizing level in cancer management, and expertise in histopathology will be required no matter what the future holds for the molecular-genetic dimensions of neoplasia. It is not only reasonable but necessary for pathologists to resist the methodological imperialism *de jour.* There will be a continuing role for surgical pathology oncopathological decision-making in the postgenomic age [33–38].

References

1. Hacking I. The taming of chance. Cambridge: Cambridge University Press; 1990.
2. Hacking I. An introduction to probability and inductive logic. Cambridge: Cambridge University Press; 2001.
3. Sox Jr HC, Blatt MA, Higgins MC, Marton KI. Medical decision making. Boston: Butterworths; 1988.
4. Howard RA. The foundations of decision analysis revisited. In: Edwards W, Miles JRF, Winterfeldt DV, (eds.) Advances in Decision Analysis. New York, NY: Cambridge University Press; 2007. p. 32–56
5. Russell S, Norvig P. Artificial intelligence: a modern approach. 3rd ed. Englewood Cliffs: Prentice-Hall; 2009.
6. Howard R. Decision analysis: practice and promise. Manage Sci. 1988;34(6):679–93.
7. Zadeh LA. Fuzzy sets. Inf Control. 1965;8:338–53.
8. Vineis P. Methodological insights: fuzzy sets in medicine. J Epidemiol Community Health. 2008;62(3):273–8.
9. Kosko B, Isaka S. Fuzzy logic. Sci Am. 1993 (July):76–81.
10. Seising R. From vagueness in medical thought to the foundations of fuzzy reasoning in medical diagnosis. Artif Intell Med. 2006;38(3):237–56.
11. Sadegh-Zadeh K. The prototype resemblance theory of disease. J Med Philos. 2008;33(2):106–39.
12. Bartels PH, Thompson D, Weber JE. Expert systems in histopathology. IV. The management of uncertainty. Anal Quant Cytol Histol. 1992;14(1):1–13.
13. Spiegelhalter DJ. Understanding uncertainty. Ann Fam Med. 2008;6(3):196–7.

14. Hájek A. Interpretations of probability. The Stanford Encyclopedia of Philosophy, In: Edward N. Zalta editor 2010. Springer; http://plata.stanford.edu/archives/spr2010/entries/probability-interpret/. Accessed 5 April 2011.
15. Goodman SN. Probability at the bedside: the knowing of chances or the chances of knowing? Ann Intern Med. 1999;130(7):604–6.
16. Hendrickson M, Longacre T. Pathology of uterine cancers. In: Gershenson D, McGuire WP, Gore M, Quinn MA, Thomas G, editors. Gynecologic cancer. controversies in management. 1st ed. Edinburgh: Elsevier Churchill Livingstone; 2004. p. 209–28.
17. Kempson RL, Fletcher CD, Evans HL, Hendrickson MR, Sibley RK. Tumors of the soft tissues (atlas of tumor pathology (AFIP)). 1st ed. Washington: American Registry of Pathology; 2001.
18. Wick MR, Bourne TD, Patterson JW, Mills SE. Evidence-based principles and practices in pathology: selected problem areas. Semin Diagn Pathol. 2005; 22(2):116–25.
19. Vollmer RT. Differential diagnosis in immunohistochemistry with Bayes theorem. Am J Clin Pathol. 2009;131(5):723–30.
20. Weir MM, Bell DA, Young RH. Grade 1 peritoneal serous carcinomas: a report of 14 cases and comparison with 7 peritoneal serous psammocarcinomas and 19 peritoneal serous borderline tumors. Am J Surg Pathol. 1998;22(7):849–62.
21. Gould SJ. Full house. The spread of excellence from Plato to Darwin. New York: Three Rivers Press; 1996.
22. Tversky A, Kahneman D. Judgment under uncertainty: heuristics and biases. Science. 1974;185(4157): 1124–31.
23. Hastie R, Dawes RM. Rational choice in an uncertain world. The psychology of judgment and decision making. Thousand Oaks: Sage Publications; 2001.
24. Gilovich T, Griffin D, Kahneman D. Heuristics and biases. the psychology of intuitive judgment. Cambridge: Cambridge University Press; 2002.
25. Nathwani BN, Clarke K, Lincoln T, et al. Evaluation of an expert system on lymph node pathology. Hum Pathol. 1997;28(9):1097–110.
26. Heckerman DE, Horvitz EJ, Nathwani BN. Toward normative expert systems: Part I. The Pathfinder project. Methods Inf Med. 1992;31(2):90–105.
27. Koller D, Friedman N. Probabilistic graphical models: principles and techniques. Cambridge: MIT Press; 2009.
28. Bartels PH. Future directions in quantitative pathology: digital knowledge in diagnostic pathology. J Clin Pathol. 2000;53(1):31–7.
29. Montironi R, Cheng L, Lopez-Beltran A, Mazzucchelli R, Scarpelli M, Bartels PH. Decision support systems for morphology-based diagnosis and prognosis of prostate neoplasms: a methodological approach. Cancer. 2009;115(13 Suppl):3068–77.
30. Forrester J. If p, then what? Thinking in cases. Hist Hum Sci. 1996;9(3):1–25.
31. Costa J. Is clinical systems pathology the future of pathology? Arch Pathol Lab Med. 2008;132(5):774–6.
32. Donovan MJ, Costa J, Cordon-Cardo C. Systems pathology: a paradigm shift in the practice of diagnostic and predictive pathology. Cancer. 2009;115 Suppl 13:3078–84.
33. Rosai J. Why microscopy will remain a cornerstone of surgical pathology. Lab Invest. 2007;87(5):403–8.
34. Natkunam Y, Mason DY. Prognostic immunohistologic markers in human tumors: why are so few used in clinical practice? Lab Invest. 2006;86(8):742–7.
35. Ladanyi M, Chan WC, Triche TJ, Gerald WL. Expression profiling of human tumors: the end of surgical pathology? J Mol Diagn. 2001;3(3):92–7.
36. Beckman M. Tumor complexity prompts caution about sequencing. J Natl Cancer Inst. 2006;98(24): 1758–9.
37. Crawford JM. Original research in pathology: judgment, or evidence-based medicine? Lab Invest. 2007;87(2):104–14.
38. Fischer AH. The evolution of tumor biology: seeking a balance between gene expression profiling and morphology studies. J Mol Diagn. 2002;4(1):65.
39. Moons KG, van Es GA, Deckers JW, Habbema JD, Grobbee DE. Limitations of sensitivity, specificity, likelihood ratio, and bayes' theorem in assessing diagnostic probabilities: a clinical example. Epidemiology. 1997;8(1):12–7.

Part II

Solutions Offered by Evidence-Based Pathology and Laboratory Medicine

11 Evidence-Based Approach to Evaluate Information Published in the Pathology Literature and Integrate It with Personal Experience

Alberto M. Marchevsky and Mark R. Wick

Keywords
Evidence-based pathology • Pathology literature evaluation • Evaluating information in pathology • Pathology interpretation of data • Personal experience in pathology

This chapter explores how to interpret and evaluate information published in the pathology literature and integrate it with personal experience using a systematic approach based on general Evidence-Based Pathology (EBP) principles [1, 2]. Previous chapters have described some of the methodological problems encountered in the current pathology literature and have explained basic concepts of EBP as a derivative of Evidence-Based Medicine. Perusal through these materials can certainly raise legitimate questions regarding whether the "EBP approach" has really introduced new concepts, a topic that is discussed in more detail in Chap. 2 [3–8]. As reviewed by Drs. Costa and Whitaker, pathologists generally believe that most information used in our daily practice is based on sound observations, the results of evaluating tissue and other body samples with the latest analytical methods, and the use of statistically significant data. It is probably not too adventurous to estimate that many pathologists probably view EBP as the "repackaging" of information under the catchy "evidence-based" logo. Yet, if we review the current literature from an epistemological point of view and using the systematic approach described in this chapter, one can argue that the quality of future pathology publications could be enhanced by the use of more precise methodology that explicitly lists the objectives of each study, considers the limitations resulting from the characteristics of the materials being investigated in the development of conclusions, and analyzes the results with an eye toward developing information that is useful for the evaluation, diagnosis, and treatment of individual patients. Greater awareness of this EBP-based process will also hopefully assist pathologists planning to perform future studies that would yield information that could be applicable for the diagnosis of pathological specimens.

Epistemology is the branch of philosophy interested in the theory of knowledge [9–14]. It promotes the analysis of the nature and limitations of various conceptual paradigms and observational methods used for the acquisition and interpretation of new information. The first

A.M. Marchevsky (✉)
Pulmonary and Mediastinal Pathology,
Department of Pathology and Laboratory Medicine,
Cedars-Sinai Medical Center, Los Angeles, CA, USA
and
David Geffen School of Medicine, University of California, Los Angeles, CA, USA
e-mail: Alberto.Marchevsky@cshs.org

A.M. Marchevsky and M.R. Wick (eds.), *Evidence Based Pathology and Laboratory Medicine*,
DOI 10.1007/978-1-4419-1030-1_11, © Springer Science+Business Media, LLC 2011

sections of the chapter will review from an epistemological standpoint the study designs that are generally being used in pathology research and teaching, as exemplified by recent publications in peer-reviewed journals, using a systematic process to evaluate the validity and clinical applicability of the results and conclusions of these studies. The various comments are not intended to judge on the quality of the articles selected for review, but to explore methodological characteristics and details in an effort to evaluate the validity of the results of each study and their applicability in current pathology practice. The last section of the chapter will introduce the problem of how to use EBP principles to integrate the information published in the literature with personal data and experience, a topic that is described in more detail in Chap. 13 and 15.

EBP Guide to Readers: Is the Information Valid and Applicable to My Cases?

The scientific method is a body of techniques designed for knowledge acquisition, based on the collection of data through observation, experimentation, and the formulation and testing of hypotheses [15–21]. The goal of the scientific method is to seek the truth. However, knowledge about elusive "truths" frequently evolves as a result of an iterative process where new information poses new questions, leading to the generation of new hypotheses that stimulate the collection of additional data that update previous knowledge. In addition, knowledge is influenced by beliefs held as a result of tradition, education, and various cultural, psychological, and sociological factors. Beliefs can alter the perception of observations and influence the interpretation of data resulting in a variety of biases that can distort the validity of presumably scientific information. The peer review system has been designed to evaluate the information and conclusions being presented in scientific studies in an effort to prevent the dissemination of erroneous information and minimize the publication of biased and scientifically unsound information [20, 22–32]. However, as expert reviewers often have their own preconceptions and biases, the fact that new information has been reported in the peer review literature offers no absolute guarantee about its scientific value, leaving the reader with the personal responsibility to evaluate the validity of published data [30]. In addition, practicing pathologists are likely to read the literature with these two general questions in mind: do these conclusions apply to my patients? and what can I learn from this study that could be applied to the evaluation of my tissue specimens or other laboratory samples?

Table 11.1 Systematic evidence-based process to evaluate published information

Does the study include comprehensive and unbiased background information?
Does the study list one or more clear hypothesis/es?
What study design is used?
Are the conditions of the study sufficient to test the hypothesis?
Are the results of the study internally valid?
Does the study test for the external validity of the results?
What is the evidence level of the study results?
What is the applicability of the study results for the evaluation and diagnosis of my individual patients?

The systematic EBP-based process listed in Table 11.1 can be useful to evaluate the quality and clinical validity of the information published in the peer review literature and other sources of medical data and integrate it with personal experience for the evaluation of tissue samples and laboratory specimens from individual patients. The questions listed in the table can then be expanded to formulate the more specific queries listed in other tables.

Does the Study Include Comprehensive and Unbiased Background Information: Narrative Reviews Versus Systematic Literature Reviews

An initial step during the evaluation of the validity of the content of pathology publications is to identify the methodology used for the selection of pertinent background information. Such information from previous literature is frequently used to justify the hypothesis being tested in a study, evaluate the results, formulate conclusions, and/or integrate them with previous knowledge. The methodology used to select background information is particularly pertinent when evaluating the content of review articles. Unfortunately, perusal through multiple articles in the recent pathology literature shows that it is generally customary to use a highly personalized approach to the selection of references and background information [33–36]. Authors, presumably based on their own experience and professional judgment, pick and choose selected information from a variable number of references usually found in the Pubmed database of the National Library of Medicine and do not explain why certain publications were included, while others may have been excluded by design or neglect. As discussed in previous chapters, this unstructured process for the selection of background information does not necessarily provide an objective and comprehensive review process or assure readers that additional studies that contradict the conclusions of the present study and/or the current beliefs of its authors were considered.

Systematic reviews are research summaries that use explicit, objective, and well-defined search criteria to perform a thorough literature search followed by critical appraisal of individual studies to identify valid and applicable evidence in multiple databases [32, 37–39]. The Centre for Evidence-Based Medicine of Oxford University and the Cochrane collaboration suggest that systematic reviews include five sections: background, objectives, methods of the review, results and conclusions. They also recommend seven steps for the preparation and maintenance of systematic reviews, as shown in Table 11.2 [22, 40–46]. Somewhat ironically, not even systematic reviews are necessarily uniform, as there are no widely agreed-upon sets of standards for the production of systematic reviews. For example, a recent review of 300 studies by Moher et al. [47] found that different strategies are being used for the preparation of systematic reviews and not all are equally reliable.

Data from systematic reviews can be integrated and analyzed with the statistical method of meta-analysis, as discussed in Chap. 9.

Table 11.2 Seven steps suggested by the Cochrane Collaboration for the preparation and maintenance of systematic literature reviews

Formulating a problem
Locating and selecting studies
Critical appraisal of studies
Evidence levels
Collecting data
Analyzing and presenting results
Meta-analysis
Interpreting results
Improving and updating reviews

Does the Study List One or More Explicit Hypotheses? What Is the Purpose of the Study?

The majority of original contributions in the pathology literature include one or more hypothesis, but it can be difficult at times to find the description of hypothesis or specific purposes of the study in the text of a publication and to fully understand why the investigators have selected particular approaches to the evaluation of their pathologic materials. For example, the recent paper by Mahajan et al. [48] is an interesting study describing gastric foveolar-type and other types of dysplasia in patients with Barrett's esophagus. Reading the article using the systematic approach shown in Table 11.1 suggests the following questions and answers: (1) Does the study include comprehensive and unbiased background information? It is difficult to answer this question as a systematic literature review was not performed. (2) Does the study list one or more clearly formulated hypotheses? The article does not list specific questions to be investigated. The Abstract describes the purpose of the paper as "The prevalence, diagnostic criteria, and natural history of gastric-type Barrett's dysplasia were systematically evaluated in 1854 endoscopic biopsies from a cohort of 200 consecutive Barrett's dysplasia patients." The Materials and Methods section of the paper describes the process of finding cases and how they were studied, but does not include explicit questions or hypothesis to be investigated. The lack of explicit questions or hypotheses to be investigated may appear to pathology readers as an unnecessary or redundant process, but often leads to questions that cannot be answered by the readers and ambiguity in the interpretation of data by pathologists other than the authors of the study. For example, reading the Materials and Methods section of the Mahajan et al. paper, we learn that the study included all cases of Barrett's esophagus and dysplasia diagnosed at their institution during a particular time span using clearly spelled out criteria for the intestinal variant of dysplasia in Barrett's esophagus. In contrast, it is less clear how the diagnosis of gastric-type dysplasia was rendered by "simultaneous consensus agreement of the two gastrointestinal pathologists and pathology resident authors." The paper does include a table with diagnostic criteria, but it is not referred to in Methods and is not referenced, so is difficult to understand whether these criteria were derived before or after evaluation of the various diagnostic criteria that were analyzed with statistics. This ambiguity can lead to respectful questions such as how did they diagnose their cases, or what is their "gold standard" other than themselves? Indeed, in our opinion, this diagnostic process raises the suspicion of a circular reasoning process that is not all that unusual in pathology publications: diagnoses are rendered because lesions look in a certain way to authors who then evaluate the prevalence of specific features in lesions that they classified in a certain manner. In contrast, the formulation of explicit tasks, hypothesis, or patient-centered questions, as proposed by EBM and EBP advocates, could have precluded some of these problems and perhaps even improve on the readability and comprehensiveness of the study. For example, the methodology could have been structured with definitions and hypothesis that could have organized the information as follows: (1) define foveolar-type dysplasia in the presence of explicit histopathologic criteria from the literature and not as "unequivocal neoplastic epithelium confined to the luminal side of the basement membrane," a definition subject to variable interpretation by readers. (2) Define the criteria for grading dysplasias, with references. (3) Discuss whether foveolar-type dysplasia and mixed foveolar-type dysplasias should be graded in a similar or distinct manner from the more common form of intestinal-type dysplasia. (4) Test with kappa statistics whether the classification and/or grading based on the explicit criteria is reproducible among all authors, including the residents who are probably not experts in gastrointestinal pathologists. (5) Divide the data into three groups: pure foveolar-type dysplasia, gastric-type dysplasia, and both. (6) Evaluate for each of these three groups how many cases evolved to higher grades of dysplasia and carcinoma. (7) Evaluate by dysplasia type and grade how many cases evolved to higher grades of dysplasia and carcinoma. (8) Evaluate the time that it took for the development of carcinoma, by dysplasia type and grade. Evaluation of each of these specific tasks could have precluded some of the questions suggested in the following section of this chapter or suggest specific questions for future research, should the currently available clinico-pathologic materials be insufficient to provide answers to all six topics.

Recent studies have explored the use of this proposed approach where specific questions are formulated and the study organized to systematically answer them [49–51]. They are discussed in more detail in Chap. 10. It remains to be explored whether a more structured study design that includes a list of specific tasks or questions improves on the quality and readability of pathology publications.

What Study Design Is Used?

It can be helpful to understand the type of study design used by the authors of a particular publication in order to estimate the potential validity of its results and conclusions [52–55]. In general, there are three categories of biomedical research: observational, experimental, and evaluation of treatment effects [55]. In addition, investigators can use meta-analysis to aggregate the results of different studies and reconcile differences.

Experimental pathology studies are generally designed using adequate control groups and tightly controlling the various experimental conditions in order to decrease the influence of covariates in the statistical analysis of the data [53, 54, 56]. However, most publications in the pathology literature are observational and are designed to correlate the relationship between laboratory findings or specific pathologic findings detected with histopathology, immunohistochemistry, molecular, and other methods and some aspect of disease, such as progression, recurrence, or death [57]. Observational studies can suggest significant associations between variables, but cannot generally used to determine cause and effect [10, 12]. The results of observational studies are often influenced by covariates that are not independent of each other [58, 59].

Different study designs can be used in observational studies (Table 11.3) [57, 60, 61]. Cohort studies are usually used in epidemiology, but have been used in pathology to describe the findings that develop prospectively or retrospectively over a period of time in a population exposed to putative carcinogens or other environmental variables [55, 62, 63]. Time-series studies and case-control studies are more commonly used in anatomic pathology [64]. Time-series studies investigate the correlation of certain findings with the development of others at various points in time. The data are best collected prospectively, but can be retrospective. In the more commonly used case-control study design format, the cases are divided into case-subjects and controls. The latter study design format can be structured as nested case-control studies where the data are stratified into various subgroups.

Table 11.3 Types of study designs

Observational studies
Cohort study
Prospective
Retrospective
Time series
Case-control study
Nested case-control
Cross-sectional study
Experimental studies
Case-control
Treatment studies
Randomized controlled trials
Double-blind randomized trial
Single-blind randomized trial
Nonblind trial
Nonrandomized trial

It is our impression that the type of study design is not customarily spelled out in most pathology publications. For example, if we query as to the study design of the Mahajan et al. [48] paper, we are not told specifically but surmise that is probably a time-series type study where certain features were described in a population that was investigated using "longitudinal follow-up information" [48]. Yet, the "statistical analysis" section of the paper does not evaluate whether the cohort had enough subjects in each category to derive forecasts or explain to nonstatisticians whether the statistical tests used to evaluate the results were appropriate for time-series type of data. The lack of this information leads nonstatisticians to become skeptical whether the study had enough subjects in the various dysplasia classes to reach clinically significant conclusions. For example, the study included "200 consecutive Barrett's dysplasia patients" followed for variable periods of time and up to 8 years. Data were collected retrospectively and prospectively. The cohort included only 11 cases of pure foveolar-type dysplasia and 19 with mixed dysplasia types, while the majority ($n=170$) of cases showed findings of the more common intestinal-type dysplasia. Twelve of the 30 patients with pure or mixed gastric-type dysplasia progressed to higher grade of dysplasia, while 13 did not progress and 5 were lost to follow up. Five of the eleven of the patients that progressed had mixed type of dysplasia. What have we learnt about the prognostic significance of pure gastric-type dysplasia in patients with Barrett's esophagus that we could use in our practice? The study probably supports our previous knowledge that patients with Barrett's esophagus and dysplasia are at a high risk of developing malignancy. Is the risk higher for patients with foveolar-type dysplasia than in patients with mixed dysplasia or intestinal-type dysplasia? The evidence in the paper is probably inconclusive to answer this question. Does the dysplasia grade predict the likelihood of the development of malignancy or when a patient is most likely to be diagnosed with malignancy? The study does not answer this question. Although the study describes a carefully evaluated group of patients with dysplasia and Barrett's esophagus, the results do not provide, in our opinion, best evidence supporting the conclusion that "the recognition of Barrett's gastric-type dysplasia and use of the proposed grading criteria should promote better diagnostic classification of the Barrett's neoplasm spectrum."

As suggested in the previous section of this chapter, the use of a more systematic study design that included a more explicit description of the goals of the study and explored which study design was most appropriate to evaluate various problems may have precluded some of these questions and perhaps temper the conclusions of this study.

Are the Conditions of the Study Sufficient to Test the Hypothesis?

Clinico-pathologic studies in anatomic pathology are frequently difficult to conduct as they are frequently designed to evaluate tissue samples with unusual conditions that are hard to collect and involve the use of expensive and time-consuming tests. It is somewhat surprising that, in contrast to the painstaking attention to detail that is routinely devoted to the description of the technical analysis of the samples, little publication space is often devoted to discussing whether the pathologic materials are sufficient in sample size and the conditions of a study are adequate to test specific hypotheses. In addition, there is a tendency to assume that because additional findings are found with new methods in various lesions, these findings are of clinical value. These problems are particularly evident in studies that evaluate the diagnostic validity of new and sophisticated diagnostic methods. For example, the recent study by Brunelli et al. [65] evaluated and beautifully illustrated the "Diagnostic usefulness of fluorescent cytogenetics in differentiating chromophobe renal cell carcinoma from renal oncocytoma." The study evaluated 11 chromophobe renal carcinomas and 12 renal oncocytomas "showing different clinical outcomes." The investigators concluded that "the study demonstrates that indeed FISH performed on formalin-fixed, paraffin-embedded tissue can provide clinically useful information more reliably than karyotyping of most of these tumors." Analyzing the study using the epistemological approach by using the questions suggested in Table 11.1, we learn that the study does not include a systematic review of the literature, listing of specific hypothesis, or a specific description of the study format. As in the study by Mahajan, the lack of a description of the explicit purposes of the study can lead to ambiguities. For example, readers could argue that 100% of the cases were diagnosed as either chromophobe renal cell carcinoma or renal oncocytoma using histopathology, so what is the diagnostic advantage of using FISH or karyotyping in the cases used to derive conclusions? Where is the evidence that FISH and karyotyping improved on the specificity and/or sensitivity of the differential diagnosis between chromophobe renal cell carcinoma and renal oncocytoma? In addition, as the study does not provide correlation between the FISH, karyotype, or other findings such as clinical stage, prognosis, or other clinical data, what is the evidence that the findings "provide clinically useful information"? The paper does not provide data to answer these questions and perhaps, more troublesome, does not elaborate on these issues that are probably of interest to practicing pathologists in its discussion. Indeed, although FISH is apparently better than karyotyping for the evaluation of these neoplasms, "uncertainty remains as to whether variations in tumor karyotype can produce confounding results that bring into question the usefulness of FISH analysis in distinguishing between these 2 tumor types."

The EBP process being described in this chapter could have obviated critiques to a paper that was conducted with exquisite attention to laboratory details. For example, the study could have been structured around four explicit questions: (1) What are the abnormalities that can be found with FISH in well-characterized cases of chromophobe renal cell carcinoma and renal oncocytoma? (2) What are the abnormalities that can be found with karyotyping in well-characterized cases of chromophobe renal cell carcinoma and renal oncocytoma? (3) Can FISH or karyotyping improve on the specificity of a differential diagnosis between renal oncocytoma and chromophobe renal cell carcinoma in difficult cases? (4) Which are the FISH and/or karyotyping abnormalities that are most helpful to improve the specificity of this differential diagnosis in difficult cases? Formulations of specific questions such as these may have suggested to the authors the need to include in the study cases that were particularly difficult to diagnose and the use of some external diagnostic "gold standard" for the diagnosis of chromophobe renal cell carcinoma such as disease progression or metastasis or the opinion of an external panel of experts.

Are the Results of the Study Internally Valid?

It is beyond the scope of this chapter to discuss in detail the various methodological details that can influence the results of observational studies. Table 11.4 suggests seven questions that can help readers evaluate whether the results of a study are supported by the data. Most of the answers to these questions are discussed in the review of the indications and limitations of various statistical tests in Chap. 4. An issue that is usually not explored in clinico-pathologic studies in the pathology literature is whether the number of samples of various conditions provides sufficient sample sizes to investigate various hypotheses. As explained in Chap. 8, power analysis can be used to estimate from preliminary data the optimal number of cases to exclude the possibility that negative results are not significant to a power of 0.80. Application of this methodology to the study of conditions, such as thymomas, that are associated with the potential to recur or metastasize many years after initial diagnosis can yield surprising results. For example, a recent study with meta-analysis of almost 1,000 thymomas estimated that over 7,000 cases would be needed to conduct a study valid to a power of 0.80 [66].

Table 11.4 Specific queries to evaluate the internal validity of a study

What study design was used?
Is it a prospective or retrospective study?
Were control cases selected appropriately?
Are the sample sizes adequate?
Was power analysis performed?
Were the findings evaluated with the appropriate statistical tests?
Do the findings support the conclusions of the study?

Does the Study Test for the External Validity of the Results?

The conclusions of observational studies in pathology are validated by analyzing the results collected from relatively small samples with descriptive statistical methods. The samples are usually samples of convenience which are generally not selected randomly from the entire population of subjects with a particular entity of interest [1]. The adequacy of sample sizes are usually not estimated. Observational studies performed under these conditions cannot adequately estimate whether their results are applicable to subjects in other population groups. These problems can be minimized by collecting large samples from multiple institutions located in different states or countries. Another approach is to test the results of a study with another "test sample" composed of specimens that were not used to derive the conclusions of the study [1, 2, 24]. These test samples can be collected retrospectively by dividing cases into two groups, training and testing or validation sets prior to the performance of the study. The results obtained from the training set are tested with "unknown" cases in the validation group.

The question as to whether external validation of classification results is really needed in well-conducted observational studies was systematically explored in an analysis of the classification of individual lung cancer cell lines based on DNA methylation markers analyzed with two multivariate statistical tests, linear discriminant analysis and artificial neural networks [67]. The conditions of this study were better controlled than the usual clinico-pathologic study as the cell lines had been previously well characterized by other studies and therefore there was no question about the correct diagnoses. In addition, classification was rendered using the "objective" process of collecting data with molecular methods and evaluated with multivariate statistical methods. Initially, the data from all cell lines were included in one data set with similar number of cell lines in the two diagnostic categories. All cell lines were classified correctly in this data set by using selected DNA methylation markers and artificial neural networks, suggesting that this technology allows for an objective diagnosis of these cell lines in all cases. However, this conclusion would have been fraught with the circular reasoning problem described above of classifying cases according to the findings in certain cases and then concluding that certain variables contributed to classification of the same samples. Indeed, when the data were divided into training and test cases and organized into ten different combinations of randomly selected paired training and test sets, the results varied considerably from the initial conclusion. The number of correctly classified test cell lines dropped from 100% to 62–87%, according to which combinations of training and test sets were analyzed. The latter results suggested that although the technology was promising as a method to classify these cell lines on the basis of DNA methylation markers and multivariate statistical tests, larger populations of cell lines and/or perhaps other molecular data were probably needed to derive more robust classifications models that would apply more consistently to test cases. If this study would have been performed according to the study format that is currently being used in most pathology studies, evaluating a particular test or tests using all cases in one data set, it would have concluded that cell lines can be diagnosed with 100% accuracy using DNA methylation markers and artificial neural network technology. The contrast in results underscores the need to validate the conclusions of studies proposing new diagnostic criteria using validation or test data that were not used to derive the classification features.

External validation of results is currently seldom used in the pathology literature and is increasingly being used in the oncology and other literature [68–70]. New diagnostic criteria are usually proposed on the basis of the analysis of a particular group of cases and it is assumed that other pathologists evaluating other specimens could reach similar conclusions, without testing this assumption. In our view, this practice can result in considerable interobserver variability diagnostic problems that increase variability and confusion in the literature. For example, a recent study reviewing the prognosis of patients with idiopathic interstitial lung disease showed that the survival of patients with a diagnosis of usual interstitial pneumonia (UIP) in the seven studies where the survival of these patients was compared with the prognosis of nonspecific interstitial pneumonia (NSIP) cases ranged from 11% (4.4–24.9 95% confidence interval) to 58% (44.6–70.3) [71]. The survival proportions of NSIP patients ranged from 39% (23.3–57.3) to 100% (85.1–100). The marked variability in prognosis may be related to differences in the clinical characteristics of patients and variable therapeutic modalities in various international hospitals, but are so considerable that they suggest that patients with UIP and NSIP are not being consistently diagnosed as such by different expert pulmonary pathologists. Indeed, a study of interobserver variability in the diagnosis of chronic diffuse lung diseases with kappa statistics has shown only moderate agreement between different investigators diagnosing UIP and NSIP, with kappa=0.590 and kappa=0.420, respectively [72]. There is a need for better diagnostic criteria for the differential diagnosis between these two conditions which is applicable to different populations of patients diagnosed by different pathologists.

Chapter 7 discusses the topic of the external validity of study results in more detail.

What Is the Evidence Level of the Study Results?

As discussed in previous chapters, the standardization of various medical procedures, evaluation of "quality" of care, and the "evidence-based" rubric are increasingly important processes in modern Medicine [73, 74]. Many medical specialties currently sponsor the development of "evidence-based" practice guidelines, but as a group pathologists have been slow to adopt a similar approach.

EBM advocates have also promoted the use of various "evidence levels" (ELs) schemes, generally aimed at an assessment of the validity and clinical applicability of therapeutic procedures [74, 75]. For example, a recent book by Straus et al. [74] codifies several ELs with level I being the best. Level 1a is the label for systematic reviews with homogeneity of randomized clinical trials (RCTs); level 1b refers to individual RCTs with narrow confidence intervals; level 2a denotes systematic homogeneous reviews of cohort studies; level 2b includes individual cohort studies including "low-quality" RCTs (e.g., with <80% follow-up); level 3a refers to systematic homogeneous reviews of case-control studies; level 3b is principally represented by individual case-control studies; level 4 denotes case series with poor-quality cohort-based and case-control studies; and level 5 is the EL represented by "expert opinion" without explicit critical appraisal or first-hand generation of data ("first principles"). Other comparable EL systems have been published by the Cochrane collaboration and similar groups [22, 40–45]. Generally, only information obtained by RCTs, or systematic review with meta-analysis of homogeneous case-control studies, has been considered as evidence in levels 1 and 2. Data derived from individual case-control assessments are usually considered to be in level 3 or higher, denoting lower quality, because it has been shown that such observational studies are affected negatively by sources of bias that result from patient selection, sample size, distribution of data, lack of independent validation, and others. Ironically, RCT often use pathologic diagnoses as rigid classifiers in their statistical analysis. However, such lesions are diagnosed pathologically by different pathologists or by "central pathology review" on the basis of criteria previously published in EL 3 or "worse" literature.

The ELs that are used for evaluation of clinical treatment protocols generally pose a somewhat unfair proposition for pathologists [76]. Because scientific studies in our specialty do not lend themselves to the use of RCT designs, clinical EL systems essentially consign most pathology literature to EL 3 or worse. However, the notion that pathologist-generated literature is, at best, mediocre undervalues the many contributions of our specialty to the body of medical knowledge. Indeed, well-designed case series and even some seminal case reports published in the pathology literature have described new diseases and clinico-pathological entities.

The classification of most information published in the pathology literature as EL 3 or higher using clinical EL scales seems to have little relevance to the particulars of our professional discipline and may act as a disincentive for pathologists to improve the quality of the design and interpretation of future studies. The notion that our literature provides at best mediocre information markedly undervalues the many contributions of pathology to medical knowledge. Indeed, many case reports and case series in pathology have provided the initial descriptions of new diseases and clinico-pathologic entities. In addition, if one accepts the proposition that studies by pathologists are only likely to produce level 3 or worse evidence, there is little incentive to improve on the use of sound EBP principles to improve on the design quality of future studies. We have proposed a scale of ELs for publications in pathology and laboratory medicine which takes into account the various issues discussed in this book and is shown in Table 11.5 [76]. This scale classified as level I the evidence derived with well-designed case-control studies with external validation of results using prospective validation sets collected at other institutions, meta-analysis of level 2 studies, and expert recommendations based on the latter. Other types of observational studies are classified as providing ELs 2–5. There is a need for professional societies such as the College of American Pathologists (CAP), Association of Directors of Anatomic and Surgical Pathology (ADASP), and others to develop more comprehensive and authoritative EL scales to evaluate the quality of evidence in the pathology literature.

Table 11.5 Proposed scale of evidence levels for publications in pathology and laboratory medicine

Level 1	Case-control studies with external validation of results, using prospective validation data sets from other institutions Meta-analyses of level 2 studies "Expert" recommendations based on meta-analyses of level 2 or 3 studies
Level 2	Case-control studies with validation of results, using prospective validation data-sets from the same institution Meta-analyses of level 3 studies "Expert" recommendations based on a systematic review of literature without formal meta-analyses
Level 3	Case-control studies with validation of results using retrospective validation data sets from the same institution
Level 4	Case-control studies without validation
Level 5	Case series without controls, or individual case reports

Table 11.6 Specific queries to evaluate what is the applicability of the results of a study for the diagnosis and prognostication of individual patients

What prior knowledge and beliefs do I have regarding the topic being investigated in this study?
How can I use the results of the study for the pathologic evaluation of my patients?
Can our laboratory perform the tests reported in the study?
What is the sensitivity and specificity of the results?
What are the positive and negative predictive values of the results?
What is the incremental diagnostic value of the proposed new tests?
How accurate is the prognostic information being offered by the results of the study?
How useful is the prognostic information offered by the results of the study for the treatment of our patients?

What Is the Applicability of the Study Results for the Evaluation and Diagnosis of Individual Patients? Guide to the Integration of Best Available Evidence from the Literature with Personal Experience

There is little current pathology literature exploring the topic of how to integrate the best available evidence with personal experience using EBP principles. As discussed before, it is well known that diagnostic criteria and laboratory details developed at other institutions may not be automatically applicable to others. Indeed, it is currently required by the CAP accreditation process that each institution issues its own technical manual for the performance and interpretation of laboratory tests, rather than using external documents without review and adaptation to local practices [77–81].

Table 11.6 suggests some specific queries that can be used to guide pathologists integrate best available evidence from the literature with personal experience. The process involves performing a systematic review of pertinent literature, identification of best available evidence and estimation of ELs, accrual of cases of personal experience, and test whether the recommendations in the literature apply to local cases and under what conditions. This EBP-based methodology was recently applied in a study "Evidence-based evaluation of the risks of malignancy predicted by thyroid fine needle aspiration biopsies" [82]. A National Cancer Institute (NCI) "Thyroid Fine-Needle Aspiration (FNA)" State of the Science Conference proposed in 2008 standardized nomenclature and "risks of malignancy" associated with various diagnostic categories. Six categories were proposed for the diagnosis of thyroid FNAs: benign, follicular lesion of undetermined significance (FLUS), follicular neoplasm, suspicious for malignancy, malignant, and nondiagnostic [7]. With the exception of nondiagnostic, each category in the proposed thyroid FNA classification scheme was associated with a "risk of malignancy" derived from data collected from the literature [8–12]. In the NCI publications, the risks of malignancy reported to be associated with the benign, FLUS, neoplasm (follicular neoplasm or Hurthle cell neoplasm), suspicious for malignancy, and malignant categories were <1, 5–10, 20–30, 50–75, and 100%, respectively [7]. We performed a systematic literature review and evaluated our experience with 879 thyroid FNA. Interestingly, the manuscript was initially written using several specific questions as explained above, but this did not conform to editorial guidelines. Systematic literature review yielded mostly EL 3 information with malignancy risks calculated on the basis of surgical follow-up. As clinical findings other than FNA results are considered during the selection of patients with a thyroid nodule that should undergo thyroidectomy, we calculated our malignancy risks using other denominators, such as total number of cases, patients with FNA follow-up, and others. Analysis of our data yielded various relative risk estimates and showed that, as suspected, the risk estimates proposed by the NCI group of experts probably overestimated the probability of thyroid malignancy for patients with FNA diagnoses of "benign" and "follicular lesions of undetermined significance." In contrast for patients with FNA diagnosed as malignant or suspicious for malignancy, the malignancy risks in our population were similar to those in the literature. Our data also showed that in our patient population, the FNA diagnoses could be grouped from five categories other than nondiagnostic to three diagnostic categories, "benign," "FLUS+neoplasm," and "suspicious+malignant," which provided nonoverlapping risks of malignancy. A more recent study showed that the three-category diagnostic scheme for thyroid FNA also decreases interobserver diagnostic variability among different cytopathologists.

Meta-analysis can also be used to integrate the results from the literature and personal experience, as exemplified by recent studies of thymomas, discussed in more detail in Chap. 15.

References

1. Marchevsky AM. Evidence-based medicine in pathology: an introduction. Semin Diagn Pathol. 2005;22:105–15.
2. Marchevsky AM, Wick MR. Evidence-based medicine, medical decision analysis, and pathology. Hum Pathol. 2004;35:1179–88.
3. Guerette PH. Managed care: cookbook medicine, or quality, cost-effective care? Can Nurse. 1995;91:16.
4. Holm RP. Cookbook medicine. S D Med. 2009;62:371.
5. Leape L. Are practice guidelines cookbook medicine? J Ark Med Soc. 1989;86:73–5.
6. Parmley WW. Practice guidelines and cookbook medicine – who are the cooks? J Am Coll Cardiol. 1994;24:567–8.
7. Steinberg KE. Cookbook medicine: recipe for disaster? J Am Med Dir Assoc. 2006;7:470–2.
8. Sackett DL, Rosenberg WM, Gray JA, et al. Evidence based medicine: what it is and what it isn't. BMJ. 1996;312:71–2.
9. Bibace R, Watzlawik M. Epistemology and values are interrelated. Fam Med. 2009;41:690–1.
10. Dellavalle RP, Freeman SR, Williams HC. Clinical evidence epistemology. J Invest Dermatol. 2007;127:2668–9.
11. Dunn M, Ives J. Methodology, epistemology, and empirical bioethics research: a constructive/ist commentary. Am J Bioeth. 2009;9:93–5.
12. Michel LA. The epistemology of evidence-based medicine. Surg Endosc. 2007;21:145–51.
13. Pena A. Personal epistemology and uncertainty. Fam Med. 2009;41:691–3.
14. Rodgers JL. The epistemology of mathematical and statistical modeling: a quiet methodological revolution. Am Psychol. 2010;65:1–12.
15. Defining the scientific method. Editorial. Nat Methods. 2009;6:237.
16. Haig BD. How to enrich scientific method. Am Psychol. 2008;63:565–6.
17. Haig BD. Scientific method, abduction, and clinical reasoning. J Clin Psychol. 2008;64:1013–8.
18. Kenkel JM. Revisiting the scientific method. Aesthet Surg J. 2009;29:167–8.
19. Levins R. Whose scientific method? Scientific methods for a complex world. New Solut. 2003;13:261–74.
20. Noseda M, McLean GR. Where did the scientific method go? Nat Biotechnol. 2008;26:28–9.
21. Satava RM. The scientific method is dead – long live the (new) scientific method. Surg Innov. 2005;12:173–6.
22. Cundiff DK. Evidence-based medicine and the Cochrane Collaboration on trial. MedGenMed. 2007;9:56.
23. DeAngelis CD, Thornton JP. Preserving confidentiality in the peer review process. JAMA. 2008;299:1956.
24. Marchevsky AM. The application of special technologies in diagnostic anatomic pathology: is it consistent with the principles of evidence-based medicine? Semin Diagn Pathol. 2005;22:156–66.
25. Miracle VA. The peer review process. Dimens Crit Care Nurs. 2008;27:67–9.
26. Molassiotis A, Richardson A. The peer review process in an academic journal. Eur J Oncol Nurs. 2004;8:359–62.
27. Moore KN. Keeping up journal integrity: the peer-review process. J Wound Ostomy Continence Nurs. 2005;32:3–5.
28. Mullins CD. The peer-review process: gifts of time. Clin Ther. 2005;27:1962.
29. Scanes CG. The peer-review process. Poult Sci. 2008;87:1–2.
30. Smith R. Peer review: a flawed process at the heart of science and journals. J R Soc Med. 2006;99:178–82.
31. Vettore MV. The peer review process in health journals. Cad Saúde Pública. 2009;25:2306–7.

32. Wright RW, Brand RA, Dunn W, et al. How to write a systematic review. Clin Orthop Relat Res. 2007; 455:23–9.
33. Adeniran AJ, Tamboli P. Clear cell adenocarcinoma of the urinary bladder: a short review. Arch Pathol Lab Med. 2009;133:987–91.
34. Laurini JA, Carter JE. Gastrointestinal stromal tumors: a review of the literature. Arch Pathol Lab Med. 2010;134:134–41.
35. Popescu OE, Landas SK, Haas GP. The spectrum of eosinophilic cystitis in males: case series and literature review. Arch Pathol Lab Med. 2009;133:289–94.
36. Ueng SH, Mezzetti T, Tavassoli FA. Papillary neoplasms of the breast: a review. Arch Pathol Lab Med. 2009;133:893–907.
37. Chen TH, Li L, Kochen MM. A systematic review: how to choose appropriate health-related quality of life (HRQOL) measures in routine general practice? J Zhejiang Univ Sci B. 2005;6:936–40.
38. Deenadayalan Y, Grimmer-Somers K, Prior M, et al. How to run an effective journal club: a systematic review. J Eval Clin Pract. 2008;14:898–911.
39. Hunt DL, Haynes RB. How to read a systematic review. Indian J Pediatr. 2000;67:63–6.
40. What does the Cochrane Collaboration say about adherence to evidence-based practice recommendations? Physiother Can. 2009;61:116.
41. Clarke M. The Cochrane Collaboration and the Cochrane Library. Otolaryngol Head Neck Surg. 2007;137:S52–4.
42. Overman VP. The Cochrane collaboration. Int J Dent Hyg. 2007;5:62.
43. Scherer RW. 2.2 Evidence-based health care and the Cochrane Collaboration. Hum Exp Toxicol. 2009; 28:109–11.
44. Summerskill W. Cochrane Collaboration and the evolution of evidence. Lancet. 2005;366:1760.
45. Tanjong-Ghogomu E, Tugwell P, Welch V. Evidence-based medicine and the Cochrane Collaboration. Bull NYU Hosp Jt Dis. 2009;67:198–205.
46. Winkelstein Jr W. The remarkable Archie: origins of the Cochrane Collaboration. Epidemiology. 2009;20:779.
47. Moher D, Tsertsvadze A, Tricco AC, et al. A systematic review identified few methods and strategies describing when and how to update systematic reviews. J Clin Epidemiol. 2007;60:1095–104.
48. Mahajan D, Bennett AE, Liu X, et al. Grading of gastric foveolar-type dysplasia in Barrett's esophagus. Mod Pathol. 2010;23:1–11.
49. Gupta R, Dastane A, McKenna Jr RJ, et al. What can we learn from the errors in the frozen section diagnosis of pulmonary carcinoid tumors? An evidence-based approach. Hum Pathol. 2009;40:1–9.
50. Gupta R, McKenna Jr R, Marchevsky AM. Lessons learned from mistakes and deferrals in the frozen section diagnosis of bronchioloalveolar carcinoma and well-differentiated pulmonary adenocarcinoma: an evidence-based pathology approach. Am J Clin Pathol. 2008;130:11–20.
51. Herbst J, Jenders R, McKenna R, et al. Evidence-based criteria to help distinguish metastatic breast cancer from primary lung adenocarcinoma on thoracic frozen section. Am J Clin Pathol. 2009;131:122–8.
52. Glasziou P, Heneghan C. A spotter's guide to study designs. Evid Based Nurs. 2009;12:71–2.
53. Lu CY. Observational studies: a review of study designs, challenges and strategies to reduce confounding. Int J Clin Pract. 2009;63:691–7.
54. Noordzij M, Dekker FW, Zoccali C, et al. Study designs in clinical research. Nephron Clin Pract. 2009;113:c218–21.
55. Ridgway PF, Guller U. Interpreting study designs in surgical research: a practical guide for surgeons and surgical residents. J Am Coll Surg. 2009;208: 635–45.
56. Li S, Dickson DW, Iacobuzio-Donahue CA, et al. The launch of international journal of clinical and experimental pathology. Int J Clin Exp Pathol. 2008;1:i.
57. Foucar E, Wick MR. An observational examination of the literature in diagnostic anatomic pathology. Semin Diagn Pathol. 2005;22:126–38.
58. Vollmer RT. Multivariate statistical analysis for anatomic pathology. Part II: failure time analysis. Am J Clin Pathol. 1996;106:522–34.
59. Vollmer RT. Multivariate statistical analysis for pathologist. Part I, The logistic model. Am J Clin Pathol. 1996;105:115–26.
60. Foucar E. Diagnostic precision and accuracy in interpretation of specimens from cancer screening programs. Semin Diagn Pathol. 2005;22:147–55.
61. Foucar E. Classification of error in anatomic pathology: a proposal for an evidence-based standard. Semin Diagn Pathol. 2005;22:139–46.
62. Li Q, Kuriyama S, Kakizaki M, et al. History of cholelithiasis and the risk of prostate cancer: The Ohsaki cohort study. Int J Cancer. 2011;128(1):185–91.
63. Silva DR, Menegotto DM, Schulz LF, et al. Mortality among patients with tuberculosis requiring intensive care: a retrospective cohort study. BMC Infect Dis. 2010;10:54.
64. Meier DS, Weiner HL, Guttmann CR. Time-series modeling of multiple sclerosis disease activity: a promising window on disease progression and repair potential? Neurotherapeutics. 2007;4:485–98.
65. Brunelli M, Delahunt B, Gobbo S, et al. Diagnostic usefulness of fluorescent cytogenetics in differentiating chromophobe renal cell carcinoma from renal oncocytoma: a validation study combining metaphase and interphase analyses. Am J Clin Pathol. 2010;133: 116–26.
66. Marchevsky A, Gupta R, Casadio C, et al. World Health Organization classification of thymomas provides significant prognostic information for selected stage III patients: evidence from an international thymoma study group. Hum Pathol. 2010;41(10):1413–21.
67. Marchevsky AM, Tsou JA, Laird-Offringa IA. Classification of individual lung cancer cell lines based on DNA methylation markers: use of linear discriminant analysis and artificial neural networks. J Mol Diagn. 2004;6:28–36.
68. Blute ML. Editorial comment on: external validation of the Mayo Clinic stage, size, grade, and necrosis

(SSIGN) score for clear-cell renal cell carcinoma in a single European centre applying routine pathology. Eur Urol. 2010;57:110–1.
69. Shariat SF, Karakiewicz PI, Godoy G, et al. Survivin as a prognostic marker for urothelial carcinoma of the bladder: a multicenter external validation study. Clin Cancer Res. 2009;15:7012–9.
70. Utsumi T, Kawamura K, Suzuki H, et al. External validation and head-to-head comparison of Japanese and Western prostate biopsy nomograms using Japanese data sets. Int J Urol. 2009;16:416–9.
71. Marchevsky A, Gupta R. Evidence-based pathology: interobserver diagnostic variability at "moderate" to "substantial" agreement levels could significantly change the prognostic estimates of clinico-pathologic studies. Ann Diagn Pathol. 2010;14(2):88–93.
72. Park JH, Kim DS, Park IN, et al. Prognosis of fibrotic interstitial pneumonia: idiopathic versus collagen vascular disease-related subtypes. Am J Respir Crit Care Med. 2007;175:705–11.
73. Straus SE, Sackett DL. Bringing evidence to the clinic. Arch Dermatol. 1998;134:1519–20.
74. Straus SE, Richardson WS, Glasziou P, et al. Evidence-based medicine. How to practice and teach EBM. New York: Elsevier; 2005.
75. Gross R. Decisions and evidence in medical practice. St. Louis: Mosby; 2001.
76. Marchevsky AM, Wick MR. Evidence levels for publications in pathology and laboratory medicine. Am J Clin Pathol. 2010;133:366–7.
77. American College of Physicians. Clinical Efficacy Assessment Project; 2010. Ref Type: Internet Communication.
78. Novis DA, Gephardt GN, Zarbo RJ. Interinstitutional comparison of frozen section consultation in small hospitals: a College of American Pathologists Q-Probes study of 18, 532 frozen section consultation diagnoses in 233 small hospitals. Arch Pathol Lab Med. 1996;120:1087–93.
79. Steindel SJ, Howanitz PJ, Renner SW. Reasons for proficiency testing failures in clinical chemistry and blood gas analysis: a College of American Pathologists Q-Probes study in 665 laboratories. Arch Pathol Lab Med. 1996;120:1094–101.
80. Tholen D, Lawson NS, Cohen T, et al. Proficiency test performance and experience with College of American Pathologists' programs. Arch Pathol Lab Med. 1995;119:307–11.
81. Wagner LR, Carson JG. The College of American Pathologists, 1946-1996: membership and its benefits. Arch Pathol Lab Med. 1997;121:427–37.
82. Marchevsky AM, Walts AE, Bose S, et al. Evidence-based evaluation of the risks of malignancy predicted by thyroid fine-needle aspiration biopsies. Diagn Cytopathol. 2010;38(4):252–9.

Evidence-Based Cell Pathology Revisited: A Personal View

12

Kenneth A. Fleming

Keywords

Evidence-based pathology • Cell pathology • Personal experience in pathology • Morphological diagnoses • Report communication • Sampling

In 1996, I argued that cell pathology for the twenty-first century needed a more rigorous evidence base for its three key components: sampling, morphological diagnosis, and report communication [1]. I suggested that the criteria used in each component should be based on evidence which showed the component to be both reproducible (for example, as in kappa value) and relevant, as expressed by an appropriate measure of accuracy in predicting clinical status (for example, sensitivity and specificity).

At that time, the evidence base for these criteria in the great majority of diseases was often rudimentary. Since then, there has been a major expansion of knowledge in many of the areas, although there is still much to be done. More importantly, understanding what is needed in terms of methodology to establish the evidence base was only beginning to be defined 15 years ago. Much work has been done on establishing standards for the reporting of diagnostic tests – for example, STARD (Standards for Reporting of Diagnostic Accuracy) [2] – and on how to assess the quality of the literature on diagnostic tests [3], although wider dissemination is needed.

Despite these advances, there is still a considerable gap between the depth of the evidence base used in, for example drug therapy, and that used in cell pathology. Thus, for example, classification of types of evidence into various levels, to rank the quality of research used to analyze a particular problem, has been a fundamental aspect of evidence-based medicine. These levels are well accepted and increasingly widely used in evidence-based therapeutics, but there are currently no uniformly accepted definitions of levels of evidence for evidence-based cell pathology. There have been several proposals and, for example, the Royal College of Pathologists (RCPath) datasets for cancer (http://www.rcpath.org/index.asp?PageID=154, see below) use a modification of the Scottish Intercollegiate Guidelines Network (SIGN) (http://www.sign.ac.uk/guidelines/fulltext/50/index.html) guidelines. These guidelines have much in common with those of the GRADE group (Grading of Recommendations Assessment Development and Evaluation) [4], particularly in their emphasis on patient-related outcomes, in addition to study design. In addition, by analogy with drug research, Gludd and Gludd [5] have proposed that studies in evidence-based diagnostics

K.A. Fleming (✉)
Director, Oxford University Clinical Academic Graduate School, Associate Dean, Oxford Post Graduate Medicine and Dental Deanery, Oxford, UK
e-mail: kenneth.fleming@medsci.ox.ac.uk

A.M. Marchevsky and M.R. Wick (eds.), *Evidence Based Pathology and Laboratory Medicine*, DOI 10.1007/978-1-4419-1030-1_12,

should have four phases, with phases III and IV determining the impact on patient outcome.

Unfortunately, however, the great majority of research in cell pathology, aimed at establishing how relevant a particular feature is in diagnosis, prognosis, or management, consists of retrospective, cohort studies, with no controls, frequently with small numbers and often of relatively short duration. Randomization and external validation are very rare, as are power calculations to assess whether the size of the study is sufficient to determine the statistical significance of a particular result. In the therapeutic field, such types of studies would be judged as among the lowest levels of evidence and carry proportionately little weight. This relative lack of rigor is a result partly of the still-developing nature of the methodology, and also of the inherent difficulty of designing, in cell pathology, the equivalent of a therapeutic randomized trial. Despite this, cell pathology needs to establish evidence levels of equivalent rigor to those used in evidence-based medicine and apply them with the same degree of universality.

In this chapter, I shall concentrate mainly on research from UK and Europe, which over the last 15 years has explored the development and application of the evidence base to each of the three key areas of cell pathology mentioned above. I shall largely, but not exclusively, use carcinoma, especially colorectal carcinoma, and hepatic pathology as exemplars from a much wider range of examples to illustrate the developments.

Sampling

As we all know, you can be using the most sophisticated diagnostic test available, but if the tissue you are provided with is not from the appropriate region, then the test is useless. So what is the evidence base for optimum sampling of an organ to establish accurate diagnosis and to guide prognostication and therapy?

One of the most systematically analyzed areas in this field is sampling in relation to malignancy. Over the last 15 years or so, there have been concentrated efforts to establish a better evidence base for appropriate sampling of a large variety of tumors. In the UK, one of the most complete of these evidence bases is a series of publications by the RCPath on data sets for tumors (http://www.rcpath.org/index.asp?PageID=154). Currently, the RCPath has produced over 30 such data sets which cover most of the common tumors. There are strictly defined rules on how the dataset should be organized, what issues should be addressed, and what types of evidence are acceptable. The aim of these data sets is wider than sampling, but significant parts of the protocols are focused on defining which parts of a tumor, including resection margins, should be sampled for accurate diagnosis, staging, prognostication, and guidance of therapy.

As an example of the approach, one of the most intensively studied areas is the adequacy of sampling in colorectal cancer (CRC). One component of this is the evidence that involvement of tumor in the nonperitoneal surgical margin – previously called the circumferential or radial margin – is a strong predictor of local recurrence. This has resulted in clear acceptance that this margin must be identified and sampled and, if positive, additional therapy such as radiation or chemotherapy, instigated.

However, despite the fact that there have been concerns about this issue for many years, the evidence of how best to identify and sample these margins is relatively recent. Thus in 1986, Quirke et al. [6], in a prospective analysis of 52 cases with a median follow-up of 23 months, showed clearly that those tumors with spread to the lateral margin, as identified by whole-specimen mounting and 5–10 mm serial tissue-sectioning, were very strongly associated with local recurrence – 92% specificity, 95% sensitivity, and 85% positive predictive value. In this paper, the proportion of local recurrences in a retrospective control group of 52 stage- and grade-matched patients, followed up for a median of 90 months, who had been staged as negative for lateral margin involvement by routine sampling, was the same as in the patients who had been staged as positive by serial sectioning. This clearly indicated that routine sampling was not detecting most cases of lateral margin involvement.

Subsequently, Ng et al. [7] published a prospective cohort study of 80 cases of rectal carcinoma with median follow-up of 26.6 months. They used whole-mounting and serial sectioning at 5–8 mm intervals. After uni- and multivariate analysis, clearance as determined by this type of examination was one of three pathological features which independently related to prognosis. Interestingly, a proportion of tumors which were staged as fully excised by this method suffered recurrence. While there are several possible explanations, this may suggest that sectioning at 5–8 mm is too great an interval, but to my knowledge, this has not been assessed.

Although these papers, and many others published on this topic, clearly indicate the importance of sampling the nonperitoneal margin properly, in general, they are of short duration and are cohort studies, with small numbers and no randomizing, and as such provide relatively low-level evidence to support their hypothesis. Furthermore, although the original papers were published over 20 years ago, it is clear that inadequate sampling is still widespread. Thus, for example, while it has been estimated that, using the technique outlined above, on average, one would expect to find evidence of extramural vascular invasion in 30% of cases of CRC, in a paper from 2007, Quirke and Morris [8] stated that, in practice, pathologists only report this finding in around 10% of cases.

Another important area of research into optimum sampling has been the attempts of recent years to identify what sampling is necessary to establish, with acceptable degrees of certainty, the presence or absence of secondary deposits of tumor in regional lymph nodes (LN). This work has largely dealt with the number of nodes to be sampled, what microscopic sampling should be performed, and the anatomical location of these nodes.

Until relatively recently, there was *no* evidence-based advice on the number of nodes which need to be sampled to provide reasonable certainty about the presence or absence of metastases. The expectation was that as many as could be found were examined. Interestingly, in the 1990s, the average number found in CRC was around 6 per case [8]. Now for many tumors, specific numbers of lymph nodes are recommended. Thus, for CRC, at least 12 lymph nodes are recommended (http://www.rcpath.org/index.asp?PageID=154).

However, what is the evidence for this? Since 1989, when Scott and Grace [9] investigated the use of fat clearance as a method of improving lymph node recovery in CRC, several papers have examined the relationship between the total number of LN recovered and the likelihood of identifying metastases in these nodes. In 2003, Swanson et al. [10] undertook a retrospective analysis of the National Cancer Data Base (which is a prospective database of more than 260,000 cases of colon cancer in the USA) to correlate clinical outcome with number of LN examined by the pathologist. They showed that less than 8 nodes were inadequate to assign node-negative status to a T3 tumor, while conversely identification of 13 nodes was sufficient to stage a tumor as node-negative. Subsequently, there has been considerable research around this topic supporting this view – see systematic review of this area [11].

However, there are dissenting views. A recent publication [12] suggested explanations other than more accurate staging for the association between higher lymph node numbers and better outcomes. Indeed, a paper from 2002 [13], using mathematical modeling, suggested that, for early-stage colonic tumors, more than 30 LNs need to be examined to ensure 85% probability of true negativity, whereas examining 12 nodes gives only a 25% probability in T3/4 tumors. In addition, given that between 1998 and 2001, fewer than 50% institutions in the US (involving only 44% patients) adhered to the current guideline of 12 LN [14], this makes the achievement of a larger LN harvest both a high priority and highly problematic.

A related and arguably more important factor in lymph node analysis is the detection (or not) of metastases. Indeed, what is the evidence of how best to detect metastatic tumor in a LN?

Despite the crucial importance of this aspect of tumor pathology, extraordinarily, there is no agreed evidence-based protocol. There is much variation in the methods used by pathologists, ranging from simple bisection and embedding of each half, face down, followed by a solitary H. and E. section, to the examination of multiple and even serial levels with immuno-histology or molecular analysis for carcinoma cells. These latter approaches have shown that the occurrence of metastases is often missed by less intensive examination and thereby that they can convert a tumor to a higher stage [15].

Putting aside the controversial issue of whether detection of micrometastases (as in breast carcinoma) is associated with poorer prognosis – for which there is an extensive and somewhat contradictory literature – most of these techniques are too labor-intensive for routine examination of a large numbers of nodes and so several recent papers have proposed focusing on the sentinel nodes and subjecting them to intensive sampling. Protocols involving elaborate modeling of dissection and sectioning of the sentinel node (involving, for example, many sections and immunochemistry) have been proposed, but to do this in a truly evidence-based manner – prospectively, at appropriate power, with external validation – even for breast carcinoma, would take tens of thousands of patients and at least 10 years [15]. This latter paper recommended that an achievable aspiration would be to use a less comprehensive, but a statistically valid sampling method, with standardized protocols for evaluation and classification of metastases and correlating these to clinical outcomes in a population-based registry or national cancer database.

Outside the arena of malignancy, there has been some investigation of the more general problem of sampling. In the liver, where a needle biopsy represents between a 30,000th and 50,000th of the organ, the question is, how representative is such a small proportion?

One way of addressing this question has been by performing two or more biopsies (either from the left and right lobes or by performing multiple passes from the same biopsy site) in a variety of conditions and comparing the appearances. This has shown variation in the appearances of the different biopsies. Thus, in noncaseating granulomas, over 50% of the multiple biopsies failed to show the abnormality, and in cirrhosis, 25% of biopsies did not show the lesion [16]. For such an important diagnosis, this is extremely worrying. Similarly, in focal diseases such as Primary Sclerosing Cholangitis, there was considerable discordance between the two biopsies – advanced disease was missed in 40% of biopsies and cirrhosis in 37% [17].

A related aspect is the adequacy of the amount of material obtained, whether by one or more passes. Again, the question is what is an adequate amount of tissue to provide a reasonable sample?

Several papers [18, 19] have examined the effect of variation of length of a liver biopsy on the grading and staging of inflammation and fibrosis in chronic viral hepatitis. Thus, Colloredo et al. [19], by masking increasing fractions of a biopsy, showed that as biopsy length decreased, mild grading increased – mild grade increased from 49.7% in tissue equal/greater than 3 cm, to 86.6% in a 1 cm long portion of the same biopsy. Similarly, the proportion of biopsies showing mild fibrosis increased from 59% in 3 cm biopsies, to 80% in 1 cm biopsies.

Bedossa et al. [18], using the METAVIR scoring system for fibrosis, image analysis, and virtual biopsies of increasing length, showed that increasing length from 15 to 25 mm decreased the coefficient of variation of fibrosis from 55 to 45%. To reach a CV of 25% required a biopsy of over 80 mm and increasing beyond this did not produce further reduction. A 15 mm biopsy correctly assigned the METAVIR score in only 65% of the biopsies, which increased to 75% in 25 mm biopsies. Further increase in length did not result in further improvement. In view of this, the authors recommended a biopsy of 25 mm length as the minimum length for fibrosis assessment.

As a result of analyses such as the above, there has been a consensus for some time that a liver biopsy of at least 20–25 mm length and containing at least 11 complete portal tracts is the minimal size needed for adequate assessment – this despite the fact that such biopsies are, at best, still nowhere near 100% accurate. Amazingly, the evidence is that even these sizes are not routinely achieved [20] and that this situation still persists. Thus, a recent paper [21] retrospectively reviewed 163 biopsies in a tertiary referral hospital in the UK and found that the median length was 13.3 mm (range 5.6–50 mm) with a median of 4 complete portal tracts (range 0–18).

Almost certainly part of this failure to obtain adequate biopsies reflects concerns about increased adverse complications resulting from increased sample size and passes. For this reason, trans-jugular liver biopsy, with four passes, has been suggested as a safer and more effective method of liver biopsy, producing material of adequate size and volume [22]. Curiously again, despite the evidence supporting this approach, it is not the norm, suggesting therefore that inadequate diagnoses are widespread. Why is this? Could it be that ignorance of the problem is the main reason, rather than safety concerns.

Summary

As can be seen from the above, the evidence base for valid sampling of many organs has still to be fully established. However, irrespective of the complexities and divergent views, the key message is that evidence-based methodologies for determination of the best methods of sampling – whatever the organ or disease – are available and can be used to establish the necessary guidance for the twenty-first century.

Morphological Diagnoses

Examining the microscopic features of tissue to obtain a diagnosis is the cornerstone of cell pathology, and in many instances, is regarded as the gold standard. To be acceptable in the twenty-first century, where molecular signatures are being developed, the microscopic features which rule in or rule out a particular diagnosis should be reproducible and relevant. Yet, when one examines the evidence base for these two components of cell pathology diagnosis 150 years or so after Virchow, it is still surprisingly limited.

Reproducibility

Reproducible means that when several pathologists look for a particular morphological feature, they should all reach the same conclusion about its presence or absence (interobserver reproducibility) and when the same pathologist looks for the feature on different occasions (intraobserver reproducibility), again she/he agrees about its presence or absence on those different occasions. Reproducibility is usually measured by kappa value, although this method of statistical analysis has some weaknesses [23].

Reassuringly, measurement of reproducibility of pathological features is being used with increasing frequency in a wide range of diseases and organs. Depressingly, when applied to many of the time-honored and traditional morphological features used in tissue diagnosis, these features are often so poorly reproducible between pathologists as to undermine the basis of their continued use [1].

In liver for example, several papers [24–26] have examined the inter-/intraobserver reproducibility of the inflammatory and fibrosis components of the various scoring systems. Almost universally, the inflammatory components have kappa values which, at best, are fair, while in comparison, fibrosis scoring is regularly more reproducible. This in [24] the kappa value for periportal necrosis was 0.36, for lobular necrosis was 0.38, and for portal inflammation was 0.25, while the kappa value for fibrosis was 0.78.

Here, inflammatory features thought to be important for diagnosis, prognosis, and management are so relatively poorly reproducible that they probably cannot be trusted. Despite this, and although scoring systems are recommended only for clinical trials, on occasions they are used in clinical service and therapeutic decisions influenced by them. It would be interesting to know what patients think of this rather unsatisfactory situation.

How do we improve this? One approach is clearer and more precise definitions of the abnormality concerned (as in IgA nephropathy – see below). Another method is the use of "good example" images which can be visualized on a computer screen and compared by the pathologist to the image she/he is seeing down their microscope. The pathologist picks the "good example" which best fits his/her own microscopic image to identify the presence or absence of a particular microscopic pathological feature. Such technology can also be combined with a computerized decision support system (DSS) (based on Bayesian belief networks) not only to measure and improve reproducibility, but also to provide a teaching tool.

To illustrate this, a recent paper [27] described this process in cervical pathology. The authors selected eight morphological features (evidence nodes) which were linked to five final diagnoses (decision nodes) via a conditional probability matrix. The latter gives a numerical probability of the likelihood of finding a particular feature in a particular diagnosis (for example, severe basal cell nuclear pleomorphism in normal equals 0.01).

How does this work? In practice, the observer views a biopsy and classifies each of the eight morphological features by comparing the microscopic image with the on-screen image. To do this, she/he positions a sliding pointer on the spectrum of images which most closely resembles the image seen down the microscope. The software automatically calculates a likelihood of finding the particular feature in each possible diagnosis. After all the features have been scored, the diagnosis with the highest probability is the final diagnosis. A cumulative probability graph is generated which shows the changes in likelihood of diagnosis as each morphological feature is assessed.

The system was tested on 50 colposcopic biopsies selected to have the full range of diagnoses and tested on two experienced pathologists, two trainee pathologists and two medical students. Intra- and interobserver reproducibility were measured using a weighted kappa value (weighted such that more serious differences are given greater weight), with and without use of the DSS. This showed that while intraobserver reproducibility was the same in both approaches, interobserver reproducibility for the consultants improved from a 0.46 to 0.54 using the DSS.

Perhaps more importantly than modestly improving interobserver reproducibility, the system allows comparison between individuals in their analysis of each feature and is thus an invaluable teaching tool. It also potentially allows, with relative ease, assessment of a particular feature by large numbers of pathologists of variable experience and competence. This will allow more informed selection of which features should be used in a diagnosis and abandonment of those that are insufficiently reproducible.

Relevance

In contrast to reproducibility, by relevant, I mean that the presence of the feature in question indicates likelihood of presence of a particular disease or clinical outcome, the degree of likelihood being expressed numerically. The latter is usually described as accuracy of diagnosis and there are several ways (all of which have particular merits and demerits) in which this can be described – sensitivity, specificity, positive and negative predictive values (PPV, NPV), odds, and hazard ratios – for the disease in question (see elsewhere in this book for definitions). The methodologies for determining the sensitivity, specificity, PPV, NPV, odds, and hazard ratios for any feature are well established. Of these, while sensitivity and specificity are being used in the cell pathology literature with increasing frequency, the other methods of measuring accuracy are used much less frequently.

However, there has been one recent example of an evidence-based approach to morphological diagnosis which combined assessment of both the reproducibility of the pathological features and their accuracy in predicting outcome. This is the Oxford classification of IgA nephropathy [28].

The authors of the paper wished to establish which of the pathological features of IgA nephropathy best correlated with clinical outcome, independent of treatment or other factors. To do this, they initially agreed a list of what morphological features can be present (divided between glomerular, tubulo-interstitial, etc.), agreed specific definitions – for example, extra capillary proliferation or cellular crescent is "extra capillary lesion comprising cells and extra-cellular matrix, with less than 50% cells and less than 90% matrix" – and tested these morphological features for reproducibility among themselves.

On the basis of these results, they refined their definitions and divided the features into several groups according to kappa value – high reproducibility, kappa value greater than 0.6, moderate reproducibility, kappa 0.4–0.6, and poor reproducibility, less than 0.4. The latter features were then excluded from further consideration. Twenty-four features were scored, and of these, fourteen were either high or moderately reproducible. The authors then established what correlations there were between each of these features (correlation coefficients) and selected one feature as representative of each correlation group, for subsequent analysis. The selection was based on reproducibility, ease of identification, and susceptibility to sampling error. This resulted in six features being identified as the evidenced-based pathological lesions of IgA nephropathy.

In an accompanying paper [29], the authors then performed analyses of the correlation of the selected pathological features with a variety of clinical features (for example, proteinuria, GFR, mean arterial pressure) and outcomes (for example, rate of decline of renal function, survival without dialysis). They then determined a measurement of the accuracy which the pathological feature had for a particular clinical feature/outcome.

Thus, the pathological features which had been shown to be reproducible were analyzed by uni- and multivariate analysis for correlation with clinical features and outcomes. For some of the pathological variables (continuous variables with skewed distribution), Receiver Operating Curves (ROC) were constructed to determine optimal cut-offs between positive or negative results. Hazard ratios were calculated, as were odds ratios.

The final result was a recommendation that four microscopic features should be assessed and given a score, each providing an independent, evidence-based, measure of likelihood of progression of disease.

While this investigation was a retrospective observational study with variable sourcing of data, it is a relatively rare example of a rigorously evidence-based analysis of the reproducibility of the microscopic features of a disease and how they predict clinical outcome. The authors recognized that validation in an independent prospective study, with data collected in a uniform manner, is necessary for confirmation of their findings, but the basic approach is a model for all histopathology in the twenty-first century.

Summary

Morphological diagnosis is the beating heart of cell pathology, but when examined systematically, many of the features we assess have relatively poor reproducibility and inadequate assessment of their relevance to clinical outcome. However, as in sampling, we know how to tackle these issues and improving this situation can be addressed by a long-term, systematic commitment to generating quantified data on the reproducibility and accuracy of the pathological features of each disease, along the lines of the IgA nephropathy papers.

Report Communication

As I said some 14 years ago, there has been very little research into the evidence-base of the best format for the composition of the cell pathology report. Since then, there has been a considerable move towards data sets, especially in cancer reporting (see above). Such data sets are structured as a proforma to list all of the features thought to be relevant to diagnosis, prognosis, and management, the role of the pathologist being to fill in the appropriate measurement and/or comment. The rationale behind such forms is twofold: first, by listing all relevant factors, the report should therefore contain all the information thought to be important. Second, by minimizing free text, it reduces the possibility of misinterpretation of the report by the clinician or patient.

Two questions arise from this transformation of the report format. First, has the completeness of the reporting increased? Second, have the new formats increased/decreased communication between the pathologist and clinician?

In answer to the first question, a number of papers have examined this question and generally the answer is yes. Thus in CRC, in one department, the completeness of the reported data set improved from 0 to 96% [30], while a randomized prospective study of the use of computerized proforma reports in 16 hospitals in Wales, for breast and CRC, involving over 2,000 reports, showed a 28.4% increase in completeness of reports, in comparison with nonproforma reports [31]. However in this latter study, 31.2% of the CRC reports still were incomplete for core data. At one level, this seems extraordinary. Why would information which is thought to be important not be reported?

Of course, some of this may simply be forgetting to fill in relevant section, perhaps because of pressure of work. Alternatively, it may be that the data are not easy to elucidate or that the pathologist does not (at least subconsciously) believe that the information is truly relevant. Presumably such causes of incompleteness can be addressed, at least in computerized reporting, by ensuring that the report cannot be signed off if data points are still missing. However, there has been little research into the causes of the missing information. Until this has been properly researched, it cannot be said that the evidence-base for the most effective report communication has been established.

What about the second question – has the adoption of data set reports improved the interpretation of pathology findings by the clinician?

There is essentially no quantified research on this matter. In the study from Wales [31], surgeons greatly welcomed the reconfiguring of reports into this type of format. Anecdotally and from personal experience, similar views have been expressed, but hard evidence that this has improved communication and decreased mistakes does not exist at present. It could be argued either that this is so self-evident that formal confirmation is not needed, or that, as the great majority of cell pathologists participate in meetings with the clinicians, at which cases are discussed, these provide a satisfactory channel for accurate communication. While this is undoubtedly true, it is also true that usually only a subset of cases is discussed at such meetings, leaving the majority of reports not considered. Furthermore, in referral cases this often does not apply. Also, increasingly in the UK at least, there are moves towards more distant provision of cell pathology in off-site labs, which will make the holding of such clinical meetings less straightforward. While potentially telepathology can provide a substitute, this underlines the need for reports to contain only relevant, accurate information, presented in as unambiguous a form as possible.

Conclusion

Evidence-based cell pathology as an approach for the twenty-first century has made considerable advances in the last 14 years or so. Most, if not all, of the appropriate methodology now exists, but the challenge is in the application of the various methodologies to particular problems.

Part of this lack of implementation reflects the inherent difficulty of designing the equivalent of a therapeutic randomized trial in cell pathology, but I suspect the greatest barrier to widespread application is not technical or methodological, but a failure by pathologists to recognize the full extent of the problems such as those outlined in this chapter and elsewhere in this book. Addressing this issue will require greater profile for the evidence-based cell pathology movement, through the usual channels of publications, conferences, and so on, but probably the most important factor will be the incorporation of the principles into curricula for pathology training.

References

1. Fleming KA. Evidence-based pathology. J Pathol. 1996;179:127–8.
2. STARD Group. Towards complete and accurate reporting of studies of diagnostic accuracy: the STARD initiative. Clin Chem. 2003;49:1–6.
3. Mariska MG, et al., on behalf of the Cochrane Diagnostic Test Accuracy Working Group. Systematic reviews of diagnostic test accuracy. Ann Intern Med. 2008;149:889–97.
4. Schunemann HJ, et al., for the GRADE Working Group. Grading quality of evidence and strength of recommendations for diagnostic tests and strategies. BMJ. 2008;336:1106–10.
5. Gludd C, Gludd LL. Evidence based diagnostics. BMJ. 2005;330:724–6.
6. Quirke P, Dixon MF, Durdey P, Williams NS, Local recurrence of rectal adenocarcinoma due to inadequate surgical resection: histopathological study of lateral tumour spread and surgical excision. Lancet. 1986;328:996–9.
7. Ng IOL et al. Surgical lateral clearance in resected rectal carcinomas. A multivariate analysis of clinicopathological features. Cancer. 1993;71:1972–6.
8. Quirke P, Morris E. Reporting colorectal cancer. Histopathology. 2007;50:103–12.
9. Scott KWM, Grace RH. Detection of lymph node metastases in colorectal carcinoma before and after fat clearance. Br J Surg. 1989;76:1165–7.
10. Swanson RS, Compton CC, Stewart AK, Bland KI. The prognosis of T3N0 colon cancer is dependent on the number of lymph nodes examined. Ann Surg Oncol. 2003;10:65–71.
11. Chang GJ, Rodriguez-Bigas MA, Skibber JM, Moyer VA. Lymph node evaluation and survival after curative

resection of colon cancer: systematic review. J Natl Cancer Inst. 2007;99:433–41.
12. Kenelly R, Winter DC. Quality assurance measures in rectal cancer: caveat utilitor. Gut. 2010;59:139–40.
13. Goldstein NS. Lymph node recoveries from 2427 pT3 colorectal resection specimens spanning 45 years: recommendations for a minimum number of recovered lymph nodes based on predictive probabilities. Am J Surg Pathol. 2002;26:179–89.
14. Baxter NN et al. Lymph node evaluation in colorectal cancer patients: a population-based study. J Natl Cancer Inst. 2005;97:219–25.
15. Weaver DL. Pathology evaluation of sentinel lymph nodes in breast cancer: protocol recommendations and rationale. Mod Pathol. 2010;23:S26–32.
16. Maharaj B et al. Sampling variability and its influence on the diagnostic yield of percutaneous needle biopsy of the liver. Lancet. 1986;1:523–5.
17. Olsson R et al. Sampling variability of percutaneous liver biopsy in primary sclerosing cholangitis. J Clin Pathol. 1995;48:933–5.
18. Bedossa P, Dargere D, Paradis V. Sampling variability of liver fibrosis in chronic hepatitis C. Hepatology. 2003;38:1449–57.
19. Colloredo G, Guido M, Sonzogni A, Leandro G. Impact of liver biopsy size on histological evaluation of chronic viral hepatitis: the smaller the sample, the milder the disease. J Hepatol. 2003;39:239–44.
20. Cholongitas E et al. A systematic review of the quality of liver biopsy specimens. Am J Clin Pathol. 2006;125:710–21.
21. Chan J, Alwahab Y, Tilley C, Carr N. Percutaneous medical liver core biopsies: correlation between tissue length and the number of portal tracts. J Clin Pathol. 2010;63:655–66.
22. Cholongitas E, Burroughs AK. Is it difficult to obtain an optimal liver biopsy specimen? Hepatology. 2009;51:355–6.
23. Altman DG. Practical statistics for medical research. London: Chapman and Hall/CRC Texts in Statistical Science; 1990.
24. Bedossa P, on behalf of the French METAVIR Study Group. Intraobserver and interobserver variations in liver biopsy interpretation in patients with chronic hepatitis C. Hepatology. 2005;20:15–20.
25. Westin J, Lagging LM, Wejstål R, Norkrans G, Dhillon AP. Interobserver study of liver histopathology using the Ishak score in patients with chronic hepatitis C virus infection. Liver. 1999;19:183–7.
26. Grønbaek K et al. Interobserver variation in interpretation of serial liver biopsies from patients with chronic hepatitis C. J Viral Hepat. 2002;9:443–9.
27. Price GJ et al. Computerised diagnostic decision support system for the classification of preinvasive cervical squamous lesions. Hum Pathol. 2003;34:1193–203.
28. Roberts ISD et al. The Oxford classification of IgA nephropathy: pathology definitions, correlations, and reproducibility. Kidney Int. 2009;76:546–56.
29. Cattran DC et al. The Oxford classification of IgA nephropathy: rationale, clinicopathological correlations, and classification. Kidney Int. 2009;76:534–45.
30. Cross SS, Feeley KM, Angel CA. The effect of four interventions on the informational content of histopathology reports of resected colorectal carcinomas. J Clin Pathol. 1998;51:481–2.
31. Branston IK et al. The implementation of guidelines and computerized forms improves the completeness of cancer pathology reporting. The CROPS project: a randomized controlled trial in pathology. Eur J Cancer. 2002;38:764–72.

13 Development of Evidence-Based Diagnostic Criteria and Prognostic/ Predictive Models: Experience at Cedars Sinai Medical Center

Alberto M. Marchevsky and Ruta Gupta

Keywords

Evidence-based diagnostic criteria • Prognostic models in pathology • Evidence-based pathology • Cedar Sinai Medical Center experience in evidence-based diagnostic criteria

Evidence-based pathology (EBP) offers a conceptual framework and analytical tools to evaluate the scientific quality and potential clinical validity of information published in the literature [1–3]. EBP general concepts and principles also suggest the specific question-data-method-Bayesian inference-appraisal (QDMBA) paradigm shown in Table 13.1. This paradigm can help guide the review of information in the pathology literature and help formulate the experimental design of clinico-pathologic studies. The paradigm is based on six general assumptions: (a) clinico-pathologic problems are best approached by explicitly formulating answerable patient-based questions that need to be investigated using the literature and personal experience, (b) data trumps authority and tradition, (c) the experimental design of studies is important to optimize the information that can be obtained from available data and generate the highest possible evidence level, (d) it is often more valuable to analyze data using a Bayesian inference approach that considers the pre-test and post-test probabilities of findings rather than analyzing it with descriptive statistics, (e) the limitations of the data and experimental design of a study need to be considered in the discussion and explicitly disclosed, and (f) the conclusions of a study need to be appraised over time with additional prospective data in a process of continuous improvement.

In this chapter, we briefly describe several studies performed in our laboratory at Cedars-Sinai Medical Center exploring different elements of the QDMBA paradigm for the evaluation of clinico-pathologic problems related mostly to our area of interest, thoracic pathology. We will review these articles and others from an epistemological viewpoint in an effort to provide examples about how the proposed "EBP" approach can potentially improve on the quality of the evidence generated by clinico-pathologic studies in anatomic pathology.

A.M. Marchevsky (✉)
Pulmonary and Mediastinal Pathology,
Department of Pathology and Laboratory Medicine,
Cedars-Sinai Medical Center, Los Angeles, CA, USA
and
David Geffen School of Medicine,
University of California, Los Angeles, CA, USA
e-mail: Alberto.Marchevsky@cshs.org

A.M. Marchevsky and M.R. Wick (eds.), *Evidence Based Pathology and Laboratory Medicine*,
DOI 10.1007/978-1-4419-1030-1_13, © Springer Science+Business Media, LLC 2011

Table 13.1 Question-data-method-Bayesian inference-appraisal (QDMBA) paradigm for the evaluation of clinico-pathologic problems

A. Frame specific patient-based *questions* regarding particular diagnoses or other problems of interest
1. What are we trying to study and why?
B. Collect *data* from literature and own experience
1. Data ("evidence") trumps eminence and tradition
C. *Methodological details* of studies are important to assess evidence levels
D. *Bayesian inference* approach to evaluation data
1. Estimate quantitatively or qualitatively the pre-test probabilities of the pathologic findings or test results of interest
2. Estimate quantitatively or qualitatively the post-test probabilities of the pathologic findings or test results of interest
E. The results and conclusions of a study need to be *appraised* over time and updated as more data becomes available

Table 13.2 Specific patient-centered questions: the first step to evaluate information using an evidence-based approach

Questions are formulated using a root (who, what, where, how, why) followed by a verb
Background questions
Query for general knowledge regarding disease, treatment, or other topic
Foreground questions
Query for specific knowledge to inform clinical decisions or actions

Questions That Address Specific Patient-Centered Problems: How to Ask Practical and Answerable Questions of Clinical Relevance

Medical knowledge is constantly evolving at an ever more rapid course. Pathologists striving to diagnose their cases using the latest classification schema and latest information regarding the latest immunostains, molecular tests, and other information need to hone their skills at asking relevant answerable clinico-pathologic questions and at developing strategies designed to find this information in the literature and integrate it with their personal experience [2, 3]. Unfortunately, these are not skills that are generally emphasized or formally taught during pathology residency training.

Various teaching tactics for the formulation of answerable clinical questions are described in detail in the excellent book on "Evidence-Based Medicine How to Practice and Teach EBM" by Straus et al. Queries are categorized as "background" and "foreground" questions (Table 13.2) [4]. "Background" questions are designed to ask for general knowledge regarding a disease, treatment, pathologic condition, or other topic. They are formulated using a *question root* such as who, what, where, when, how, why, *followed by a verb.* Background questions generally *address a specific* disease, pathologic entity, test, or other aspect of health care. Examples of background type question are as follows: What is the etiology of diffuse alveolar damage? How do carcinomas of the prostate usually disseminate? Why is there necrosis in cases of invasive aspergillosis?

"Foreground" questions according to Straus et al. [4] query for specific knowledge to inform clinical decisions or actions. They have four essential components: (1) patient-specific problem, (2) intervention or exposure, (3) comparison if relevant, and (4) clinical outcomes, including time frame if relevant. In anatomic pathology, the four components of foreground questions can probably be simplified into three: patient-specific problem, pathologic examination or laboratory test, and relevance for patient care (prognosis or prediction of response to specific therapy). Examples of background type question are as follows: Which immunostains should be used during the evaluation of transbronchial biopsy to differentiate adenocarcinoma from squamous cell carcinoma? How many immunostains should be used to distinguish malignant mesothelioma from adenocarcinoma? What is the prognosis of a non-smoking woman with a stage I lung adenocarcinoma that shows the EGFR gene mutation?

Why Bother Formulating Clear Questions?

Straus et al. [4] suggest that formulating well-designed patient-centered questions can help practitioners in seven ways: (1) help focus scarce learning time into gathering knowledge that is relevant to our patients needs, (2) help focus learning on evidence that addresses specific aspects of practice, (3) suggest high-yield search strategies to find relevant information in the literature, (4) suggest how the answers can be formatted to provide clinically useful information, (5) help in communication with other physicians, (6) provide a teaching tool to help train students, residents, and others, and (7) help grow our knowledge base as the questions are answered. Most of these concepts probably apply to the practice and learning of anatomic pathology and laboratory medicine.

Data ("Evidence") Trumps Eminence and Tradition

The evidence-based medicine (EBM) literature reveals some ongoing tension between the data-based approach favored by EBM advocates and the more traditional teaching and practice of medicine that reveres personal experience and clinical expertise [5–10]. This debate has resulted in the use of some colorful acronyms. For example, EBM advocates have proposed the term "Eminence-based Medicine" to deride the practice of medicine based on the opinion and advice of recognized experts, while some of the latter physicians grumble about "Evidence-Slaved Medicine," "Economy-Based Medicine," and "Cookbook Medicine" [11–19]. A detailed discussion of the arguments for each of these competing views of the current practice of medicine is beyond the scope of this chapter. Briefly, one can conclude that: (1) the "best evidence" collected by randomized clinical trials and revered by EBM aficionados as the best type of available knowledge has some limitations and/or is often nonexistent, (2) there are many medical interventions that have never been validated in randomized clinical trials but are yet very valuable for patient care, and (3) there are various widely used medical practices that are either wasteful, ineffectual and/or not supported by current knowledge.

Pathologists, a particularly conservative group of physicians, have generally ignored this debate and continued pursuing the testing of various specimens with the latest available technology and using in their daily practice various disease classification schemas developed years ago by groups of experts and updated over time. Diagnostic classes tend to be split over into multiple subclasses with limited debate regarding their diagnostic reproducibility and clinical applicability. In addition, schemas such as the current World Health Organization (WHO) classifications of lung neoplasms, sarcomas, and other neoplasms do not generally incorporate current information regarding the results of immunostains and/or molecular studies as definitional criteria, although these tests are being widely used and probably variably interpreted by different pathologists [20, 21].

EBP advocates the critical evaluation of the purpose of classification models, and the evidence levels of the data supporting various classification models and other practices. These efforts will hopefully advance anatomic pathology and laboratory medicine into more scientific endeavors, although it is fully recognized that there is a considerable "art" component in the practice of pathology related to the nature of the field and the variable ability and clinical experience of different practitioners.

Widely Accepted and/or Long-Held Practices and "Traditions" Need to Be Changed When Not Supported by Current Best Evidence

In instances where the best available evidence does not support widely accepted and/or long-held practices, EBP advocates for a change. Recent studies of thymomas performed in our laboratory using various elements of the QDMBA paradigm can be used to illustrate this problem [22–24]. Generations of pathologists have been trained by eminent experts to evaluate thymomas very carefully for the presence of microscopic transcapsular invasion [25]. Indeed, a previous classification schema of thymomas advocated the classification of the tumors into benign or malignant thymomas based on the absence or presence of local invasion [25]. In addition, thymomas that exhibit microscopic transcapsular invasion have been classified by Masaoka et al. [26] and others since the early 1980s as stage II disease. These concepts were accepted for many years and advocated by one of us (AM) in the 1980s in two subsequent editions a book devoted to the surgical pathology of mediastinal lesions and in other publications [27–29]. However, after becoming interested in EBP, we decided to evaluate, following some of the methods described in this book, whether these widely accepted concepts are actually supported by best evidence [24]. We formulated two simple background type questions: Is there a significant difference in prognosis between patients with stages I and II thymoma? What level of evidence is available to answer the previous question? A systematic review of the literature was performed and only level III data were found. The systematic review did not find any randomized clinical trials or level II studies in the English literature evaluating the prognostic significance of transcapsular invasion in thymoma patients. The level III data from 2,451 thymomas reported in 21 studies were analyzed with meta-analysis, showing no significant survival differences between patients with Masaoka stages I and II thymomas (Fig. 13.1a, b). The lack of significant differences in the prognosis of patients with stages I and II thymomas supports the notions that (1) evaluation of transcapsular invasion is of limited clinical value in tumors that lack invasion of neighboring organs or the pleura and (2) the staging schema for thymomas needs to be updated. Interestingly, review of the seminal study of 27 patients with stage I thymomas and 7 patients with stage II disease by Masaoka et al. [26] showed that while patients with clinical stages I and II thymoma had slightly different 92.6 and 85.7% 5-year survival rates, respectively, these apparent survival differences were not statistically significant. In summary, this is a simple example of how certain concepts that had been taught by eminent physicians for many years to the point of becoming a "tradition" are found to lack best evidence to support them.

a

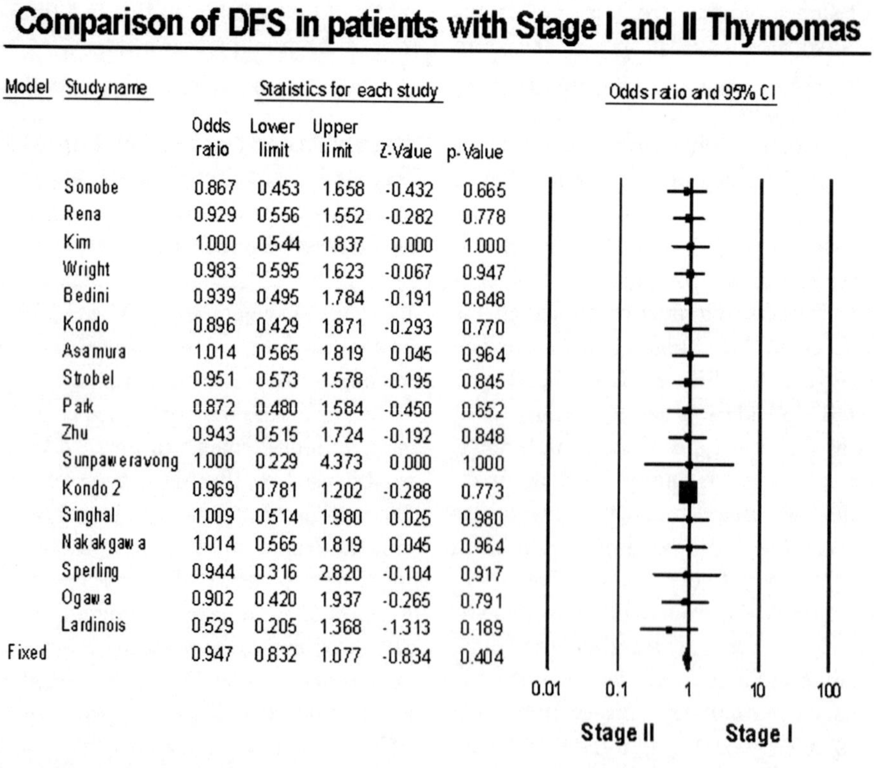

Fig. 13.1 (**a, b**) The level III data from 2,451 thymomas reported in 21 studies were analyzed with meta-analysis, showing no significant survival differences between patients with Masaoka stages I and II thymomas (From Gupta et al. [24]; with permission)

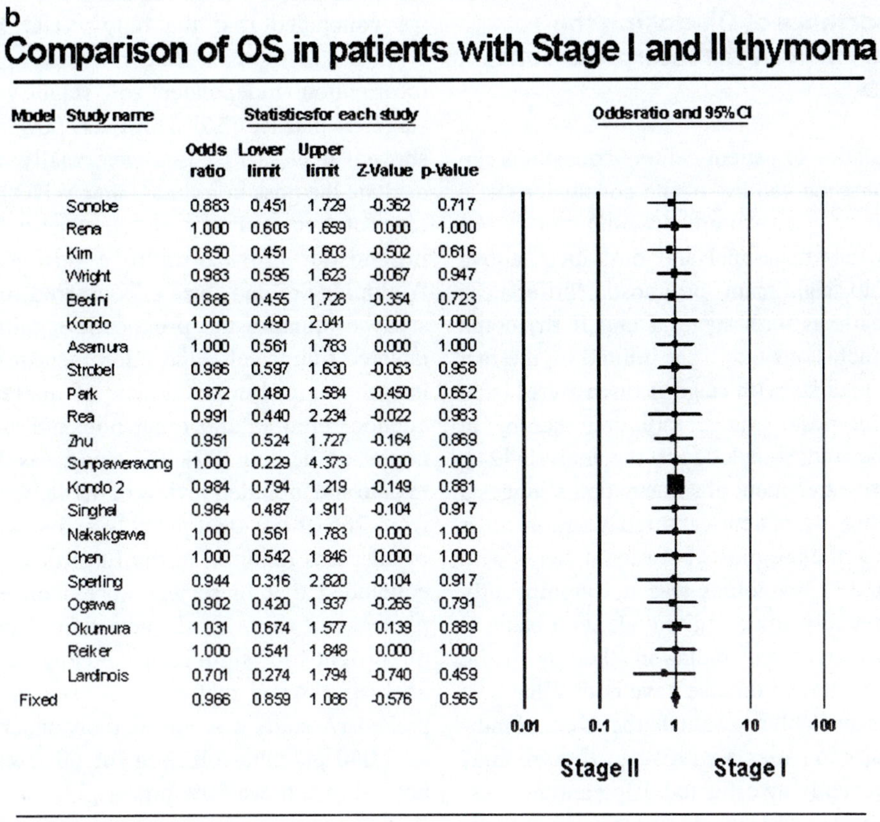

Fig. 13.1 (continued)

The Experimental Design of Studies Is Important: Evidence Levels

The importance of selecting the correct methodological approach to particular clinico-pathologic problems and the evaluation of the quality of the information published in the literature using "evidence levels" is discussed in detail in Chap. 11 [30]. The discussion included the pathology-specific scale of evidence levels shown in Table 13.3. In summary, well-designed prospective studies that validate their results using prospective data that was not used to develop the proposed diagnostic criteria or other results are given the best marks as level I or II evidence [30]. By contrast, clinicians generally classify the information published in well-designed randomized prospective clinical trials as level I evidence [4, 10, 31–34].

Table 13.3 Proposed scale of evidence levels for publications in pathology and laboratory medicine

Level 1	Case-control studies with external validation of results, using prospective validation data-sets from other institutions Meta-analyses of level 2 studies "Expert" recommendations based on meta-analyses of level 2 or 3 studies
Level 2	Case-control studies with validation of results, using prospective validation data-sets from the same institution Meta-analyses of level 3 studies "Expert" recommendations based on a systematic review of literature without formal meta-analyses
Level 3	Case-control studies with validation of results using retrospective validation datasets from the same institution
Level 4	Case-control studies without validation
Level 5	Case series without controls, or individual case reports

The Importance of Disclosing the Potential Flaws of the Interpretations of Results

The formulation of patient-centered questions can help evaluate the validity of the conclusions of a study and suggest future investigations. For example, the meta-analysis described above showing no significant prognostic differences between patients with stages I and II thymoma yielded conclusions that were limited by the fact that some patients with stage II disease had been treated with postoperative radiation therapy in some of the studies included in the analysis [24]. This selective treatment of some patients suggests the following two patient-centered questions: Is it possible that the prognosis between patients with stages I and II thymomas was not significantly different because some individuals with stage II disease had received radiation therapy while patients with stage I disease have not? What best evidence is available to evaluate the effect of radiation therapy in patients with stage II thymoma? This was recently investigated using another systematic review of best evidence with meta-analysis [35]. The study showed that radiation therapy does not significantly change the prognosis of patients with stage II thymomas, supporting the concept that the lack in significant prognostic differences between patients with stages I and II thymomas does not result from treatment effect.

The Importance of Evaluating Whether a Study Analyzed a Sufficient Sample Size

As explained in Chap. 8, sample size estimations and power analysis are currently routinely performed in clinical trials and other clinical studies but are seldom performed in studies published in the anatomic pathology literature. This can lead to overly optimistic or pessimistic evaluations of negative results. For example, in a recent meta-analysis of 905 thymomas classified by WHO and staged by Masaoka staging, collected from multiple hospitals in Asia, Europe, and California, we concluded that the only WHO histologic type of thymomas that provided prognostic information independent of stage was A in stage III disease [36]. However, power analysis showed that 7,077 cases were really needed to exclude the possibility that other WHO histologic types of thymoma may provide stage-independent prognostic information to a power of 80%. A similar problem was encountered in a recent study evaluating the prognostic significance of isolated tumor cells and micrometastases in the intrathoracic lymph nodes of patients with adenocarcinoma and other nonsmall cell carcinomas of the lung [37]. The study was the largest to date and included review of 4,148 lymph nodes from 266 of our own patients and meta-analysis of all cases reported in the English literature. It concluded that there was no evidence that the presence of these small metastatic deposits was of prognostic significance. However, power analysis showed that even this seemingly comprehensive study was considerably underpowered, as 3,060 patients followed for 60 months were needed to achieve 80% power [37].

Bayesian Inference Can Be More Useful for Clinical Purposes than Analysis of Data with Descriptive Statistics: The Importance of Distinguishing Prior Probabilities from Posterior Probabilities

Bayesian inference is an analytical method based on the principles of Bayesian statistics that involves evaluating how the degree of belief in a hypothesis changes as additional data or evidence is collected [38–44]. Bayes' theorem adjusts probabilities given new data using the formula

$$P(A\backslash B) = \frac{P(B\backslash A)P(A)}{P(B)}$$

where, $P(A\backslash B)$: posterior probability given prior probability A probability from event B. $P(A)$ = prior probability of A that does not take into account event B. $P(B)$ probability after collecting information from event B. Pathologists certainly do not need to estimate Bayesian statistics in daily practice but would probably benefit from an understanding of the differences between *prior probabilities*, the likelihood of certain diagnoses or other events prior to the evaluation of pathologic specimens or laboratory samples, from *posterior probabilities*, the likelihood of certain conclusions after the pathologic or laboratory samples are examined [45–49]. Surprisingly, this simple distinction is often lost in the anatomic pathology literature when studies reporting the diagnostic value of a new test are designed following the format: "cases classified as either A or B by histopathology were tested with new test C. New test C was positive in 95% of A cases, therefore test C is very useful for the differential diagnosis between A and B." One could argue that the prior probability of correct diagnoses of either A or B by histopathology in this group of patients was 1.0. It is not possible for a new test C to provide posterior probabilities higher than 1.0 in the same population.

Ironically, many anatomic pathologists have probably been trained not to use a qualitative Bayesian inference process. For example, it is often recommended that histologic slides should be looked at without prior clinical information, not to "bias" the observations, although to our knowledge there are no studies showing that learning about the clinical history of a patient prior to pathologic examination decreases the quality of diagnostic interpretations. The process of Bayesian inference that analyzes how the results improve sequentially as additional evidence is available is also not usually recommended during the utilization process of immunostains or other tests. By contrast, use of the concept of prior and posterior probabilities can be helpful in daily practice. For example, in a recent review of the pathology of metastatic lesions, we explained how estimating the prior probabilities of the most probable diagnoses in a particular patient, based on gender, age and location of the lesions, and the development of a short list of the most likely diagnoses *prior* to the evaluation of histologic slides and/or the performance of immunostains or others tests can improve on the diagnostic process and guide the selection of appropriate immunohistochemical tests [50].

Utilization of the Bayesian inference process could also probably improve on the quality of future clinico-pathologic studies in anatomic pathology. Indeed, most studies in anatomic pathology have evaluated their results by comparing the data in two or more populations with univariate and multivariate statistics and/or survival statistics. The results of these studies often provide important insights regarding the clinical significance of particular findings in different populations of interest, but it is often difficult to apply their conclusions to the evaluation of tissue specimens or clinical laboratory samples from individual patients, as there is often some overlap in values, as explained in the next section.

Use of Probabilities, Odds, and Various Ratios to Sort Out Overlapping Diagnostic Criteria

Most pathologic entities exhibit a spectrum of pathologic findings that overlap to some extent with those present in other entities that need to be considered in a differential diagnosis. A similar problem is present during evaluation of the results of immunostains, molecular and other tests, as there are few ancillary tests that provide 100% specificity for a particular diagnosis. Seasoned pathologists usually interpret the presence of overlapping diagnostic criteria and test results using a qualitative approach that places available information "in context" based on prior clinical experience, and decide whether a particular diagnosis is more likely than others based on prior experience. Somewhat surprisingly, there have been relatively few studies where a similar approach has been applied in a more formal, quantitative manner using the mathematical concepts of probabilities, odds, probability ratios, odds ratios, and likelihood ratios. By contrast, these metrics have been widely used in laboratory medicine.

Recent studies from our laboratory evaluating the diagnosis of bronchioloalveolar carcinoma (BAC), well-differentiated pulmonary adenocarcinoma, and carcinoid tumor on frozen sections can be used to illustrate the potential value of using the Bayesian inference process in anatomic pathology [51, 52]. Table 13.4, taken from the study comparing BAC and well-differentiated adenocarcinoma with reactive epithelial atypia, shows the incidence of 11 histopathologic features that in our clinical experience can be helpful to distinguish well-differentiated adenocarcinomas of the lung and BAC from reactive atypia on frozen section [52]. They include histopathologic features such as the abrupt transition, nuclear cytoplasmic ratio and others that are more frequent in BAC and adenocarcinomas than in reactive type II pneumocyte atypia and others, and other criteria that are more frequent in the latter condition, such as the presence of granulomas (Fig. 13.2). However, most of these histopathological features are present in significantly different proportions in the two populations of interest (malignant vs. benign) as shown in Table 13.5. How can a pathologist use this variable information to diagnose a single lung biopsy? One possible approach is to rely on the sensitivity and specificity of each pathological feature, by diagnosis, shown in Table 13.5. This type of information poses interpretation conundrums as it is difficult to reconcile variable sensitivities and specificities. Looking at Table 13.5, taken from the same study, how can a pathologist decide whether "grossly evident nodule/lesion" with sensitivity of 0.95 and specificity of 0.52 is better or worse for the diagnosis of malignancy than "anisocytosis" with a sensitivity of 0.56 and

Table 13.4 Incidence of 11 statistically significant parameters in cases of reactive atypical epithelial hyperplasia and BAC or well-differentiated adenocarcinomas of the lung

Parameter	RA (%)	AC (%)
Grossly evident nodule or lesion	50	93.1
Abrupt transition	62.5	88.46
Multiple patterns of growth	18.5	61.5
Granuloma	30.90	3.8
Anisocytosis	16.98	57.69
Proportion of atypia	33.9	80.76
Nuclear pseudoinclusion	44	73.91
Macronucleoli	0	8.5
N/C >80	44.6	84.61
Irregular nuclear membrane	53.7	84.61
Atypical mitoses	0	25.7

From Gupta et al. [52]. © 2003–2010 American Society for Clinical Pathology. © 2003–2010 American Journal of Clinical Pathology

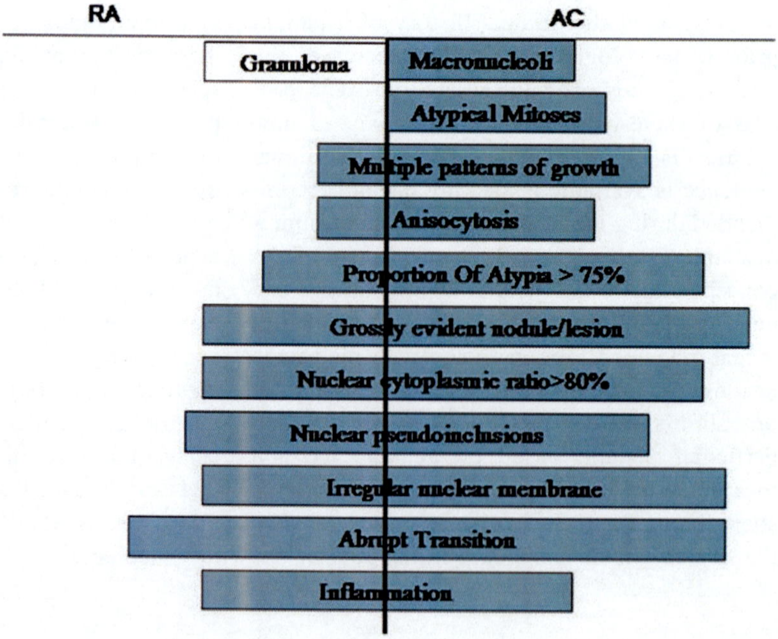

Fig. 13.2 They include histopathologic features such as the abrupt transition, nuclear cytoplasmic ratio and others that are more frequent in bronchioloalveolar carcinoma (BAC) and adenocarcinomas than in reactive type II pneumocyte atypia and others, and other criteria that are more frequent in the latter condition, such as the presence of granulomas (From Gupta et al. [24]; with permission)

Table 13.5 Analysis of "statistically significant" diagnostic features for the diagnosis of pulmonary BAC or well-differentiated adenocarcinoma using Bayesian statistics

Feature	Chi square test (*p* value)	Sensitivity[a]	Specificity[a]	Odds ratio[a]	Relative risk[a]	Likelihood ratio[a]
Grossly evident nodule/lesion	0.00	0.95	0.52	19.25	7.75	1.99
Abrupt transition	0.016	0.88	0.37	0.217	3.172	1.40
Multiple growth patterns	0.00	0.64	0.83	7.04	0.301	3.77
Granuloma	0.006	0.004	0.70	0.089	0.140	0.13
Anisocytosis**	0.00	0.56	0.83	0.150	3.125	3.21
Proportion of atypia	0.00	0.81	0.65	0.129	4.2	2.30
Nuclear pseudoinclusions	0.017	0.74	0.56	0.277	2.470	1.68
Macronucleoli	0.011	0.12	1.00		3.348	9,999
N/C ratio >80%	0.001	0.85	0.54	0.157	3.862	1.83
Irregular nuclear membrane	0.007	0.85	0.46	4.74	3.125	1.58
Atypical mitoses	0.00	0.38	1.00	0.00	3.528	9,999

[a] Bayesian statistics

** Anisocytosis was noted when the size of atypical epithelial cells varied by 3 times or more the size of the neighboring epithelial cells

From Gupta et al. [52].

specificity of 0.83? Another approach to the interpretation of overlapping data is to use simple statistics favored in the EBM literature, such as probability ratios, odds ratios, and likelihood ratios. These metrics, also shown in Table 13.5, allow sorting out the diagnostic value of each histopathological criteria or combinations of features by diagnosis and for use of the information for the diagnosis of single patients. Probability ratio or relative risk (RR) is the ratio of the probability of an event occurring in a population versus the probability of taking place in another. For example, if a particular diagnostic feature is present in 80% of A cases and 20% of B cases, the probabilities of such as features being present in populations A and B are 0.8 and 0.2 respectively. The RR is 4 for population A as compared to B, indicating that the feature is 4× more probable to be present in the first of the two populations. As explained in Chap. 4, odds are estimated by the simple formula: odds = probability/(1−probability). For example of a probability of 0.8, the odds would be 0.8/(1−0.8) = 4. OR offer a measure of effect size that describes the strength of association between two binary data values. RRs are easier to interpret and offer more intuitive data. OR is usually used with logistic regression and in situations where RR cannot be readily estimated. RR and OR do not take into account the prevalence of different populations. LR is based on sensitivity and specificity and therefore takes into account the prevalence of different conditions. LR+ = sensitivity/(1−specificity) and provides of the presence of a particular finding in a population that combines both the sensitivity and specificity of such feature. LR− = 1−sensitivity/specificity and provides an estimate of the potential validity of a negative test.

Table 13.5 and Fig. 13.2 show how the information provided by these ratios can be used in a more intuitive manner for the diagnosis of individual frozen sections as more closely resemble the reasoning process that is usually used by pathologists for a differential diagnoses: "diagnosis A is more likely than diagnosis B because of the presence of a combination of particular histologic features." If we look at the various LR+ listed in Table 13.5, the presence of macronucleoli and atypical mitoses strongly supports the possibility of malignancy, while others such as N/C ratio > 80% and irregular nuclear membrane are less valuable. Figure 13.2 shows this information in a simple graphical manner. In this figure, the vertical line separates the two diagnoses, reactive atypia to the left and adenocarcinoma to the right. Features with high LR+ such as macronucleoli and atypical mitosis show almost no overlap in the two diagnoses, while others such as the irregular nuclear membranes and abrupt transition show considerable overlap. Although the information in Fig. 13.2 does not provide a pathologist with absolute diagnostic criteria for the diagnosis of reactive atypia or adenocarcinoma, it can be helpful to evaluate the likelihood of any of the two diagnoses based on the presence of features with the highest LR+.

Use of Probability, Odds, and Likelihood Ratios for the Selection of Cost-Effective Immunohistochemistry and Other Ancillary Tests

There are no widely used methodologies to help develop evidence-based guidelines for the cost-effective utilization of immunostains and other diagnostic and prognostic tests in anatomic pathology. Pathologists have to rely on the information, usually presented in tables, included in books and other publications. However, as there are few antibodies or other tests that are 100% specific for any one diagnosis, these tables frequently show results using variable number of +/– or listing the sensitivity and specificity data of each test. Tables 13.6 and 13.7 show an example of the variable sensitivity and specificity of different immunostains in cases of malignant mesothelioma and adenocarcinoma, collected in a recent systematic review [53]. In the presence of such variability, pathologists often rely on the advice of recognized experts in the field to select which markers are more helpful and how many markers should be used, although experts often do not completely agree with each other. Surprisingly, there has been little interest in the application of simple statistics such as probability ratios (risk ratios), odds ratios, and likelihood ratios that can be very helpful to sort out the information that is more likely to provide a particular answer of interest. For example, a systematic review of 88 publications provided information about the use of 15 antibodies for the differential diagnosis between pulmonary adenocarcinoma and malignant mesothelioma and listed the opinions of various experts [53]. The review showed that while most studies identified that certain antibodies such as calretinin, Wilm's tumor-1 (WT-1), Ber-EP4, and others were most helpful in this differential diagnosis, various experts did not agree about how many immunohistochemical tests were necessary and which antibodies needed to be included in a panel. Analysis of OR (Table 13.8) clearly showed that the use of a large number of antibodies was considerably worse than the use of even 1 marker and that 7 antibodies provided optimal sensitivity and specificity for this differential diagnosis: MOC-31, BG8, CEA, TTF-1, CK5/6, WT-1, and HBME-1 [53]. Table 13.9 shows that the OR provided by selected panels of immunostains for the diagnosis of epithelioid malignant mesothelioma. For example use of all 15 markers provides OR = 9.46 while

Table 13.6 Summary of data from the literature averaging the results from multiple studies: sensitivity and specificity of carcinoma markers for identifying pulmonary adenocarcinomas during the differential diagnosis with malignant mesothelioma

Marker	Sensitivity (%)	Specificity (%)
CEA (n = 1,524)	83	95
Ber-EP4 (n = 702)	80	90
B72.3 (n = 769)	80	93
LEU-M1 (p = 1,473)	72	93
MOC-31 (n = 213)	93	93
E-Cadherin (n = 183)	86	82
TTF-1 (n = 366)	72	100
Lewis-BG8 (n = 213)	93	93

From Westfall et al. [54], with permission of Wiley

Table 13.7 Summary of data from the literature averaging the results from multiple studies: sensitivity and specificity of mesothelial markers for identifying epithelioid malignant mesothelioma during the differential diagnosis with adenocarcinoma

Marker	Sensitivity (%)	Specificity (%)
CK5/6 (n = 402)	83	85
Vimentin (n = 773)	62	75
Calretinin (n = 885)	82	85
HBME-1 (n = 769)	85	43
Thrombomodulin (n = 831)	61	80
N-Cadherin (n = 151)	78	84
WT-1 (n = 264)	77	84

From Westfall et al. [54], with permission of Wiley

Table 13.8 Odds ratios of negative immunoreactivity in malignant mesothelioma

Epitope	Proportion of negative MM*	MM # cases	Proportion of negative AC**	AC # cases	Odds ratio
CEA	0.95	1,818	0.17	1,524	92.76
Ber-EP4	0.9	899	0.20	702	36.00
B72.3	0.93	700	0.20	769	53.143
LEU-M1	0.93	1,204	0.28	1,473	34.16
MOC-31	0.93	276	0.07	213	176.51
E-Cadherin	0.82	218	0.14	183	27.98
TTF-1	0.82	240	0.28	366	1,233.19
Lewis-BG8	1.00	197	0.07	231	176.51
CK5/6	0.17	402	0.85	402	0.036
Vimentin	0.38	773	0.75	815	0.204
Calretinin	0.18	885	0.85	912	0.04
HBME-1	0.15	769	0.43	676	0.23
Thrombomodulin	0.39	831	0.8	964	0.16
N-Cadherin	0.22	151	0.84	121	0.54
WT-1	0.23	264	0.96	213	0.01

*Malignant mesothelioma
**Adenocarcinoma

Table 13.9 Odds ratios of selected panels of immunostains for the diagnosis of epithelioid malignant mesothelioma

Panel		Odds ratio
A	All 15 markers reviewed in the study by King and associates	9.46
B	7 Markers selected for their superior specificity and specificity (CEA, MOC-31, TTF-1, BG8, CK5/6, WT-1, and HBME-1)	27.01
C	2 Mesothelial markers with the best individual OR (CK5/6 and WT-1)	34.44
D	2 Epithelial markers with the best individual OR (MOC-31 and TTF-1)	198.18
E	Combination of the "best" two mesothelial and epithelial markers (MOC-31, TTF-1, CK5/6, and WT-1)	48.63
F	Combination of the "best" mesothelial and epithelial markers (TTF-1 and WT-1)	96.34

use of the best mesothelial and epithelial markers yields OR = 96.34.

Similar methodology helped optimize the selection of antibody panels for the evaluation of pleural effusions with malignant epithelioid cells [54]. Table 13.10 shows that while presentation of data using the sensitivity and specificity for each antibody used for the diagnosis of mesothelioma and carcinoma by site of origin shows considerable overlap, analysis of the data. Analysis of this data using post-test odds helps stratify the results by differential diagnosis. As a result of this information, we were able to select antibody panels for male (calretinin, TTF-1, PSA, and CDX2) and female patients (calretinin, TTF-1, ER, and CA125) that provided the most optimal information to evaluate the site of origin of a metastatic carcinoma in a pleural effusion.

Back to the Future: Is Molecular Pathology Going to Replace Pathologic Diagnoses? Classification and Prognostic/Predictive Models Based on Multivariate Data Analysis

Rapid advances in molecular pathology suggest the possibility that molecular tests will be able to identify in the near future various conditions that are currently being diagnosed by pathologists using microscopy. From an epistemological standpoint, these claims are somewhat reminiscent of the interest 2 or 3 decades ago at developing image analysis systems that could diagnose pathologic and cytologic samples objectively and reliable [49]. These investigations led to the development of image analysis systems for the semi-automatic

Table 13.10 Post-test odds of positive immunoreactivity by antibody and diagnosis in pleural effusions with malignant mesothelioma or metastastic carcinomas

	Diagnosis (post-test odds)						
Antibody	Mesothelioma	Lung	Breast	Müllerian	Stomach	Colon	Prostate
Ber-EP4	0.0	0.6	0.5	0.2	0.1	0.0	0.0
MOC-31	0.0	0.6	0.6	0.2	0.1	0.0	0.0
CEA	0.0	1.7	0.1	0.0	0.1	0.1	0.0
Calretinin	4.0	0.0	0.0	0.2	0.0	0.0	N/A
CK5/6	3.0	0.3	N/A	0.0	N/A	0.0	N/A
WT-1	0.2	0.0	0.7	0.7	N/A	N/A	N/A
CK7	0.0	1.4	0.4	0.1	0.0	0.0	0.0
CK20	N/A	0.2	0.0	0.0	0.2	1.5	0.0
TTF-1	0.0	∞	0.0	0.0	0.0	0.0	0.0
ER	N/A	0.1	4.0	0.2	N/A	N/A	N/A
PR	N/A	0.0	∞	0.0	N/A	N/A	N/A
CA125	N/A	0.3	N/A	3.5	N/A	N/A	N/A
CDX2	N/A	0.0	N/A	0.0	0.5	2.0	N/A
PSA	N/A	0.0	N/A	N/A	0.0	N/A	∞

N/A Not applicable

screening of pap tests that evaluate multiple features with multivariate statistics, neural networks, or other mathematical tools for reasoning with uncertainty [55–57]. Some of these instruments are currently approved by the Food and Drug Administration (FDA) for clinical use. However, the road to the development of automated image analysis systems for diagnosis was difficult, not because of the lack of resolution of the image analysis systems or of computer power, but partly because of the difficulties at validating the results of studies so that they would be applicable to the population at large of pap tests. The analysis of data in these systems is based on the analysis of multivariate data using methods that apply probability theory. Small errors due to chance that are acceptable within the limits of the statistical test tend to become magnified as a large number of variables are analyzed, resulting in occasional spurious outputs derived from data over fit or shrinkage. For example, if a feature is statistically significant to $p=0.001$ in two different entities, there is 1 in 100 chance that it will be encountered in the wrong end of a differential diagnosis. When this 1% is propagated through hundreds of features, it can lead to spurious results. Validation of these systems requires large numbers of test cases that are often difficult and very costly to gather and analyze [56, 57]. In general, a ratio of ten test cases per variable is recommended to minimize the probability of errors due to data overfit [47].

Molecular Classifications Based on Multivariate Data

Molecular classifications and prognostic/predictive models using information from multiple genes analyzed with high-throughput methods will likely face similar problems when the data is analyzed with bioinformatics techniques [58–60]. Our previous study exploring the development of classification models for lung cancer cell lines based on DNA methylation markers can help illustrate the problem of attempting to classify pathologic lesions using molecular data [61]. We evaluated well-characterized cells lines of small cell lung cancer and nonsmall cell lung cancer for the presence of DNA methylation levels at 20 loci, using the real time PCR assay MethyLight. Cell lines were divided into various training set and test sets. Cases were rotated to be included in some of the training and test sets, using jackknife techniques. The data were analyzed with linear discriminant analysis and neural networks. The initial results were excellent, and neural network models could apparently classify all the cell lines with 100%

Table 13.11 Classification of test cases ($n=16$) by linear discriminant models and artificial neural networks

	Linear discriminant analysis		Linear discriminant analysis after logarithmic transformation of the data		Artificial neural network	
Model (training cell lines $n=71$)	Number of correctly classified cell lines	Kappa coefficient	Number of correctly classified cell lines	Kappa coefficient	Number of correctly classified cell lines	Kappa coefficient
Models trained with all variables						
1	12	0.50	12	0.5	16	1
2	10	0.25	12	0.5	16	1
3	12	0.50	14	0.75	16	1
4	10	0.25	11	0.35	16	1
5	10	0.25	13	0.62	16	1
Models trained with five variables (ESR1, MTHFR, PTGS2, CDKN2A, CALCA)						
6	13	0.62	13	0.62	16	1
7	10	0.25	10	0.25	14	0.75
8	14	0.75	13	0.62	14	0.75
9	13	0.62	13	0.62	14	0.75
10	13	0.62	13	0.62	15	0.88

specificity. However, when the same data were split into different training and test sets, the results varied, as shown in Table 13.11 [61]. Interestingly, some of the same cell lines were classified as either small cell or nonsmall cell by different neural networks or linear discriminant analysis when the models were trained using slightly different data subsets. These results suggest that future studies attempting to classify tumors using multivariate molecular or other data will need to be validated with large sets of test data before their clinical validity is established, a process that is likely to be expensive and time consuming, unless better data analysis methods are developed as a result of advances in bioinformatics.

Forecasting Models Based on Multivariate Data: Beyond Cell Type and Stage as Predictors of Prognosis and Response to Therapy

Linear discriminant analysis, multivariate logistic regression, neural networks, and Bayesian belief networks can also be used to model prognostic systems that estimate prognosis or other clinical variable using data collected with histopathology, immunohistochemistry, and other methods [61–64]. These methods have been used experimentally in our laboratory to estimate the likelihood of positive regional lymph nodes in patients with breast cancer and colon cancer, the prognosis of lung cancer patients and other conditions [65–67]. It is beyond the scope of this chapter to discuss this topic in detail, but if pathologists are willing to explore beyond the standard considerations of using cell type and survival statistics to predict prognosis and predict therapy response, there is a wealth of bioinformatics techniques for the analysis of multivariate data that could be used to combine clinico-pathologic data with that obtained with new IHC and molecular tests. These models could be specifically designed to estimate the prognosis of various diseases and likely response to selected therapies and could help reestablish the traditional role of pathologists guiding the hands of surgeons and other physicians in the bioinformatics era.

Appraisal and Integration of Published Evidence with Personal Experience

Previous chapters of this book, particularly Chap. 11, have described various methods that can be used by pathologist to evaluate the probable quality and validity of information published in the literature. However, it is well known that the results of a study performed on a particular patient cohort may not apply to other patients, because of diagnostic variability, demographics, and other factors. While clinical laboratories have developed various methods of proficiency testing to ensure that different laboratories will yield similar results on the same blood or other samples, there is relatively scanty literature in anatomic pathology dealing with the problem of how best to standardize diagnosis and integrate best evidence from the literature with personal experience [68, 69].

Appraisal of Classification Schema Proposed by Groups of Experts and Integration into Personal Practice

Classification schema proposed by groups of experts could and probably should be evaluated by practicing pathologists before they are implemented in routine practice by reviewing the best evidence that supports various recommendations. As there is variability among different patient populations, it is probably advisable that some preliminary testing be performed to evaluate how well the new schema can be applied to the diagnosis and management of local patients. To explore this subject, we recently evaluated the risks of malignancy predicted by thyroid fine-needle aspiration (FNA) biopsies published by a group of experts sponsored by the National Cancer Institute [70]. A review of the publications listed in the NCI document revealed that the experts had relied mostly on level III evidence based on surgical follow-up. Such information is probably biased toward higher risk of malignancy estimates, as patients who undergo thyroidectomy do so because of the FNA results and/or other clinical findings. To test this hypothesis, we analyzed our own data from 879 patients who underwent thyroid FNA at our hospital during a 2-year period, using different denominators to estimate malignancy risks: surgery, repeat FNA, both surgery or repeat FNA, and all patients as a surrogate for clinical follow-up [70]. As expected, the risk estimates for patients with malignant or suspicious for malignant categories by thyroid FNA were similar for calculations performed using all four denominators. By contrast, for the benign category, the risk estimates calculated using surgical follow-up were considerably higher than for those using surrogate clinical follow-up as the denominator. The study showed that NCI recommendations were generally valid for our patients with a diagnosis of "suspicious for malignancy" and "malignant" categories, while they probably variably overestimated the risk of malignancy for our patients with other diagnoses. It also demonstrated that stratifying the diagnostic categories into three groups other than nondiagnostic: "benign," "follicular lesion of undetermined significance or neoplasm," and "suspicious or malignant" resulted in better, non-overlapping risk predictions.

What Is the Purpose of Classifications in Anatomic Pathology: Should Lesions Be Grouped by Histogenesis, Morphology, or Their Forecasting Value?

Various classes of classifiers have been used to organize classification schema of tumors and other lesions in pathology. Schemas are generally based on the presumed histogenesis of the neoplasms, their morphologic features and/or their ability to forecast the prognosis of patients and/or the efficacy of various therapeutic measures. There is no general agreement regarding which classifiers are preferable. For example, the WHO classifies tumors of soft tissue and bone using a histogenetic or cell type approach, lung neoplasms using a mixed histogenetic and histomorphological approach, and pleural neoplasms using a histomorphological approach [20, 21]. In addition, some classification schemas of neoplasms attempt to correlate "cell type" or "histologic type" with prognosis while others use tumor grade for this purpose. Reviewing the classifiers used in various schemas from an epistemological point of view, one could propose that classifications based on morphology should strive to be very descriptive with clear and explicit diagnostic features so that they can be reproducibly applied by different pathologists with excellent agreement levels as measured by kappa statistics. By contrast, schema designed to forecast prognosis or predict response to therapy should provide precise estimates of the future. In addition, often both types of classifiers are considered in the organization of lesions in pathologic classifications, although it is often very difficult to optimize the schema to achieve both diagnostic reproducibility and excellent forecasting ability. Classifications optimized for the latter frequently need to incorporate features beyond morphology, such as the results of tumor markers and other tests, disease stage, and other clinical considerations and effects of therapy.

Recent studies of thymomas can also be used to illustrate the concept that, as the specific purposes of various classification schemas are often not explicitly listed by their authors, there is some confusion in the way pathologists currently tend to organize and use classification schema. Thymic epithelial neoplasms are currently classified by WHO based on their histomorphology into thymomas types A, B1, B2, B3, AB, and thymic carcinomas [22, 23, 71]. We explored the forecasting ability of this classification schema by performing a systematic review with meta-analysis of available best evidence for patients with thymomas classified by WHO criteria. As in the previous study, only level III data from 2,192 thymomas reported in 15 studies were identified [36]. Such best available evidence showed considerable variability in the proportions of WHO thymoma cell types in different studies, suggesting interobserver variability problems. For example, the proportion of type A thymomas varied from 5 to 24% while the proportion of B3 thymomas varied from 6 to 34%. This variability suggested that the subclassification of thymomas according to current WHO criteria may not be entirely reproducible among different pathologists. This conclusion is supported by the study by Rieker et al. [72] showing in a large multicenter study that interobserver agreement for the subclassification of WHO type B thymomas into B1, B2, and B3 lesions was only at the low moderate level with kappa = 0.49. Analyzing the classification scheme from the view point of how well it forecasts survival, our meta-analysis showed no significant survival differences for patients with thymomas A, AB, and B1 [36]. By contrast, there were significant survival differences between patients with A/AB/B1 thymomas and those with B2 and B3 thymomas (Fig. 13.3a, b), suggesting that only three categories of thymic epithelial lesions other than carcinomas are of prognostic value. The results of the meta-analysis raise interesting questions about how to modify the WHO classification of thymomas in the future. Should these neoplasms continue to be classified into five histologic types, because of the way they look to at least some observers under the microscope, and in spite of interobserver variability problems? If WHO continues to recommend a classification scheme including five histologic types should they be organized into three grades that appear to predict survival? Should the classification schema be collapsed into only three histologic types based on prognosis? This may reduce the possibility of interobserver variability as pathologists will have fewer diagnostic choices but would involve aggregating thymomas A, AB, and B1 that in typical cases look different from each other under the microscope. To our knowledge, there is no consensus among the intellectual leaders in pathology about how to approach these types of questions in a consistent manner. In our view, it would be sensible to develop two types of classifications for lesions such as thymomas and other neoplastic and non-neoplastic conditions: (1) diagnostic classification schema and (2) multivariate forecasting models. The diagnostic classification schema would serve to stratify various conditions in a manner that continues to take advantage from the extensive clinico-pathologic knowledge collected by physicians over many years. These classifications would use very explicit diagnostic criteria identifiable with gross pathology, histopathology, immunohistochemistry and molecular techniques, and would be designed to provide the best possible interobserver diagnostic agreement levels, so that patients would be consistently classified with the same disease or entity at different medical facilities. The gold standard for this type of classifications would be very high kappa coefficients of interobserver agreement. Multivariate

a

Thymoma A vs. AB

Study name	Odds ratio	Lower limit	Upper limit	Z-Value	p-Value
Rena	2.273	0.249	20.741	0.728	0.467
Kim	1.596	0.069	37.077	0.291	0.771
Bedini	2.072	0.102	42.210	0.474	0.636
Park	1.531	0.066	35.526	0.265	0.791
Rea	3.561	0.172	73.703	0.822	0.411
Okumura	5.756	0.322	102.868	1.190	0.234
Reiker	0.078	0.004	1.400	-1.732	0.083
Chalabreysse	0.533	0.029	9.708	-0.425	0.671
	1.366	0.499	3.742	0.606	0.544

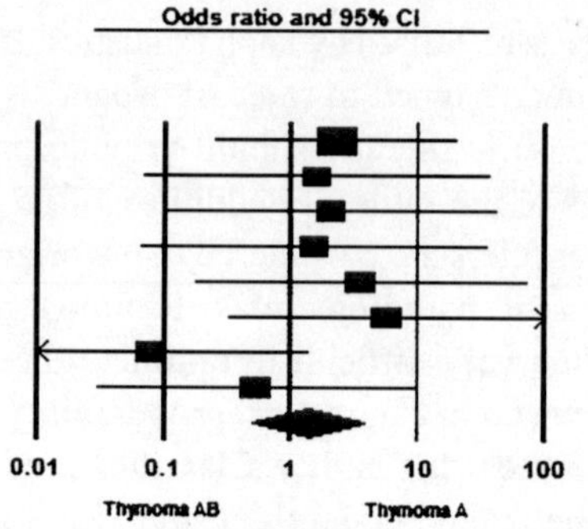

Thymoma A vs. B1

Study name	Odds ratio	Lower limit	Upper limit	Z-Value	p-Value
Rena	3.684	0.423	32.078	1.181	0.238
Wright	4.216	0.192	92.659	0.913	0.361
Bedini	5.261	0.245	113.125	1.061	0.289
Kondo	1.667	0.073	38.277	0.319	0.749
Park	1.800	0.065	50.097	0.346	0.729
Rea	7.909	0.392	159.769	1.349	0.177
Nakakgawa	6.852	0.304	154.606	1.210	0.226
Chen	1.545	0.057	42.147	0.258	0.796
Okumura	4.030	0.212	76.504	0.928	0.353
Reiker	0.660	0.182	2.387	-0.633	0.526
Chalabreysse	0.800	0.043	14.886	-0.150	0.881
	1.828	0.860	3.885	1.568	0.117

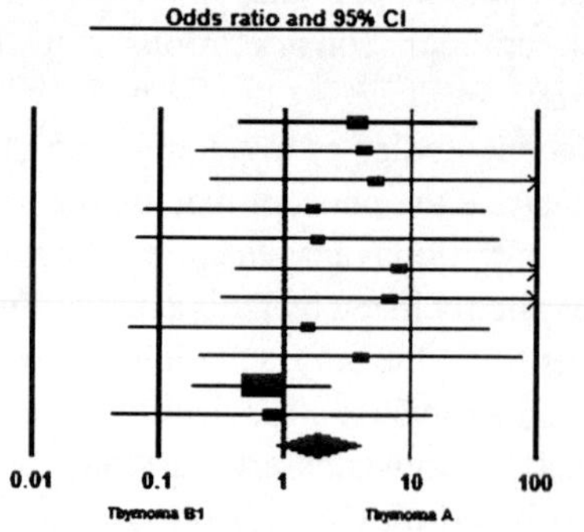

b

Thymoma B1 vs. B2

Study name	Odds ratio	Lower limit	Upper limit	Z-Value	p-Value
Sonobe	19.138	1.006	363.495	1.965	0.049
Rena	2.327	0.849	6.374	1.642	0.101
Wright	1.136	0.147	8.757	0.123	0.902
Bedini	0.990	0.265	3.698	-0.015	0.988
Kondo	1.786	0.140	22.700	0.447	0.655
Strobel	2.776	0.144	53.350	0.677	0.498
Park	2.595	0.294	22.917	0.858	0.391
Rea	8.444	2.184	32.658	3.092	0.002
Singhal	5.069	0.193	132.816	0.974	0.330
Nakakgawa	1.040	0.168	6.450	0.042	0.966
Chen	46.400	5.436	396.086	3.507	0.000
Okumura	7.018	2.571	19.157	3.803	0.000
Reiker	1.119	0.334	3.757	0.183	0.855
Chalabreysse	1.000	0.081	12.399	0.000	1.000
	2.924	1.900	4.499	4.880	0.000

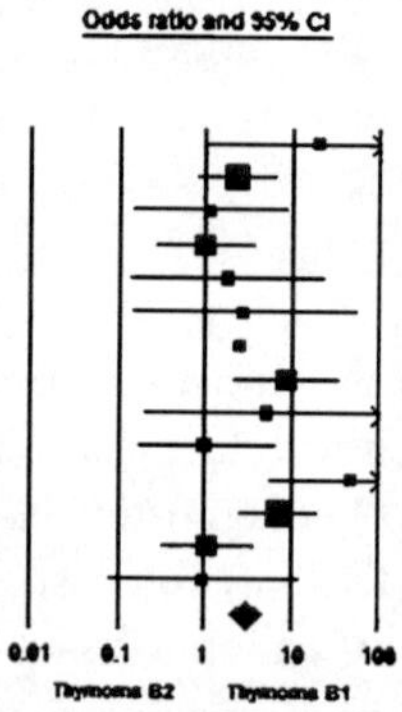

Thymoma B1 vs. B3

Study name	Odds ratio	Lower limit	Upper limit	Z-Value	p-Value
Sonobe	31.000	1.725	557.209	2.330	0.020
Rena	8.686	2.190	34.449	3.075	0.002
Wright	4.730	0.988	22.645	1.945	0.052
Bedini	2.200	0.520	9.299	1.072	0.284
Kondo	1.136	0.093	13.886	0.100	0.920
Strobel	6.231	0.309	125.527	1.194	0.232
Park	5.333	0.589	48.300	1.489	0.136
Rea	7.600	1.997	28.929	2.974	0.003
Singhal	16.333	0.570	467.761	1.632	0.103
Nakakgawa	9.100	1.389	59.619	2.303	0.021
Chen	6.737	0.760	59.754	1.713	0.087
Okumura	18.889	5.555	64.230	4.706	0.000
Reiker	1.250	0.190	8.233	0.232	0.817
Chalabreysse	2.500	0.224	27.940	0.744	0.457
	6.090	3.754	9.878	7.320	0.000

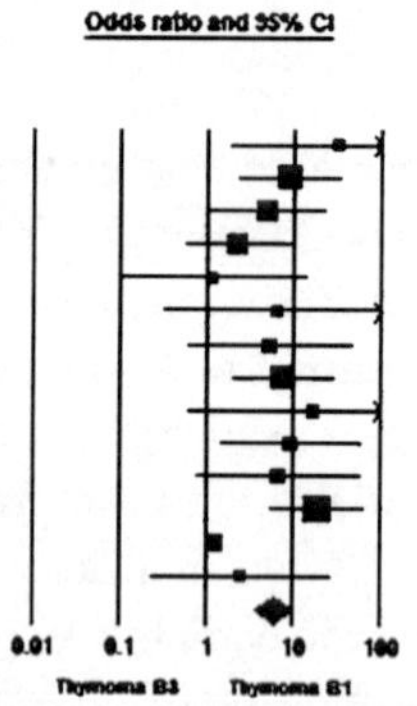

Thymoma B2 vs. B3

Study name	Odds ratio	Lower limit	Upper limit	Z-Value	p-Value
Sonobe	1.667	0.535	5.195	0.881	0.379
Rena	3.733	1.048	13.301	2.032	0.042
Wright	4.162	0.864	20.061	1.777	0.076
Bedini	2.222	0.632	7.808	1.245	0.213
Kondo	0.636	0.034	11.909	-0.302	0.762
Strobel	2.232	0.542	9.190	1.112	0.266
Park	2.056	0.664	6.365	1.249	0.212
Rea	0.900	0.299	2.710	-0.187	0.851
Singhal	3.500	0.177	69.339	0.822	0.411
Nakakgawa	8.750	1.840	41.606	2.727	0.006
Chen	0.145	0.049	0.434	-3.454	0.001
Okumura	2.692	1.091	6.643	2.148	0.032
Reiker	1.117	0.215	5.800	0.131	0.896
Chalabreysse	2.500	0.364	17.173	0.932	0.351
	1.671	1.170	2.387	2.824	0.005

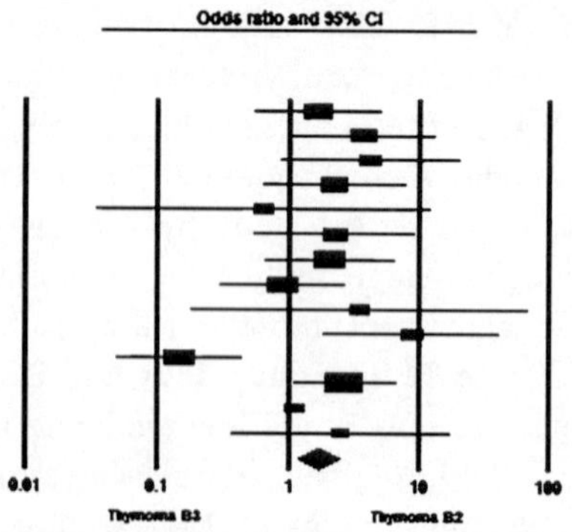

Fig. 13.3 (**a**) Significant survival differences exist between patients with A/AB/B1 thymomas and (**b**) those with B2 and B3 thymomas (From Gupta et al. [52]. © 2003–2010 American Society for Clinical Pathology. © 2003–2010 American Journal of Clinical Pathology)

forecasting models are not really classification schemas and, should probably be based on multivariate statistical analysis or other tools for reasoning with uncertainty such as decision tree analysis, neural networks, Bayesian belief networks, and others. Forecasting models would be optimized to predict survival and/or response to selected treatment options with the highest possible precision and at the lowest possible cost. These forecasting models could include selected information provided by the diagnostic classifications, stage and other clinical information, laboratory, molecular, and other data optimized in a multivariate analysis designed to best provide the information that surgeons and oncologists need to treat patients in a cost-effective manner.

How Valid Is the Prognostic Information Provided by Pathologic Diagnoses? The Inconvenient Problem of Interobserver Variability

A discussion of the appraisal of information from the literature and integration with personal experience cannot be complete without a brief discussion of the problem of interobserver variability and its influence on prognostic estimates and on the definition of new entities [73]. Clinico-pathologic entities are usually described when a significant statistical association is found between a set of diagnostic features and survival or other outcome variables. The new entity is thereafter integrated into the appropriate classification schema. Pathologic classifications are regularly published without evaluation of whether pathologists other than the authors can reproducibly diagnose cases of the new entity. Depending on how distinct particular histopathologic features are and how often they are present in different entities that need to be included in a differential diagnosis, different pathologists can arrive at different conclusions, resulting in interobserver diagnostic variability. This problem has been documented in multiple studies involving neoplasms of the lung, gynecologic tract, and others [74, 75]. It is less understood how these diagnostic variability could influence the statistical significance of the data that is used to define new clinico-pathologic entities. We recently explored this problem using the distinction between usual interstitial pneumonia (UIP) and nonspecific interstitial pneumonia (NSIP), two closely related forms of chronic diffuse lung disease that can be difficult to distinguish from each other on wedge lung biopsies [73]. Using the QDMBA process described in this chapter, we formulated specific questions and performed a systematic review of the literature. Seven retrospective level III studies were found that had evaluated patients with both UIP and NSIP and provided survival information. As shown in Table 13.12, there is considerable interstudy variability in the prognosis of patients diagnosed as either UIP or NSIP. In addition, 95% confidence intervals of the data showed considerable overlap in survival proportions among patients with UIP and NSIP in several of the studies reviewed. Although all studies confirmed the general concept that NSIP patients have significantly better survival than those with UIP, the survival proportions reported for UIP and NSIP patients ranged from 11–58% to 39–100% respectively. This variability showed that the survival proportions of patients diagnosed with UIP at some centers was 5× better than in others. Variability for NSIP patients was in the order of 3×. As all these studies were retrospective cases series, it is possible that the results were influenced by demographics, the severity of disease at diagnosis, and treatment effect. Interestingly, a simulation performed using the data from each study, keeping the number of patients surviving the disease as a constant and increasing or decreasing at 5–30% intervals the number of patients with either UIP or NSIP, to simulate interobserver diagnostic variability, showed that changing approximately 10% of the diagnoses would have changed the statistical significance of all the studies. Analysis of the data generated by the various simulations with kappa statistics showed that kappa values at moderate agreement levels could significantly change the prognostic estimates of studies reporting the prognosis of patients with UIP and NSIP. The results of the study strongly underscore the need to develop pathologic classifications that minimize the problem of interobserver variability and the importance of testing for possible interobserver variability before new pathologic classifications are disseminated.

Table 13.12 Evidence summary from studies evaluated with the simulation tool

Author	Number of cases	Number of usual interstitial pneumonia (UIP) patients	UIP survival % and 95% CI[a]	Number of nonspecific interstitial pneumonia (NSIP) patients	NSIP survival % and 95% CI[a]
Parra	109	55	36.3 (24.9–49.5)	22	77.3 (56.6–89.9)
Riha	70	53	58 (44.6–70.3)	7	80 (43.3–95.4)
Park	362	203	49 (42.2–55.8)	66	73 (61.3–82.2)
Bjoraker	104	63	28 (18.4–40.1)	14	80 (53.9–93.2)
Flaherty	109	51	30 (19.2–43.6)	30	90 (74.4–96.5)
Travis	101	56	43 (30.9–56.0)	22	100 (85.1–100)
Nicholson	78	37	11 (4.4–24.9)	28	39 (23.3–57.3)
Total	697	518	40.9 (36.7–45.2)	189	75.1 (68.5–80.7)

[a]95% confidence intervals (CI) were estimated from published data
From Marchevsky and Gupta [73], with permission of Elsevier

Field Testing New Pathologic Classifications Before They Are Published

A logical approach to minimize the influence of interobserver diagnostic variability would be for the authors of new classifications that are likely to be used by many pathologists worldwide, such as those published by WHO, to field-test the diagnostic reproducibility of the proposed schema with an adequate sample of pathologists to evaluate whether they could apply them consistently in their practices. This process could lead to modifications in the proposed classification schema or definitions of various diagnostic criteria prior to publication, in an effort to decrease possible interobserver diagnostic variability. Currently, it is sometimes disturbing that even the authors of diagnostic classifications disagree among themselves, a problem that is sometimes highlighted when various experts render variable diagnoses during slide symposia at national and international teaching conferences. We recently explored the concept of testing the validity of proposed diagnostic before publication in a recent study suggesting several evidence based criteria to help distinguish metastastic breast cancer from primary lung adenocarcinoma on thoracic frozen sections [76]. The study of 129 frozen sections was conducted using the QDMBA paradigm and initially showed, somewhat to our surprise, that in most patient populations, including ours, primary lung adenocarcinomas were approximately twice more frequent than metastatic breast cancer, a somewhat counterintuitive finding in patients with a previous history of breast cancer. Using these pre-test probabilities and the incidence of various pathologic features in the two populations we identified, using post-test OR several significant pathologic criteria that favored the diagnosis of primary lung adenocarcinoma. They include the presence of acini, lepidic growth, nuclear pseudoinclusions, and central scar. By contrast, the presence of comedonecrosis, solid nests of tumor cells, trabecular architecture, and cribriform growth favored the probability of metastastic breast cancer (Fig. 13.4). Once these diagnostic criteria were obtained, they were explained to a group of attending pathologists and residents, and their validity tested using exams administered before and after the training session. The exercise showed that most participants were able to significantly improve the accuracy of the diagnosis of either primary lung adenocarcinoma or metastastic breast carcinoma using the proposed criteria. Feedback from the exercise was used to improve on the definition of various criteria and the way they were grouped prior to publication.

Conclusion

It is apparent from the epistemological review of current practices provided in this book that pathologists have been much more interested in

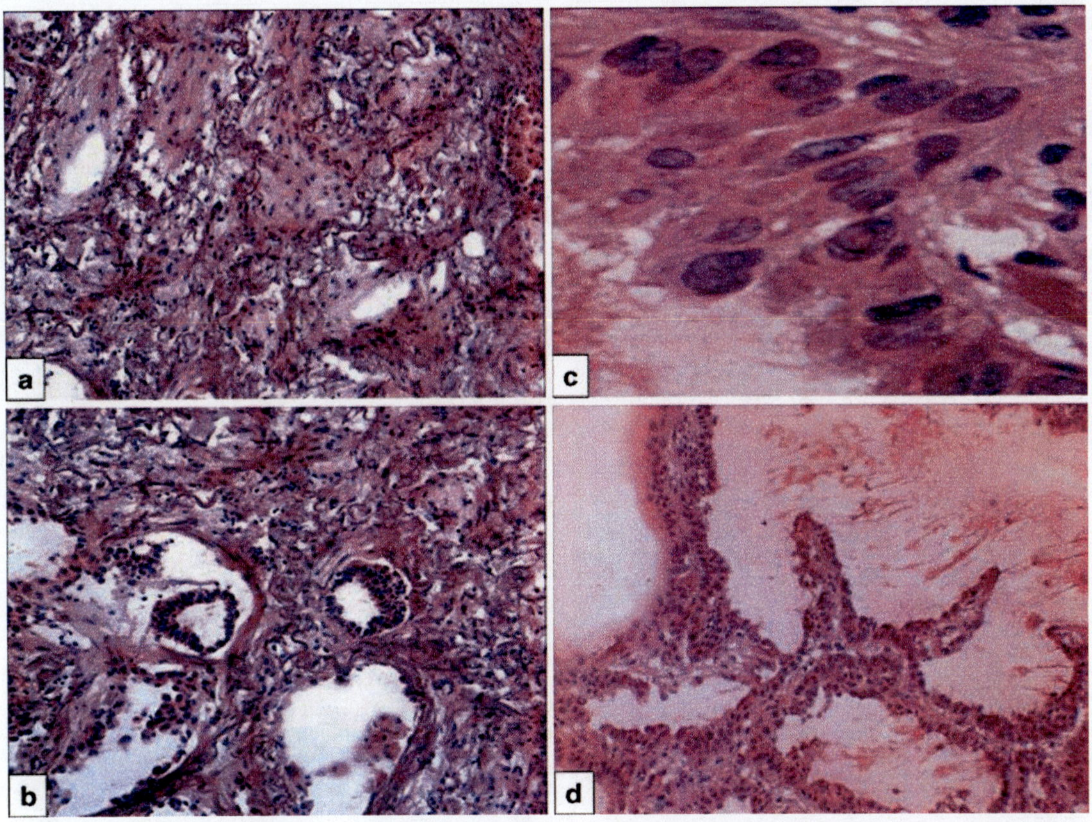

Fig. 13.4 (a–d) The presence of comedonecrosis, solid nests of tumor cells, trabecular architecture, and cribriform growth favors the probability of metastastic breast cancer (From Herbst et al. [76], © 2003–2010 American Society for Clinical Pathology. © 2003–2010 American Journal of Clinical Pathology)

collecting new information that to consider its validity and/or clinical applicability. This chapter suggests a systematic approach to the evaluation of data that could advance the specialty to the next level. The proposed systematic approach does not offer any new analytical concepts but merely organizes the process of collecting and evaluating data in a manner that reflects basic elements of the scientific method. The chapter also discusses the fact that, unfortunately, pathologists have been reluctant to develop novel paradigms that integrate new data with preexistent knowledge taking advantage of statistical and other analytical methods that are currently being use in clinical medicine, business, engineering, and other fields of interest. In an era where evidence levels, quality of care, cost-effectiveness, and other quantitative yardsticks are being increasingly used to evaluate the added value being provided by different physicians to the continuum of patient care, the application of some of the concepts being illustrated in this chapter will hopefully stimulate some interest in the application of EBP concepts to their research and practice.

References

1. Fleming KA. Evidence-based pathology. J Pathol. 1996;179:127–8.
2. Marchevsky AM. Evidence-based medicine in pathology: an introduction. Semin Diagn Pathol. 2005;22:105–15.
3. Marchevsky AM, Wick MR. Evidence-based medicine, medical decision analysis, and pathology. Hum Pathol. 2004;35:1179–88.
4. Straus SE, Richardson WS, Glasziou P, et al. Evidence-based medicine. How to practice and teach EBM. New York: Elsevier; 2005.

5. Kenkel JM. Revisiting the scientific method. Aesthet Surg J. 2009;29:167–8.
6. Michel LA. The epistemology of evidence-based medicine. Surg Endosc. 2007;21:145–51.
7. Sackett D. Evidence-based medicine. Lancet. 1995; 346:1171.
8. Sackett DL, Rosenberg WM. The need for evidence-based medicine. J R Soc Med. 1995;88:620–4.
9. Sackett DL, Rosenberg WM, Gray JA, et al. Evidence based medicine: what it is and what it isn't. BMJ. 1996;312:71–2.
10. Treadwell JR, Tregear SJ, Reston JT, et al. A system for rating the stability and strength of medical evidence. BMC Med Res Methodol. 2006;6:52.
11. Guerette PH. Managed care: cookbook medicine, or quality, cost-effective care? Can Nurse. 1995;91:16.
12. Holm RP. Cookbook medicine. S D Med. 2009; 62:371.
13. Leape L. Are practice guidelines cookbook medicine? J Ark Med Soc. 1989;86:73–5.
14. Parmley WW. Practice guidelines and cookbook medicine – who are the cooks? J Am Coll Cardiol. 1994; 24:567–8.
15. Steinberg KE. Cookbook medicine: recipe for disaster? J Am Med Dir Assoc. 2006;7:470–2.
16. Bhandari M, Zlowodzki M, Cole PA. From eminence-based practice to evidence-based practice: a paradigm shift. Minn Med. 2004;87:51–4.
17. Leppaniemi A. From eminence-based to error-based to evidence-based surgery. Scand J Surg. 2008;97: 2–3.
18. Petri E, Kolbl H. Eminence, or rather eloquence, or rather economy-based medicine? Int Urogynecol J Pelvic Floor Dysfunct. 2004;15:147–8.
19. Marchevsky D. Predicting violence. Br J Psychiatry. 1999;175:585.
20. Brambilla E, Travis WD, Colby TV, et al. The new World Health Organization classification of lung tumours. Eur Respir J. 2001;18:1059–68.
21. Fletcher DM, Unni K, Mertens F. World Health Organization classification of tumors. Tumors of soft tissue and bone. Lyon, France: IARC Press; 2002.
22. Marchevsky AM, McKenna Jr RJ, Gupta R. Thymic epithelial neoplasms: a review of current concepts using an evidence-based pathology approach. Hematol Oncol Clin North Am. 2008;22:543–62.
23. Marchevsky AM, Gupta R, McKenna RJ, et al. Evidence-based pathology and the pathologic evaluation of thymomas: the World Health Organization classification can be simplified into only 3 categories other than thymic carcinoma. Cancer. 2008;112: 2780–8.
24. Gupta R, Marchevsky AM, McKenna RJ, et al. Evidence-based pathology and the pathologic evaluation of thymomas: transcapsular invasion is not a significant prognostic feature. Arch Pathol Lab Med. 2008;132:926–30.
25. Shimosato Y, Mukai K. Atlas of tumor pathology. Tumors of the mediastinum. Washington, DC: AFIP Press; 1997.
26. Masaoka A, Monden Y, Nakahara K, et al. Follow-up study of thymomas with special reference to their clinical stages. Cancer. 1981;48:2485–92.
27. Marchevsky A. The mediastinum. Pathology (Phila). 1996;3:339–48.
28. Marchevsky A, Kaneko M. Surgical pathology of the mediastinum. New York: Raven Press; 1991.
29. Marchevsky AM, Hammond ME, Moran C, et al. Protocol for the examination of specimens from patients with thymic epithelial tumors located in any area of the mediastinum. Arch Pathol Lab Med. 2003; 127:1298–303.
30. Marchevsky AM, Wick MR. Evidence levels for publications in pathology and laboratory medicine. Am J Clin Pathol. 2010;133:366–7.
31. Straus SE, Sackett DL. Bringing evidence to the clinic. Arch Dermatol. 1998;134:1519–20.
32. Dellavalle RP, Freeman SR, Williams HC. Clinical evidence epistemology. J Invest Dermatol. 2007;127: 2668–9.
33. Overman VP. The Cochrane collaboration. Int J Dent Hyg. 2007;5:62.
34. Summerskill W. Cochrane Collaboration and the evolution of evidence. Lancet. 2005;366:1760.
35. Marchevsky AM, Parakh RS, Hakimian B. Radiation therapy does not improve the prognosis of patients with stage II thymoma, supporting previous evidence suggesting that the presence of transcapsular invasion is not a significant prognostic feature. Mod Pathol. 2010;23(1S):409A. Ref Type: Abstract.
36. Marchevsky AM, Gupta R, Casadio C, et al. The World Health Organization classification of thymomas provides significant prognostic information for selected stage III patients: evidence from an international thymoma study group. Hum Pathol. 2010; 41:1413–21.
37. Marchevsky AM, Gupta R, Kusuanco D, et al. The presence of isolated tumor cells and micrometastases in the intrathoracic lymph nodes of lung cancer patients is not associated with decreased survival. Hum Pathol. 2010;41(11):1536–43.
38. Evans JS, Handley SJ, Over DE, et al. Background beliefs in Bayesian inference. Mem Cognit. 2002; 30:179–90.
39. Friston KJ, Penny W, Phillips C, et al. Classical and Bayesian inference in neuroimaging: theory. Neuroimage. 2002;16:465–83.
40. Kersten D, Mamassian P, Yuille A. Object perception as Bayesian inference. Annu Rev Psychol. 2004;55: 271–304.
41. Schmid CH. Using Bayesian inference to perform meta-analysis. Eval Health Prof. 2001;24:165–89.
42. Tenenbaum JB, Griffiths TL. Generalization, similarity, and Bayesian inference. Behav Brain Sci. 2001;24: 629–40.
43. Xu F, Tenenbaum JB. Word learning as Bayesian inference. Psychol Rev. 2007;114:245–72.
44. Zelen M, Parker RA. Case-control studies and Bayesian inference. Stat Med. 1986;5:261–9.

45. Marchevsky AM, Hauptman E, Shepard C, et al. Computerized interactive morphometry of brushing cytology specimens. Acta Cytol. 1988;32:341–6.
46. Marchevsky AM, Klapper E, Gil J. Computerized classification of nuclear profiles in non-Hodgkin's lymphomas. Am J Clin Pathol. 1987;87:561–8.
47. Marchevsky AM, Gil J, Jeanty H. Computerized interactive morphometry in pathology: current instrumentation and methods. Hum Pathol. 1987;18:320–31.
48. Marchevsky AM, Hauptman E, Gil J, et al. Computerized interactive morphometry as an aid in the diagnosis of pleural effusions. Acta Cytol. 1987; 31:131–6.
49. Marchevsky AM, Gil J. Applications of computerized interactive morphometry in pathology. II. A model for computer generated diagnosis. Lab Invest. 1986;54: 708–16.
50. Marchevsky AM, Gupta R, Balzer B. Diagnosis of metastatic neoplasms: a clinicopathologic and morphologic approach. Arch Pathol Lab Med. 2010;134: 194–206.
51. Gupta R, Dastane A, McKenna Jr RJ, et al. What can we learn from the errors in the frozen section diagnosis of pulmonary carcinoid tumors? An evidence-based approach. Hum Pathol. 2009;40:1–9.
52. Gupta R, McKenna Jr R, Marchevsky AM. Lessons learned from mistakes and deferrals in the frozen section diagnosis of bronchioloalveolar carcinoma and well-differentiated pulmonary adenocarcinoma: an evidence-based pathology approach. Am J Clin Pathol. 2008;130:11–20.
53. Marchevsky AM, Wick MR. Evidence-based guidelines for the utilization of immunostains in diagnostic pathology: pulmonary adenocarcinoma versus mesothelioma. Appl Immunohistochem Mol Morphol. 2007;15:140–4.
54. Westfall DE, Fan X, Marchevsky AM. Evidence-based guidelines to optimize the selection of antibody panels in cytopathology: pleural effusions with malignant epithelioid cells. Diagn Cytopathol. 2010;38: 9–14.
55. Cengel KA, Day SJ, vis-Devine S, et al. Effectiveness of the SurePath liquid-based Pap test in automated screening and in detection of HSIL. Diagn Cytopathol. 2003;29:250–5.
56. Godfrey SE. The Pap smear, automated rescreening, and negligent nondisclosure. Am J Clin Pathol. 1999;111:14–7.
57. Keyhani-Rofagha S, Palma T, O'Toole RV. Automated screening for quality control using PAPNET: a study of 638 negative Pap smears. Diagn Cytopathol. 1996;14:316–20.
58. Garcia JJ, Folpe AL. The impact of advances in molecular genetic pathology on the classification, diagnosis and treatment of selected soft tissue tumors of the head and neck. Head Neck Pathol. 2010;4:70–6.
59. Greco FA, Erlander MG. Molecular classification of cancers of unknown primary site. Mol Diagn Ther. 2009;13:367–73.
60. Tang P, Skinner KA, Hicks DG. Molecular classification of breast carcinomas by immunohistochemical analysis: are we ready? Diagn Mol Pathol. 2009;18: 125–32.
61. Marchevsky AM, Tsou JA, Laird-Offringa IA. Classification of individual lung cancer cell lines based on DNA methylation markers: use of linear discriminant analysis and artificial neural networks. J Mol Diagn. 2004;6:28–36.
62. Marchevsky A, Gil J, Silage D. Computerized interactive morphometry as a potentially useful tool for the classification of non-Hodgkin's lymphomas. Cancer. 1986;57:1544–9.
63. Marchevsky AM, Shah S, Patel S. Reasoning with uncertainty in pathology: artificial neural networks and logistic regression as tools for prediction of lymph node status in breast cancer patients. Mod Pathol. 1999;12:505–13.
64. Marchevsky AM, Patel S, Wiley KJ, et al. Artificial neural networks and logistic regression as tools for prediction of survival in patients with Stages I and II non-small cell lung cancer. Mod Pathol. 1998;11: 618–25.
65. Bellotti M, Elsner B, De Paez LA, et al. Neural networks as a prognostic tool for patients with non-small cell carcinoma of the lung. Mod Pathol. 1997;10: 1221–7.
66. Esteva H, Marchevsky A, Nunez T, et al. Neural networks as a prognostic tool of surgical risk in lung resections. Ann Thorac Surg. 2002;73:1576–81.
67. Singson RP, Alsabeh R, Geller SA, et al. Estimation of tumor stage and lymph node status in patients with colorectal adenocarcinoma using probabilistic neural networks and logistic regression. Mod Pathol. 1999;12:479–84.
68. Steindel SJ, Howanitz PJ, Renner SW. Reasons for proficiency testing failures in clinical chemistry and blood gas analysis: a College of American Pathologists Q-Probes study in 665 laboratories. Arch Pathol Lab Med. 1996;120:1094–101.
69. Tholen D, Lawson NS, Cohen T, et al. Proficiency test performance and experience with College of American Pathologists' programs. Arch Pathol Lab Med. 1995;119:307–11.
70. Marchevsky AM, Walts AE, Bose S, et al. Evidence-based evaluation of the risks of malignancy predicted by thyroid fine-needle aspiration biopsies. Diagn Cytopathol. 2010;38:252–9.
71. Marchevsky A, Gupta R, Casadio C, et al. World Health Organization classification of thymomas provides significant prognostic information for selected stage III patients: evidence from an international thymoma study group. Hum Pathol. 2010;41(10): 1413–21.
72. Rieker RJ, Hoegel J, Morresi-Hauf A, et al. Histologic classification of thymic epithelial tumors: comparison of established classification schemes. Int J Cancer. 2002;98:900–6.
73. Marchevsky AM, Gupta R. Interobserver diagnostic variability at "moderate" agreement levels could

significantly change the prognostic estimates of clinicopathologic studies: evaluation of the problem using evidence from patients with diffuse lung disease. Ann Diagn Pathol. 2010;14:88–93.
74. Baak JP. The role of computerized morphometric and cytometric feature analysis in endometrial hyperplasia and cancer prognosis. J Cell Biochem Suppl. 1995;23:137–46.
75. Travis WD, Gal AA, Colby TV, et al. Reproducibility of neuroendocrine lung tumor classification. Hum Pathol. 1998;29:272–9.
76. Herbst J, Jenders R, McKenna R, et al. Evidence-based criteria to help distinguish metastatic breast cancer from primary lung adenocarcinoma on thoracic frozen section. Am J Clin Pathol. 2009;131:122–8.

Evaluation and Reduction of Diagnostic Errors in Pathology Using an Evidence-Based Approach

14

Raouf E. Nakhleh

Keywords
Diagnostic errors in pathology • Evidence-based pathology • Evaluation of diagnostic errors in pathology • Human error in diagnostic pathology

A substantial proportion of patients' diagnoses and treatments are dependent on reliable tissue diagnoses in surgical pathology and cytopathology. This can easily be demonstrated in cases of cancer as well as many inflammatory conditions such as organ rejection [1–4]. In cancer management, tissue diagnosis and staging are the most important determinants of prognosis and therapy. Likewise, determining the level of rejection in allograft biopsies is the main determinant of immunosuppressive therapy. The importance of a correct diagnosis in these situations cannot be overemphasized.

In attempting to reduce errors many advocate a systems approach [5]. At the heart of this approach is the admission that humans are fallible and will make mistakes and therefore the systems around them should be designed to minimize errors while at the same time continuously checking to identify errors and correcting them at the earliest point in the process.

In this scheme of error reduction a handful of reasons are cited as the primary causes of errors. They include; lack of communication, variable input, complexity, inconsistency, human intervention, tight time constraints, and a hierarchical culture. The literature on pathology errors is far from comprehensive and has not for the most part taken this approach but does offer clues of how errors occur and how they could be addressed. In this chapter, I will discuss how errors occur in surgical pathology and then attempt to adapt to pathology existing proven knowledge used in many industries to reduce errors.

Errors in Surgical Pathology

Part of the problem in addressing errors is the various ways that errors can occur and the various ways that they may be reported (Table 14.1). While the literature is variable in measuring the level of errors that exist in anatomic pathology, it is safe to say that errors exist and have been reported in a range up to 40% of cases, hence the need to evaluate and determine ways to reduce errors [6]. A study by Meier et al. focuses on the development and validation of a taxonomy of defects [7]. This report derived its information from review of amended reports from seven institutions. Errors are categorized into four broad categories; misinterpretations, misidentifications, specimen defects, and report defects. Using these categories, Meier et al. were able to estimate the

R.E. Nakhleh (✉)
Department of Pathology, Mayo Clinic Florida,
4500 San Publo Road, Jacksonville, FL 32224, USA
e-mail: Nakhleh.raouf@mayo.edu

A.M. Marchevsky and M.R. Wick (eds.), *Evidence Based Pathology and Laboratory Medicine*,
DOI 10.1007/978-1-4419-1030-1_14,

Table 14.1 Evidence-based approach to error reduction: where do errors occur?

1. Where in the test cycle do errors occur?	**Quality assurance data** Preanalytic – up to 40% Analytic – 25% Postanalytic – 29–44%
2. Where do the most significant errors occur?	**Legal claims** Preanalytic – 8–9% Analytic – 90% Postanalytic – 1%
3. What are the most significant errors?	Analytic error Specimen identification Report defects

Table 14.2 Classification of errors

Error types	Error subtypes
Misinterpretation	False-negative False-positive Misclassification
Misidentification	Patient Tissue Laterality
Specimen defects	Lost Inadequate Absent or discrepant measurements Nonrepresentative sampling Absent or inappropriate ancillary studies
Report defects	Typographical errors Missing or wrong demographic or procedural information Electronic transmission or format defects

occurrence of errors within the framework of the surgical pathology test cycle (Table 14.2). About a fourth of errors occur within the analytic phase (misinterpretation and some specimen defects) of the test cycle. The remaining errors occur about equally within the preanalytic (misidentification and some specimen defects) and postanalytic (report defects) phases of the test cycle.

There are other means of evaluating the existence of error which can focus on significant errors or errors that have the potential for patient harm. Evaluation of errors from a legal perspective yields a completely different picture [8, 9]. Reports of legal judgments and settlements against pathologists demonstrate that the vast majority (>90%) of these cases are analytic errors, and 60–70% of these errors are false-negative results. Since legal judgments and settlements usually result because of patient harm, it may be safe to say that these represent significant diagnostic errors. Error reduction efforts, therefore, should be focused on the analytic phase of the test cycle and the factors in the pre- and postanalytic phase that have a strong influence on determining an accurate diagnosis.

Errors Within the Different Phases of the Test Cycle

In this section, errors are discussed in relationship to where they occur within the test cycle. In the next section, most of these errors will be discussed as to the reason they occur and possible remedies to help reduce errors.

Preanalytic Errors

While all errors in the preanalytic phase of the test cycle are potentiality significant, by virtue of its potential for catastrophe, specimen misidentification stands out as the most important potential error [10]. Misidentified specimens have resulted in surgical procedures being performed on the wrong site and even on the wrong patient. Specimen identification errors not only occur principally within the preanalytic phase of the test cycle but are also well documented within the analytic and postanalytic phases of the test cycle.

The responsibility of initial specimen identification is shared between the laboratory and every other department where specimens are generation. This includes operating rooms, endoscopy suits, physicians' offices, outpatient surgical centers, and interventional radiology among others. Problems occur because the vast majority of individuals that label specimens are usually not trained by pathology and are not accountable to pathology. The system is extremely complex when you consider the number of locations and individuals involved. To get a handle on this problem, an institution has to bring focus on the problem. The Joint Commission has focused on patient identification as a patient safety goal and specimen identification is part of this goal [11]. It is recommended that specimen identification be made an institutional goal and not simply a laboratory goal [10, 12, 13]. In this light, the responsibility of specimen identification is shared equally between clinical departments and pathology. Factors that have been shown to improve specimen identification are twofold [14]. First is the introduction of redundant checks such as remote order entry for inclusion of patients into the laboratory system, checks of patient identity at every hand-off such as at specimen pick-up and at accessioning and checking the patient identity before release of reports. Second, over time continuous monitoring has been shown to improve specimen identification. The reason is not clear, but it is thought the continuous monitoring keeps the focus on the problem that results in long-term improvement.

Analytic Errors

Analytic errors or diagnostic errors occur for a variety of reasons, some of which are addressed blow. While analytic errors are not insignificant, if one considers the complexity of systems needed to arrive at a correct diagnosis, it is a wonder that more errors do not occur. To arrive at a correct diagnosis three systems must operate adequately to achieve the desired result. (1) A lesion must be clinically identified and adequately sampled. (2) The laboratory must be able to appropriately process the tissue and have the ability to provide all necessary ancillary tests. (3) A pathologist must have sufficient knowledge, experience, and judgment to arrive at the appropriate diagnosis. The first system resides in the preanalytic realm and is mostly beyond the control of the laboratory, and therefore will not be addressed here. The second system speaks to the optimal operation of the laboratory. Error reduction in laboratory systems is discussed below by using lean design, automation, reducing complexity, and by incorporating multiple checks into the system [15, 16]. One further step that should be addressed regarding ancillary tests is the establishment of appropriate validation procedures and the prudent use of proficiency testing material where available [17]. The third system includes the pathologists' individual training, specialization, organization, and individual traits. Error reduction in this area is addressed collectively with the use of consensus diagnostic criteria, prudent use of redundant sign-out including the use of specialists, the use of ancillary testing when appropriate, and the use of checklists. Many of these topics are also addressed below.

Postanalytic Errors

The two most often cited postanalytic errors are incomplete reports and lack of communication for significant and unexpected (critical) findings [18, 19]. Effectively addressing incomplete reports has been demonstrated with the use of computer based checklist reports [20]. Occasionally, however, reports are incomplete because the wrong or incomplete history is given. This can be established with simple examples; colonic biopsies are performed for multiple reasons including colonic polyps or to rule out inflammatory processes. If the biopsy is accompanied by the history of polyp, the pathologist will address the differential diagnosis of a mass and if no findings of a polyp are identified, the diagnosis will most likely be "benign colonic mucosa." However, if the history is "diarrhea" then the pathologist will examine the biopsy tissue more carefully for inflammatory conditions and if none are found the diagnosis is likely to be something akin to "no inflammatory changes identified." Sometimes a clinician has a specific diagnosis to rule out such as amyloidosis. If this is not conveyed, it may be easily missed and ancillary studies may not be performed to identify or exclude the specific finding.

Reasons for Diagnostic Errors and Potential Remedies

Variable Input: Lack of Communication

Many studies have demonstrated that communication failure is a key element in many errors in medicine [21, 22] (Tables 14.3–14.5). One of the

Table 14.3 What are the causes of errors?

What are the factors that contribute to errors in medicine?	Can an example be found in pathology that demonstrates each factor?
Variable input – communication	Absent or incomplete clinical history
Complexity	There are potentially over 100 steps in reaching a diagnosis
Inconsistency	Use of diagnostic criteria, report formatting and content, training, and experience
Human intervention	The entire process is dependent on human handling of specimens
Hand-offs	Tissue is transferred multiple times with the need to maintain ID
Tight time constraints	Batch mode is pervasive in surgical pathology
Hierarchical culture	Lack of questioning of authority

Table 14.4 Potential remedies or solution to errors

What are the factors that contribute to errors in medicine?	What are the potential solutions for pathology?
Variable input – communication	Electronic medical record, remote order entry with forced functions, automate clinical history retrieval, multidisciplinary clinical teams
Complexity	Lean production redesign, automate were possible, standardize
Inconsistency	Standardization of diagnostic criteria, Standardize procedures, Standardize report content and layout, continuous education
Human intervention	Use checklists to assure compliance, automate were possible, remove distractions
Hand-offs	Use of tools such as ink, barcodes, RFID, remote order entry, redundant checks to assure correct ID
Tight time constraints	Continuous processing as much as possible, emphasize doing the job well vs. doing the job fast, remind all of the pitfalls
Hierarchical culture	Change the culture, take away fear of reporting problems

Table 14.5 Additional error prevention strategies

Continuous monitoring	Continuous monitoring has been shown to improve a measure over time. Two areas relevant to surgical pathology include specimen identification and frozen section – permanent section correlation
Report formatting	1. Use of diagnostic headlines to emphasize key points 2. Maintenance of layout continuity with other reports and over time 3. Optimization of information density 4. Reduction of extraneous information

most important communications that has been shown to affect diagnostic accuracy and completeness in the clinical information provided with the specimen. Variability in the content and accuracy of clinical information provided to surgical pathology with the biopsy tissue has been shown in multiple studies to affect diagnostic accuracy [23–26]. In a study of amended reports, 10% of cases were amended because additional information was obtained beyond the requisition slip [25]. An additional 20% of cases were amended because the clinician asked for review of the case, presumably because of an apparent clinical-pathologic discrepancy. In a study focused on clinical history provided by clinicians, 6.0% of cases in which additional history was obtained lead to a change of diagnosis [24]. And in a study of malpractice claims against pathologists, up to 20% of cases were due to the pathologist's ability to obtain all the pertinent information [26]. A recent study of atypical melanocytic lesions showed a significant increase in diagnostic agreement with the inclusion of pertinent clinical information [23]. Unfortunately, there are no good studies that have attempted to improve on the clinical input to pathologists. The increasing availability of electronic medical records, although not proven, seems to have alleviated some problems. The pathologist still has to take the initiative to find the desired information. Adoption of electronic medical records appears to be underway in medium and large hospitals and laboratory systems. Significant gaps remain particularly for specimens that are obtained at doctors' offices and outpatient centers beyond a defined healthcare system or institution. Over time, developments of secure internet based technology solutions are likely to facilitate the electronic medical record. One method that has been shown to improve patient identification and could improved clinical information is remote order entry [14]. Functionality that would force the inclusion of the clinical history before a specimen can be entered into the laboratory system could be adopted. Another potential solution could be the automatic inclusion of the clinical note of the physician that obtains the tissue. Of course these solutions are not possible without the presence of robust computer systems.

Complexity

There is a greater chance of mishap with greater complexity. Intuitively, it seems obvious that a process with many steps has a greater chance of error than a similar process with only one or two steps. This can actually be demonstrated mathematically in hypothetical and real situations. If a process has one step in it and has a 1% chance of error, a similar process with 25 steps and a 1% error at each step bring that total error risk to 22% [5]. This can be demonstrated in real life with measured errors as well.

Surgical pathology errors have not been measured at every step, but surgical pathology is a complex process requiring numerous steps within the laboratory to complete tissue processing and diagnosis with endless variations that may lead to error. This is the reason why many have used lean production techniques to improve histologic processes, gain efficiency, and reduce errors. Using lean methodology, Zarbo et al. reduced the overall misidentification case rate and histological slide misidentification rate by 62 and 95%, respectively [15].

Although variable results have been achieved, at this time, lean redesign with selective introduction of automation appears to offer the best opportunity for improvement in the histology laboratory [15, 27, 28]. Lean redesign addresses three potential error prone processes. First, lean aims to either eliminate steps when possible or better alien steps so that processes are smoother and less disruptive (reduce complexity). Second, lean redesigns of surgical pathology introduces the judicial use of technology with the use of barcodes or other technologies to eliminate redundant steps such as reentry of identification data on slides and blocks. The introduction of technology addresses issues of inconsistency in hand writing or data reentry and in other processes such as staining with the introduction of automatic stainers. Third, lean redesign results in standardization of processes and the elimination of conflicting procedures and the need to train in multiple procedures.

Inconsistency

Inconsistency can be demonstrated as a source of error in at least two ways in surgical pathology. The first is in the effect of diagnostic criteria on diagnostic reproducibility and the second is in the pathologists' ability to provide more complete reports with the use of synoptic reports. During the past couple of decades dramatic improvements have been made in the adoption of standardization in diagnostic criteria and in the adoption of standardized cancer reports.

The following example demonstrates the effect of the use of standardized diagnostic criteria on the level of diagnostic agreement. In 1991, Dr. Rosai conducted a study which strongly suggested that inter-observer concordance in the classification of breast ductal proliferative disease was unacceptably low [29]. In this study, Dr. Rosai asked a panel of experts to review the same set of cases and render their diagnoses. Soon after publication of this study, Schnitt et al. published a similar study that demonstrated high concordance among a panel of the same experts in the diagnosis of proliferative ductal lesions [30].

In the study by Schnitt et al., the experts were instructed to use standardized criteria for the diagnosis of lesions. The difference is a stark demonstration of the power of standardization. This has been shown in other areas of surgical pathology such as urothelial neoplasia, Barrett's dysplasia and organ rejection [1, 2, 31, 32].

The other aspect of standardization is that of report content. This is particularly important in oncology where different treatment options are available and are dependent on pathologic grading, staging, and tumor marker expression [33, 34]. This is easily demonstrated using the example of breast cancer where a variety of treatment options are considered based on tumor grade, stage, and the expression of ER, PR and HER2. The adoption of national standards in the form of standard grading and staging of tumors has greatly facilitated and accelerated national treatment trials in the evaluation of potential therapies. This has been further accentuated with the use of standardized computer based forms that have been shown in multiple studies but none as eloquently as in a randomized prospective examination of pathology reports in a study by Branston et al. [20]. The control arm of the study included eight hospitals that did not use computer based cancer reports (checklists) and the study arm included eight hospitals that used computer based cancer reports (checklists). This study concluded that reports in the hospitals with the computer checklists were more complete 28% of the time. The study also found that clinicians found these reports preferable while pathologists found them acceptable.

One aspect of reports that should be considered is the ability of clinicians to derive the information that they need to treat the patient from the report. Powsner demonstrated that clinicians routinely misinterpreted pathologists' reports 30% of the time [35]. Factors that were cited to be associated with improvement of this gap included familiarity with report format and clinical experience. Dr. Valenstine in a review of pathology report formatting suggests that four evidence-based and time-tested principles may be helpful in formatting reports for more effective communication. These include: (1) the use of diagnostic headlines to emphasize key points, (2) maintenance of layout continuity with other reports and over time, (3) optimization of information density, and (4) reduction of extraneous information [36]. Dr. Valenstine based his conclusion by extension of research performed in other fields outside of medicine including cockpit design in aviation and newspaper print effectiveness.

Human Intervention

Surgical pathology remains a process that is heavily dependent on human physical and intellectual activity. With the exception of very short segments of the test cycle, surgical pathology is most assuredly dependent on humans doing their jobs. As such, surgical pathology is subject to human error. As in other areas of health care, a systems approach to quality management in surgical pathology has been recommended to reduce errors [37, 38]. At its core, this management style advocates design of processes with two features in mind; prevention of errors and detection of errors.

In design of systems that prevent errors, two methods have prevailed. First, introduction of automation whenever possible works well where information must be re-inputted into the system [15]. The use of slide and block labelers as well as the use of barcode technology are good examples where human intervention in the form of reentering information may be avoided with the use of automated equipment thus reducing the potential for error. Automation may be used to simplify a process in the sense that a machine will do multiple steps, whereas from the human perspective the process is reduced to one or two steps. Machines also have the added advantage of reducing procedural variations because machines operate at a tight range of specification and are not subject to distraction. Automatic stainers and coverslipers demonstrate this utility well.

Reducing cognitive errors at the point of diagnosis has been challenging, but methods have emerged that reduce or detect error. The principle method of error prevention has been redundancy in the form of review of cases before or after cases are verified or signed out.

In three publications it has been shown that review of cases by more than one pathologists helps lower the number of amended reports and possibly the error rate [25, 39, 40]. In a multi-institutional study of amended reports, cases that were reviewed before a case was signed out had an amended report rate of 1.2/1,000, vs. 1.6/1,000 for cases that were reviewed after they were signed out. Renshaw and Gould demonstrated that cases reviewed by greater than one pathologist resulted in a lower disagreement rate and amended report rate. Dr. Novis also presented evidence that review of cases by two pathologists vs. one resulted in lower error rates. The best strategy for case review has not been formulated, but may be dependent on the type of material seen at any one institution and the number of pathologists participating in case sign-out. Review of cases after they have been verified is an extension of the same principle, but falls into the realm of error detection, since this process would occur beyond the point of error prevention.

The use of checklists has been advocated as a tool to control the extent of human intervention. This can easily be demonstrated with the use of cancer checklists for reporting all necessary parameters in cancer reports [20, 33, 34, 41]. With the use of checklists, a pathologist is reminded of all the items that should be in that report. Indeed, a computer system can be built to force individuals to complete a report before a report can be verified or signed out. Checklists can also be used for a whole host of tasks in the laboratory to assure that things get done [42]. An example of this includes a list of tasks that a technologist or clerk must perform to prepare an accessioning station at the beginning of the day and a list of tasks that must be done at the end of the day to make sure nothing is forgotten.

Updated Knowledge on Diagnostic Criteria and Staging

Various subspecialty groups have expended a great deal of effort to establish diagnostic criteria for various diseases and conditions with the intent of standardization. But pathologists still have to update themselves and their systems in the use of these diagnostic criteria. Part of the problem is the great diversity of specimen types that pathologists have to address. Some larger pathology practice groups have adopted complete subspecialization for their case sign outs. In this situation, a GI pathologist takes care of the GI cases, a hematopathologist signs out the hematologic cases and so on. Individuals in each subspecialty are responsible for updating themselves on the current literature in that field and often are reasonably knowledgeable on the treatment options and other clinical scenarios. In this type of practice the pathologists communicate frequently with their clinician counter parts in conferences and on specific cases. Also, in larger groups there tends to be multiple specialists in the same field and so there is ample depth and opportunity to discuss and work though complex cases. In intermediate sized pathology groups, a similar strategy has taken form, although not to the same extent. In these groups, most pathologists are generalists, but have subspecialty interests. Each pathologist with subspecialty interest takes on the responsibility of keeping up with a particular field and is responsible for updating their pathology colleagues while at the same time serves as the point person with their clinical colleagues in that field. For a small practice, it is much more difficult to be up to date in all subspecialty fields. For this reason, smaller practices tend to liberally use expert consultation in areas outside their comfort zone. Therefore, we have at least three practice systems that attempt to address the knowledge needs of pathologists. It is not clear which system is best or produces the least amount of errors. I am unaware of any studies that have attempted to directly measure the efficacy of these practice settings. Reports that have attempted to study differences between generalists and specialists in clinical practice offer some generality that may apply to pathology as well. These studies suggest that specialists were generally more knowledgeable in their area of interest and were quicker to adopt new treatments, but also used more resources [43, 44]. There is a suggestion that the quality of care by specialists exceeded care by generalist for selected conditions.

Tight Time Constraints

A number of external pressures focus the need to have time constraints in surgical pathology. Regulatory mandates, while not strict, are often cited as a main reason to have good turnaround time. However, pressure from clinical colleagues and an inherent need to please our customers (patients and clinicians) have greater influence on our desire to produce a diagnostic result in the least amount of time possible.

The total turnaround time is usually not the real issue leading to errors, the problem is in batch work and time constraints. In an ideal environment work would be evenly spaced and maintained at regular intervals with sufficient time to accomplish each task. Surgical pathology is prone to batch work and time constraints; specimens are typically delivered in batches and are accessioned and processed in batches. After dissection and placement in cassettes, the tissue typically must be placed onto processors that begin at a certain point in time thus providing time constraints. This has a greater impact when the workload is heavier than usual or when fewer employees are available. This problem also applies to the pathologist at sign-out where cases are usually brought in batches. While the pathologist rarely has a definitive deadline to complete the work, there is pressure to get those cases done that day and maintain an adequate turn-around time. This pressure may be intensified if the pathologist has other commitments that occupy a portion of the day and the work should be completed before a long weekend or a vacation.

The net effect of batch work and time constraints is that people may skip over critical steps that assures proper handling, processing, and interpretation. This could include quality checks that were instituted to prevent errors such as double checking two patient identifiers.

Hierarchical Culture

A hierarchical culture is one in which authority is not questioned for fear of retribution or more commonly to avoid the unpleasant consequence of such episodes. While this type of behavior frequently is generational and cultural, it is frequently encouraged or accentuated by the behavior of leadership. While this is often unintentional, the pathologist's mood and response to a simple event such as technologist bringing in additional tray of slides on a busy day may be sufficient to initiate a technologist's avoidance behavior. It takes only a few similar episodes for a technologist to decide that avoidance is the best strategy for a harmonious work day. So when problems occur that may be addressed quickly as they occur, the choice is made to avoid communication and to let things stand. To alleviate this situation the pathologist or others in a position of authority have to remove that element of fear and discomfort that comes with bringing forth problems. This way, problems are managed in real time and are not allowed to fester.

References

1. Racusen LC, Solez K, Colvin RB, et al. The Banff 97 working classification of renal allograft pathology. Kidney Int. 1999;55:713–23.
2. Demetris AJ, Batts KP, Dhillon AP, et al. Banff schema for grading liver allograft rejection: an international consensus document. Hepatology. 1997;25: 658–63.
3. Edge SB, Byrd DR, Compton CC, Fritz AG, Greene FL, Trotti A, editors. AJCC cancer staging manual. 7th ed. New York: Springer; 2009.
4. Raab SS, Grzybicki DM, Janosky JE, et al. Clinical impact and frequency of anatomic pathology errors in cancer diagnoses. Cancer. 2005;104:2205–13.
5. Spath PL. Reducing errors through work systems improvement. In: Spath PL, editor. Error reduction in health care. Chicago: AHA Press; 1999. p. 199–234.
6. Weiss MA. Analytic variables: diagnostic accuracy. In: Nakhleh RE, Fitzgibbons PL, editors. Quality management in anatomic pathology: promoting patient safety through systems improvement and error reduction. Northfield: The College of American Pathologists; 2005. p. 55–61.
7. Meier FA, Zarbo RJ, Varney RC, et al. Amended reports: development and validation of a taxonomy of defects. Am J Clin Pathol. 2008;130:238–46.
8. Kornstein MJ, Byrne SP. The medicolegal aspect of error in pathology; A search of jury verdicts and settlements. Arch Pathol Lab Med. 2007;131:615–8.
9. Troxel DB. Medicolegal aspects of error in pathology. Arch Pathol Lab Med. 2007;130:617–9.

10. Nakhleh RE. Lost, mislabeled and unsuitable surgical pathology specimens. Pathol Case Rev. 2003;8: 98–102.
11. The Joint Commission. Accreditation Program; Laboratory National Patient Safety goals. http://www.jointcommission.org/GeneralPublic/NPSG/gp_npsg.htm. Accessed 1 May 2010.
12. Simpson JB. A unique approach for reducing specimen labeling errors: combining marketing techniques with performance improvement. Clin Leadership Manag Rev. 2001;15:401–5.
13. Makary MA, Epstein J, Pronovost PJ, Millman EA, Hartmann EC, Freischlag JA. Surgical specimen identification errors: a new measure of quality in surgical care. Surgery. 2007;141(4):450–5.
14. Valenstine PN, Raab SS, Walsh MK. Identification errors involving clinical laboratories: a College of American Pathologists Q-Probes study of patient and specimen identification errors at 120 institutions. Arch Pathol Lab Med. 2006;130:1106–13.
15. Zarbo RJ, Tuthill M, D'Angelo R, et al. The Henry Ford Production System; reduction of surgical pathology in-process misidentification defects by bar code-specific work process standardization. Am J Clin Pathol. 2009;131:468–77.
16. D'Angelo R, Zarbo RJ. The Henry Ford Production System; Measures of process defects and waste in surgical pathology as a basis for quality improvement initiatives. Am J Clin Pathol. 2007;128:423–9.
17. Wolf AC, Hammond EH, Schwartz JN, et al. American Society of Clinical Oncology/College of American Pathologists guideline recommendations for human epidermal grown factor receptor 2 testing in breast cancer. Arch Pathol Lab Med. 2007; 131(1):18–43.
18. Nakhleh RE. Patient safety and error reduction in surgical pathology. Arch Pathol Lab Med. 2008;132: 181–5.
19. Nakhleh RE, Souers R, Brown RW. Significant and unexpected, and critical diagnosis in surgical pathology: a college of American Pathologists' survey of 1130 laboratories. Arch Pathol Lab Med. 2009;133: 1375–8.
20. Branston LK, Greening S, Newcombe RG, et al. The implementation of guidelines and computerized forms improves the completeness of cancer pathology reporting. The CROPS project: a randomized controlled trial in pathology. Eur J Cancer. 2002;38: 764–72.
21. Lingard L, Espin S, Whyte S, et al. Communication failures in the operating room: an observational classification of recurrent types and effects. Qual Saf Health Care. 2004;13(5):330–4.
22. Krautscheild LC. Improving communication among healthcare providers: preparing student nurses for practice. Int J Nurs Educ Scholarsh. 2008;5:1–13.
23. Ferrara G, Argenyi Z, Argenziano G, et al. The influence of clinical information in the histopathologic diagnosis of melanocytic skin neoplasms. PLoS One. 2009;4:e5375.
24. Nakhleh RE, Gephardt G, Zarbo RJ. Necessity of clinical information in surgical pathology: a College of American Pathologists Q-Probes Study of 771,475 surgical pathology cases from 341 institutions. Arch Pathol Lab Med. 1999;123:615–9.
25. Nakhleh RE, Zarbo RJ. Amended reports in surgical pathology and implications for diagnostic error detection and avoidance: a College of American Pathologists' Q-Probes Study of 1, 667, 547 accessioned cases in 359 laboratories. Arch Pathol Lab Med. 1998;22:303–9.
26. Troxell DB, Sabella JD. Problem areas in pathology practice: uncovered by review of malpractice claims. Am J Surg Pathol. 1994;18:821–31.
27. Raab SS, Grzybicki DM, Condel JL, et al. Effect of lean method implementation in the histopathology section of an anatomical pathology laboratory. J Clin Pathol. 2008;61:1193–9.
28. Condel JL, Sharbaugh DT, Raab SS, et al. Error free pathology: applying lean production methods to anatomic pathology. Clin Lab Med. 2004;24:865–99.
29. Rosai J. Borderline epithelial lesions of the breast. Am J Surg Pathol. 1991;15:209–21.
30. Schnitt SJ, Connolly JL, Tavassoli FA, et al. Interobserver reproducibility in the diagnosis of ductal proliferative breast lesions using standardized criteria. Am J Surg Pathol. 1992;16(12):1133–43.
31. Montgomery E, Bronner MP, Goldblum JR, et al. Reproducibility of the diagnosis of dysplasia in Barrett esophagus: a reaffirmation. Hum Pathol. 2001;32(4):368–78.
32. Yin H, Leong AS. Histologic grading of noninvasive papillary urothelial tumors: validation of the 1998 WHO/ISUP system by immunophenotyping and follow-up. Am J Clin Pathol. 2004;121(5):679–87.
33. Ruby SG, Henson DE. Practice protocols for surgical pathology: a communication from the Cancer Committee of the College of American Pathologists. Arch Pathol Lab Med. 1994;118:120–1.
34. Fielding LP, Henson DE. Multiple prognostic factors and outcome analysis in patients with cancer: communication from the American Joint Committee on Cancer. Cancer. 1993;17:2426–9.
35. Powsner SM, Costa J, Homer RJ. Clinicians are from Mars and pathologists are from Venus: clinician interpretation of pathology reports. Arch Pathol Lab Med. 2000;124:1040–6.
36. Valenstein PN. Formatting pathology reports: applying four design principles to improve communication and patient safety. Arch Pathol Lab Med. 2008;132: 84–94.
37. Norris B. Human factors and safe patient care. J Nurs Manag. 2009;17(2):203–11.
38. D'Addessi A, Bongiovanni L, Volpe A, Pinto F, Bassi P. Human factor in surgery: from Three Mile Island to the operation room. Urol Int. 2009;83(3): 249–57.
39. Novis D. Routine review of surgical pathology cases as a method by which to reduce diagnostic errors in a community hospital. Pathol Case Rev. 2005;10:63–7.

40. Renshaw AA, Gould EW. Measuring the value of review of pathology material by a second pathologist. Am J Clin Pathol. 2006;125:737–9.
41. Association of Directors of Anatomic and Surgical Pathology. Standardization of the surgical pathology report. Am J Surg Pathol. 1992;16(1):84–6.
42. Brown RW. Quality management in the histology laboratory. In: Nakhleh RE, Fitzgibbons PL, editors. Quality management in anatomic pathology: promoting patient safety through systems improvement and error reduction. Northfield: The College of American Pathologists; 2005. p. 77–92.
43. Harrold LR, Field TS, Gurwitz JH. Knowledge, pattern of care and outcomes of care for generalists and specialists. J Gen Intern Med. 1999;14:499–511.
44. Donohoe MT. Comparing generalist and specialist care; discrepancies, deficiencies and excesses. Arch Intern Med. 1998;158:1596–608.

Meta-Analysis 101 for Pathologists 15

Ruta Gupta and Alberto M. Marchevsky

Keywords

Meta-analysis in pathology, evidence-based pathology • Data collection in pathology • Odds ratios • Effect sizes • Forest plots • Funnel plots • Publication Bias

Meta-analysis is a statistical procedure that integrates the results of independent studies with a similar research hypothesis, explores data heterogeneity and synthesizes summaries if appropriate [1]. Well conducted meta-analysis allows for objective integration and comparison of multiple study results and can also be used to explain the heterogeneity between study results [1]. The basic principles, applications, construction, and statistical methods of meta-analysis are discussed in more detail in Chap. 9 by Dr. Vamvakas. This statistical method has been applied to the integration of randomized controlled clinical trials in an attempt to estimate overall effects. Meta-analysis has been used in epidemiology to investigate the reasons for differences in risk estimates between observational studies and to discover patterns of differences among study results. In this chapter, we attempt to provide pathologists potentially interested in applying meta-analysis in their research with a simplified "how-to" guide to the performance of meta-analysis, using examples from our previous experience.

Evidence-based medicine (EBM) has advocated the use of meta-analysis for systematic and quantitative analysis of randomized control trials for over a decade [2]. Three general applications of meta-analysis include: (1) integration of the findings of studies with varying sample size but demonstrating treatment effect operating in the same direction, (2) investigation of the reasons for disagreements among studies reporting contradictory treatment effects, and (3) integration of the findings of different studies with similar research hypothesis but not attaining statistical significance due to small sample sizes or other factors that influence statistical power [3–5]. The results of the first type of studies are usually used for the design of definitive randomized controlled clinical trials (RCT) with an optimal cohort size that can provide level I evidence. The results of the second type of studies can be very helpful to explain the reasons for contradictory results in studies using similar hypotheses. The use of meta-analysis to integrate the results of underpowered, nonsignificant studies as an alternative to RCT in clinical research is controversial [5].

R. Gupta (✉)
Department of Anatomic Pathology,
The Canberra Hospital, ACT Pathology, Garran,
Australian Capital Territory 2606, Australia
e-mail: rutagupta@gmail.com

A.M. Marchevsky and M.R. Wick (eds.), *Evidence Based Pathology and Laboratory Medicine*,
DOI 10.1007/978-1-4419-1030-1_15,

Applications of Meta-Analysis in Anatomic Pathology

Anatomic pathologists have been slow to accept the basic tenets of EBM, although there is a recent increasing interest in their application to the specialty, so-called evidence-based pathology (EBP) [3–6]. The traditional apprenticeship based teaching in anatomical pathology emphasizes the learning from the "experience of one's teachers." This learning model has great strengths as it helps transmit information in an interactive manner and provides students with the role models offered by various teachers, but it also has some of the disadvantages that EBM advocates have attributed to so-called Eminence-Based Medicine [6–9]. In particular, anatomic pathologists place great confidence in the opinion and publications of their teachers and tend to disregard findings or recommendations published by others that contradict them. In addition, the majority of literature in anatomical pathology comprises of case control studies, case series, case reports, and opinion based narratives where the importance of variables such as study design, sample size, patient selection bias, length of follow-up, treatment effect, and others is not emphasized [10]. Systematic reviews and meta-analysis provide the methodology to integrate information from the literature in a manner that is potentially more comprehensive and less subjective than ad-hoc literature reviews prepared by experts.

Only a few studies have attempted to use meta-analysis in Anatomic Pathology [11–16]. For example, Faraji et al. evaluated renal epithelioid angiomyolipomas with meta-analysis in an attempt to identify various prognostic factors for this newly defined relatively unusual entity using the data available in 69 studies in the literature and demonstrated that male gender, large tumor size, marked cytologic atypia, and extensive tumor necrosis portend an unfavorable outcome [14]. Anderson et al. used meta-analysis to evaluate the utility of immunohistochemical panels in determining the site of origin of metastatic malignancies. The results of their meta-analysis showed that studies evaluating the utility of immunohistochemistry using both primary as well as metastatic tumors provided correct identification in 82.3% cases as against 65.6% in the studies using only metastatic tumors. The authors thus confirmed that there exists an unmet need for additional definitive immunomarkers and also emphasized the importance of minimum performance measures while evaluating newer diagnostic modalities [15]. Several novel prognostic markers are being evaluated for melanoma, however none of these are incorporated into clinically relevant guidelines, staging systems, or standard of care for melanoma patients. Gould Rothberg et al. evaluated the reasons for this disconnects using meta-analysis. Their conclusions reflect the current state of literature in anatomic pathology and emphasize the need for stringent adherence to reporting guidelines, test validation, and cohort selection [16]. We recently used meta-analysis to evaluate a variety of problems related to anatomic pathology and some of these materials are used to illustrate various aspects of the techniques in this chapter [11–13].

Meta-Analysis Methodology: A Step by Step Guide to the Analysis

The application of meta-analysis to the evaluation of data from the literature and/or own experience is relatively simple with the use of modern software. We have performed our studies using Comprehensive Meta-analysis 2.0 (Biostat, Inc. Englewood, New Jersey). Several other commercial softwares are available, including Clin Tool software (http://www.clintools.com/contact.html), Meta-analyst (http://tuftscaes.org/meta_analyst/) providing free online calculators for meta-analysis of binary, continuous and diagnostic data, Metastat (http://echo.edres.org:8080/meta/metastat.htm) and others.

Data Collection: Systematic Literature Review and Evidence Summaries

Meta-analysis is usually well suited for comparing the effects of a particular variable of interest in a test group using a well-matched control group to estimate odds ratios (OR). The first and usually most difficult and time consuming step in the application of meta-analysis to published data is the performance of a systematic literature review to collect comprehensive data from the literature. As explained in previous chapters, systematic literature reviews include a specific time period and explicit listings of database/s searched and search terms, in contrast to ad-hoc reviews that allow investigators to select references from the literature based on subjective criteria not specified in a manuscript. The data elements of interest for study with meta-analysis could be, for example, the effect of a particular treatment, the prognostic value of a test (e.g., survival, recurrence rate, other) or others. The data is organized in evidence summaries in a manner that is suitable for analysis and as explained below. It is often practical to insert it into spreadsheets such as Excel (Microsoft, Redmond WA), in a manner that can be pasted directly into Comprehensive Meta-analysis 2.0 (Biostat, Inc. Englewood, New Jersey) or other software.

Unfortunately, it is often quite difficult to extract information that is suitable for meta-analysis from the medical literature because of the lack of reporting standards. Indeed, attempts at performing meta-analysis on published data can provide investigators with an eye-opening experience regarding the extensive variability in the manner that results are often reported in the anatomic pathology and other medical literature [16]. For example, the data collected in various studies is frequently embedded in different areas of a manuscript, such as "Methods," "Results", and "Discussion." Presence of protein expression by immunohistochemistry is often variably defined in different studies with lower limits for positivity ranging from 5 to 20% [17–20]. Outcomes such as survival and response to treatment are reported using variable definitions (e.g., overall survival, or disease specific survival), and using variable lengths of follow-up [21, 22]. Use of ambiguous terminology in medical publications is one of the most difficult to overcome barriers during the collection of data for meta-analysis [16].

Another common problem during the collection of data for meta-analysis is that medical publications frequently describe only secondary data such as p values, sensitivity, specificity, or other selected results rather than listing the data collected during the study and used by the investigators in their statistical analysis. This type of secondary data does not permit reviewers or a reader to double check on the accuracy of the results reported in publications and does not make available to other investigators the data originally collected in a study that could be combined with the results of other studies reporting similar effects and analyzed with meta-analysis. With the advent of relatively inexpensive storage capability in computer networks, the widespread use of the Web and the progressive migration of publications into electronic formats, it may be possible in the near future to develop new publication standards that encourage the storage of the primary data used by the authors of a publication in their calculations in "electronic appendices" that are made available to reviewers and readers and that could be used by investigators in future studies. This data would probably need to be copyright protected, as currently text and tables are.

We will illustrate the performance of a systematic review, collection of data, and preparation of evidence summaries for meta-analysis using examples from our recent study evaluating the prognostic value of the 2004 World Health Organization (WHO) histologic classification of thymomas [13, 23]. In our study, we elected to query the English literature for the period 1999–2007, as a previous classification scheme for thymomas proposed by WHO in 1999 was quite similar to the 2004 version being investigated, using the PubMed database of the National Library of Medicine and the following search terms: thymomas, pathology, prognosis, and/or stage. We arbitrarily elected as an inclusion criteria in the meta-analysis, availability of 5 years minimum of clinical follow-up. The search identified 15 studies with 2,192 thymoma patients classified according to WHO histologic type and followed postoperatively for longer than 5 years [13]. Survival and recurrence, by WHO histologic type, were selected as the variables of interest.

As the study was not designed to investigate the effect of particular treatment on a test group, the usual application of Comprehensive Meta-analysis 2.0 (Biostat, Inc. Englewood, New Jersey) software, we compared the number of patients being alive or dead at follow-up, by two histologic types at a time, one representing a "test group" and the other a "control group." As the meta-analysis was performed comparing the prognosis of patients with two different WHO histologic types of type at a time, for example those of thymomas A and AB, and the software needs the number of patients in each category to estimate odds and OR, we collected four data points from each study: total number of thymoma A patients, number of thymoma A patients alive at follow-up, number of thymoma AB patients, and number of thymoma AB patients alive at follow-up. The evidence summary of these data is shown in Table 15.1.

Data Analysis – Calculation of Odds Ratios, Preparation of Forest Plots, and Selection of Model to Be Used for Meta-analysis

Selected columns from Table 15.1 were readily imported into Comprehensive Meta-analysis 2.0 (Biostat, Inc. Englewood, New Jersey) software and OR, log OR, and standard errors were automatically estimated for each study, as shown in Fig. 15.1. Please note that the software estimates OR and other statistics only for studies that include an "event." In this example, an "event" requires that a study report some patients that did not survive, resulting in smaller numbers of "survived patients" than "total number of patients" in either the thymoma A or AB groups. Studies such as those by Kim, Bedini, and others that do not report "events" for these particular subsets of thymoma patients, resulting in OR = 1, are not included in the meta-analysis [24, 25]. The investigator can also elect to exclude from meta-analysis the data from selected studies that are considered inadequate because of their design characteristics, small sample sizes, or other technical flaws. In our example, we included all 15 studies identified by the systematic review, to avoid introducing another source of potential bias.

Once the information is entered in the software, the software eliminates from analysis the data from studies that report events, weighs the data of the remaining studies according to the cohort size evaluated in each publication, and performs the statistical analysis, as shown in Fig. 15.2. The figure shows, from left to right, the model used for the analysis, as explained below, the studies evaluated, statistics for each study including OR, lower limit, upper limit, *Z*-value and *p*-value and a forest plot showing in a graphical manner the OR, and 95% confidence intervals for all studies. It is beyond the scope of this chapter to explain the rationale behind the use of fixed or random models to evaluate data in meta-analysis. In general, the fixed model assumes that the effect size of all the studies is within a range that does not need to be normalized, so the effect size of each study is left as constant. In the random model it is assumed that there is some variability in the effect sizes of different studies due to variables such as different sample sizes and others. The analysis of effect sizes using random models applies a mathematical formula that normalizes the effects sizes of all studies toward an overall mean effect size, in an attempt to minimize the effect of design differences between studies. In our study of thymomas and others we have analyzed the data using both fixed models and random models and have generally obtained similar results [11–13].

Figure 15.2 shows that there are no significant survival differences between patients with A and AB thymomas, in any of the studies with p values >0.05. The bottom row shows the statistics for the entire population of patients from all the selected studies, calculated using a fixed model; it also shows a nonsignificant result with $p = 0.544$. The same data can be viewed using high resolution graphics that exhibit in more detail the characteristics of the forest plot, as shown in Fig. 15.3. Each horizontal line represents a study. The vertical lines show different OR, 0.01, 0.1, 1, 10, and 100. The OR from each study is summarized by a square. The size of each square is proportional to the weight being assigned to the results of each

Table 15.1 Evidence summary of data pertaining to thymoma patients available in literature

	Thymoma A			Thymoma AB			Thymoma B1			Thymoma B2			Thymoma B3		
References	SP	TNC	%Surv	SP	TNC	%Surv	SP	TNC	%Surv	SP	TNC	%Surv	SP	TNC	%Surv
Sonobe et al. [26]	10	10	100	15	15	100	18	18	100	14	21	66.70	18	33	54.50
Rena et al. [27]	20	21	95	44	49	90	38	45	85	35	50	71	5	13	40
Kim et al. [24]	7	7	100	2	25	92	12	12	100	NA	32	NA	NA	20	NA
Wright et al. [28]	21	21	100	52	52	100	25	27	92	22	24	92	37	51	73
Bedini et al. [25]	5	5	100	34	40	84.6	11	16	68.18	20	29	68.14	8	16	50
Kondo et al. [29]	8	8	100	17	17	100	25	27	94	7	8	94	11	12	92
Strobel [30]	21	21	100	48	48	100	13	13	100	53	58	91	19	23	81
Park et al. [31]	7	7	100	24	26	93.2	12	13	88.90	37	45	82.40	18	26	71.30
Rea et al. [32]	14	14	100	28	31	90	16	20	78	9	28	33	10	29	35
Singhal et al. [33]	10	10	100	7	7	100	24	24	100	14	15	95	4	5	80
Nakagawa et al. [34]	18	18	100	56	56	100	13	15	86	25	29	85	5	12	38
Chen et al. [35]	8	8	100	68	68	100	16	17	94.10	10	39	75	19	27	70
Okumura et al. [36]	18	18	100	67	77	87	50	55	91	57	97	59	9	26	36
Rieker et al. [37]	33	43	76	20	20	100	20	24	84	67	82	82	8	10	78
Chalabreysse et al. [38]	8	9	88.88	15	16	93.8	10	11	90.90	20	22	90.90	12	15	80
Total number or range	208	220	76–100	497	547	92–100	303	337	78–100	390	579	59–92	183	318	38–92

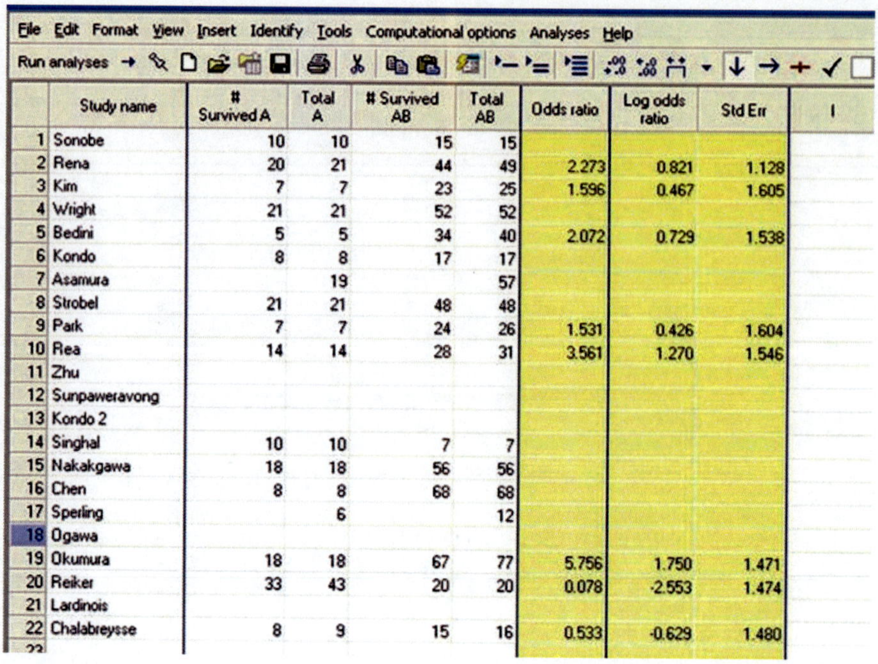

	Study name	# Survived A	Total A	# Survived AB	Total AB	Odds ratio	Log odds ratio	Std Err
1	Sonobe	10	10	15	15			
2	Rena	20	21	44	49	2.273	0.821	1.128
3	Kim	7	7	23	25	1.596	0.467	1.605
4	Wright	21	21	52	52			
5	Bedini	5	5	34	40	2.072	0.729	1.538
6	Kondo	8	8	17	17			
7	Asamura		19		57			
8	Strobel	21	21	48	48			
9	Park	7	7	24	26	1.531	0.426	1.604
10	Rea	14	14	28	31	3.561	1.270	1.546
11	Zhu							
12	Sunpaweravong							
13	Kondo 2							
14	Singhal	10	10	7	7			
15	Nakakgawa	18	18	56	56			
16	Chen	8	8	68	68			
17	Sperling		6		12			
18	Ogawa							
19	Okumura	18	18	67	77	5.756	1.750	1.471
20	Reiker	33	43	20	20	0.078	-2.553	1.474
21	Lardinois							
22	Chalabreysse	8	9	15	16	0.533	-0.629	1.480

Fig. 15.1 Tabulation of survival data of thymoma patients stratified by WHO histologic type in the meta-analysis software (Comprehensive Meta-analysis 2.0 [Biostat, Inc. Englewood, NJ]). The *left hand side columns* list the names of various studies, the total number of patients, and the number of patients surviving in each histologic type. The *right hand side columns* provide the odds ratio, the log odds ratio with standard error for survival differences in patients with thymoma type A vs. patients with thymoma type AB. The software computes statistics only for those studies in which an event (death or recurrence) has occurred (from Marchevsky et al. [13], with permission of John Wiley and Sons)

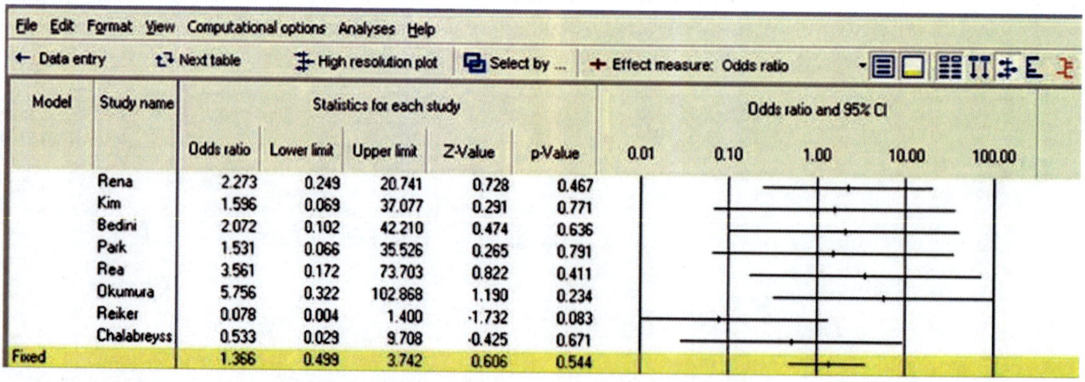

Model	Study name	Odds ratio	Lower limit	Upper limit	Z-Value	p-Value
	Rena	2.273	0.249	20.741	0.728	0.467
	Kim	1.596	0.069	37.077	0.291	0.771
	Bedini	2.072	0.102	42.210	0.474	0.636
	Park	1.531	0.066	35.526	0.265	0.791
	Rea	3.561	0.172	73.703	0.822	0.411
	Okumura	5.756	0.322	102.868	1.190	0.234
	Reiker	0.078	0.004	1.400	-1.732	0.083
	Chalabreyss	0.533	0.029	9.708	-0.425	0.671
Fixed		1.366	0.499	3.742	0.606	0.544

Fig. 15.2 Statistical analysis computed by the software. The figure shows, from *left* to *right*, the model used for the analysis, as explained below, the studies evaluated, statistics for each study including OR, lower limit, upper limit, Z-value and *p*-value, and a forest plot showing in a graphical manner the OR and 95% confidence intervals for all studies

study, usually as a result of the cohort size. The bottom of the forest plots show a diamond summarizing the integrated odds ratio and 95% confidence intervals for all studies in the analysis. The width of the diamond is proportional to the overall 95% CI. Please note that all squares and the diamond are close to the vertical line representing an OR of 1.

Study name	Statistics for each study				
	Odds ratio	Lower limit	Upper limit	Z-Value	p-Value
Rena	2.273	0.249	20.741	0.728	0.467
Kim	1.596	0.069	37.077	0.291	0.771
Bedini	2.072	0.102	42.210	0.474	0.636
Park	1.531	0.066	35.526	0.265	0.791
Rea	3.561	0.172	73.703	0.822	0.411
Okumura	5.756	0.322	102.868	1.190	0.234
Reiker	0.078	0.004	1.400	–1.732	0.083
Chalabreysse	0.533	0.029	9.708	–0.425	0.671
	1.366	0.499	3.742	0.606	0.544

Odds ratio and 95% CI

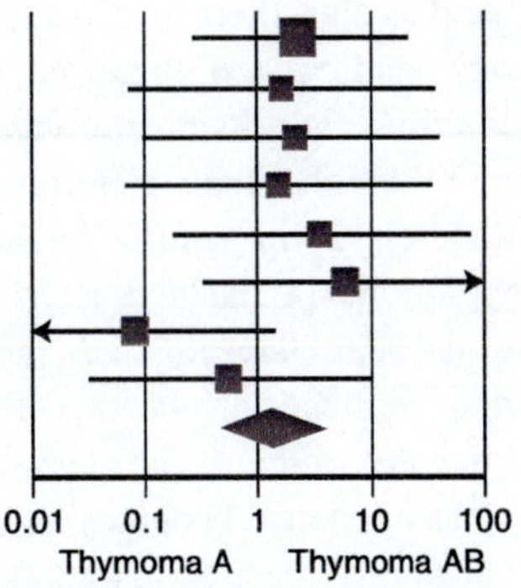

Meta Analysis

Fig. 15.3 Forest plot as computed by the software. The right hand side of the figure shows the Forest plot comprising of *vertical lines* which represent odds ratios (OR) of 0.01, 0.1, 1, 10, and 100. Each *horizontal line* represents the 95% confidence interval (CI) for each study. The *square* size represents the cohort size of each study. The *diamond* at the *bottom* of the graph represents the overall odds ratio. The width of the diamond is proportional to the overall 95% CI. All the *horizontal black lines* corresponding to the CI of each individual study cross the *vertical black line* corresponding to the OR of 1 indicating lack of significant survival difference between patients with thymoma type A and type AB. Also the diamond giving the integrated odds ratio intersects the vertical line corresponding with odds ratio of 1

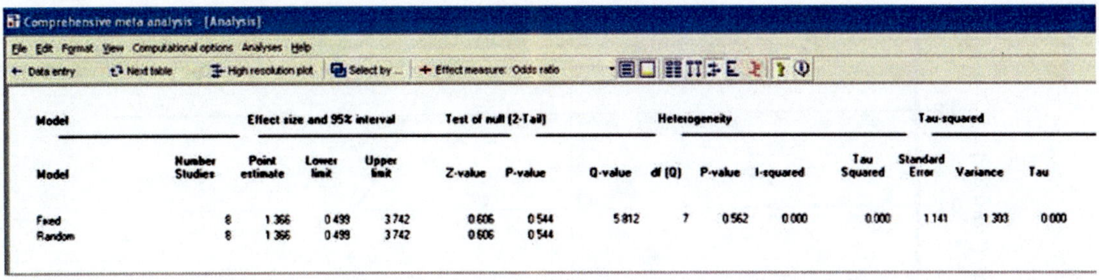

Model		Effect size and 95% interval			Test of null (2-Tail)		Heterogeneity				Tau-squared			
Model	Number Studies	Point estimate	Lower limit	Upper limit	Z-value	P-value	Q-value	df (Q)	P-value	I-squared	Tau Squared	Standard Error	Variance	Tau
Fixed	8	1.366	0.499	3.742	0.606	0.544	5.812	7	0.562	0.000	0.000	1.141	1.303	0.000
Random	8	1.366	0.499	3.742	0.606	0.544								

Fig. 15.4 Range of statistics computed by meta-analysis softwares

Data Analysis: Evaluation of the Statistical Significance of the Results Using Various Statistical Tests

In addition to the *p* values shown in Fig. 15.3 and the forest plot, the software provides more detailed statistics in various tables. For example, Fig. 15.4 shows the effect sizes of the data using fixed and random models, with 95% CI, results of 2-tailed *t*-test and other statistics. Pathologists attempting to evaluate the significance of meta-analysis beyond a simple understanding of *p* values probably need to enlist help from professional statisticians.

Evaluation of Potential Data Heterogeneity and Publication Bias

Meta-analysis integrates the results of data collected by other investigators under somewhat variable conditions, raising questions as to whether the results obtained with this methodology are reliable. This is a particular problem in anatomic pathology as diagnoses are frequently used as classifiers or dependent variables in various studies and there is a certain degree in interobserver diagnostic variability, as discussed in other chapters. Heterogeneity is defined as differences in results between studies due to variations in the characteristics of the populations being investigated, methodology used for data collection, various forms of bias, and how the outcome is measured and interpreted. Heterogeneity becomes significant when data variability between studies is greater than it would be expected from sampling variation alone. Publication bias occurs when the publication of research results depend on their nature and direction [39]. It often results from the tendency for researchers to report the results of studies that are "positive," and show a statistically significant finding and for reviewers to reject results that do not conform with what has been previously been reported. Publication bias results in the so-called file drawer problem, that many studies are conducted but not published because they did not produce statistically significant results, potentially resulting in information that is uknown in the literature and skewed toward positive results.

Various statistical methods have been designed to evaluate for data heterogeneity and publication bias. Heterogeneity can be explored with graphical methods such as forest plots and radial plots and various statistical tests such as the *Q*-test, meta-regression, and others. Forest plots allow readers to compare the results of all studies at a glance, as shown in Fig. 15.3.

Publication bias is explored with funnel plots and various tests designed to test for funnel test of asymmetry, such as the rank correlation method, Egger's linear regression, trim and fill and others. An example of funnel plot is shown in Fig. 15.5. The plot shows a vertical line, two

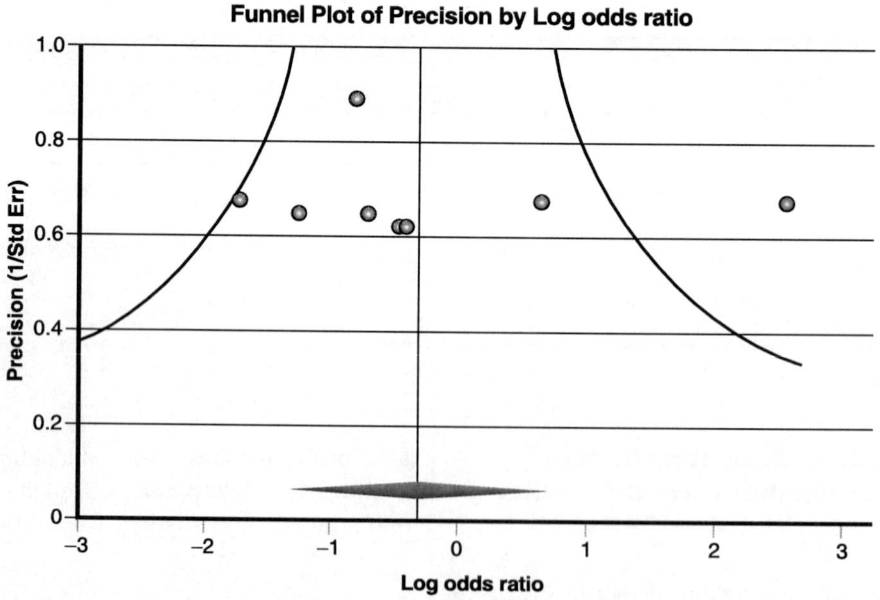

Fig. 15.5 Evaluation of heterogeneity between study results by Funnel plot. Comparison of Thymomas A and AB amongst various studies shows the data to be heterogenous. The plot shows a *vertical line*, two lateral *curves,* and multiple small *circles*. Each circle represents a single study. The height of each circle represents the weight being assigned to the results of the study. In instances when the data from various studies is homogeneous, the curves are close to the vertical line and all circles are clustered near the vertical line in a symmetrical distribution. In this analysis, the plot shows six studies to the left of the vertical line and only two in the opposite direction, indicating marked heterogeneity of the data

lateral lines and multiple small circles. Each circle represents the results of a single study. The height of each circle represents the weight being assigned to the results of the study. Funnel plots of homogeneous data usually show the lateral lines close to the vertical line and all circles clustered near the central vertical line in a symmetrical distribution balanced in height and number of circles on both sides of the vertical line. In contrast, Fig. 15.5, resulting from the meta-analysis comparing thymomas A with thymomas AB shows considerable data heterogeneity: six circles are to the right of the vertical line and one other to the left of the vertical line. Figure 15.6 shows a composite of the various statistical tests provided by Comprehensive Meta-analysis 2.0 (Biostat, Inc. Englewood, New Jersey) software to evaluate for funnel test asymmetry.

It is beyond the scope of this chapter to review in detail the theory and applications of various statistical tests for the evaluation of data heterogeneity and publication bias during meta-analysis. In our previous research, we have used funnel plots and the Egger's regression intercept test to evaluate our data.

Brief Review of Our Experience with the Use of Meta-analysis for the Evaluation of Selected Problems in Anatomic Pathology

We have used meta-analysis in our laboratory for the evaluation of the prognostic role of micrometastases and isolated tumor cells in patients

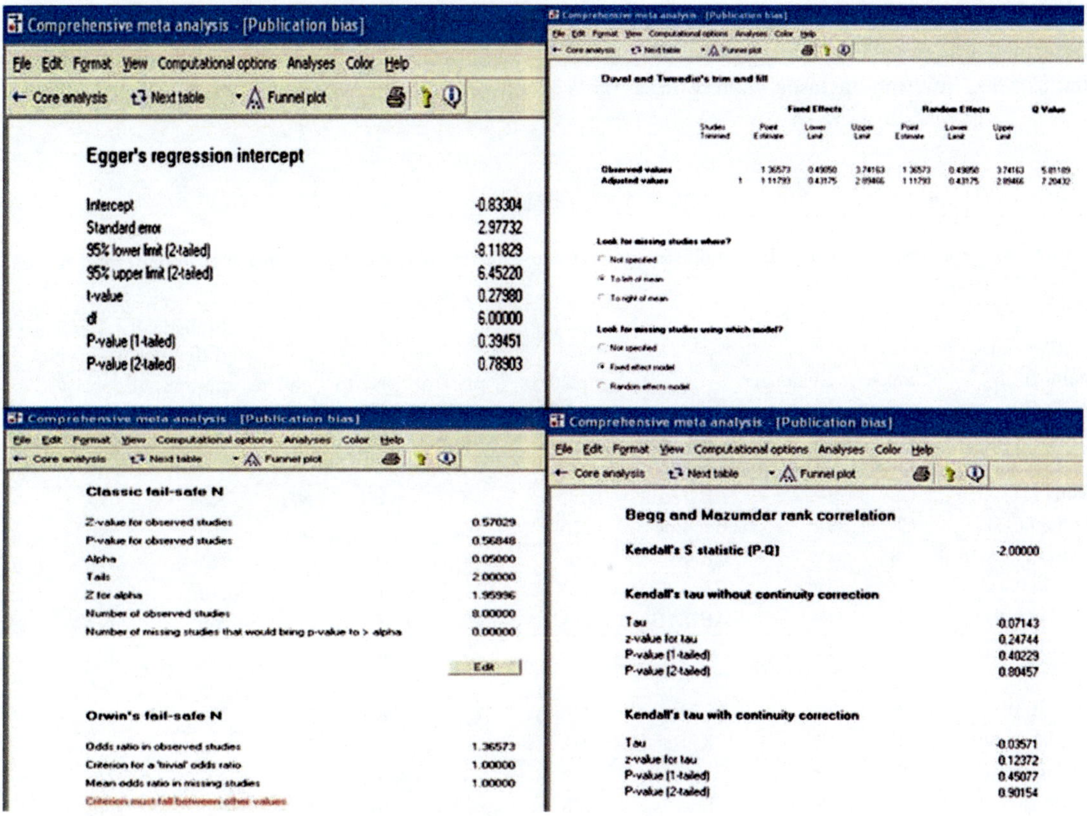

Fig. 15.6 Examples of statistics computed by meta-analysis software

with lung cancer, the clinical applicability of various tests for the evaluation of epidermal growth factor receptor (EGFR) in lung cancer patients, and the study of the prognosis of patients with thymomas, relatively infrequent neoplasms that are associated with indolent clinical behavior [11–13].

Use of Meta-analysis for the Evaluation of Prognostic and Predictive Features and for the Integration of Personal Experience with Published Data

Our recent study of the prognostic role of isolated tumor cells and micrometastases in the intrathoracic lymph nodes of lung cancer patients provides an example of how to use this statistical method for the evaluation of prognostic features in anatomic pathology, integrating data from own experience with that previously published in the literature [40]. A few studies of the prognostic role of these small nodal deposits, described under various names such as occult metastases, micrometastases, and others have suggested that they are associated with poor prognosis and decreased survival rates. In contrast, several other studies, including one from our laboratory, have not been able to demonstrate a significant association between the presence of isolated tumor cells or micrometastases and survival [41] (Table 15.2). To evaluate this topic in a more formal way we reviewed our experience, performed a systematic literature review and analyzed all available results with meta-analysis. Our recent experience consisted of 4,148 intrathoracic lymph nodes from 266 consecutive clinical stage I non-small lung cancer patients evaluated with hematoxylin and eosin stained slides and keratin immunostains for the presence of isolated tumor cells and micrometastases. The systematic literature review identified 13 studies providing data on the prognostic role of micrometastases in 835 patients detected with either immunohistochemistry or molecular methods, including our current data, with non-small cell carcinomas. Table 15.2 shows the evidence summary of the data. Meta-analysis of data from the 835 non-small cell carcinoma of the lung patients showed that there was no significant correlation

Table 15.2 Evidence summary: immunohistochemical detection of micrometastases in the regional lymph nodes of NSCLC patients

Author and number of cases (*n*)	Study design	Evidence level	IHC	pN0 to PN0 (I+)	pN0 to pN1mi	pN0 to pN2mi	pN1 to pN2mi	Statistically significant difference in survival	
								pN0 vs. pN1mi	pN1 vs. pN2mi
Melphi (16)	CS	IV	CK, CK7, CK 19	NA	2	NA	NA	NA	NA
Rena (87)	CS	IV	AE1/AE3	11	3	1	NA	No	NA
Izbicki (93)	CS	IV	Ber-Ep4	NA	16	NA	6	No	No
Marchevsky (60)	CS	IV	CK	7	3	0	1	No	No
Ishiwa (54)	CS	IV	CK	NA	11	7	1	No	No
Osaki (115)	CS	IV	AE1/AE3	NA	19	13	NA	Yes	NA
Passlick (54)	CS	IV	Ber-Ep4	NA	5	8	2	No	NA
Gu (49)	CS	IV	CK, p53	NA	9	13	NA	Yes	NA
Wu (103)	CS	IV	AE1/AE3	NA	13	8	NA	Yes	NA
Goldstein (80)	CS	IV	CK, Ber-Ep4	NA	2	1	NA	No	NA
Hashimoto (31)	CS	IV	Cam 5.2	NA	8	9	5	No	No
Nicholson (49)	CS	IV	CK	NA	3	NA	NA	No	No
Maruyama (44)	CS	IV	Cam 5.2	NA	19	12	NA	Yes	NA

between the presence of micrometastases detected with either immunohistochemistry or molecular methods and prognosis and that there was no sufficient data to evaluate for the prognostic role of isolated tumor cells in patients with non-small cell carcinoma of the lung. The results of the meta-analysis performed with the micrometastases data collected using immunohistochemistry, with the corresponding forest plot are shown in Fig. 15.7. Figure 15.8 shows the forest plot of results from the literature using molecular methods for the detection of micrometastases, also nonsignificant. The results of both meta-analysis indicate that detection of micrometastases does

Study name	Statistics for each study				
	Odds ratio	Lower limit	Upper limit	Z-Value	p-Value
Rena	0.936	0.151	5.801	−0.071	0.943
Mineo	0.168	0.009	3.300	−1.174	0.240
Hashimoto	0.500	0.056	4.473	−0.620	0.535
Marchevsky	0.800	0.124	5.171	−0.234	0.815
Osaki	0.910	0.431	1.921	−0.247	0.805
Goldstein	0.295	0.014	6.275	−0.782	0.434
Ishiwa	0.923	0.189	4.499	−0.099	0.921
Wu	0.622	0.235	1.644	−0.958	0.338
Gu	0.840	0.272	2.594	−0.303	0.762
Nicholson	1.400	0.267	7.349	0.398	0.691
CSMC	1.115	0.570	2.184	0.319	0.750
	0.873	0.608	1.254	−0.735	0.462

Odds ratio and 95% CI

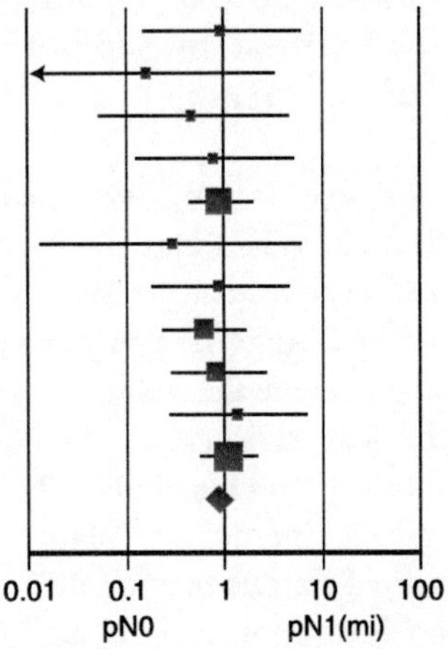

Meta Analysis

Fig. 15.7 Results of meta-analysis evaluating the prognostic value of micrometastases detected with immunohistochemistry in patients with non-small cell carcinoma of the lung. The meta-analysis allowed for the quantitative integration of our own results with those identified in the literature by a systematic review. Please note that the results are not significant, as shown by the forest plot and summary statistics

Study name	Statistics for each study				
	Odds ratio	Lower limit	Upper limit	Z-Value	p-Value
Hashimoto	0.429	0.096	1.910	−1.111	0.266
Nosotti	0.741	0.209	2.621	−0.466	0.642
Wang	0.593	0.218	1.615	−1.023	0.306
	0.591	0.295	1.185	−1.482	0.138

Odds ratio and 95% CI

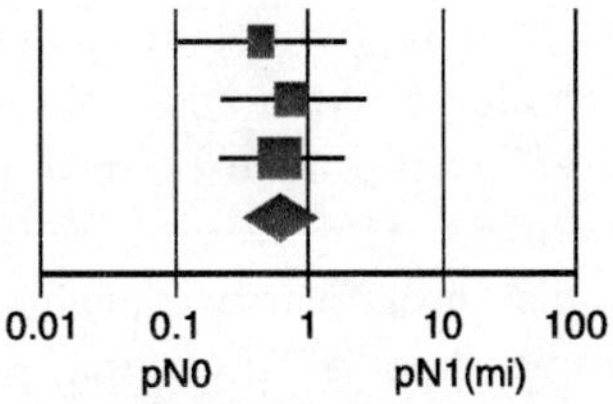

Meta Analysis

Fig. 15.8 Results of meta-analysis evaluating the prognostic value of micrometastases detected with molecular methods in patients with non-small cell carcinoma of the lung. Please note that the results are not significant, as shown by the forest plot and summary statistics not portend prognostic significance. However, evaluation of the results of our meta-analysis with power analysis demonstrated that 3,060 patients followed for 60 months would be needed to achieve 80% power in a study designed to detect survival differences between patients with negative nodes and micrometastases.

Use of Meta-analysis for the Study of Infrequent Diseases that are Associated with Indolent Clinical Course: Opportunities for National and International Collaborations

Our recent study with meta-analysis showing that the WHO classification of thymomas provides significant prognostic information for selected stage III thymoma patients can be used to illustrate the value of this methodology for the integration of data collected at different international hospitals [42]. Thymomas and thymic carcinomas are relatively uncommon mediastinal lesions that are difficult to study because no institution can collect the large number of patients required to achieve significant statistical power and the survival effect size is small because the tumors usually follow an indolent clinical course, with only some tumors recurring and/or metastasizing 10 years or longer after initial treatment. It is very difficult to organize a randomized clinical trial to study thymomas. Indeed, our systematic literature review showed that no such studies have been reported [12, 13]. Previous studies of thymoma patients, including two studies with meta-analysis performed in our laboratory, showed that WHO histologic type and Masaoka stage provide significant prognostic information for thymoma patients. However, there is only one study where prognosis was evaluated by WHO histologic type of thymoma previously stratified by Masaoka stage [30]. This information is important as therapy is usually selected on the basis of stage rather than histology. As information about thymoma patients stratified by both WHO histologic type and stage are not available in the literature, we contacted by email the authors of recent studies reporting the prognosis of thymoma patients categorized using the WHO scheme and were able to collect data from 905 patients treated at hospitals in Japan, Korea, Italy, Germany, and the United States, formatted in a manner suitable for meta-analysis. Table 15.3 shows the evidence summary listed in these data. Meta-analysis showed than when stratified by stage, significant survival differences could be estimated in patients with stage III disease, between thymomas A and B2 and A and B3. Figure 15.9 shows the meta-analysis comparing the survival of stage III patients with thymomas A and B2, with the corresponding forest plot. The latter shows that most studies show OR < 1 and that evaluation of the data with the fixed model yields $p = 0.003$.

Does Meta Analysis have a Future as a Useful Statistical Tool in Anatomic Pathology?

As illustrated with the previous examples, meta-analysis could be used more widely in anatomic pathology to integrate the results of multiple studies in a more precise manner than with currently used ad-hoc summary tables. Experience with this methodology will hopefully persuade pathologists about the need to report data in a more consistent and explicit manner so that it could be readily extracted in the future by other investigators. Meta-analysis could also be used more often to estimate effect sizes across multiple studies in efforts at integrating the results from current studies with those previously published in the literature.

Table 15.3 Evidence summary: number of patients who survived their thymoma for a minimum of 5 years, stratified by WHO histologic type and Masaoka stage

	WHO type A				WHO type AB				WHO type B1				WHO type B2				WHO type B3			
References	I	II	III	IV	I	II	III	IV	I	II	III	IV	I	II	III	IV	I	II	III	IV
Okumura (n=271)	71	100	100	NA	68	60	83	0	65	73	70	50	76	84	73	0	50	70	70	50
Kim (n=117)	100	100	NA	NA	83	57	NA	100	100	100	0	NA	95	85	50	33	67	92	80	33
Rena (n=180)	100	100	100	NA	100	100	100	0	100	100	100	100	100	100	100	82	NA	100	100	87
Yoshida (n=94)	67	100	NA	NA	100	94	100	NA	100	100	NA	NA	100	100	100	50	100	100	100	100
CSMC (n=56)	NA	100	NA	NA	100	100	0	NA	50	75	50	67	100	67	50	100	100	100	50	100
TMH (n=20)	100	100	NA	NA	100	50	NA	0	100	100	NA	NA	NA	NA	NA	NA	NA	NA	100	NA
Strobel (n=168)	100	100	50	50	93	100	100	NA	100	100	NA	NA	100	100	91	83	NA	86	90	75

Study name	Statistics for each study					Odds ratio and 95% CI
	Odds ratio	Lower limit	Upper limit	Z-Value	p-Value	
Okumura	1.145	0.043	30.400	0.081	0.935	
Rena	0.012	0.000	0.347	−2.571	0.010	
Strobel	0.033	0.002	0.491	−2.478	0.013	
	0.070	0.012	0.415	−2.932	0.003	

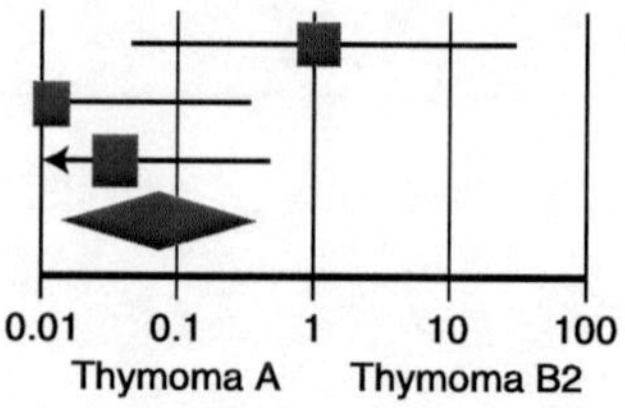

Meta Analysis

Fig. 15.9 The forest plots of the meta-analysis of patients with stage III thymomas with histologic type A vs. histologic types B2. The software estimates the odds (odds = probability/1 − probability) for each outcome, weighs the data from various institutions according to their cohort size, estimates the overall OR for all cases, and calculates *p* values. The *vertical lines* represent the levels of OR. The *small squares* represent the results of each study. The size of each square is proportional to the weight assigned to the results of each study. The rhomboid represents the results of the overall data. The horizontal lines represent the 95% CI of each study

References

1. Egger M, Smith GD, Phillips AN. Meta-analysis: principles and procedures. BMJ. 1997;315(7121): 1533–7.
2. Antman EM, Lau J, Kupelnick B, Mosteller F, Chalmers TC. A comparison of results of meta-analyses of randomized control trials and recommendations of clinical experts. Treatments for myocardial infarction. JAMA. 1992;268(2):240–8.
3. L'Abbe KA, Detsky AS, O'Rourke K. Meta-analysis in clinical research. Ann Intern Med. 1987;107(2): 224–33.
4. Jenicek M. Meta-analysis in medicine. Where we are and where we want to go. J Clin Epidemiol. 1989;42(1):35–44.
5. Goodman SN. Have you ever meta-analysis you didn't like? Ann Intern Med. 1991;114(3):244–6.
6. Steinberg KE. Cookbook medicine: recipe for disaster? J Am Med Dir Assoc. 2006;7(7):470–2.
7. Guerette PH. Managed care: cookbook medicine, or quality, cost-effective care? Can Nurse. 1995; 91(7):16.
8. Holm RP. Cookbook medicine. S D Med. 2009; 62(9):371.
9. Leppaniemi A. From eminence-based to error-based to evidence-based surgery. Scand J Surg. 2008;97(1):2–3.
10. Crawford JM. Original research in pathology: judgment, or evidence-based medicine? Lab Invest. 2007;87(2):104–14.
11. Gupta R, Dastane AM, McKenna Jr R, Marchevsky AM. The predictive value of epidermal growth factor receptor tests in patients with pulmonary adenocarcinoma: review of current "best evidence" with meta-analysis. Hum Pathol. 2009;40(3):356–65.
12. Gupta R, Marchevsky AM, McKenna RJ, et al. Evidence-based pathology and the pathologic evaluation of thymomas: transcapsular invasion is not a significant prognostic feature. Arch Pathol Lab Med. 2008;132(6):926–30.
13. Marchevsky AM, Gupta R, McKenna RJ, et al. Evidence-based pathology and the pathologic evaluation of thymomas: the World Health Organization classification can be simplified into only 3 categories other than thymic carcinoma. Cancer. 2008;112(12):2780–8.
14. Faraji H, Nguyen BN, Mai KT. Renal epithelioid angiomyolipoma: a study of six cases and a meta-analytic study. Development of criteria for screening the entity with prognostic significance. Histopathology. 2009;55(5):525–34.
15. Anderson GG, Weiss LM. Determining tissue of origin for metastatic cancers: meta-analysis and literature review of immunohistochemistry performance. Appl Immunohistochem Mol Morphol. 2010;18(1):3–8.
16. Gould Rothberg BE, Bracken MB, Rimm DL. Tissue biomarkers for prognosis in cutaneous melanoma: a systematic review and meta-analysis. J Natl Cancer Inst. 2009;101(7):452–74.
17. Alonso SR, Ortiz P, Pollan M, et al. Progression in cutaneous malignant melanoma is associated with distinct expression profiles: a tissue microarray-based study. Am J Pathol. 2004;164(1):193–203.
18. Niezabitowski A, Czajecki K, Rys J, et al. Prognostic evaluation of cutaneous malignant melanoma: a clinicopathologic and immunohistochemical study. J Surg Oncol. 1999;70(3):150–60.
19. Straume O, Sviland L, Akslen LA. Loss of nuclear p16 protein expression correlates with increased tumor cell proliferation (Ki-67) and poor prognosis in patients with vertical growth phase melanoma. Clin Cancer Res. 2000;6(5):1845–53.

20. Florenes VA, Maelandsmo GM, Faye R, Nesland JM, Holm R. Cyclin A expression in superficial spreading malignant melanomas correlates with clinical outcome. J Pathol. 2001;195(5):530–6.
21. Dziadziuszko R, Witta SE, Cappuzzo F, et al. Epidermal growth factor receptor messenger RNA expression, gene dosage, and gefitinib sensitivity in non-small cell lung cancer. Clin Cancer Res. 2006; 12(10):3078–84.
22. Pugh TJ, Bebb G, Barclay L, et al. Correlations of EGFR mutations and increases in EGFR and HER2 copy number to gefitinib response in a retrospective analysis of lung cancer patients. BMC Cancer. 2007;7:128.
23. Travis WD, Brambilla E, Muller-Hermelink HK, et al. Tumors of the lung, pleura, thymus and heart. Lyon: IARC Press; 2004.
24. Kim DJ, Yang WI, Choi SS, Kim KD, Chung KY. Prognostic and clinical relevance of the World Health Organization schema for the classification of thymic epithelial tumors: a clinicopathologic study of 108 patients and literature review. Chest. 2005;127(3): 755–61.
25. Bedini AV, Andreani SM, Tavecchio L, et al. Proposal of a novel system for the staging of thymic epithelial tumors. Ann Thorac Surg. 2005;80(6): 1994–2000.
26. Sonobe S, Miyamoto H, Izumi H, et al. Clinical usefulness of the WHO histological classification of thymoma. Ann Thorac Cardiovasc Surg. 2005;11:367–73.
27. Rena O, Papalia E, Maggi G, et al. World Health Organization histologic classification: an independent prognostic factor in resected thymomas. Lung Cancer. 2005;50:59–66.
28. Wright CD, Wain JC, Wong DR, et al. Predictors of recurrence in thymic tumors: importance of invasion, World Health Organization histology, and size. J Thorac Cardiovasc Surg. 2005;130:1413–21.
29. Kondo K, Yoshizawa K, Tsuyuguchi M, et al. WHO histologic classification is a prognostic indicator in thymoma. Ann Thorac Surg. 2004;77:1183–8.
30. Strobel P, Marx A, Zettl A, Muller-Hermelink HK. Thymoma and thymic carcinoma: an update of the WHO Classification 2004. Surg Today. 2005;35: 805–11.
31. Park MS, Chung KY, Kim KD, et al. Prognosis of thymic epithelial tumors according to the new World Health Organization histologic classification. Ann Thorac Surg. 2004;78:992–97; discussion 997–8.
32. Rea F, Marulli G, Girardi R, et al. Long-term survival and prognostic factors in thymic epithelial tumours. Eur J Cardiothorac Surg. 2004;26:412–8.
33. Singhal S, Shrager JB, Rosenthal DI, et al. Comparison of stages I-II thymoma treated by complete resection with or without adjuvant radiation. Ann Thorac Surg. 2003;76:1635–41; discussion 1641–1632.
34. Nakagawa K, Asamura H, Matsuno Y, et al. Thymoma: a clinicopathologic study based on the new World Health Organization classification. J Thorac Cardiovasc Surg. 2003;126:1134–40.
35. Chen G, Marx A, Wen-Hu C, et al. New WHO histologic classification predicts prognosis of thymic epithelial tumors: a clinicopathologic study of 200 thymoma cases from China. Cancer. 2002;95:420–9.
36. Okumura M, Ohta M, Tateyama H, et al. The World Health Organization histologic classification system reflects the oncologic behavior of thymoma: a clinical study of 273 patients. Cancer. 2002;94:624–32.
37. Rieker RJ, Hoegel J, Morresi-Hauf A, et al. Histologic classification of thymic epithelial tumors: comparison of established classification schemes. Int J Cancer. 2002;98:900–6.
38. Chalabreysse L, Roy P, Cordier JF, et al. Correlation of the WHO schema for the classification of thymic epithelial neoplasms with prognosis: a retrospective study of 90 tumors. Am J Surg Pathol. 2002;26:1605–11.
39. Dickersin K. The existence of publication bias and risk factors for its occurrence. JAMA. 1990;263(10): 1385–9.
40. Marchevsky AM, Gupta R, Kusuanco D, Mirocha J, McKenna RJ. The presence of isolated tumor cells and micrometastases in the intrathoracic lymph nodes of patients with lung carcinomas is not associated with decreased survival. Hum Pathol. 2010;41:1536–43.
41. Marchevsky AM, Qiao JH, Krajisnik S, Mirocha JM, McKenna RJ. The prognostic significance of intranodal isolated tumor cells and micrometastases in patients with non-small cell carcinoma of the lung. J Thorac Cardiovasc Surg. 2003;126(2):551–7.
42. Marchevsky AM, Gupta R, Casadio C, et al. World Health Organization classification of thymomas provides significant prognostic information for selected stage III patients: evidence from an International Thymoma Study Group. Hum Pathol. 2010;41: 1413–21.

Evidence-Based Practices in Applied Immunohistochemistry: Dilemmas Caused by Cross-Purposes

16

Mark R. Wick, Paul E. Swanson, and Alberto M. Marchevsky

Keywords

Evidence-based pathology • Immunohistochemistry • Evidence-based immunohistochemistry • Prognostic-predictive immunohistochemistry • Diagnostic immunohistochemistry

Immunohistochemistry (IHC) has existed as an area of scientific inquiry for 70 years, and it truly has changed the way in which anatomic pathology is practiced during that span of time [1, 2]. Conventional histochemistry antedated IHC by almost a century, and had itself been a huge technological breakthrough. However, until the availability of IHC, scientists and physicians were limited in their ability to identify cellular products in situ, as histochemical methods were limited in their capacity to identify many cellular products that may have diagnostic, prognostic, or predictive value in the practice of Medicine [3–6]. The same comment can be made for another adjunctive histomorphological procedure, transmission electron microscopy (TEM) [7–10], which had been introduced by Ernst Ruska – a physicist – in 1931 [11].

Surprisingly, and rather inexplicably as there is little doubt that TEM significantly extended the analytic potentials of light microscopy and histochemistry, both TEM and IHC were only slowly integrated into the clinical (hospital-based) practice of pathology. Indeed, ultrastructural analysis was still being "introduced" as a useful procedure for patient care 50 years after its inception [8], and IHC did not enjoy widespread interest or application by practitioners until around 1980 [2].

Perhaps because of this protracted evolution, little attention was given, until relatively recently, to the role of quality assurance (QA) in either TEM or diagnostic IHC (DIHC). In particular, pathologists and other physicians especially tended to have a naïve expectation that immunostains were merely formulaic – in other words, if one used appropriate reagents and followed prescribed procedural steps, an optimal result was expected to obtain. That attitude likely derived from experience with histochemistry, where such provisions *would* typically produce the expected outcome. In addition, there is limited consensus about how to use IHC tests for the work-up of various clinicopathologic entities. Different investigators propose the use of various IHC tests based on the results of selected studies, and there are few expert- consensuses or evidence-based guidelines to guide practitioners during the selection of the antibodies that should be tested during the work-up of specific differential diagnoses. There is also a lack of guidelines suggesting how to interpret the results, particularly when there is some overlap in findings, as IHC results are often not included as diagnostic

M.R. Wick (✉)
Department of Pathology, University of Virginia Medical School, Charlottesville, VA, USA
e-mail: mrw9c@virginia.edu

A.M. Marchevsky and M.R. Wick (eds.), *Evidence Based Pathology and Laboratory Medicine*, DOI 10.1007/978-1-4419-1030-1_16,

criteria in the various classification schema proposed by widely respected groups of experts selected by the World Health Organization (WHO) and other professional groups.

As we shall consider shortly, DIHC is anything but mechanical. Many biological and chemical factors have a meaningful impact on the final results of this method, and these must be addressed individually wherever possible. The topic of how to select the most effective antibodies that need to be tested for various differential diagnoses, problems related to the over utilization of IHC, and the fervent but misdirected hope that this methodology can be employed in a nondiagnostic setting to provide prognostic and predictive data will be discussed. Finally, technical alternatives to immunohistologic evaluation will be summarized.

Diagnostic Immunohistochemistry: An Historical Perspective

The concept of adding a detectable chemical "tag" to target-specific reagent antibodies seems today to be a straightforward, if not simple, idea. Nevertheless, such a conclusion is purely contextual. In 1940, the structure of antibodies was only rudimentarily understood, and the notion of attaching a visible chromophore to them was completely novel. A 27-year-old medical resident from Boston, MA – Dr. Albert Hewett Coons (Fig. 16.1) – developed the idea while on vacation in Europe [12]. At least one German colleague – Dr. Kurt Apitz of Charite' Hospital in Berlin – thought little of it, for good reasons [12]. The necessary process of joining chemicals to antibodies had never been attempted, and synthesis of the chemical "tags" that Coons had in mind – fluorescent molecules – also was a fledgling area. Finally, no microscope capable of visualizing fluorophores then existed.

Undeterred, Coons returned to Boston to work out each of these problems. By 1941, he and his colleagues had demonstrated not only the feasibility but also the applicability of fluorescent immunohistology for the localization of particular protein targets in human tissues [13, 14] (Fig. 16.2). That development launched the entire scientific discipline of IHC and earned Coons the prestigious Albert Lasker Award in 1959 [15].

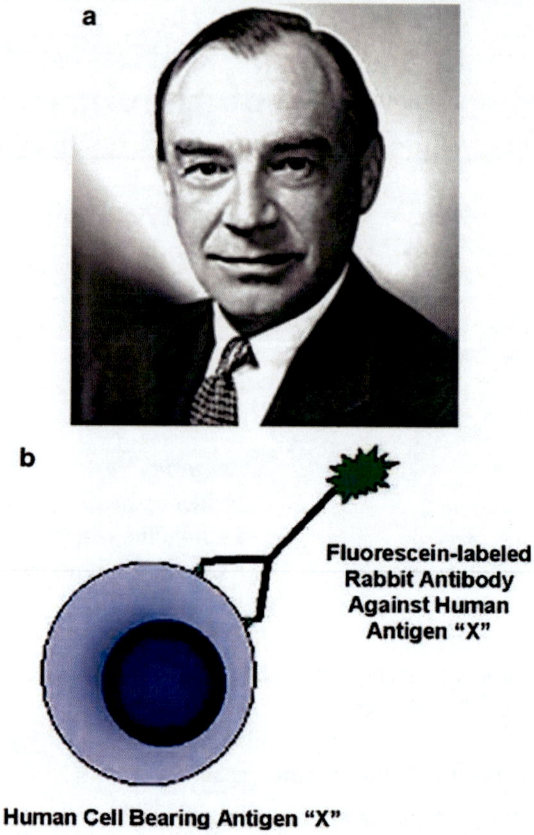

Fig. 16.1 (**a**) Albert Hewett Coons, M.D. (1912–1978), the originator of immunohistochemistry. Dr. Coons was given the Lasker Award in 1959 for that contribution. (**b**) In direct immunofluorescence methods, as devised by Coons, a fluorophore is attached to a reagent antibody, which is specific for a polypeptide epitope in substrate tissue

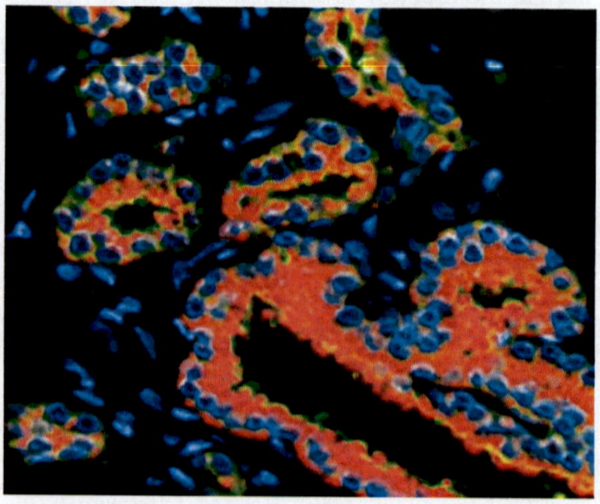

Fig. 16.2 Immunofluorescence study for alpha-methylacyl-CoA-racemase, seen as a *red-orange* signal in this section of prostatic adenocarcinoma

Probably because immunofluorescence microscopy does not allow for a simultaneous appreciation of morphological detail, the procedure did not enjoy widespread clinical use and was primarily regarded as a research tool. There were exceptions to that statement, however, principally represented by the diagnostic use of fluorophores in renal pathology and dermatopathology [16–19]. Fundamentally, and especially in the practice of hospital-based pathology, an expanded application of DIHC depended on further development of visible chemical "partners" for reagent antibodies.

The next step in this evolution was taken in the area of TEM, where it was realized that certain electron-dense (and therefore visible) chemical moieties – such as ferritin, osmium, and gold salts – could be bound directly to reagent antibodies, as fluorescein isocyanate had been [20–23]. Hence, those reagents provided another method for localizing protein targets in substrate tissues, but at an ultrastructural level. An additional development involved the use of a gold-protein-A adduct as an indicator in TEM, preceded by incubation of target tissues with unlabeled reagent antibody (*n.b.*: protein-A is a proteinaceous product of *Staphylococcus aureus*, and is capable of binding to the Fc portion of all immunoglobulins) [24]. Once again, however, ultrastructural IHC was impractical for most practicing anatomic pathologists, because they did not have access to electron microscopes and the technique in question was quite tedious.

Finally, in the late 1960s, Ludwig Sternberger (Fig. 16.3) and colleagues developed an effective immunohistological procedure that could be used with formalin-fixed, paraffinized tissue sections and the light microscope [25, 26]. Three molecules of horseradish peroxidase were complexed with two antiperoxidase antibodies by precipitation from a mixture of enzyme and crude serum. This pentagonal structure, dubbed peroxidase-antiperoxidase (PAP) complex by Sternberger, had the intriguing attribute of being thermodynamically stable independent of antiperoxidase serum quality or affinity (and thus easy and cheap to prepare). The utility of PAP as a delivery vehicle for the reporter enzyme was also independent of affinity, since linkage of PAP to a specific tissue-bound reagent antibody depended solely on the affinity of the secondary (bridge) antibody for the free Fc fragments of PAP and the primary reagent (Fig. 16.4). Antibodies comprising the PAP complex were raised in the same animal hosts as those which produced the primary reagent antibodies, whereas the secondary "bridge" antibody derived from another species. The most common early example of such a construct was a rabbit primary antibody-sheep antirabbit "bridge" antibody-rabbit PAP complex [26].

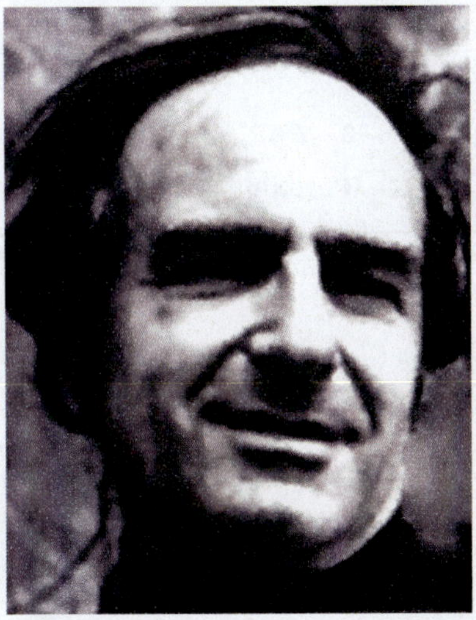

Fig. 16.3 Ludwig Sternberger, M.D., who, along with colleagues, devised the first practical light microscopic technique in immunohistochemistry in the late 1960s – the peroxidase-antiperoxidase method

Peroxidases are redox enzymes that catalyze reactions between electron donors and recipients, according to the following equations:

$$ROOR' + \text{electron donor } (2e^-) + 2H^+ \rightarrow ROH + R'OH,$$

or

$$\text{Acceptor} + H_2O_2 \rightarrow \text{oxidized acceptor} + H_2O.$$

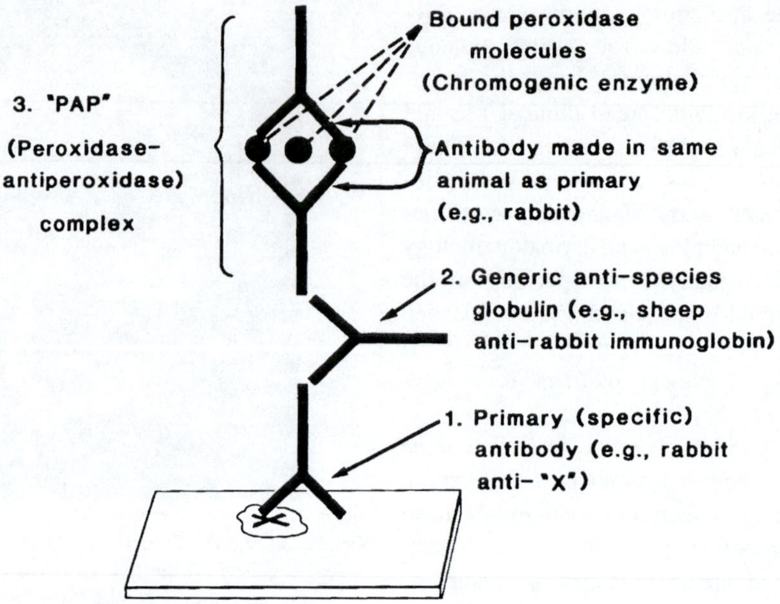

Fig. 16.4 In the peroxidase-antiperoxidase method, an unlabeled reagent primary antibody is linked to a tertiary reporter complex comprising two antibodies and several peroxidase molecules. The first and third antibodies are raised in the same animal species, whereas the second "bridge" antibody is a generic reagent raised against animal immunoglobulins representing the primary reagent and PAP complex (e.g., rabbit primary – sheep antirabbit – rabbit PAP)

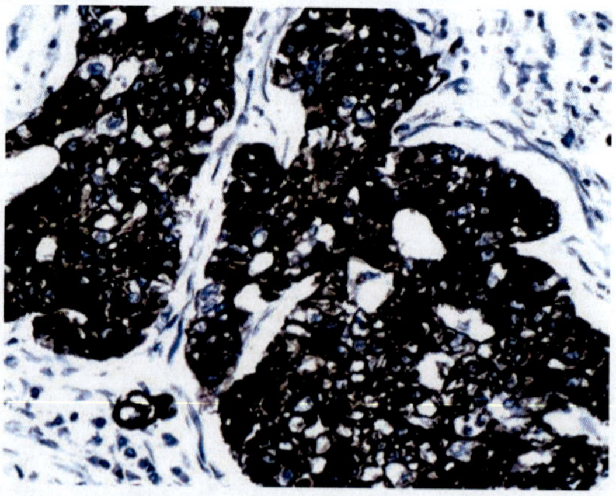

Fig. 16.5 Dense *brown-black* precipitates of diaminobenzidine-HCl are seen at sites in formalin-fixed human tissue where anti-human keratin primary antibodies have bound in a paraffin section. The peroxidase-antiperoxidase method was employed as the detection system

In the classical PAP technique, hydrogen peroxide (H_2O_2) is used as the electron donor, and 3-3′-diaminobenzidine tetrahydrochloride – which forms a colored precipitate when oxidized – is the electron recipient. The final result is a light-microscopic preparation in which brown-black labels mark the sites of specific primary antibody binding, where target proteins reside in the tissue (Fig. 16.5). That construct is responsible for the slang term "brown stains," in reference to DIHC.

Finally, pathologists and other scientists had a practical, relatively rapid (24 h), and ecumenical alternative technique to immunofluorescence microscopy that could be used in everyday practice. It seemingly remained only for an increasing number of specific primary antibodies to be raised and marketed, before the entire panoply of human proteins could be localized in tissue sections.

Realities and limitations of the PAP technique soon lessened that grand expectation. It became evident that some proteinaceous targets existed in only low densities in various tissues. Moreover, the standard process of formalin-fixation and paraffin-embedding appeared to denature, mask, or cross-link some proteins in such a way that primary antibodies could not bind to them [27, 28]. Depending upon the particulars of tissue procurement and processing, PAP stains for any given target in any given specimen might be strongly reactive, weakly positive, or altogether negative, in an unpredictable way.

This chain of events brings us to a crucial watershed in the development of DIHC as a method, and philosophies about how the technique should be used. *For practicing pathologists, the aim of immunohistology was, and is, to visualize molecular constituents of tissue that have* diagnostic *importance*. Inexplicable variability in staining intensity, as mentioned in the previous paragraph, threatens that goal and was quickly recognized as a serious potential source of interpretative error. For example, if S100 protein were to be found in a metastatic undifferentiated large-cell malignancy, in the absence of keratin, the probable diagnosis would be one of metastatic melanoma. However, keratin might actually be present in the tumor cells but missed because of technical problems in tissue processing or immunohistochemical procedure. Keratin-positive, S100-positive neoplasms are represented by *carcinomas* that originate in selected sites [29]. Therefore, failure to detect keratin – or other similarly dispositive markers – in such lesions would produce a significant mistake in the generation of *categorical data*, an issue related ultimately to poor method sensitivity. On the other hand, given that small quantities of a given marker of diagnostic importance might be expressed in diagnostically problematic settings (keratins in melanoma, to extend the argument), there also needs to be an appreciation for the relationship between high method sensitivity and errors in categorical data.

With this in mind, it is important to realize that *quantification* of results in DIHC is meaningful *only* in a binary context – i.e., immunostains are ideally either positive or negative. As a consequence of that premise, a cardinal objective for diagnostic pathologists became the maximization of specific immunolabeling, through a variety of methods, while at the same time maintaining minimal background "noise" in IHC preparations [30]. To a large extent, that intent and practice remain in place today.

In line with our earlier comment that masking, degradation, or cross-linking of available epitopes may occur in formalin-fixed tissue, compensatory efforts at signal amplification were two-pronged. One mode of attack on the problem was to devise ever more sensitive IHC techniques, in the hope of recognizing low levels of an available protein target. The best known of higher-sensitivity alternatives to the PAP procedure was developed in the late 1970s by Hsu (Fig. 16.6) and colleagues [31–33]; namely, the avidin-biotin-peroxidase complex (ABC) procedure. That innovative technique capitalized on the ability to attach biotin molecules to secondary antibodies, and also the capacity to build large reporter complexes which include avidin, biotin, and horseradish peroxidase. The latter composites can be attached to the biotinylated secondary antibody, which is, in turn, bound to the Fc portion of a specific primary reagent antibody. The result compounds the number of peroxidase molecules that are associated with any one protein target, far beyond the biochemical capability of the PAP technique (Fig. 16.7).

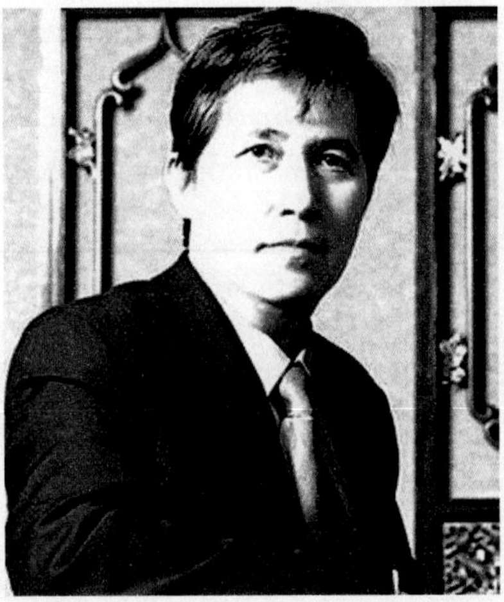

Fig. 16.6 Su-Ming Hsu, M.D., Ph.D., the principal developer of the avidin-biotin-peroxidase complex (ABC) procedure in immunohistochemistry

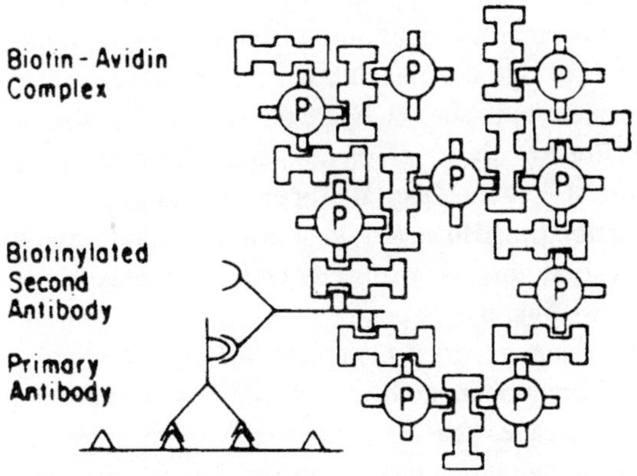

Fig. 16.7 The avidin-biotin-peroxidase complex method offers a high level of sensitivity because of the multimeric nature of the peroxidase-bearing "reporter" molecule

Therefore, an amplification of the immunostaining signal is the predictable outcome.

Later variations on that theme included labeled streptavidin-biotin-peroxidase (LSAB), ABPAP (serially combined PAP and ABC procedures), and alkaline phosphatase-antialkaline phosphatase (APAAP) methods [34–38], and, more recently, a paradigm in which approximately 20 secondary antibodies from more than one animal source are attached polymerically to a dextran backbone that also carries >100 peroxidase molecules [37, 39] (Fig. 16.8). That approach, called dextran-polymer-based (*Envision*[R]), and other proprietary formulations, IHC obviates the need for separate labeled secondary antibodies from differing animals. At the same time, it greatly increases final immunostaining intensity in most applications.

All of those approaches for signal maximization center on the notion of increasing the numbers of signal molecules that are bound to a target protein in tissue. They are all effective in visualizing low densities of antigens whose epitopes are still at least partially open to bind to primary antibodies. However, what could be done about desired targets with *completely* "masked" or cross-linked epitopes?

Trading, perhaps, on pathologists' experiences in immunohematology – where it has been known for decades that controlled enzymatic digestion could unmask certain antigens on erythrocytes [40, 41] – the same procedure was applied to paraffin sections in DIHC in the late 1970s. Pepsin, trypsin, proteinase-3, ficin, pronase, papain, and bromelain were, and still are, employed in this setting [42–47]. Predictably, the results demonstrated that different enzymes affected various targets differently. In other words, one catalyst might enhance immunoreactivity for protein "A" but decrease labeling for protein "B." Another offshoot of this work was the realization that certain classes of tissue constituents were *routinely* masked by formalin fixation; a prime example is represented by the intermediate-filament proteins, including keratin, vimentin, desmin, neurofilament, and glial fibrillary acidic protein [28]. Those

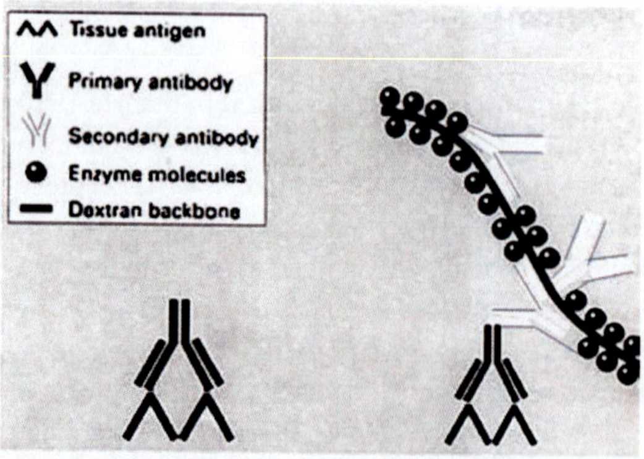

Fig. 16.8 In the dextran-polymer-based system of immunohistochemistry, several secondary "link" antibodies, from different animal hosts, are bound to a dextran carrier that also carries multiple peroxidase molecules

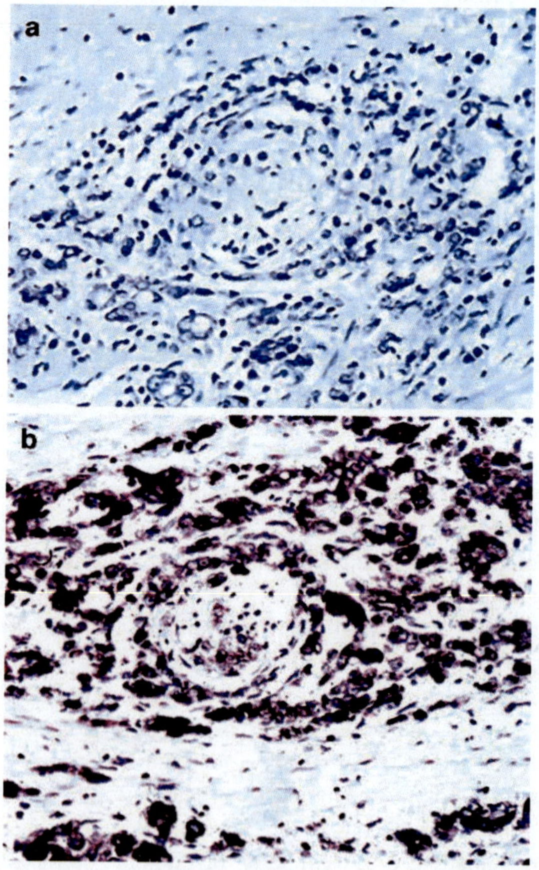

Fig. 16.9 (**a**) Immunostaining of a formalin-fixed, poorly differentiated, prostatic adenocarcinoma for pankeratin, with no epitope-retrieval techniques. There is no discernible reactivity. (**b**) Prior treatment of the sections with ficin "unmasks" the target antigen and allows the antikeratin antibody to bind

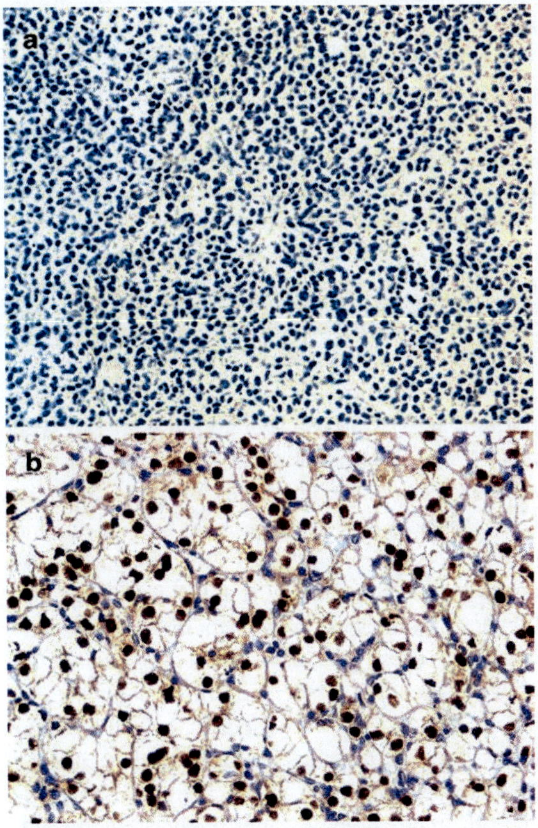

Fig. 16.10 (**a**) Immunostaining of a paraffin section for PAX2, a nuclear marker, in renal cell carcinoma with no epitope retrieval. (**b**) Heat-induced antigen retrieval with citrate buffer allows for antibody recognition of the target

markers can only be visualized optimally using some type of unmasking procedure (Fig. 16.9). The same statement applies to virtually all intranuclear proteins [48] (Fig. 16.10).

The next major advance in this area of DIHC occurred in the early 1990s. Empirical experience showed that the controlled heating of paraffin sections, when immersed in ionic solutions in a microwave oven or a steamer, could accomplish the same results as proteolytic unmasking methods [49–55]. Thus, the term "heat-induced epitope retrieval" (HIER) was coined. Today, this process is a *de rigueur* element of practical immunohistology. In similarity to enzymatic digestion, HIER augments the intensity of immunolabeling for some markers and decreases it for others, vis-à-vis IHC procedures that omit an unmasking step [55].

But, what, exactly, is being "undone" by proteolysis or HIER? To this day, the answer to that question is still vague. Several hypotheses have been advanced to account for epitope unmasking. These include the breakage of fixation-induced coupling of "irrelevant" but sterically interfering large proteins to peptide epitopes; the abrogation of electrostatic, van der Waal-like charges between epitopes and Fab fragments of reagent antibodies; dissolution of cagelike calcium complexes around epitope sequences; and a reversal of Mannich reactions between proteins [56–59]. The latter are organic reactions featuring the amino-alkylation of acidic protons, placed next to carbonyl groups during formaldehyde fixation [58]. On the other hand, there is an increasing understanding that the tertiary structure of the target epitope (liner vs. conformational) may greatly influence the ability of retrieval methods to improve immunoreactivity in routinely processed materials.

Other tissue fixatives have been evaluated as alternatives to formalin, including solutions based on methyl alcohol, ethyl alcohol, acetone, or combinations thereof [60–65]. These are either expensive or unwieldy for use in routine hospital pathology; moreover, they produce their own peculiar alterations in epitope preservation and are not necessarily any "kinder" to certain target proteins than formalin.

All of these considerations may seem arcane in regard to the standardization of immunohistology. However, they are, in fact, key preanalytical and intra-analytical elements that affect the latter process. It is not possible to obtain perfect control of the concentrations and pH of fixatives and buffers, the duration of fixation, the dimensions of tissue blocks and histologic sections used for IHC, the biological activities of various proteolytic enzymes, and the nature of heat distribution during HIER procedures. We do not mean to say that pathologists must not *try* to accomplish that task, but a more realistic goal is to aim for an end result of consistent and functionally binary (positive or negative) results in DIHC. Undeniably, an element of artificiality accompanies that approach, because one externally controls the ranges of reactivity in any immunostaining procedure through the subjective process of antibody titration against target tissues and, by extension, specific target diagnoses. Nevertheless, *as long as technical parameters are maintained within narrow confines, even an artificial system can be effectively used diagnostically.* The Canadian Association of Pathologists has recently published a set of guidelines that are useful in this specific context [66]. They also include a discussion of proper "positive" and "negative" controls in DIHC, as well as a consideration of cross-validating techniques (see http://ajcp.ascpjournals.org/content/133/3/354.full). Furthermore, a series of other papers, written over a 20-year period, has also outlined methods for QA in diagnostic immunohistology [67–73].

Specific Methods for Quality Control in DIHC

"Validation" and "verification" are terms that are often used in reference to DIHC. In a pure sense, the first of them – validation – refers to the process of testing putatively reactive and nonreactive tissues for the target antigen, to document the absence of false-positive and false-negative results. The second, verification, relates to proper performance of an immunohistochemical assay in a specific setting – e.g., in paraffin sections as opposed to frozen tissue [66].

There are alternative meanings to one of these two terms that are also appropriate. *Chronological* validation of immunostains can and should be done over time in any given laboratory; here, known positive and negative test cases are studied over and over to monitor the consistency of results. *Procedural* validation (or "cross"-validation) implies that a "positive" immunostain is confirmed by data generated through another testing method. A representative example is electron microscopic evidence of epithelial differentiation in the same tissue sample that showed immunoreactivity for epithelial markers. *Extramural* validation applies when tissue samples show the same immunoreactivity patterns in at least two laboratories, with one acting as a reference [67]. All three of these procedures should be a part of QA measures in any DIHC laboratory. If vendors or lots are changed at some point for a particular antibody reagent, or there is an alteration in procedural platforms (e.g., manual vs. automated staining), internal QA assessments should reflect those facts. It is particularly important to give an extramural reference laboratory a detailed description of one's own IHC methods, so that its personnel can apply the same procedures to monitor reproducibility of results.

Unfortunately, because these techniques take time, effort, and money to do regularly, many hospital laboratories have abridged or ignored them. Nevertheless, that is a prescription for performance problems over time. The Canadian experience is relevant here. After well-publicized problems with intra- and inter-laboratory reproducibility for selected biomarkers, provincial efforts to standardize laboratory practice through guidelines and through centralized external QA have prompted considerable attention to test validation/verification and significant improvement in lab-to-lab concordance. These processes, now being centralized under a Canadian Association of Pathologists initiative called cIQc (www.ciqc.ca), have the potential to provide realtime feedback to participating laboratories regarding best practices in tissue preparation, methodology (and method platforms), controls, reagent selection, and interpretation. Similar programs exist in the UK as well, and perhaps the most robust external QA program available to pathology labs worldwide is NordiQC (www.nordiqc.org). By contrast, centralized external QC in the United States has its only meaningful expression in College of American Pathologists IHC surveys, and despite well over a decade of experience, this program provides little meaningful feedback to participating labs. More recent attention on test validation has prompted the development of recommended guidelines for performance of selected biomarkers (*Her2/neu, estrogen receptor protein [ERP] and progesterone receptor protein [PRP]) and more specific guidelines for test validation, but these guidelines lack a clear evidence-based argument for many of the core recommendations. Perhaps the requirement of initial and ongoing test validation for these biomarkers will focus laboratory attention on the value of external and internal QA, but at the time of this writing, it is likely that fewer than half of American laboratories have meaningful validation procedures in place for most immunohistochemical tests.

Published Literature on DIHC: How Should It Be Used?

Medical publications concerning IHC span at least 40 years, with many variations in technique as well as results. Even today, some readers of the literature miss the fact that differences in reagents and protocols will have potentially striking influences on the final staining "product." This is due, in part, to a lack of complete methodologic information in some reports, making selected elements of the published literature unreproducible. Recent consensus work on IHC, fluorescent in situ hybridization, and other techniques may help mitigate this shortcoming.

Even so, in our current working environment, if one wishes to achieve a reliable, workable structure of diagnostic immunohistology in any given laboratory, one of two requirements must be met. The first, and the most onerous, demands that extensive "catalog" testing be done with each antibody one wishes to use, probably by analysis of tissue "microarrays" (Fig. 16.11). Parenthetically, "microarray" is simply a new name for an old concept introduced by Dr. Hector Battifora, who described the use of "multitumor ['sausage'] tissue blocks" 25 years ago [74]. In this approach, one records the immunoreactivity of each particular antibody, with a particular staining platform, against many examples of many tumor types, generating a statistical matrix to be used in interpretation [75–77]. The time and resources necessary to accomplish this task are daunting. Alternatively, and more expeditiously, one can use the literature to see which reagents and procedures have been used by reference IHC laboratories that have published their results widely. Those reagents and procedures can then be replicated – exactly – with the expectation that the results of the external laboratory will be mirrored in one's own experience.

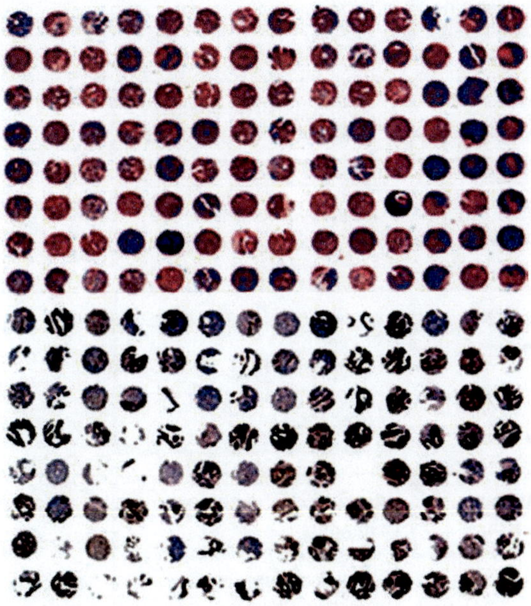

Fig. 16.11 A tissue microarray, comprising many samples of neoplastic tissue from a variety of human tumor types, stained with hematoxylin and eosin (*top*) and an antibody to pankeratin (*bottom*)

The principal error that enters into this process is focused on attempts to compare things that are incomparable. If reagents or procedures are not the same in laboratory A as in laboratory B, their results will not be parallel over time [78].

Does DIHC Conform to the Principles of Evidence-Based Medicine?

The foregoing discussion begs a question – is DIHC a truly evidence-based area of pathology? The response is necessarily equivocal, depending on supporting information. If one accepts the premise that DIHC is best used as a binary, somewhat artificial but reproducible practical tool, the reply is a qualified "yes." However, even that response has a major caveat, focused on the unswerving need to copy and control the reagents and procedures used by investigators with wide and published experiences. And, in this context, the literature (the evidentiary basis for DIHC) may unintentionally mislead those who consult uncensored studies, data sets, or meta-analyses of existing information. Indeed, without a clear understanding of the shortcomings of selected studies (aggravated by the lack of complete methodologic detail noted earlier), a casual reader of the literature might conclude that few, if any, markers of putative diagnostic interest are reliable. At issue is the value of the extant literature taken as a whole. It does not escape our attention that a dichotomous (and diagnostically useful) stain result, when based on reliable literature sources or external QA, will assume a more continuous (and less useful) expression across a targeted differential diagnosis when uncensored literature is employed. But the pathologist is not merely responsible for being able to access the most reliable evidence for a given test. As one of us has stated in an earlier communication:

> Surgical pathologists and cytopathologists must, by consensus or by mandate, use only validated standardized methods for DIHC, to the absolute exclusion of others. This statement seems simple, but it is far from that. Many variables, including the size and thickness of tissue blocks used for immunohistology, the nature and length of fixation, methods used for epitope 'retrieval,' antibody binding-detection technique, choice of chromogenic substrate, and the use of intensifiers of immunoprecipitation, are all included under the rubric of immunohistochemical 'method' [71].

In referring to the flow diagram of evidence-based medicine (EBM) devised by Friedland et al. [79] (Fig. 16.12), one finds additional points of potential departure between the fields of DIHC and pristine EBM. These come under the heading of "medical decision-making techniques," and are represented by probability assessments, decision analysis, and evaluation of cost-effectiveness. In specific reference to immunohistology, pathologists (and other physicians) are commonly oblivious to the concepts of prior diagnostic probability, posterior diagnostic probability, and likelihood ratios. They often obtain immunostains with little or no attention to how (or if) the results will alter their morphological diagnostic impressions. Are the tests likely to be dispositive, will they substantially narrow the field of possibilities, or might they merely cause confusion? The answers to those questions must come from a combination of empirical experience and data obtained from the pertinent literature [80]. *An immunostain should not be procured simply based on its availability, because, with a probability of >0, results may not conform to the "expected" product.* An example follows.

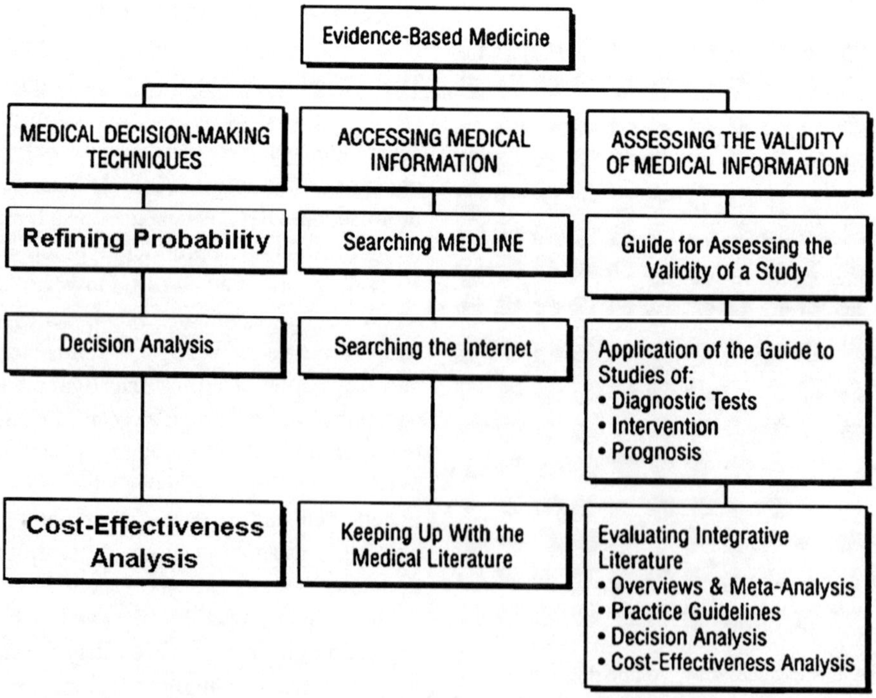

Fig. 16.12 Organization diagram depicting the elements of evidence-based medicine, as conceptualized by Friedland et al. [79]

Immunohistochemical Results: Relationship to Prior and Posterior Probability

An irregular mass was detected mammographically in the left breast of a 57 year old woman (Fig. 16.13). An excisional biopsy of the lesion demonstrated an infiltrative carcinoma featuring the linear growth of small polygonal cells with regular, round nuclei; only small nucleoli; and a low mitotic rate (Fig. 16.14). Profiles of tumor cells tended to surround preexisting interlobular and intralobular ducts. The attending pathologist obtained an immunostain for E-cadherin, which yielded positive results (Fig. 16.15). There was also reactivity for estrogen and progesterone receptor proteins, and a lack of *HER-2* gene amplification, a diagnosis of Nottingham grade II invasive ductal adenocarcinoma was therefore made (erroneously).

The scenario just described is not rare, in our experience, and it illustrates problems that accompany an ignorance of probability refinement. Essentially, all pathologists would accept the microscopic image of the breast tumor in the exemplary case as completely diagnostic for invasive lobular carcinoma (ILC). Thus, the prior diagnostic probability approximates 100%, and is not lessened appreciably by a single unexpected immunohistochemical result. Da Silva et al. [81] have shown that approximately 20% of ILCs manifest aberrant immunoreactivity for E-cadherin; hence, that test is far from determinative, in and of itself. In short, an expert knowledge of morphology still provides very high prior diagnostic probabilities. Procuring unnecessary immunostains in that circumstance is more likely to produce confusion than certainty. This reality, in turn, feeds directly into "medical decision analysis." Surgical pathologic diagnoses never exist in a vacuum – the attending physician will use such information to structure a plan of treatment, and pathologists' mistakes may well become clinicians' mistakes. Da Silva et al. reached similar conclusions, stating:

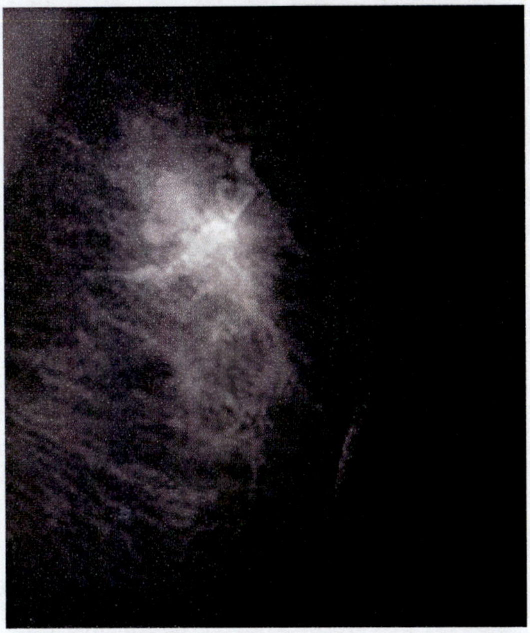

Fig. 16.13 Mammographic image of the left breast, showing an irregular mass density having the morphologic features of a malignancy

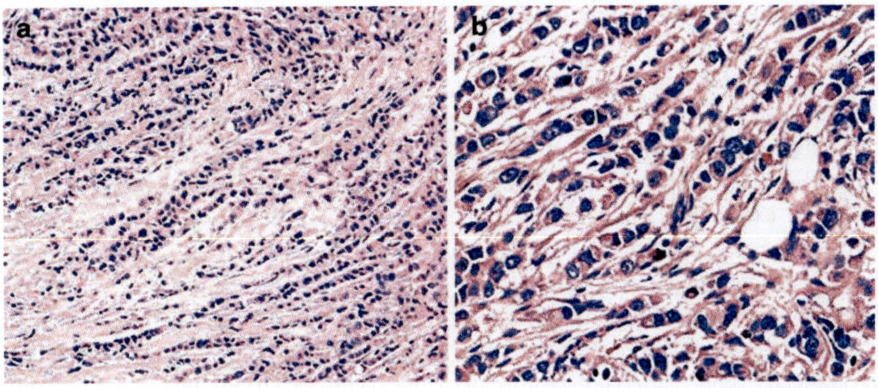

Fig. 16.14 (a, b) Linear profiles are seen of an invasive breast carcinoma exhibiting cellular monomorphism and relatively bland nuclear features. The images are diagnostic of infiltrating lobular mammary adenocarcinoma

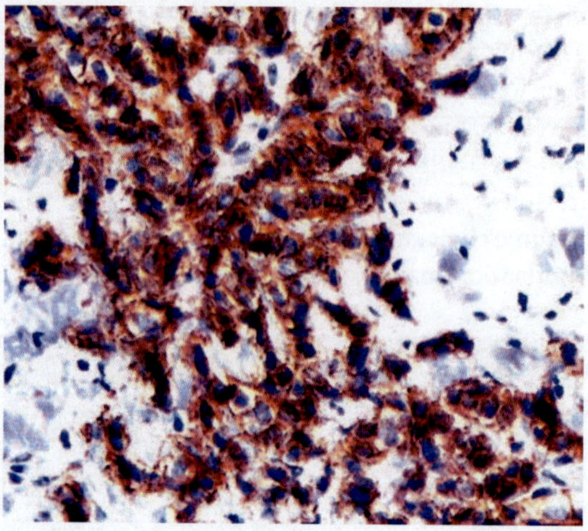

Fig. 16.15 Aberrant immunoreactivity in lobular breast carcinoma for E-cadherin. The latter marker is by no means determinative of ductal differentiation in breast cancers, as supposed by some observers

> Positive staining for E-cadherin should not preclude a diagnosis of lobular in favor of ductal carcinoma. Molecular evidence suggests that even when E-cadherin is expressed, the cadherin-catenin complex maybe nonfunctional. Misclassification of tumors may lead to mismanagement of patients in clinical practice… [81]

Revisionistic approaches to histopathologic diagnosis, based exclusively on information from nonmorphological adjunctive techniques, are unscientific and nonbiological. In fact, they typically reflect a kind of circular reasoning.

Use and Abuse of DIHC for Diagnostic Purposes in Routine Pathology Practice

When and How Should DIHC Be Used During the Diagnostic Process?

Readers may consider that it is silly to discuss when and how to use DIHC in daily practice in 2010, but it is our anecdotal experience from consultations that there is considerable variability and confusion in the pathology community about which antibodies should be used for certain differential diagnoses, how many antibodies should be tested, and how to interpret IHC results that do not conform to diagnoses that would otherwise be rendered on the basis of histopathologic criteria. Indeed, many pathologists and reference laboratories appear to apply DIHC using a "shotgun approach," perhaps reasoning that "the more the better" and without full consideration of what they are planning to do with the results. This practice results not only in unnecessary costs but also in diagnostic dilemmas that lead to further testing, potential confusion, and/or diagnostic errors.

It is well known that there are few if any entirely specific IHC results for any one diagnosis. In addition, the definitions of various clinico-pathologic entities provided by WHO, Armed Forces Institute of Pathology (AFIP), and other standard textbooks and publications do not generally include various potential DHIC results as diagnostic criteria [82–86]. Except for hematologic and lymphoproliferative disorders and selected other conditions, pathology publications generally define a variety of entities on the basis of clinico-pathologic criteria, describe their gross pathology and histopathologic features, and include in a subsequent section a description of the characteristic immunophenotype of the lesion and sometimes the sensitivity and specificity of various antibodies [87, 88]. These descriptions do not generally provide specific information regarding when and how to use selected antibodies to confirm or disprove the diagnosis of the entity being described. This practice raises the question of how best to use immunophenotypic information obtained by testing antibodies that are usually less than 100% specific for the diagnosis of entities that have been previously defined on the basis of clinical features, gross pathology, and H&E histopathology. In particular, in which cases should the DHIC test results override the diagnostic impressions collected from the clinical findings, gross pathology, and H&E histopathology? In daily practice, it is often comforting to observe that the immunophenotype of a lesion conforms with the description provided in the literature, "confirming the diagnosis," but it can be equally discomforting to render a particular diagnosis in the presence of negative results after the tests have been performed. In these instances, practicing pathologists are expected to interpret the puzzling DIHC results based solely on their "clinical judgment," a paradigm that has been somewhat discredited in the Evidence-Based Medicine literature [89, 90].

For example, one of us (AM) recently consulted two separate internationally respected experts regarding the diagnosis of a spindle cell lung neoplasm that had histomorphologic features of solitary fibrous tumor (SFT) but exhibited negative tumor cell immunoreactivity for CD34, in the presence of positive immunoreactivity for that antibody in tumor blood vessels. One of the experts opined that the tumor was indeed an SFT while the other did not. Who rendered the correct diagnosis? Should we continue using the CD34 test during the diagnostic process of a presumed SFT if we are not certain about how to interpret negative DIHC results? In our view, if more detailed information regarding how to interpret CD34 immunoreactivity during the diagnostic process of an SFT were explicitly addressed in pathology textbooks and other publications, either as formal recommendations or as a definitional criteria, the need to worry about the diagnosis of this case and/or generate a consultation at additional cost to the patient would be obviated.

Another example from AM's consultation practice illustrates some of the problems generated by the use of unnecessary DIHC tests. A pneumonectomy specimen showed two nodules of carcinoid tumor involving the lung and N2 mediastinal lymph nodes. The consult materials included 15 different immunostains, including neuroendocrine markers, CK7, CK20 and TTF-1, and others. DIHC for Ki-67, an immunostain that is being routinely used for the evaluation of neuroendocrine neoplasms in our laboratory was not performed. The tumor cells exhibited cytoplasmic immunoreactivity for chromogranin, synaptophysin, CK7, and CK20 but only weak and patchy nuclear immunoreactivity for TTF-1. Does this patient have a metastatic carcinoid tumor from the gastrointestinal (GI) tract or a primary pulmonary carcinoid tumor? Literature review showed a few studies of a small number of carcinoid tumors arising in the lung and GI tract [91]. Primary pulmonary carcinoid tumors were uniformly negative for CK20 and positive for CK7 while most GI primaries exhibited cytoplasmic immunoreactivity for CK20 and variable CK7 immunoreactivity. Is this enough evidence to diagnose the case as a metastatic carcinoid tumor to the lung from a primary GI lesion? If neither the original pathologist nor the consultant is certain about how to interpret the information provided by the CK7 and CK20 tests, what is their diagnostic value or clinical applicability?

Further questions can be asked regarding the use of Ki-67 IHC for the work-up of pulmonary neuroendocrine neoplasms. Should we really perform this test routinely, as we currently do at Cedars-Sinai Medical Center based on requests from our oncologists? In reality, the WHO diagnostic criteria for pulmonary neuroendocrine neoplasms do not include the use of the Ki-67 test, and there are no widely accepted guidelines in the literature about what specific cut-off values should be used to distinguish typical from atypical pulmonary carcinoid tumors and these tumors from high-grade neuroendocrine carcinomas [92, 93]. We are being asked to perform and provide an interpretation of the relevance of the percentage of nuclear Ki-67 immunoreactivity in the tumor cells based on our overall pathologic impression about a pulmonary neuroendocrine tumor. The Ki-67 DIHC test is being used for the evaluation of GI neuroendocrine tumors and cut-off ranges of <2, 2–20, and >20% have been proposed by the American Joint Commission on Cancer for the distinction between low-grade, intermediate-grade, and high-grade lesions, based on very limited available data [94].

Review of the various principles of Evidence-Based Pathology discussed in this volume and some of the problems illustrated in this chapter strongly suggests that there is a need for more specific guidelines for the use of DIHC in daily practice that will explicitly describe which antibodies should be used to render particular diagnoses and how to interpret respective positive and negative results.

Should DIHC Be Used to Distinguish Benign from Malignant Lesions?

Certain DIHC tests are useful to help distinguish benign from malignant lesions, such as the expression of racemase in prostate biopsies that exhibit atypical epithelial lesions or of myoepithelial markers in breast biopsies with sclerosing adenosis [95, 96]. However, as certain immunophenotypes are more frequently expressed than others in selected benign or malignant lesions, pathologists can be tempted to use a variety of antibodies that have been described for other purposes to help diagnose malignant lesions. For example, AM periodically receives lung biopsies that have been tested for p53 to help distinguish benign reactive atypical pneumocytes from bronchioloalveolar carcinoma of the lung (BAC) or reactive mesothelial hyperplasia from malignant mesothelioma. Although p53 immunoreactivity has been described in BAC, malignant mesothelioma, and some presumably premalignant conditions, these descriptive observations were probably not intended as a diagnostic test of malignancy, and have not been prospectively validated for this purpose [97, 98]. Indeed, when we receive these cases, we often wonder why we were consulted if p53 was positive after being ordered by a pathologist who presumably believes in its diagnostic value. Internationally renowned experts can also disagree on when and how to use DHIC to help distinguish benign from malignant lesions. For example, AM periodically submits in consultation difficult thyroid lesions that could represent an encapsulated papillary carcinoma, follicular variant, or a follicular adenoma with some cells exhibiting nuclear folds or equivocal chromatin clearing. Some experts appear to favor the use of HMBE1 and CK19 testing for this differential diagnosis while others rely solely on the interpretation of the cytologic features of the lesion [99]. To our knowledge, there is limited information regarding the clinical validity of using DHIC in this differential diagnosis and no accepted gold standard to validate the results.

Which Antibodies Should Be Used for a Particular Differential Diagnosis? Use of Positive Likelihood Ratios to Help Select the Most Cost-Effective Components of an Antibody Panel

Evidence-Based Medicine and EBP principles favor the use of a systematic probabilistic approach for the interpretation of information and the selection of antibody panels and other tasks that aid in diagnosis, as discussed in more detail in Chaps. 4 and 13. In anatomic pathology, the general approach involves identification of the particular group of diagnoses that need to be sorted out in a particular specimen, evaluation of the relative pretest probabilities of various diagnoses based on the incidence of the various entities being considered, query for the presence of selected pathological features that can identify the most likely diagnoses, identification of the "best" antibodies based on the +likelihood ratio (+LR) of each test, and selection of the smallest panel of DHIC or other tests that can help sort out the "final" differential diagnosis using probability ratios (PR) or odds ratios (OR). Table 16.1 shows a series of questions that can guide pathologists in their use of DHIC using this systematic probabilistic approach.

Different sets of statistics are available, but +LR probably provides the most useful statistical tool to help identify the most effective antibody for a particular diagnosis, as they incorporate information regarding the prevalence of various diagnoses and information regarding the effectiveness of a test as illustrated by its true-positive, true-negative, false-positive, and false-negative results. They can be calculated using the formula +LR = sensitivity/1 − specificity.

Table 16.1 Questions that can help pathologists navigate the process of evaluating specimens with diagnostic immunohistochemistry using a systematic probabilistic approach

What is my differential diagnosis?
Which are the most likely clinico-pathological entities in the differential diagnoses, based on their prevalence in my patient population (pretest probabilities of various diagnoses)?
Which are the gross pathology features or imaging findings, if available, that can help me narrow the differential diagnosis?
What is my postgross pathology/radiology test differential diagnosis?
Which are the histopathological features that can help me narrow the previous differential diagnosis?
What is my posthistology test differential diagnosis?
Which are the most effective antibodies to help me work out the previous differential diagnosis, by their +likelihood ratios (+LR)?
Which panel of antibodies with best available +LR that would give the best probability ratios (PR) or odds ratios (OR) of rendering a final diagnosis?
What is my final diagnosis after consideration of all the available information?

A recent study by Westfall et al. used this general methodology to develop evidence-based guidelines to optimize the selection of antibody panels in pleural cytology specimens with malignant epithelioid cells [100]. The study evaluated retrospectively the use of DHIC in 153 consecutive pleural effusions diagnosed at Cedars-Sinai Medical Center. Cases were randomly divided into training and test cases as explained in Chaps. 10 and 11. The prevalence of different malignancies in the training set was identified; the most frequent diagnoses were carcinomas of the lung, breast, Mullerian tract, stomach, and colon. Thereafter, the percentage of cases that were positive for various antibodies, by diagnosis, was identified. These data were used to calculate the sensitivity and specificity of each DHIC result and their +LR. The clinical usefulness of each antibody was then stratified according to each +LR, as the most sensitive and specific test DHIC result provides the highest ratios. On the basis of these data, antibody panels for the study of pleural effusions in male (calretinin, TTF-1, and CDX-2) and female (TTF-1, ER, and CA125) patients were selected. The diagnostic value of these panels was then tested using the test set of cases and showed that they provided 100% specificity, and 77% and 50% sensitivity for male and female patients, respectively. The study also showed that the use of additional antibodies such as CK5/6, CK7, Ber-EP4, CK20, and many others did not improve the results obtained with the panels.

How Many Antibodies Should Be Used for a Particular Differential Diagnosis? Use of Probability Ratios and Odds Ratios to Help Select the Optimal Number of Antibodies that Should Be Incorporated in an Antibody Panel

Probability theory can also be used to help identify how many antibodies should be incorporated in an antibody panel to provide the most cost-effective results. Different statistical tools are available, but PR and OR probably provide the simplest and most effective tools for this task. For example, if TTF-1 is positive in 85% of pulmonary adenocarcinomas, the probability of a positive finding is 0.85 and the probability of a negative finding is 0.15. The PR is 0.85/0.15=5.7. These data can also be transformed into odds and OR using the formulas odds=probability/1−probability and OR=Odd1/Odd2 resulting in values of 5.7, 0.17, and 33.5, respectively. Probabilities of multiple tests can be combined by multiplication, and the PR and OR of various panels can be calculated.

Marchevsky and Wick used this approach for evaluation of the use of DHIC for the differential diagnosis between pulmonary adenocarcinoma and malignant mesothelioma, using data from a systematic literature review [101]. The results clearly showed that the OR of a mesothelioma diagnosis rendered by using only one antibody were superior to those obtained by using antibody panels composed with as many as 15 antibodies, disproving in this situation the theory that "the more the better." Indeed, although a pathologist may intuitively think that the larger the number of IHC tested, the more comprehensive and precise the evaluation of a lesion, in reality each test is associated with a certain number of false-positive and negative results that in aggregate progressively decrease the accuracy of the diagnosis as more antibodies are tested. For example, the OR provided by 1 antibody, 2 antibodies (MOC-31 and TTF-1), and 15 antibodies for the diagnosis of epithelioid malignant mesothelioma were 80.35, 198.18, and 9.46, respectively. The study did not advocate using only one or two antibodies for the diagnosis of malignant mesothelioma, but suggested that OR information should be considered during the selection of sensible and cost-effective antibody panels.

Prognostic-Predictive Immunohistology and EBM

At this point in our discussion, we now come to a "parting of the ways" from diagnostic immunohistology, and will, hereafter, consider the related but quite dissimilar discipline of prognostic-predictive immunohistochemistry (PPIHC). Some, but not all, of the information presented hereafter is comparable to material in the chapter of this book that is specifically directed at prognostication and prediction.

DIHC and PPIHC differ in important ways. The sole purpose and chief clinical application of DIHC are the production of reproducible categorical data, based on groups of binary test results. By contrast, PPIHC concerns an attempt to generate semiquantitative data that often are substituted for information from molecular studies, and which are used in an attempt to forecast overall case-outcomes and responses to specific therapies [102].

"Windows" of Immunoreactivity

As mentioned earlier, an integral part of antibody testing in DIHC is the setting of arbitrary but definable ranges for the detectability of target antigens in tissue. That goal is accomplished by studying a group of related specimens, e.g., prostatic adenocarcinomas with low, medium, and high Gleason scores, labeled with an antibody to prostate-specific antigen, which approximate, as closely as possible, samples with fixation characteristics like those which will be studied in one's own laboratory prospectively. An antibody titer is chosen that will recognize antigen densities within a "window" defined by the lowest grade tumor on one hand and the highest grade tumor on the other. At the same time, attention must be paid to unwanted, nonspecific "background" labeling (as well as unexpected "true" expression in diagnostically confounding cell types or patterns), with the aim of minimizing it. The process just described reflects a kind of contrivance or artifice, but it is needed in order to include the desired diagnosis and exclude others. This is a relatively straightforward procedure, and establishes a platform for binary interpretations of "positive" and "negative."

The situation pertaining to PPIHC is different, because that technique aims to detect intracellular protein concentrations over a complete continuum starting at zero and ending at infinity. In other words, it is not sufficient to determine categorically whether a target protein is present or not; instead, one must provide a semiquantitative or quantitative estimation of its density in PPIHC, instead of working within a predetermined "window" [103]. Moreover, a scientific leap of faith is attached; it is usually assumed in PPIHC that the antibody specifically recognizes the target antigen (and only this target) and that cellular protein concentrations are a direct, linear reflection of gene transcription and translation (including gene amplification), or, alternatively, a sign of crucial gene mutation [104–107]. These paradigms are often incorrect, because they tend to oversimplify the molecular pathways in which the genes of interest participate (Figs. 16.16 and 16.17).

The notion of quantitative IHC has been extant for many years, as a holy grail that is intended to provide a substitute for actual molecular assessments [103, 108–112]. This quest has persisted because IHC is relatively "easy" to perform vis-à-vis the demands of nucleic acid blotting techniques, polymerase chain reaction-based assays, and gene sequencing. PPIHC is also much less expensive and much more available to hospital practitioners. Nonetheless, there are two principal reasons that it fails in its ultimate mission, the prognostication and prediction of disease progress. The first reason is that variations in tissue fixation and processing, immunohistological technique, and ultimate visual interpretation may easily shift the result from one place to nother on a continuous scale [103]. That is not nearly so true in the "windowed" environment of DIHC.

Intralaboratory efforts at controlling preanalytic variables may enjoy a certain level of success in PPIHC; nevertheless, when samples are traded *between* laboratories (as in protocol studies of various therapies, or patient referrals from one hospital to another), distinct differences in results are often seen. Second, one must consider the concept of "dynamic range" (DR) in evaluating PPIHC preparations, as well summarized by Rimm [102].

Dynamic Range: A Physical Concept with Relevance to PPIHC

DR is a concept from the discipline of physics. It is defined as the ratio between the smallest and largest possible values of a changeable quantity

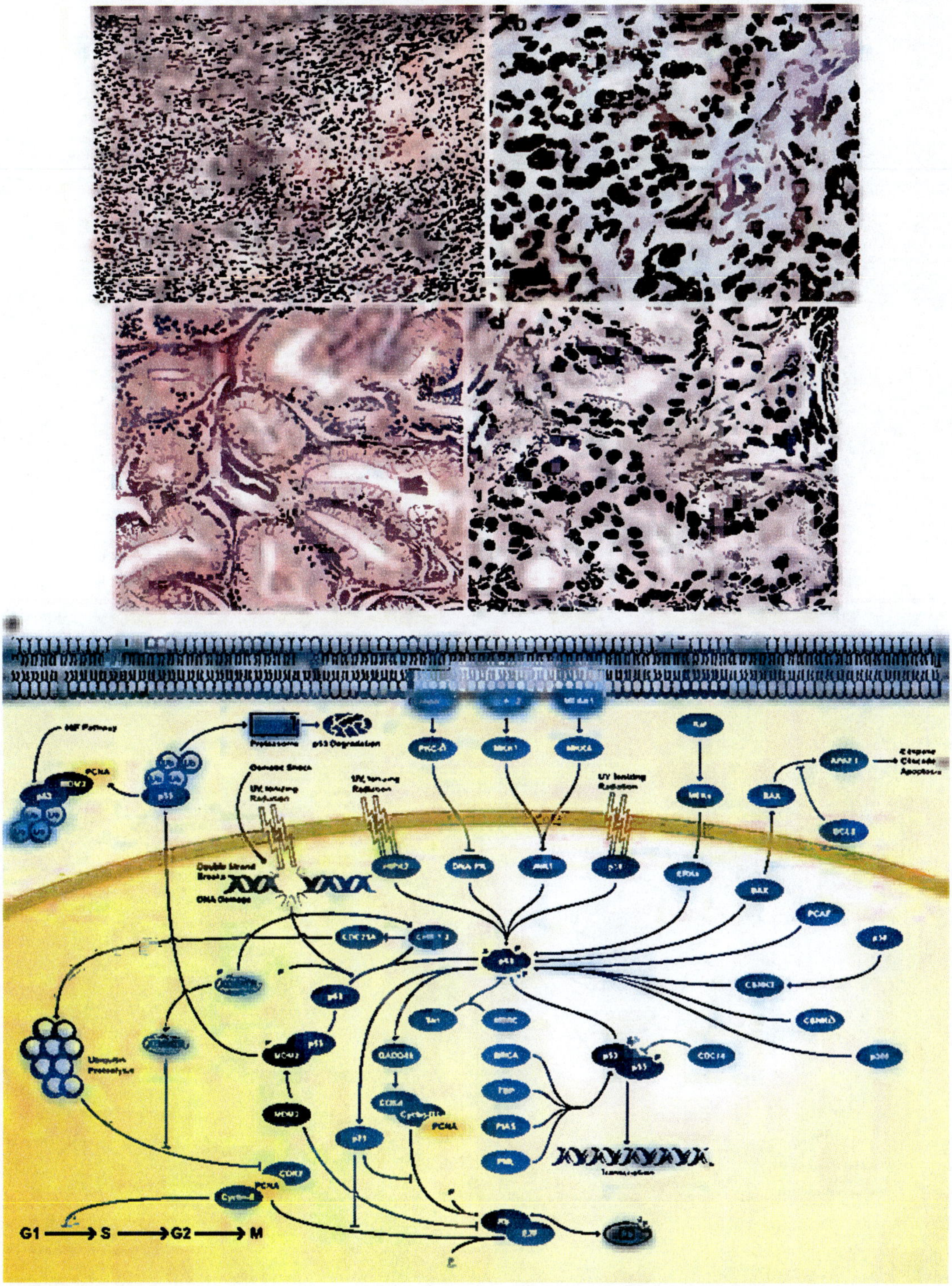

Fig. 16.16 (**a**) Glioblastoma multiforme of the frontal cerebral cortex, immunostained (**b**) for putatively mutant p53 protein. (**c**) Gleason score-6 prostatic adenocarcinoma, also immunolabeled for p53 protein (**d**). The complexity of the p53 pathway is shown here, providing several other explanations for p53 immunostaining besides actual gene mutation (**e**)

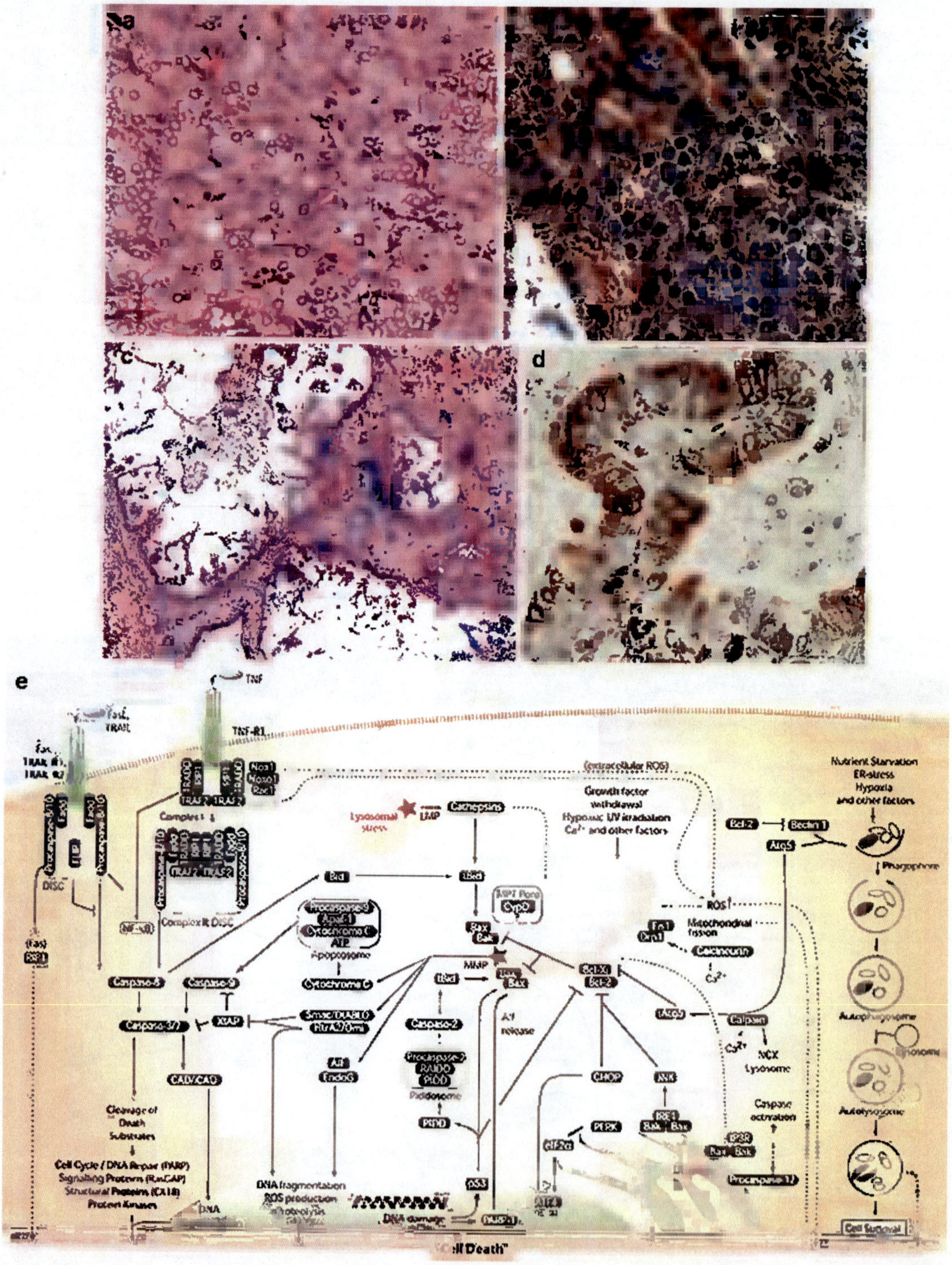

Fig. 16.17 (**a**) Gleason score 9 adenocarcinoma of the prostate, labeled for *bcl*-2 protein (**b**). Micropapillary adenocarcinoma of the lung (**c**), immunostained for *bcl*-2 (**d**). The pertinent genetic pathway impacting *bcl*-2 is also complicated (**e**)

such as sound or light [113]. DR is closely related to "signal-to-noise ratios," and both are usually measured in a base-10 logarithmic context, using the term "base-doublings" (dB). This approach yields the following equation for signals with a wide DR, where SNR = signal-to-noise ratio and P = average signal power [30]:

$$SNR_{dB} = 10_{\log 10}(P_{signal} / P_{noise}).$$

In DIHC, one aims to maximize the SNR_{dB}, and the desired staining product is represented by a dense, dark precipitate over the target antigen. In other words, almost all of the transmissible light in a microscopic preparation is absorbed by the chromogen, leaving approximately 1% for analysis by the eye or another sensor [102]. That is a good system for binary data generation, as in DIHC, but *not* for quantitative-continuous analysis as desired in PPIHC. The observer is forced to parse the remaining 1% signal into even-smaller units if a scaled result is the goal. If attempts are made to lessen the target-signal power, the signal of the *noise* assumes proportionately greater significance. That point is illustrated by Fig. 16.18, taken from the field of photography; the greater the signal power, the shorter the exposure (F-stop setting) is on a camera, and the lower the noise. However, as F-stops increase because signal intensity drops, noise steadily increases as well.

The latter construct explains why one has serious problems in trying to subdivide the mid-portion of a DR plot based on 1% residual signal power in PPIHC. Very slight alterations in the system, such as increasing the antibody concentration, adding a chromogen-intensifier, or substituting one chromogen for another, predictably change the DR results, sometimes markedly. As Rimm indicated:

> ...highly-expressing cancers may not be resolved from the majority of moderately-expressing cancers when using a high antibody concentration, owing to saturation of the assay. Using these types of observations, an investigator **[A]** might resolve only the low expressors... The reverse could be the case for an investigator **[B]** who uses a very low concentration of antibody [102].

The end result of those dichotomous outcomes is that observer A would likely group mid-range

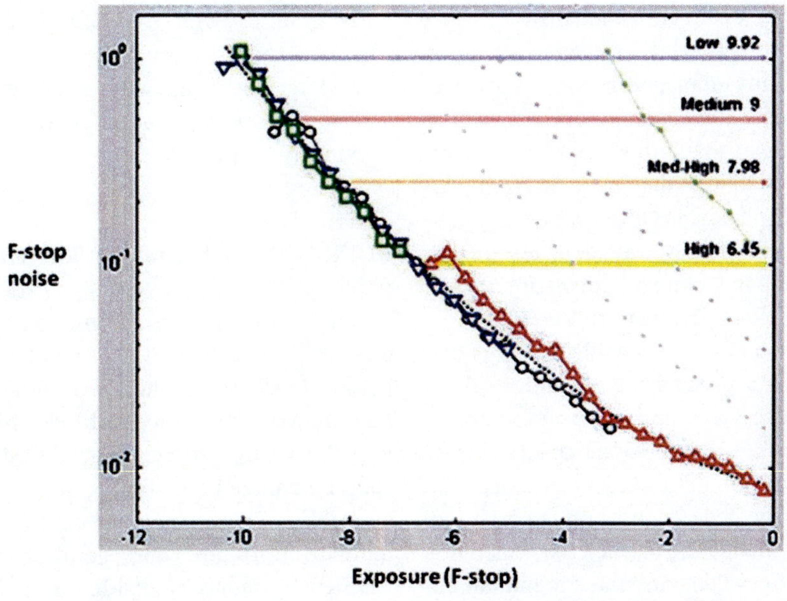

Fig. 16.18 This plot of photographic dynamic range (DR) shows that as exposure (f-stop) times increase, noise also increases and DR (low-medium-medium/high-high) decreases. In immunohistochemistry, a parallel paradigm obtains – the lower the quantity of light transmitted through an absorbing moiety (an immunostained slide), the lower the DR

cases with "high" expressors, and observer B would place them among "low" expressors. In turn, these mishaps could lead the two observers to conclude contradictorily that *both* low and high immunoexpression of the same analyte in PPIHC are prognostically associated with the same (good or bad) outcome. As stressed earlier, any other factor that affects final immunostaining intensity could potentially change the DR of the technique as well. Some examples are out-of-range pH in a given lot of formalin fixative, inappropriate fixation, inadequate epitope retrieval, or inconsistency of immunodetection methodology over time. This is likely also relevant to the apparent dichotomization of ERP and PRP by the use of altered tissue preservation techniques, or maximally sensitivity methodology.

Examples of Failure in Attempts at Quantitative PPIHC

A truism in biomedical technology is that *when one substitutes a vicarious technique for first-hand evaluation of any particular analyte, errors will result.* Looking at the "genuine article" directly is always the best course of action. Nonetheless, that statement is idealistic. Proper assessment of biochemical moieties is often tedious, technically demanding, and expensive, and it may well require special processing of tissue or fluid samples that will serve as substrates. By contrast, even though they have all been educated in science, physicians often seek the quickest, cheapest, and easiest way to a test result. Indeed, that is the most direct explanation for the current state of affairs in regard to PPIHC.

Typically, soon after a mechanistic link is discovered between a particular gene and a salient intracellular process – especially in reference to malignant diseases – attempts are made to integrate the observation into clinical practice. No matter whether the gene in question is amplified, overexpressed, mutated, or deleted, methods quickly evolve to evaluate its status in human tissue. Obviously, based on the foregoing comments, the best mode of analysis would be a direct one; i.e., first-hand assessment of the integrity of the gene itself with procedures such as Southern blotting, polymerase chain reaction-based assays, in situ hybridization, and nucleotide sequencing [114–116]. Nonetheless, because those methods are demanding ones in comparison with PPIHC, the "default" position often has been to utilize a "quantitative" immunohistochemical substitute, whenever possible, for the technical "real McCoy." This problem, of course, would be lessened if laboratories carefully validated the PPIHC method against the clinically validated marker analysis method. A prescription for success in this regard was proposed by McGuire in 1991 [117].

Moreover, a great deal of scientific naïvete has tainted such undertakings. Simply because a polypeptide gene product is detectable immunohistologically, many observers are ready to leap to the conclusion that biological inhibitors of the protein will have an inevitable effect on its role in the cell. Principal examples of that flawed line of reasoning include PPIHC testing for epidermal growth factor receptor (EGFR), *HER-2*, and c-*kit* (CD117) in human neoplasms [118–120]. Prospective attention to the principles of EBM would likely have obviated such problems. Other, slightly less troublesome analytes in PPIHC are the ERPs and PRPs in breast carcinoma.

Difficulties with the clinical evaluation of *HER*-2 status in human tumors have been discussed in Chap. 5 and are not recounted here. We will subsequently examine the other topics cited previously in more detail.

EGFR

EGFR is a member (along with *HER*-2) of the *ErbB* gene family, a group of transmembrane proteins that function as tyrosine kinase receptors and are activated by several extracellular ligands [121]. In the late 1990s, biological agents that showed the ability to block the binding of EGFR to its ligands were introduced, and several such humanized anti-EGFR antibodies now are available. These include cetuximab, panitumumab, erlotinib, and gefitinib [122, 123]. EGFR is immunodetectable on the cell surfaces of several tumors, but those of clinical interest mainly include squamous cell carcinomas of the head and neck; adenocarcinomas of the lung

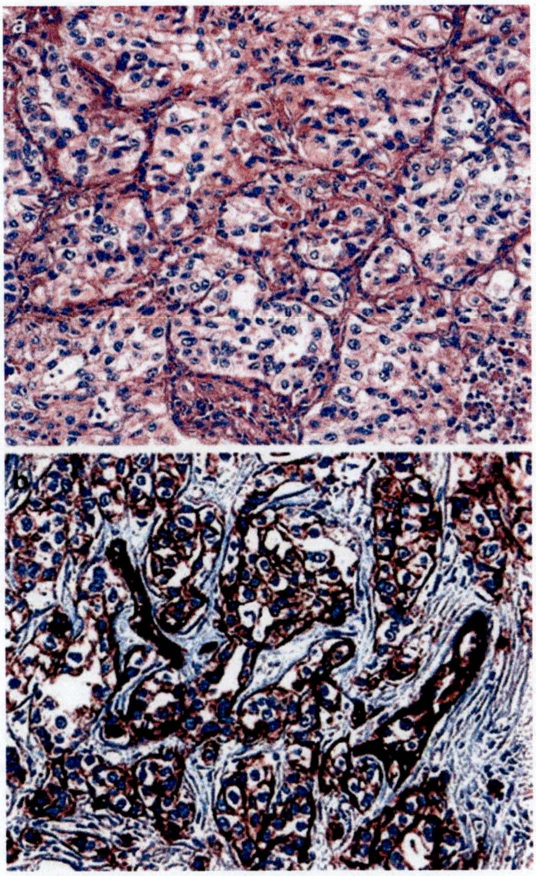

Fig. 16.19 (**a**) Adenocarcinoma of the lung, immunostained for epidermal growth factor receptor protein (**b**)

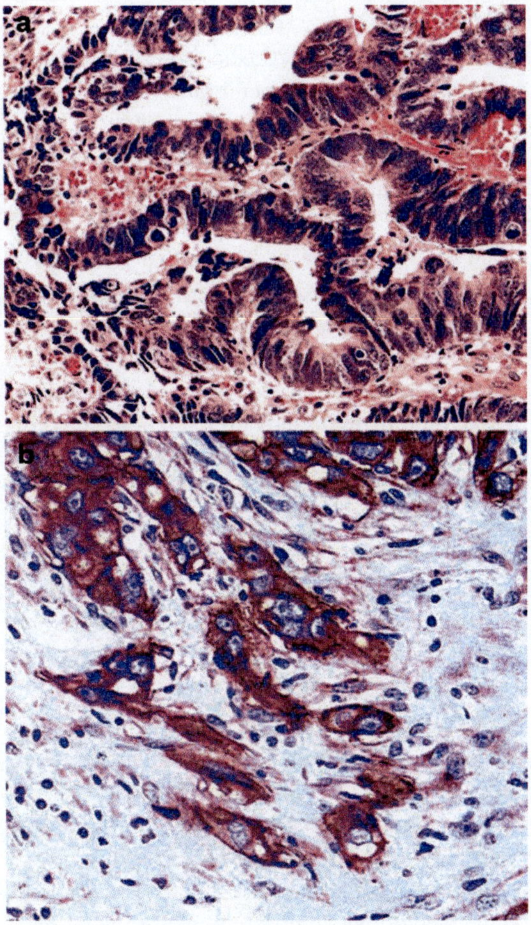

Fig. 16.20 (**a**) Adenocarcinoma of the colon, immunostained for epidermal growth factor receptor protein (**b**)

(Fig. 16.19); and colorectal adenocarcinomas [122] (Fig. 16.20).

Early treatment protocols with EGFR inhibitors required that PPIHC procedures show the presence of EGFR protein in neoplastic cells, in order for patients to be eligible for therapy. Biomedical companies with laboratory-medicine arms were quick to respond, marketing EGFR immunostaining "kits" that were approved for use by the U.S. Food and Drug Administration. However, the antibody reagents in those kits were questionably specific. For example, essentially all colorectal carcinomas were labeled with one commercial kit, making IHC testing superfluous [124]. In addition, comparisons with other (nonkit-based) anti-EGFR antibodies often produced strikingly dissimilar immunohistochemical results in the same tumors [125, 126].

After years of data accrual and analysis, virtually all recent publications have concluded that the immunohistologic EGFR status of human neoplasms has no predictive value for their possible therapeutic response to biological inhibitors [120, 124, 127–129]. It now appears that the dispositive piece of information in that regard is the presence or absence of selected EGFR gene *mutations* [129], particularly in lung adenocarcinoma, or the concomitant activating mutation of downstream elements, such as K-ras mutations in colorectal carcinoma. Indeed, in the latter setting, K-ras mutation is an independent predictive marker of kinase inhibitor therapy in metastatic colon carcinoma. Neither EGFR/K-ras mutation nor treatment response appears to have any meaningful relationship to immunoreactivity for EGFR protein.

CD117

CD117 (c-*kit* protein; "Steele factor"; "stem cell factor") is another cell membrane-based tyrosine kinase with a similar function to that of *ErbB* proteins. In the late 1990s, studies on gastrointestinal stromal tumors (GISTs) showed that the vast majority of them were immunoreactive for CD117 [130–132] (Fig. 16.21), and it became a virtual *conditio sine qua non* for that neoplasm. In keeping with the theme described above, the assumption was made that all CD117-positive tumors should, and would, respond to inhibitors of c-*kit* binding to its activating ligands. The principal biological agent in this category, imatinib, did prove to be spectacularly effective in treating metastatic GIST, as well as chronic myelogenous leukemia (CML) [133]. In the latter of those conditions, an activation of the *abl* gene (another tyrosine kinase protein) occurs because of a *bcr-abl* gene fusion relating to the t(9;22) chromosomal translocation in CML [134].

Once again, misdirected hopes of therapeutic success with imatinib arose in reference to *all* tumors that were immunoreactive for CD117. They comprised a considerable group, including primitive neuroectodermal tumor, extraskeletal myxoid chondrosarcoma, melanotic schwannoma, melanoma, angiosarcoma, uterine leiomyosarcoma, seminoma-dysgerminoma, mast cell proliferations, adenoid cystic carcinoma, some nasopharyngeal carcinomas, chromophobe renal cell carcinomas, high-grade neuroendocrine carcinomas, epithelial-myoepithelial salivary gland carcinoma, ovarian carcinomas, and some ductal breast carcinomas [135] (Fig. 16.22). Nonetheless, only GIST and CML demonstrated any meaningful clinical response to imatinib-mediated inhibition of tyrosine kinase. Further analysis has demonstrated once more that critical, activating mutations in the CD117 gene (Fig. 16.23) are required to realize a biological response to c-*kit*-inhibiting agents [136].

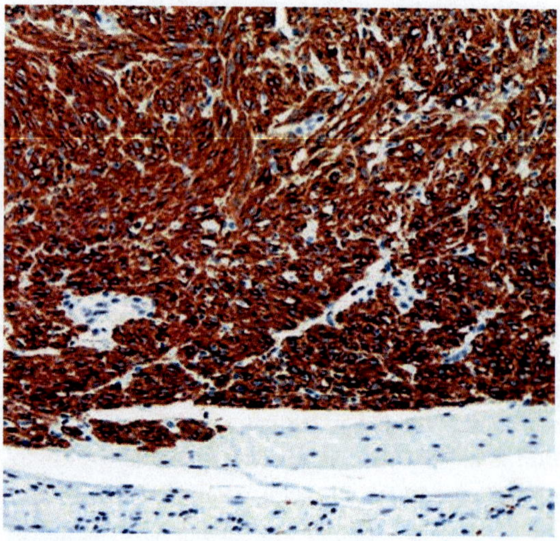

Fig. 16.21 Intense immunoreactivity is present in a gastrointestinal stromal tumor, labeled for CD117 (c-*kit* protein)

Hormone Receptors in Breast Carcinoma

In the 1970s, McGuire and others developed a chemical competitive binding assay (CCBA) for ERP and PRP, which was principally used in the evaluation of breast carcinomas [137–140]. The goal of that assessment was to study a possible relationship between quantitative ERP/PRP status and a response to hormone-modulating drugs. Many studies over several years did indeed show such an association. Breast cancers with a quantitative ERP content over a level of 10 fmol/mg protein were classified as "positive," because they showed a uniform response to the administration of tamoxifen, an estrogen antagonist [138, 139]. Indeed, the statistical level of clinical benefit from that agent was a linear one; the higher the ERP content of the tumor cells, the greater the effect was of tamoxifen [141].

Problems with the use of CCBAs for ERP and PRP centered on the need for a critical volume of fresh tumor tissue to perform the tests. Accordingly, other investigators began to evaluate tissue section-based immunoassays as alternatives, in the 1980s. These involved both immunofluorescence and immunoenzyme techniques, as applied to frozen sections of breast cancers [142]. Good – but not perfect – correlation was observed between results in CCBAs and immunohistologic methods [143, 144]. The ability to study very small biopsies with IHC was regarded as a substantial benefit, and the use of chemical competitive assays began to disappear. By the advent of the twenty-first century, they

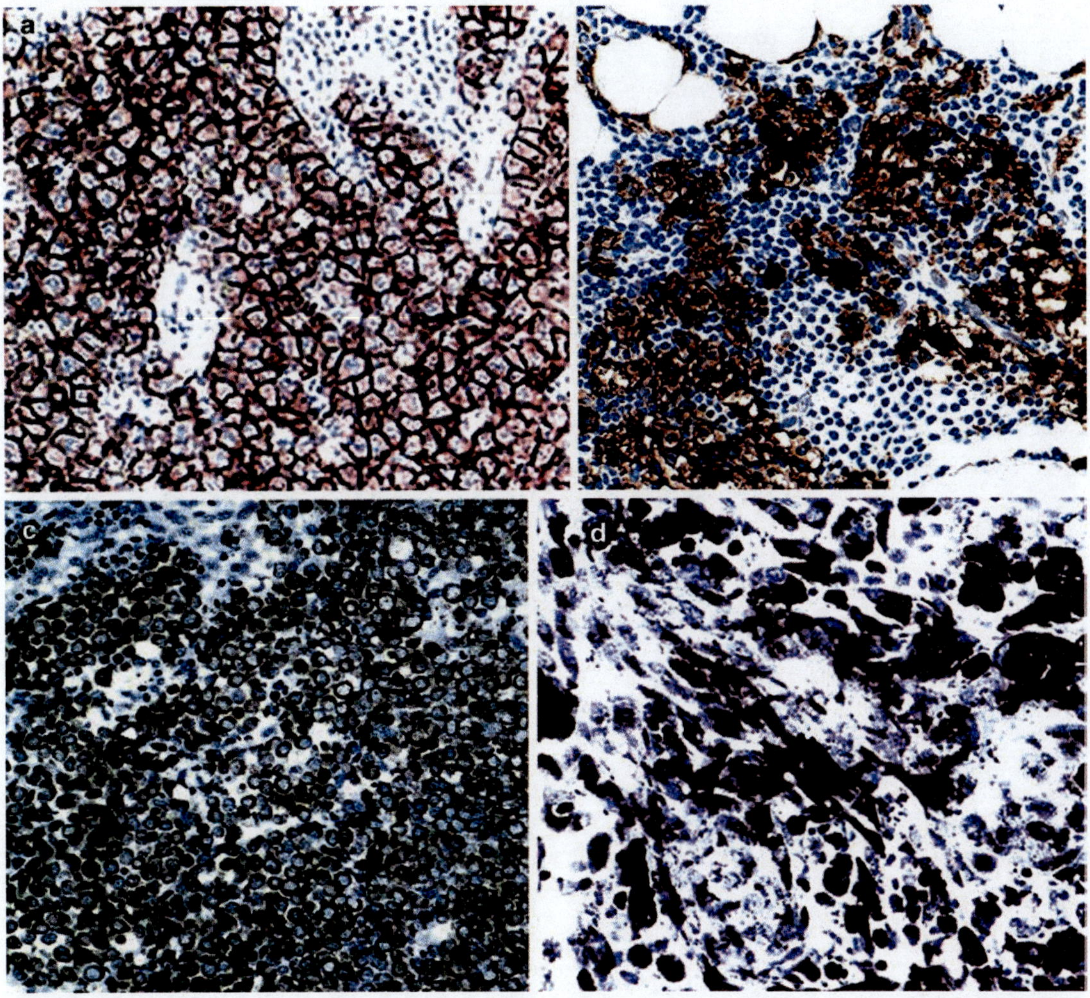

Fig. 16.22 CD117 immunoreactivity is present in (**a**) testicular seminoma; (**b**) mastocytosis of the bone marrow; (**c**) small-cell neuroendocrine carcinoma of the lung; and (**d**) metastatic melanoma. Despite their immunolabeling, none of these tumors responds to targeted anti-CD117 biological therapy

were all but extinct, and advances in HIER had made studies of *paraffin* sections for ERP and PRP routine [145] (Fig. 16.24).

Nevertheless, potentially valuable data were lost in this transition. Recent evaluations have shown a bimodal distribution [145, 146] of ERP in mammary carcinomas that was not present in the CCBA era, where a linear model obtained [139, 141]. As suggested earlier, this bimodality is almost certainly an artifact of technique and the limitations of PPIHC in delineating mid-range biochemical results, particularly when increasingly sensitive techniques are employed. Accordingly, there may be no way of knowing how close an immunohistologically "positive" ERP result is to the previous 10 fmol/mg threshold in CCBAs in many laboratories today.

This need not necessarily be the case, however. In their initial validation of estrogen receptor PPHIC, Harvey and associates (147) analyzed several anti-ER antibodies, including 6F11, and compared their immunohistochemical results with both existing validated CCBA data and survival in over 1,000 patients. Using a modified H-scoring

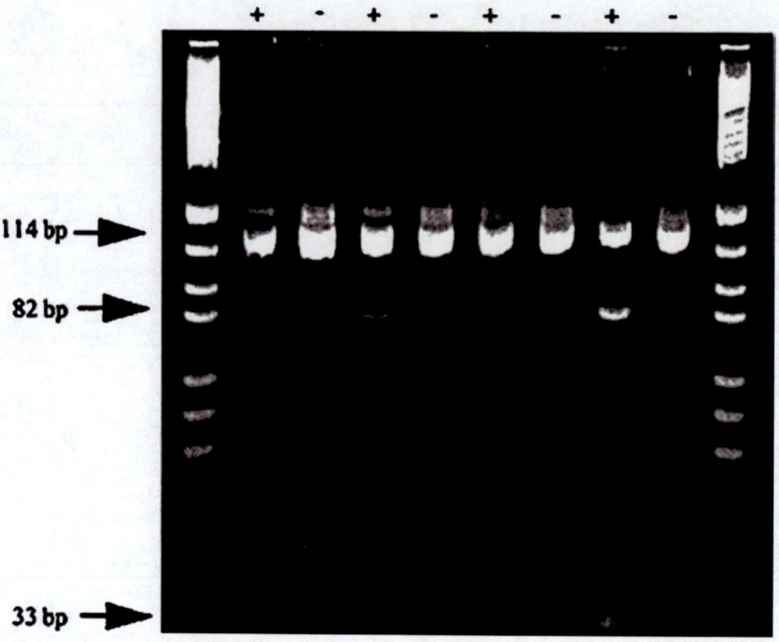

Fig. 16.23 Activating mutations in the CD117 gene, corresponding to PCR products marked by *arrows* in this blot preparation, are necessary in order for patients with CD117-immunoreactive tumors to realize beneficial effects from anti-tyrosine kinase medications

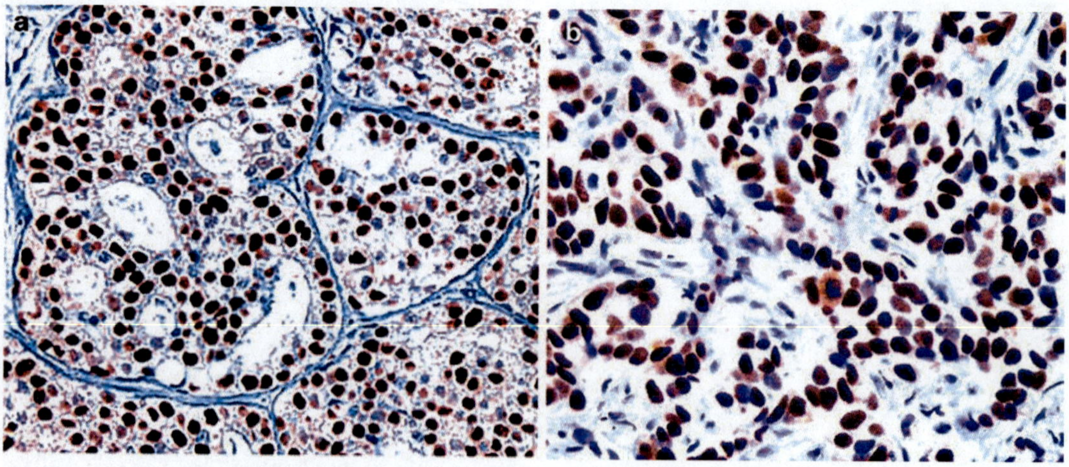

Fig. 16.24 Immunostaining for estrogen receptor protein (**a**) and progesterone receptor protein (**b**) in ductal breast carcinomas. These analytes show a bimodal distribution in paraffin sections that is likely an artifact of immunohistochemical detection

system we now know as the Allred score, a relationship approximating linearity between overall stain score and outcome, as well as Allred score and CCBA values, was demonstrated. It is also important to note that the distribution of scores was not dichotomous, but more evenly distributed over all stain outcome possibilities, with a distinct cut-point (Allred score 3) between clinical responders and nonresponders. It might be argued that the Allred score (by measuring tissue distribution and stain intensity) is merely a best-fit solution to the problem of correlation with CCBA data and survival, rather than a direct measure of true biological variation. It might also be argued that the apparent linearity of the assay with respect to CCBA and outcome was due to the use of an inferior reagent in an insensitive system (antibody 6F11 using protease/DNAse retrieval). Also, as Nadji has sagely observed:

> ...in the case of ER, immunohistochemical methods only identify a segment or epitope of ER protein that is immunologically-reactive with the used antibody. Hence, as it is, an immunohistochemical technique gives no information about the functional status of the ER molecule, and/or that of the complex downstream ER pathways. This may be one of the reasons why one-third of patients with ER-positive breast cancers initially, and another one-third eventually, do not respond to endocrine treatment modalities [148].

Those comments also raise an important secondary topic in this context. Puristically, one should only use cross-validated, ERP-positive breast cancer specimens from patients who were proven to benefit from endocrine therapy, as biological controls in clinical PPIHC. That provision is virtually never heeded today by most laboratories, but clearly was by others [117, 147, 149].

Ideally, one should employ antibody reagents whose binding to tissue targets is known to correlate with in vivo activity of the substrate. With regard to breast cancer, the active isoform of ERP appears to be phosphorylated ERP-alpha (PERPA), which reflects the presence of an intact intracellular signaling pathway [150, 151]. Nevertheless, the great majority of laboratories doing PPIHC for ERP do not utilize anti-PERPA antibodies.

Whereas an increasing number of ERP antibodies have entered the commercial market, and some of them show suboptimal specificity for functional ERP epitopes [149], attention to appropriate clinical validation using tenets proposed by McGuire may provide a basis for reproducible and meaningful PPIHC and address, at least, some of Nadji's concerns [148]. Practically speaking, without careful and appropriate validation, the true relationship between antibody specificity for functional ERP epitopes and treatment failure alluded to by Nadji cannot be understood.

Alternatives to Immunohistology for Prognostication and Prediction

In light of the deficiencies and distortions attached to PPIHC as a reflection of actual tumor-related "biopredictor" distributions, other methods have been evaluated as alternatives to traditional paraffin-section immunohistology. Four of them – the automated quantitative analysis (AQUA) system, polymerase chain reaction (PCR)-based assays, fluorescent and chromogenic in situ hybridization (FISH), and gene-chip arrays – show particular utility.

The AQUA Technique

Developed at Yale University, the AQUA method is, in a way, a return to a technique of the past, but with new dimensions [152–154]. This procedure uses immunofluorescence as its principal antigen-detection system with paraffin sections, and can vary antibody concentrations over a predefined range in the study of each test sample. Fluorescent emission data are recorded by image acquisition and software-mediated analysis, and matched to a subcellular compartment of interest (e.g., nucleus, cytoplasm, cell membrane, etc.) [152]. Results of the AQUA technique parallel those of enzyme-linked immunosorbent assays (ELISAs) in clinical chemistry, and are much better than traditional IHC at portraying linear biomarker activities over a continuous range of values [102].

Recent publications on AQUA by the Yale group of investigators have shown that ERP density in breast cancer does indeed maintain a linear association with the biological response to tamoxifen, just as it did in the past [152, 154]. Interestingly, they also demonstrate that both low and high levels of *HER*-2 protein in breast carcinomas are linked with adverse clinical behavior. p53 protein had neither of those characteristics [152].

Polymerase Chain Reaction-Based Analyses

PCR-based analyses, which have been available for over 15 years, have two potential uses in the setting being discussed. First, if it is known that one or more particular mutations in a specified gene have a prognostic significance, they can be relatively easily demonstrated by conventional PCR or "real-time" PCR (RT-PCR) [155]. In the latter case, the presence of the target nucleic acid sequence(s) is "reported" as it is detected [156]. Examples of prognostic analytes that can be studied in this way are represented by p53 mutations and activating mutations in the EGFR and CD117 genes [157]. Only a small amount of tissue is required for PCR, and the study can even be done on fine needle aspiration biopsies (Fig. 16.25) or effusion cytology specimens.

Secondly, in RT-PCR, complementary deoxyribonucleic acid (cDNA) derived from the clinical sample is analyzed in parallel with "housekeeping" genes. Comparison of the two, and standardization of final results, allows for a quantitative measurement of specific patient-related nucleic acid sequences [158]. Thus, potential gene amplification can be detected with this method [159, 160].

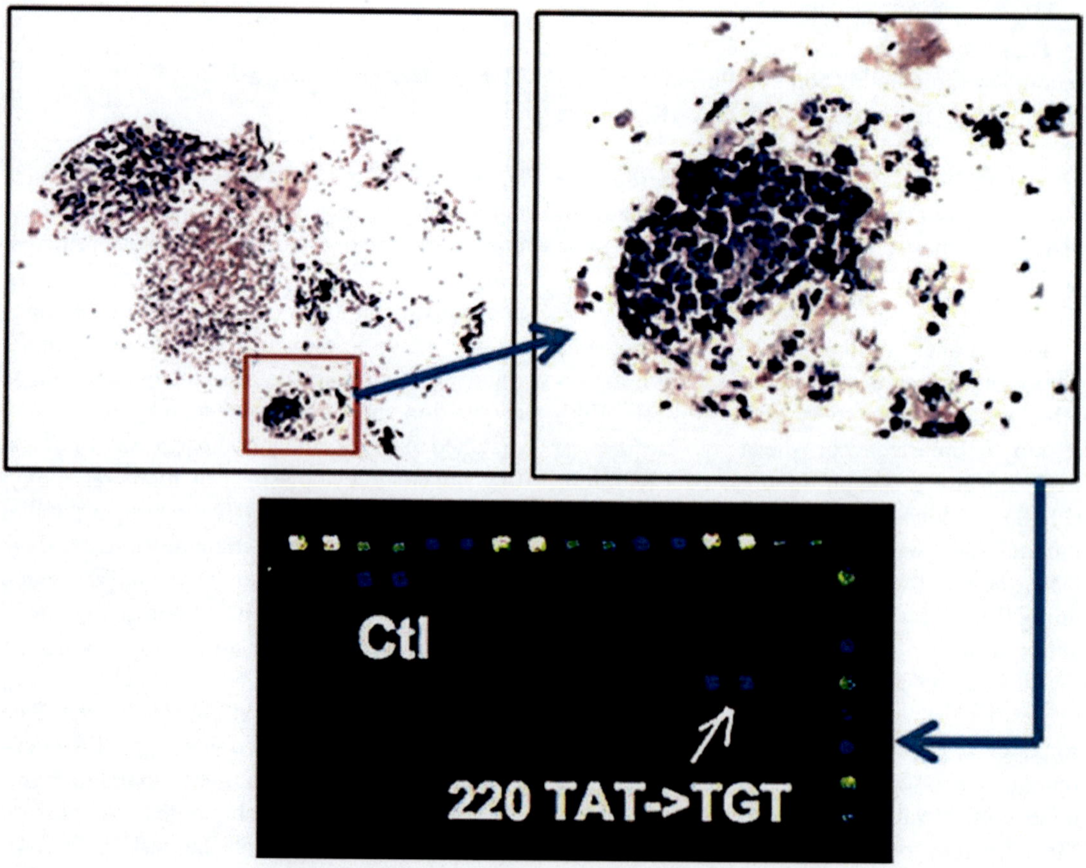

Fig. 16.25 Polymerase chain reaction-based assays for mutations in the p53 gene can be performed on specimens of limited volume, as true of this fine-needle aspiration biopsy of a nonsmall-cell lung carcinoma

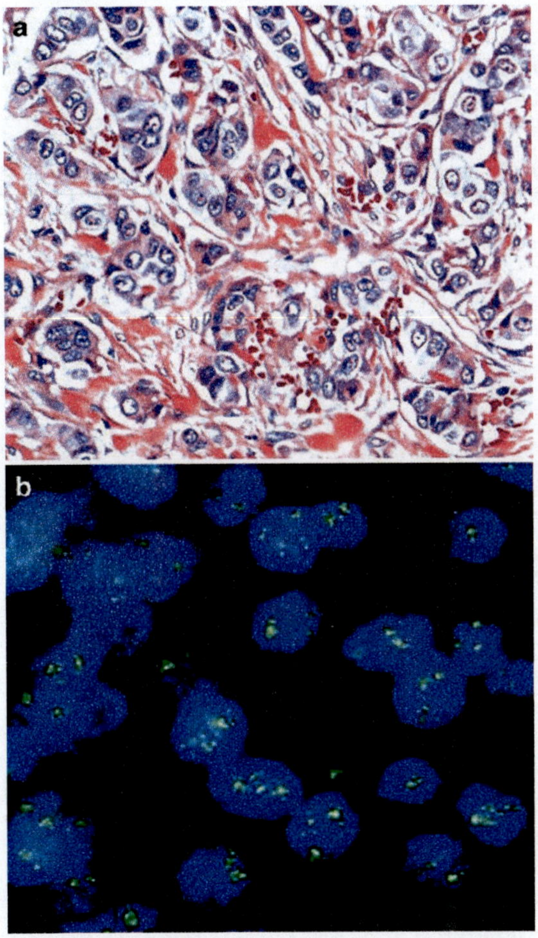

Fig. 16.26 The cells in this ductal mammary adenocarcinoma (**a**) show multiple copies of the *HER-2* gene, as depicted by the fluorescent in situ hybridization method (**b**)

Fluorescent and Chromogenic In Situ Hybridization (FISH and CISH)

FISH methods for studying the number of gene copies or the presence of specific gene mutations in human cells are now widespread [161]. Indeed, many laboratories have foregone "surrogate" testing (usually with IHC) for prognostic-predictive gene alterations and moved to exclusive use of in situ hybridization [162]. That is certainly true for *HER-2* in the current practice of surgical pathology [163]. In this technique, labeled nucleic acid probes are hybridized with native single-stranded DNA (following a denaturation step) or ribonucleic acid (RNA)

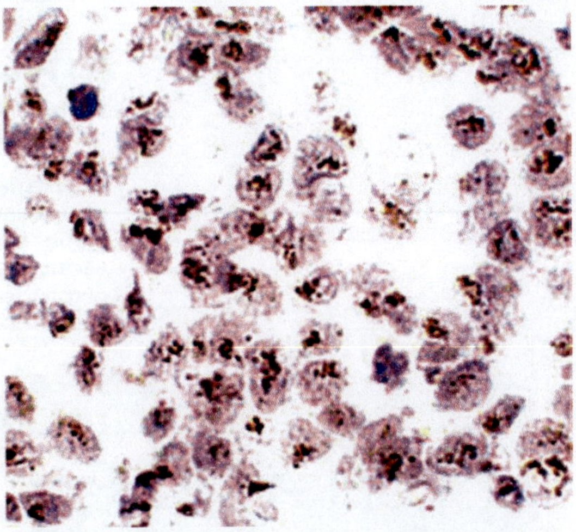

Fig. 16.27 The tumor shown in Fig. 16.26 also manifests several intranuclear signals in a chromogenic in situ hybridization study for *HER-2*

from the specimen. Detection methods depend on the nature of the probe label; it can be a radionuclide, a heavy-metal complex, a fluorophore (FISH) (Fig. 16.26), or a chromogenic dye (CISH) [159, 161, 164] (Fig. 16.27). Once again, the advantage of in situ hybridization over PPIHC is that the former method is direct, whereas the latter is indirect. In situ hybridization can be employed to assess the number of gene copies, the presence of mutant gene sequences, or the amount of intracellular messenger RNA related to a particular gene.

Nucleic Acid Microarrays

Nucleic acid microarrays are "multiplex" (multiple simultaneous test-capable) platforms that are used in the analysis of gene copies in a clinical sample, relative to integrated reference controls [165–169]. They comprise arrayed series of thousands of microscopic oligonucleotide spots, called "features." Each feature contains picomoles of specific nucleic acid sequences, known as probes or reporters (Fig. 16.28). Hybridized probe-target complexes are detected and quantified with fluorophores, heavy metals, or chemiluminescence labels, to assess the relative numbers

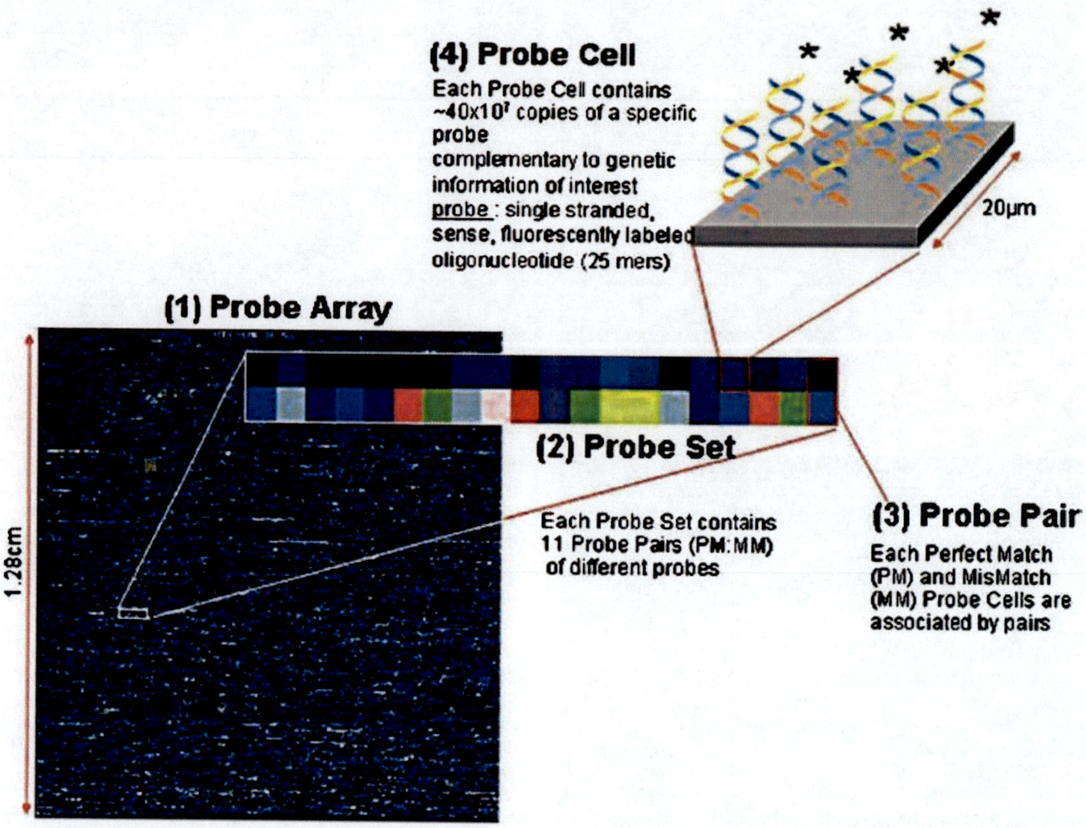

Fig. 16.28 Gene chip structure is based on the presence of many predetermined oligonucleotide spots ("features"), with which controlled and labeled nucleic acid probes can be hybridized. The results present a multifaceted picture that can show increased, decreased, or unchanged gene copy numbers as compared with integrated controls

of nucleic acid sequences in the target tissue. Because each array can contain >10^4 probes, it allows for many assays to be done in parallel. Probes are attached to a solid surface by covalent bonds; the solid component can be glass or a silicon chip [168, 169].

After hybridization with reporter probes, the chip is scanned with an appropriate detector device, and the signals are quantified. A "heat map" is then generated by associated computer software that shows which nucleic acid sequences are increased in number, which are unchanged, and which are decreased, relative to controls [169, 170] (Fig. 16.29). Depending on whether a chip comprises DNA or RNA sequences, the presence of either gene amplification or overexpression in the clinical sample can be determined with this technology.

Gene chips are powerful tools in prognostication and prediction because of their multiplex capabilities. Rather than providing information on only one gene or gene product, chips paint a broad picture of nucleic acid composition or expression in any given sample [171, 172].

Should PPIHC Have a Future, Based on EBM Principles?

This discussion has focused on the good and the not-so-good aspects of applied IHC. Casting diplomacy aside, we conclude that more of the latter elements exist than the former in reference to PPIHC. The principal reasons accounting for the persistence of "forecast"-oriented immunohistology seem to relate to its general

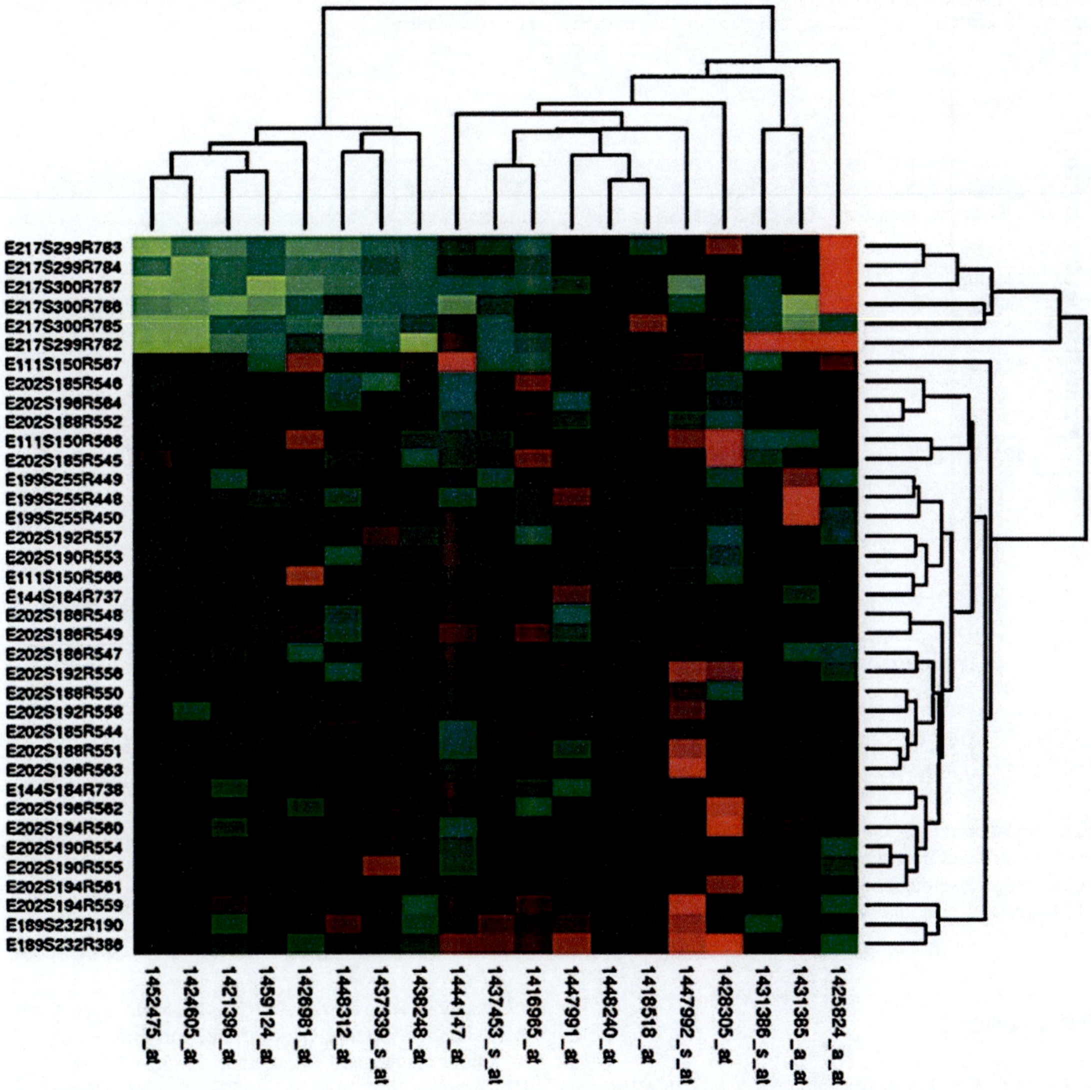

Fig. 16.29 A "heat map" of gene chip results, showing increased (*green*), unchanged (*black*), or decreased (*red*) individual gene-related signals as compared with controls

availability and relatively low cost, and *not* to its superior performance in relation to other testing methods.

Ultimately, whether the healthcare system in the United States or other countries continues to use PPIHC will depend on a comprehensive analysis of its cost-effectiveness. Other specialties have begun to use that approach with beneficial results [173, 174] (Fig. 16.30). If a test is inexpensive but it is mediocre, overused, and may produce misleading information, it logically should be abandoned. On the other hand, alternative assays that cost more, but have excellent predictive values and low rates of error, are those that best serve patients and the system at large. In that context, we believe that the future of PPIHC is, or should be, in doubt on evidence-based scientific grounds. At this stage in its evolution, medical economists are very likely better judges of its eventual fate than are pathologists or other physicians.

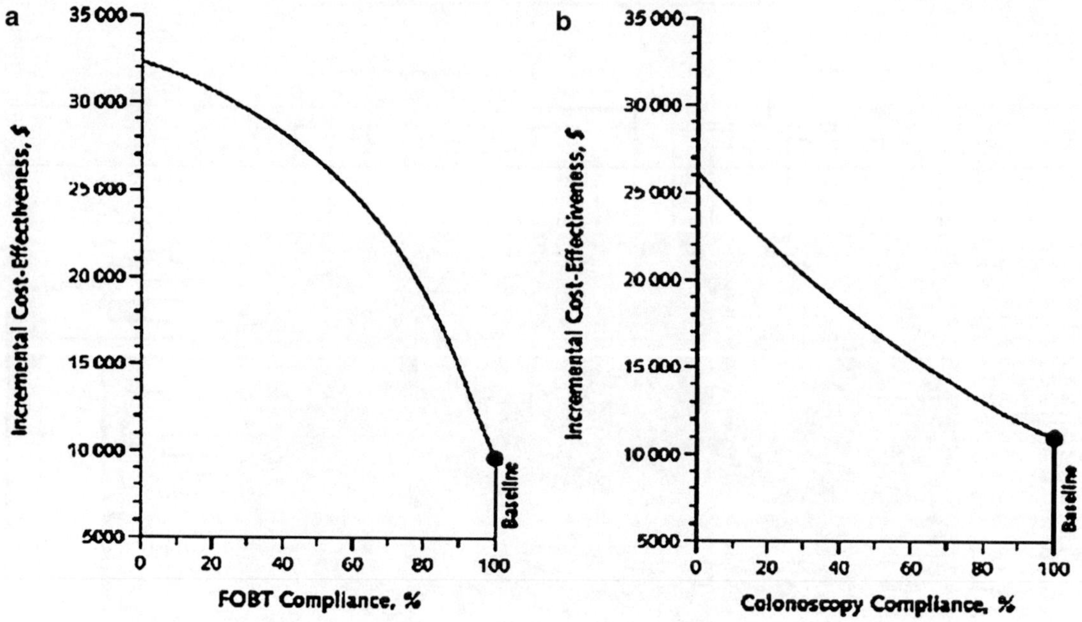

Influence of compliance with repeated fecal occult blood testing (FOBT) once per year (left) and repeated colonoscopy (right) once per decade on the incremental cost-effectiveness ratio compared with no screening.

Fig. 16.30 Graphic comparison of cost-effectiveness analyses of fecal occult blood testing (**a**) and systematic colonoscopic examination over time (**b**), for the detection of colorectal carcinoma. The area under the curve of (**b**) is less than that seen in (**a**), indicating greater cost-effectiveness of colonoscopy. This same technique can be applied to immunohistochemical evaluations

References

1. Taylor CR. Immunohistological approach to tumor diagnosis. Oncology. 1978;35:187–97.
2. Taylor CR. Immunoperoxidase techniques: practical and theoretical aspects. Arch Pathol Lab Med. 1978;102:113–21.
3. Pearse AGE. A review of modern methods in histochemistry. J Clin Pathol. 1951;4:1–36.
4. Pearse AGE. Histochemistry and its application to the basic sciences. Lect Sci Basis Med. 1955;4:358–86.
5. Lillie RD. Problems of fixation in histochemistry. J Histochem Cytochem. 1958;6:301–2.
6. Bennett HS. A perception of histochemistry. J Histochem Cytochem. 1983;31(Suppl):127–30.
7. Rosai J, Rodriguez HA. Application of electron microscopy to the differential diagnosis of tumors. Am J Clin Pathol. 1968;50:555–62.
8. Kuzela DC, True LD, Eiseman B. The role of electron microscopy in the management of surgical patients. Ann Surg. 1982;195:1–11.
9. Fisher C, Ramsay AD, Griffiths M, McDougall J. An assessment of the value of electron microscopy in tumor diagnosis. J Clin Pathol. 1985;38:403–8.
10. Ordonez NG, Mackay B. Electron microscopy in tumor diagnosis: indications for its use in the immunohistochemical era. Hum Pathol. 1998;29:1403–11.
11. Ruska E. Ernst Ruska: autobiography. Stockholm: Nobel Foundation Press; 1986.
12. McDevitt HO. Albert Hewett Coons, 1912–1978. New York: National Academies Press; 1979.
13. Coons AH, Creech HJ, Jones R. Immunological properties of an antibody containing a fluorescent group. Proc Soc Exp Biol. 1941;47:200–2.
14. Coons AH. The beginnings of immunofluorescence. J Immunol. 1961;87:499–503.
15. Lasker Foundation. 1959 Winners – Albert Lasker basic medical research award. http://www.laskerfoundation.org/awards/1959basic.htm. Accessed 7 Dec 2010.
16. Beutner EH, Jordon RE. Demonstration of skin antibodies in sera of pemphigus vulgaris patients by indirect immunofluorescent staining. Proc Soc Exp Biol Med. 1964;117:505–10.

17. Tan EM, Kunkel HG. An immunofluorescence study of the skin lesions in systemic lupus erythematosus. Arthritis Rheum. 1966;9:37–46.
18. Nagasawa T, Miyakawa Y, Shibata S. New fluorescent staining method for renal biopsy: introduction of anti-glomerular basement membrane labeled antibody. Saishin Igaku (Modern Medicine). 1968;23: 2656–63.
19. Wilson CB, Dixon FJ, Fortner JG, Cerilli GJ. Glomerular basement membrane-reactive antibody in anti-lymphocyte globulin. J Clin Invest. 1971;50: 1525–35.
20. Hall CE, Nisonoff A, Slayter HS. Electron microscopy observations of rabbit antibodies. J Biophys Biochem Cytol. 1959;6:407–12.
21. Singer SJ, Schick AF. The properties of specific stains for electron microscopy prepared by the conjugation of antibody molecules with ferritin. J Biophys Biochem Cytol. 1961;9:519–37.
22. Slot JW, Posthuma G, Chang LY, Crapo JD, Geuze HJ. Quantitative aspects of immunogold labeling in embedded and in nonembedded sections. Am J Anat. 1989;185:271–81.
23. Sternberger LA. Electron microscopic immunocytochemistry: a review. J Histochem Cytochem. 1967;15:139–59.
24. Roth J, Heitz PU. Immunolabeling with the protein A-gold technique: an overview. Ultrastruct Pathol. 1989;13:467–84.
25. Sternberger LA, Cuculis JJ. Method for enzymatic intensification of the immunocytochemical reaction without use of labeled antibodies. J Histochem Cytochem. 1969;17:190.
26. Sternberger LA, Hardy Jr PH, Cuculis JJ, Meyer HG. The unlabeled antibody-enzyme method of immunohistochemistry: preparation and properties of soluble antigen-antibody complex (horseradish peroxidase-anti-horseradish peroxidase) and its use in identification of spirochetes. J Histochem Cytochem. 1970;18:315–33.
27. Tornehave D, Folkersen J, Teisner B, Chemnitz J. Immunohistochemical aspects of immunological cross-reaction and masking of epitopes for localization studies on pregnancy-associated plasma protein A. Histochem J. 1986;18:184–8.
28. DeLellis RA, Kwan P. Technical considerations in the immunohistochemical demonstration of intermediate filaments. Am J Surg Pathol. 1988;12(Suppl): 17–23.
29. Drier JK, Swanson PE, Cherwitz DL, Wick MR. S100 protein immunoreactivity in poorly-differentiated carcinomas: immunohistochemical comparison with malignant melanoma. Arch Pathol Lab Med. 1987;111:447–52.
30. Anonymous. Signal-to-nose ratio. http://en.wikipedia.org/wiki/signal-to-noise_ratio. Accessed 7 Dec 2010.
31. Hsu SM, Raine L, Fanger H. The use of antiavidin antibody and avidin-biotin-peroxidase complex in immunoperoxidase techniques. Am J Clin Pathol. 1981;75:816–21.
32. Hsu SM, Raine L, Fanger H. Use of avidin-biotin-peroxidase complex (ABC) in immunoperoxidase techniques: a comparison between ABC and unlabeled antibody (PAP) procedures. J Histochem Cytochem. 1981;29:577–80.
33. Guesdon JL, Ternynck T, Avrameas S. The use of avidin-biotin interaction in immunoenzyme techniques. J Histochem Cytochem. 1979;27:1131–6.
34. Bratthauer GL. The avidin-biotin complex (ABC) method and other avidin-biotin bindings methods. Methods Mol Biol. 2010;588:257–70.
35. Miller RT, Groothuis CL. Improved avidin-biotin immunoperoxidase method for terminal deoxyribonucleotidyl transferase and immunophenotypic characterization of blood cells. Am J Clin Pathol. 1990;93:670–4.
36. Elias JM, Margiotta M, Gaborc D. Sensitivity and detection efficiency of the peroxidase-antiperoxidase (PAP), avidin-biotin-peroxidase complex (ABC), and peroxidase-labeled avidin-biotin (LAB) methods. Am J Clin Pathol. 1989;92:62–7.
37. Mokry J. Versatility of immunohistochemical reactions: comprehensive survey of detection systems. Acta Medica. 1996;39:129–40.
38. Swanson PE, Kagen KA, Wick MR. Avidin-biotin-peroxidase-antiperoxidase (ABPAP) complex: an immunocytochemical method with enhanced sensitivity. Am J Clin Pathol. 1987;88:162–76.
39. Kammerer U, Kapp M, Gassel AM, et al. A new rapid immunohistochemical staining technique using the Envision antibody complex. J Histochem Cytochem. 2001;49:623–30.
40. Masouredis SP, Sudora E, Mahan L, Victoria EJ. Quantitative immunoferritin microscopy of Fya, Fyb, Jka, U, and Dib antigen site numbers on human red cells. Blood. 1980;56:969–77.
41. Ripoche J, Sim RB. Loss of complement receptor type 1(CR1) on aging of erythrocytes: studies of proteolytic release of the receptor. Biochem J. 1986; 235:815–21.
42. Andrade RE, Hagen KA, Swanson PE, Wick MR. The use of proteolysis with ficin for immunostaining of paraffin sections: a study of lymphoid, mesenchymal, and epithelial determinants in human tissues. Am J Clin Pathol. 1988;90:33–9.
43. Hajdu I. The immunohistochemical detection of J-chain in lymphoid cells in tissue sections: the necessity of trypsin digestion. Cell Immunol. 1983;79:157–63.
44. Dell'Orto P, Viale G, Colombi R, Braidotti P, Coggi G. Immunohistochemical localization of human immunoglobulins and lysozyme in epoxy-embedded lymph nodes: effect of different fixatives and of proteolytic digestion. J Histochem Cytochem. 1982;30: 630–6.
45. Miller RT, Swanson PE, Wick MR. Fixation & epitope retrieval in diagnostic immunohistochemistry: a concise review with practical considerations. Appl Immunohistochem Mol Morphol. 2000;8: 228–35.

46. Hiort O, Lwan PW, DeLellis RA. Immunohistochemistry of estrogen receptor protein in paraffin sections: effects of enzymatic pretreatment and cobalt chloride intensification. Am J Clin Pathol. 1988;90:559–63.
47. Pileri S, Serra L, Martinelli G. The use of pronase enhances sensitivity of the PAP method in the detection of intracytoplasmic immunoglobulins. Basic Appl Histochem. 1980;24:203–7.
48. Taylor CR, Shi SR, Chaiwun B, et al. Strategies for improving the immunohistochemical staining of various intranuclear prognostic markers in formalin-paraffin sections: androgen receptor, estrogen receptor, progesterone receptor, p53 protein, proliferating cell nuclear antigen, and Ki-67 antigen revealed by antigen retrieval techniques. Hum Pathol. 1994;25:263–70.
49. Shi SR, Key ME, Kalra KL. Antigen retrieval in formalin-fixed paraffin-embedded tissues: an enhancement method for immunohistochemical staining based on microwave oven heating of tissue sections. J Histochem Cytochem. 1991;39:741–8.
50. Suurmeijer AJH. Microwave-stimulated antigen retrieval: a new method facilitating immunohistochemistry of formalin-fixed, paraffin-embedded tissue. Histochem J. 1992;24:597.
51. Gown AM, deWever N, Battifora H. Microwave-based antigenic unmasking: a revolutionary new technique for routine immunohistochemistry. Appl Immunohistochem. 1993;1:256–66.
52. Norton AJ, Jordan S, Yeomans P. Brief high temperature heat denaturation (pressure cooking): a simple and effective method of antigen retrieval for routinely-processed tissues. J Pathol. 1994;173:371–9.
53. Cattoretti G, Suurmeijer AJH. Antigen unmasking on formalin-fixed paraffin-embedded tissues using microwaves: a review. Adv Anat Pathol. 1995;2:2–9.
54. Miller RT, Estran C. Heat-induced epitope retrieval with a pressure cooker: suggestions for optimal use. Appl Immunohistochem. 1995;3:190–3.
55. Pileri S, Roncador G, Ceccarelli C, et al. Antigen retrieval techniques in immunohistochemistry: comparison among different methods. J Pathol. 1997;183:116–23.
56. Bogen SA, Vani K, Sompuram SR. Molecular mechanisms of antigen retrieval: antigen retrieval reverses steric interference caused by formalin-induced cross-links. Biotech Histochem. 2009;84:207–15.
57. Boenisch T. Heat-induced antigen retrieval: what are we retrieving? J Histochem Cytochem. 2006;54:961–4.
58. Leong TY, Leong ASY. How does antigen retrieval work? Adv Anat Pathol. 2007;14:129–31.
59. Werner M, Von Wasielewski R, Komminoth P. Antigen retrieval, signal amplification, and intensification in immunohistochemistry. Histochem Cell Biol. 1996;105:253–60.
60. Puchtler H, Meloan SN. On the chemistry of formaldehyde fixation and its effects on immunohistochemical reactions. Histochemistry. 1985;82:201–4.
61. Paterson DA, Reid CP, Anderson TJ, Hawkins RA. Assessment of estrogen receptor content of breast carcinoma by immunohistochemical techniques on fixed and frozen tissue and by biochemical ligand-binding assay. J Clin Pathol. 1990;43:46–51.
62. Fisher CJ, Gillett CE, Vojtesek G, Barnes DM, Millis RR. Problems with p53 immunohistochemical staining: the effect of fixation and variation in the methods of evaluation. Br J Cancer. 1994;69:26–31.
63. Battifora H, Kopinski M. The influence of protease digestion and duration of fixation on the immunostaining of keratins: a comparison of formalin and ethanol fixation. J Histochem Cytochem. 1986;34:1095–100.
64. Elias JM, Gown AM, Nakamura RM, et al. Quality control in immunohistochemistry: report of a workshop sponsored by the Biological Stain Commission. Am J Clin Pathol. 1989;92:836–43.
65. Werner M, Chott A, Fabiano A, Battifora H. Effect of formalin tissue fixation and processing on immunohistochemistry. Am J Surg Pathol. 2000;24:1016–9.
66. Torlakovic EE, Riddell R, Banerjee D, et al. Canadian Association of Pathologists-Associatio canadienne des pathologists National Standards Committee/Immunohistochemistry: best practice recommendations for standardization of immunohistochemistry tests. Am J Clin Pathol. 2010;133:354–65.
67. Reynolds GJ. External quality assurance and assessment in immunocytochemistry. Histopathology. 1989;15:627–33.
68. Wick MR. Technologic anarchy? Am J Clin Pathol. 1989;91(Suppl):S1.
69. Swanson PE. HIERanarchy: the state of the art in immunohistochemistry. Am J Clin Pathol. 1997;107:139–40.
70. Seidal T, Balaton A, Battifora H. Interpretation and quantification of immunostains. Am J Surg Pathol. 2001;25:1204–7.
71. Wick MR, Mills SE. Consensual interpretive guidelines for diagnostic immunohistochemistry. Am J Surg Pathol. 2001;26:1208–10.
72. Wick MR, Swanson PE. Targeted controls in clinical immunohistochemistry: a useful approach to quality assurance. Am J Clin Pathol. 2002;117:7–8.
73. Shi SR, Liu C, Pootrakul L, et al. Evaluation of the value of frozen tissue sections used as "gold standards" for immunohistochemistry. Am J Clin Pathol. 2008;129:358–66.
74. Battifora H. The multitumor (sausage) tissue block: novel method for immunohistochemical antibody testing. Lab Invest. 1986;55:244–8.
75. Bubendorf L, Nocito A, Moch H, Sauter G. Tissue microarray (TMA) technology: miniaturized pathology archives for high-throughput in-situ studies. J Pathol. 2001;195:72–9.
76. Horvath L, Henshall S. The application of tissue microarrays to cancer research. Pathology. 2001;33:125–9.
77. Rimm DL, Camp RL, Charette LA, Costa J, Olsen DA, Reiss M. Tissue microarrays: a new technology for amplification of tissue resources. Cancer J. 2001;7:24–31.

78. Wick MR. Quality assurance in diagnostic immunohistochemistry: a discipline coming of age. Am J Clin Pathol. 1989;92:844.
79. Friedland DJ, Go AS, Davoren JB, et al. Evidence-based medicine: a framework for clinical practice. Stamford: Appleton & Lange; 1998. p. 1–246.
80. Marchevsky AM, Wick MR. Evidence-based medicine, medical decision-analysis, and pathology. Hum Pathol. 2004;35:1179–88.
81. Da Silva L, Parry S, Reid L, et al. Aberrant expression of E-cadherin in lobular carcinomas of the breast. Am J Surg Pathol. 2008;32:773–83.
82. Tavassoli FA, Eusebi V. Tumor of the mammary glands. AFIP atlas of tumors series 4. Washington: Armed Forces Institute of Pathology; 2009.
83. Ellis GL, Auclair PL. Tumors of the salivary glands. AFIP atlas of tumors series 4. Washington: Armed Forces Institute of Pathology; 2008.
84. Fletcher CDM, Unni KK, Mertens F, editors. Pathology and genetics. World Health Organization classification of tumours. Tumours of soft tissue and bone. Lyon: IARC Press; 2002.
85. Mills SE, Carter D, Greenson JK, Reuter VE, Stoer MH. Sternberg's diagnostic surgical pathology. 5th ed. Philadelphia: Lippincott Williams & Wilkins; 2009.
86. Dabbs DJ. Diagnostic immunohistochemistry: theranostic and genomic applications, expert consults: online and print. Philadelphia: W.B. Saunders; 2010.
87. Swerdlow SH, Campo E, Harris NL, et al. World Health Organization classification of tumours of haematopoietic and lymphoid tissues. 4th ed. Lyon: IARC Press; 2008.
88. Louis DN, Ohgaki H, Wiestlier OD, Cavenoo WK. World Health Organization classification of tumours of the central nervous system. 4th ed. Lyon: IARC Press; 2007.
89. Montgomery K. How doctors think: clinical judgment and the practice of medicine. Oxford: Oxford University Press; 2005.
90. Downie RS. Clinical judgment: evidence in practice. Oxford: Oxford University Press; 2000.
91. Cai Y-C, Banner B, Glickman J, Ooze RD. Cytokeratins 7 and 20 and thyroid transcription factor 1 can help distinguish pulmonary from gastrointestinal carcinoid and pancreatic endocrine tumors. Hum Pathol. 2001;32:1087–93.
92. Brambilla E, Travis WD, Colby TV, et al. The new World Health Organization classification of lung tumours. Eur Respir J. 2001;18:1059–68.
93. Granberg D, Wilander E, Oberg K, Skogseid B. Prognostic markers in patients with typical bronchial carcinoid tumors. J Clin Endocrinol Metab. 2000; 85:3425–30.
94. Edge SB, Byrd DR, Compton CC, et al. AJCC cancer staging handbook from the AJCC cancer staging manual. 7th ed. New York: Springer; 2010. p. 234.
95. Evans AJ. Alpha-metylacyl CoA racemase (P504S): overview and potential uses in diagnostic pathology as applied to prostate needle biopsies. J Clin Pathol. 2003;56:892–7.
96. Reis-Filho JS, Milanezi F, Amendoeira I, et al. Distribution of p63, a novel myoepithelial marker, in fine-needle aspiration biopsies of the breast: an analysis of 82 samples. Cancer. 2003;99(3):172–9.
97. Saad RS, Liu Y, Han H, et al. Prognostic significant of HER2/neu, p53 and vascular endothelial growth factor expression in early stage conventional adenocarcinoma and bronchioloalveolar carcinoma of the lung. Mod Pathol. 2004;17:1235–42.
98. Cagle PT, Brown RW, Lebovitz RM. p53 immunostaining in the differentiation of reactive processes from malignancy in pleural biopsy specimens. Hum Pathol. 1994;25:443–8.
99. Mukhopadhyay N, Zhang S, Katzenstein AL. Immunohistochemical markers in diagnosis of papillary thyroid carcinoma: utility of HBME1 combined with CK19 immunostaining. Mod Pathol. 2006;19(112):1631–7.
100. Westfall DE, Fan X, Marchevsky AM. Evidence-based guidelines to optimize the selection of antibody panels in cytopathology: pleural effusions with malignant epithelioid cells. Diagn Cytopathol. 2010;38:9–14.
101. Marchevsky AM, Wick MR. Evidence-based guidelines for the utilization of immunostains in diagnostic pathology: pulmonary adenocarcinoma versus mesothelioma. Appl Immunohistochem Mol Morphol. 2007;15(2):140–4.
102. Rimm DL. What brown stains cannot do for you. Nature Biotechnol. 2006;24:914–6.
103. Taylor CR, Levenson RM. Quantification of immunohistochemistry – issues concerning methods, utility, and semiquantitative assessment. Histopathology. 2006;49:411–24.
104. Ellis CM, Dyson MJ, Stephenson TJ, Maltby EL. HER-2 amplification status in breast cancer: a comparison between immunohistochemical staining and fluorescence in-situ hybridization using manual techniques. J Clin Pathol. 2005;58:710–4.
105. Cuadros M, Villegas R. Systematic review of HER-2 breast cancer testing. Appl Immunohistochem Mol Morphol. 2009;17:1–7.
106. Prives C, Hall PA. The p53 pathway. J Pathol. 1999;187:112–26.
107. Hall PA, McCluggage WG. Assessing p53 in clinical contexts: unlearned lessons and new perspectives. J Pathol. 2006;208:1–6.
108. Gusterson BA, Hunter KD. Should we be surprised at the paucity of response to EGFR inhibitors? Lancet Oncol. 2009;10:522–7.
109. Cregger M, Berger AJ, Rimm DL. Immunohistochemistry and quantitative analysis of protein expression. Arch Pathol Lab Med. 2006;130: 1026–30.
110. Fritz P, Wu X, Tuczek H, Multhaupt H, Schwarzmann P. Quantitation in immunohistochemistry: a research method or a diagnostic tool in surgical pathology? Pathologica. 1995;87:300–9.
111. Fritz P, Multhaupt H, Hoenes J, et al. Quantitative immunohistochemistry: theoretical background and its application in biology and surgical pathology. Prog Histochem Cytochem. 1992;24:1–53.

112. Bahr GF. Frontiers of quantitative cytochemistry: a review of recent developments and potentials. Anal Quant Cytol. 1979;1:1–19.
113. Anonymous. Dynamic range. http://en.wikipedia.org/wiki/dynamic-range. Accessed 7 Dec 2010.
114. Faratian D, Clyde RG, Crawford JW, Harrison DJ. Systems pathology – taking molecular pathology into a new dimension. Natl Rev Clin Oncol. 2009; 6:455–64.
115. De Alava E. Molecular pathology in sarcomas. Clin Transl Oncol. 2007;9:130–44.
116. He YD. Genomic approach to biomarker identification and its recent applications. Cancer Biomarkers. 2006;2:103–33.
117. McGuire WL. Breast cancer prognostic factors: evaluation guidelines. J Natl Cancer Inst. 1991;83:154–5.
118. Krug LM, Crapanzano JP, Azzoli CG, et al. Imatinib mesylate lacks activity in small-cell lung carcinoma expressing c-*kit* protein: a phase-II clinical trial. Cancer. 2005;103:2128–31.
119. Bezwoda WR. c-*erbB*-2 expression and response to treatment in metastatic breast cancer. Med Oncol. 2000;17:22–8.
120. Rogers SJ, Box C, Chambers P, et al. Determinants of response to epidermal growth factor receptor tyrosine kinase inhibition in squamous cell carcinoma of the head and neck. J Pathol. 2009;218:122–30.
121. Atkins D, Reiffen KA, Tegtmeier CL, Winther H, Bonato MS, Storkel S. Immunohistochemical detection of EGFR in paraffin-embedded tumor tissues: variation in staining intensity due to choice of fixative and storage time of tissue sections. J Histochem Cytochem. 2004;52:893–901.
122. Ponz-Sarvise M, Rodriguez J, Viudez A, et al. Epidermal growth factor receptor inhibitors in colorectal cancer treatment: what's new? World J Gastroenterol. 2007;13:5877–87.
123. Heist RS, Christiani D. EGFR-targeted therapies in lung cancer: predictors of response and toxicity. http://www.medscape.com/viewarticle/589343. Accessed 7 Dec 2010.
124. Saltz L. Epidermal growth factor receptor-negative colorectal cancer: is there truly such an entity? Clin Colorectal Cancer. 2005;5 Suppl 2:S98–100.
125. Mathieu A, Weynand B, Verbeken E, et al. Comparison of four antibodies for immunohistochemical evaluation of epidermal growth factor receptor expression in non-small-cell lung cancer. Lung Cancer. 2010;69:46–50.
126. Buffet W, Geboes KP, Dehertogh G, Geboes K. EGFR-immunohistochemistry in colorectal cancer and non-small-cell lung cancer: comparison of 3 commercially-available EGFR antibodies. Acta Gastroenterol Belg. 2008;71:213–8.
127. Yamatodani T, Ekblad L, Kjellen E, Johnsson A, Mineta H, Wennerberg J. Epidermal growth factor receptor status and persistent activation of *Akt* and p44/42 *MAPK* pathways correlate with the effect of cetuximab in head and neck and colon cancer cell lines. J Cancer Res Clin Oncol. 2009;135:395–402.
128. Khambata-Ford S, Harbison CT, Hart LL, et al. Analysis of potential predictive markers of cetuximab benefit in BMS099, a phase-III study of cetuximab and first-line taxane/carboplatin in advanced non-small-cell lung cancer. J Clin Oncol. 2010;28:918–27.
129. Dacic S, Yousem SA. Molecular testing in lung carcinoma: *quo vadis*? Am J Clin Pathol. 2010; 134:7–9.
130. Hirota S, Isozaki K, Moriyama Y, et al. Gain-of-function mutations of c-*kit* in human gastrointestinal stromal tumors. Science. 1998;279:577–80.
131. Sarlomo-Rikala M, Kovatich AJ, Barusevicius A, Miettinen M. CD117: a sensitive marker for gastrointestinal stromal tumors that is more specific than CD34. Mod Pathol. 1998;11:728–34.
132. Tazawa K, Tsukada K, Makuuchi H, Tsutsumi Y. An immunohistochemical and clinicopathological study of gastrointestinal stromal tumors. Pathol Int. 1999;49:786–98.
133. Wisniewski D, Lambek CL, Liu C, et al. Characterization of potent inhibitors of the *bcr-abl* and the c-*kit* receptor tyrosine kinases. Cancer Res. 2002;62:4244–55.
134. Ben-Neriah Y, Daley GQ, Mes-Masson AM, Witte ON, Baltimore D. The chronic myelogenous leukemia-specific P210 protein is the product of the *bcr/abl* hybrid gene. Science. 1986;233:212–4.
135. Gibson PC, Cooper K. CD117 (c-*kit*): a diverse protein with selective applications in surgical pathology. Adv Anat Pathol. 2002;9:65–9.
136. De Silva CM, Reid R. Gastrointestinal stromal tumors (GISTs): c-*kit* mutations, CD117 expression, differential diagnosis, and targeted cancer therapy with imatinib. Pathol Oncol Res. 2003;9:13–9.
137. Knight III WA, Livingston RB, Gregory EJ, McGuire WL. Estrogen receptor as an independent prognostic factor for early recurrence in breast cancer. Cancer Res. 1977;37:4669–71.
138. McGuire WL. Hormone receptors: their role in predicting prognosis and response to endocrine therapy. Semin Oncol. 1978;5:428–33.
139. Hull III DF, Glark GM, Osborne CK, Chamness GC, Knight III WA, McGuire WL. Multiple estrogen receptor assays in human breast cancer. Cancer Res. 1983;43:413–6.
140. Barbanel G, Borgna JL, Bonnafous JC, Mani JC. Development of a microassay for estradiol receptors. Eur J Biochem. 1977;80:411–23.
141. Bezwoda WR, Esser JD, Dansey R, Kessel I, Lange M. The value of estrogen and progesterone receptor determinations in advanced breast cancer: estrogen receptor level but not progesterone receptor level correlates with response to tamoxifen. Cancer. 1991;68:867–72.
142. Pertschuk LP, Tobin EH, Gaetjens E, et al. Histochemical assay of estrogen and progesterone receptors in breast cancer: correlation with biochemical assays and patients' response to endocrine therapies. Cancer. 1980;46(Suppl):2896–901.

143. Seymour L, Meyer K, Esser J, MacPhail AP, Behr A, Bezwoda WR. Estimation of PR and ER by immunocytochemistry in breast cancer: comparison with radioligand binding methods. Am J Clin Pathol. 1990;94(Suppl):S35–40.
144. Tesch M, Shawwa A, Henderson R. Immunohistochemical determination of estrogen and progesterone receptor status in breast cancer. Am J Clin Pathol. 1993;99:8–12.
145. Nadji M, Gomez-Fernandez C, Ganjei-Azar P, Morales AR. Immunohistochemistry of estrogen and progesterone receptors reconsidered: experience with 5,993 breast cancers. Am J Clin Pathol. 2005;123:21–7.
146. Collins LC, Botero ML, Schnitt SJ. Bimodal frequency distribution of estrogen receptor immunohistochemical staining results in breast cancer: an analysis of 825 cases. Am J Clin Pathol. 2005;123:16–20.
147. Harvey JM, Clark GM, Osborne CK, Allred DC. Estrogen receptor status by immunohistochemistry is superior to the ligand-binding assay for predicting response to adjuvant endocrine therapy in breast cancer. J Clin Oncol. 1999;17:1474–81.
148. Nadji M. Quantitative immunohistochemistry of estrogen receptors in breast cancer: "much ado about nothing!". Appl Immunohistochem Mol Morphol. 2008;16:105–7.
149. Gomez-Fernandez C, Mejias A, Walker G, Nadji M. Immunohistochemical expression of estrogen receptor in adenocarcinomas of the lung: the antibody factor. Appl Immunohistochem Mol Morphol. 2010;18: 137–41.
150. Fuqua SA, Chamness GC, McGuire WL. Estrogen receptor mutations in breast cancer. J Cell Biochem. 1993;51:135–9.
151. Murphy LC, Skliris GP, Rowan BG, et al. The relevance of phosphorylated forms of estrogen receptor in human breast cancer in vivo. J Steroid Biochem Mol Biol. 2009;114:90–5.
152. McCabe A, Dolled-Filhart M, Camp RL, Rimm DL. Automated quantitative analysis (AQUA) of in-situ protein expression, antibody concentration, and prognosis. J Natl Cancer Inst U S A. 2005;97:1808–15.
153. Moeder CB, Giltnane JM, Moulis SP, Rimm DL. Quantitative, fluorescence-based in-situ assessment of protein expression. Methods Mol Biol. 2009;520:163–75.
154. Harigopal M, Barlow WE, Tedeschi G, et al. Multiplexed assessment of the Southwest Oncology Group-directed Intergroup Breast Cancer Trial S9313 by AQUA shows that both high and low levels of HER-2 are associated with poor outcome. Am J Pathol. 2010;176:1639–47.
155. Steel JH, Poulson R. Making sense out of in-situ PCR. J Pathol. 1997;182:11–2.
156. Lambros MB, Natrajan R, Geyer FC, et al. PPM1D gene amplification and overexpression in breast cancer: a qRT-PCR and chromogenic in-situ hybridization study. Mod Pathol. 2010;23:1334–45.
157. Ross JS. Multigene classifiers, prognostic factors, and predictors of breast cancer clinical outcome. Adv Anat Pathol. 2009;16:204–15.
158. Mocellin S, Rossi CR, Pilati P, Nitti D, Marincola FM. Quantitative real-time PCR: a powerful ally in cancer research. Trends Mol Med. 2003;9:189–95.
159. Van de Vijver M. Emerging technologies for HER-2 testing. Oncology. 2002;63(Suppl):33–8.
160. Susini T, Bussani C, Marini G, et al. Preoperative assessment of HER-2/*neu* status in breast carcinoma: the role of quantitative real-time PCR on core-biopsy specimens. Gynecol Oncol. 2010;116:234–9.
161. Wilcox JN. Fundamental principles of in-situ hybridization. J Histochem Cytochem. 1993;41:1725–33.
162. Naber SP, Tsutsumi Y, Yin S, et al. Strategies for the analysis of oncogene overexpression: studies of the *neu* oncogene in breast carcinoma. Am J Clin Pathol. 1990;94:125–36.
163. Ross JS. Saving lives with accurate HER-2 testing. Am J Clin Pathol. 2010;134:183–4.
164. Scartozzi M, Bearzi I, Mandolesi A, et al. Epidermal growth factor receptor (EGFR) gene copy number (GCN) correlates with clinical activity of irinotecan-cetuximab in k-*ras* wild-type colorectal cancer: a fluorescence in-situ (FISH) and chromogenic in-situ (CISH) analysis. BMC Cancer. 2009;9:303.
165. Guo QM. DNA microarrays and cancer. Curr Opin Oncol. 2003;15:36–43.
166. Churchill GA. Fundamentals of experimental design for cDNA microarrays. Nat Genet. 2002;32(Suppl): 490–5.
167. Murphy D. Gene expression studies using microarrays: principles, problems, and prospects. Adv Physiol Educ. 2002;26:256–70.
168. Iida K, Nishimura I. Gene expression profiling by DNA microarray technology. Crit Rev Oral Biol Med. 2002;13:35–50.
169. Ross JS, Mazumder A. Tissue microarrays and gene chips. In: Wick MR, editor. Metastatic carcinomas of unknown origin. New York: Demos Publishing; 2008. p. 177–90.
170. Wu W, Noble WS. Genomic data visualization on the Web. Bioinformatics. 2004;20:1804–5.
171. Roepman P, Horlings HM, Krijgsman O, et al. Microarray-based determination of estrogen receptor, progesterone receptor, and HER-2 receptor status in breast cancer. Clin Cancer Res. 2009;15:7003–11.
172. Idikio HA. Immunohistochemistry in diagnostic surgical pathology: contributions of protein life-cycle, use of evidence-based methods, and data normalization on interpretation of immunohistochemical stains. Int J Clin Exp Pathol. 2010;3:169–76.
173. Khandker RK, Dulski JD, Kilpatrick JB, Ellis RP, Mitchell JB, Baine WB. A decision model and cost-effectiveness analysis of colorectal cancer screening and surveillance guidelines for average-risk adults. Int J Technol Assess Health Care. 2000;16:799–810.
174. Sonnenberg A, Delco F, Inadomi JM. Cost-effectiveness of colonoscopy in screening for colorectal cancer. Ann Intern Med. 2000;133:573–84.

Evidence-Based Pathology and Laboratory Medicine in the Molecular Pathology Era: Transition of Tests from the Research Bench into Practice

17

Jia-Perng Jennifer Wei and Wayne W. Grody

Keywords
Evidence-based pathology • Molecular pathology • Genomics in pathology • ACCE test evaluation • Evidence levels analysis

As our knowledge of genomics expands, medical practice is slowly moving toward a new era of genomic medicine, with promises of personalized care and disease prevention based on genomic tools and technologies. As a result, molecular pathology has become fundamental to almost every aspect of healthcare delivery. Molecular pathology, a rapidly evolving discipline within pathology, incorporates the principles, techniques, and tools of molecular biology into diagnostic medicine in the clinical laboratory. To provide additional information for various clinical inquiries, molecular pathology integrates and applies knowledge from anatomic and clinical pathology, molecular biology, biochemistry, proteomics, and genetics. Therefore, it is strategically positioned at the interface between basic science and medicine.

With the completion of the human genome sequence and the advent of the "postgenomic era," there is increasing demand to translate genomic knowledge into clinical testing applications that have the potential to improve healthcare. However, a major hurdle in this process is the fact that standards for evaluating the clinical utility of a genetic test are not well developed. For the majority of emerging genetic tests, the goals of testing are often poorly defined or understood due to uncertain penetrance of causative mutations, prolonged time-lag between diagnosis and onset of symptoms, lack of knowledge about the natural history of newly discovered or rare disorders, and absence of effective therapeutic interventions. In addition, the underlying technologies are elaborate and constantly evolving. The newer whole-genome technologies produce such huge masses of data that interpretation of test results becomes highly complex and time consuming. Distinguishing between novel mutations and benign sequence variants is difficult and often highly speculative, depending upon a priori assumptions that may or may not be correct. Most importantly, the number and quality of studies addressing these issues are limited. As a result, test applications are being proposed and marketed based on descriptive evidence and pathophysiologic reasoning, without the appropriate data provided by well-designed clinical trials or observational studies to back them up [1].

J.-P.J. Wei (✉)
Ambry Genetics, 100 Columbia #200,
Aliso Viejo, CA 92656, USA
e-mail: jwei@ambrygen.com

A.M. Marchevsky and M.R. Wick (eds.), *Evidence Based Pathology and Laboratory Medicine*,
DOI 10.1007/978-1-4419-1030-1_17, © Springer Science+Business Media, LLC 2011

Structured Approaches for Test Evaluation: ACCE and EGAPP

To address the need for evidentiary standards in genomic medicine, the Centers for Disease Control and Prevention (CDC) sponsored the ACCE project (http://www.cdc.gov/genomics/gtesting/ACCE/acce_proj.htm#T1). The ACCE acronym denotes the four aspects of evaluation: *A*nalytic validity, *C*linical validity, *C*linical utility, and associated *E*thical, legal, and social implications [2, 3]. The ACCE project strives to establish a framework for assessing data on emerging genetic tests. To refine and test this review process for applications of genomic technology that are in transition from research to clinical practice, the National Office of Public Health Genomics (NOPHG) at the CDC launched the *E*valuation of *G*enomic *A*pplications in *P*ractice and *P*revention (EGAPP) initiative in 2004. The EGAPP effort has applied the ACCE framework to five genetic testing applications, providing evidence reports for others to use in formulating recommendations [4–8]. The EGAPP initiative continues to support timely and efficient translation of genomic applications into clinical practice by developing data collection, synthesis, and review capacity. Since strict adherence to the ACCE methodology is expensive and time consuming, we recommend using it as a general guide for decision-makers to appraise the readiness of a new genetic test for transition from discovery into clinical practice.

Formulation of the Central Question that the Test Is Supposed to Answer

According to the ACCE framework, the problem of interest needs to be carefully defined before the evidentiary review process. Depending on the purpose of the genetic test, the problem of interest may pertain to a specific medical disorder or a desired outcome. In the case of a medical disorder, it should be defined based on its clinical manifestations, rather than the laboratory tests employed for its detection. For pharmacogenomic testing, the clinical problem relates to the outcome of interest. It may be a reduction of adverse drug events, treatment optimization, or identification of patients most likely to benefit from a specific drug. The next step involves the characterization of test properties. It may entail specifying the genetic variant, the assay chosen to detect this genetic variant, reliability of the assay, consistency from laboratory to laboratory, and the complexity of test interpretation. Since the performance characteristics of a given test may vary depending on the intended use of the test, it is imperative to delineate the clinical scenario. Aspects of the clinical scenario that need to be addressed include the clinical setting (e.g., primary or specialty care; presence or absence of pre- and posttest genetic counseling), test application (e.g., diagnosis or screening), and test subjects (e.g., the general healthy population, selected high-risk individuals, or patients who are already symptomatic).

Systematic Literature Review of Available Evidence

After establishing the central question that the test is supposed to answer, one can proceed to a systematic, comprehensive search for relevant information in the scientific literature. This approach is considered acceptable, and indeed most often imperative, since it is recognized that ascertainment of clinical predictive value and genotype-phenotype correlations for most molecular tests is beyond the scope and capabilities of any one laboratory or center [9]. The strategy employed in the systematic literature review to identify relevant papers should be stipulated. Prior to the evaluation process, data sources, criteria for the inclusion or exclusion of a study, and criteria for quality assessment of a study need to be established as well.

Evaluation of the Quality of Available Evidence: Evidence Levels

The United States Preventive Services Task Force's *Guide to Community Preventive Services* has developed a sound basis for evaluating the quality of relevant studies [10]. In general, studies are characterized in terms of their design and execution. Suitability of design depends on the degree to which study design characteristics affect the validity of the results of a study. For example, prospective studies with concurrent comparison groups such as randomized controlled trials are considered of superior quality relative to observational studies without concurrent comparison groups. However, for many genetic tests, especially those for rare disorders, the prevalence of a specific genotype is so low that randomized trials are not feasible, and observational studies may provide better evidence. Assessment of study execution for a genetic test depends on several features: descriptions of the study population, sampling of the study population, measurement of genotype(s) and associated phenotype(s), data analysis, interpretation of results, and other confounding factors. If a study fails to adequately address specific aspects of these characteristics, it is considered a limitation.

Analytic Validity: Sensitivity, Specificity, Quality Control, and Assay Robustness

Subsequent to formulating the clinical problem and collecting the available best evidence from the literature, assessment of the four ACCE components can begin. EGAPP defines the analytic validity of a genetic test as its ability to accurately and reliably measure the genotype of interest [2]. Integral elements of analytic validity include analytic sensitivity, analytic specificity, quality control, and assay robustness. Analytic sensitivity reflects the detection rate, and it is the probability that a test will be positive when a target DNA sequence is present. Alternatively, analytic sensitivity can be defined as the limit of detection of an assay, namely the lowest amount of target sequence that can be detected in a specimen with confidence. The likelihood that a test will be negative in the absence of a target DNA sequence establishes the analytic specificity. Quality control encompasses a set of procedures designed to ensure the appropriate performance of a method and the quality of the resulting data. To assess the precision of a method within a laboratory, quality control usually involves the inclusion of positive and negative controls, reagent blanks, and duplicates in analytical runs. Proficiency testing (PT) is another essential component of quality assurance. For example, the College of American Pathologists (CAP) and the American College of Medical Genetics (ACMG) jointly administer PT programs for the more widely performed genetic tests. These surveys provide information regarding the consistency and accuracy of a specific test among laboratories. Finally, assay robustness examines magnitude of changes in test results secondary to small changes in preanalytic and analytic variables.

Since the technologies employed in molecular diagnostic testing are complex and constantly evolving, it is necessary to conduct a formal evaluation of analytic validity. To accomplish this task, a variety of data sources need to be used to obtain objective and reliable information. The best information derives from collaborative studies using a large panel of well-characterized samples (both cases and controls) that are exchanged between laboratories, blindly tested and reported, with the results independently analyzed [11]. Unfortunately, such optimal studies rarely exist for any genetic test, especially for a rare disease, prior to its introduction into clinical practice. Less optimal sources of data include well-designed method comparison and validation studies, data from PT programs, and FDA summaries of test kits or reagents that have been reviewed and approved by that agency.

Evaluation of the Analytic Sensitivity and Specificity of Different Molecular Tests

Most genetic variants can be tested by a variety of protocols. For example, accumulating evidence indicates that specific mutations in the tyrosine kinase domain of EGFR confer an improved response to EGFR inhibitors, such as gefitinib and erlotinib, in patients with non-small cell lung cancers [12]. The methodologies utilized to detect these mutations range from traditional Sanger sequencing to high-resolution melting analysis to allele specific real-time PCR to pyrosequencing. The test performance characteristics may differ greatly depending on the instruments and methodologies employed. The limit of detection, or analytic sensitivity, for traditional Sanger sequencing is approximately 20%, since minority nucleotide signals below that level (relative to the major nucleotide at that position) begin to blend in with the general background "noise" of the technique [13]. In practical terms, this translates into a limit of detection of the mutation of interest in a specimen no less than 20% of tumor cells carrying the specific mutation in a background of wild type cells. In contrast, utilizing allele specific real-time PCR, the analytic sensitivity may approach 1%. However, there is a paucity of studies one can rely on to determine the degree of impact (if any) on clinical outcomes caused by these differences in analytic sensitivity. Needless to say, this dearth of published studies on analytic validity limits the strength of conclusions regarding the clinical validity and utility of the test.

Clinical Performance Characteristics of Molecular Tests: Sensitivity and Predictive Value

The clinical validity of a genetic test establishes its accuracy at predicting a phenotype of interest or a clinical outcome. According to the ACCE evaluation process, clinical validity builds on analytic validity by examining five more elements: clinical sensitivity, clinical specificity, prevalence, positive and negative predictive values, and penetrance [2]. In contrast to analytic sensitivity, where the goal is to correctly identify a genotype, clinical sensitivity measures the proportion of individuals who have (or will develop) the disorder of interest and whose test results are positive; these results are considered true-positive (TP). If an individual with the phenotype of interest renders a negative result, it is considered false-negative (FN). Thus, clinical sensitivity is defined as the number of TP results divided by the sum of the TP and FN results [TP/(TP+FN)]. Clinical specificity determines the proportion of subjects with negative test values and who do not have (or will not develop) the phenotype; these results are considered true-negative (TN). If a subject lacks the phenotype of interest but yields a positive result, it is considered a false-positive (FP) result. Mathematically, clinical specificity is the quotient between the number of TN results and the sum of the TN and FP results [TN/(TN+FP)]. Prevalence refers to the number of individuals within the specified testing population who have (or will develop) the phenotype. As a result, prevalence can affect the positive and negative predictive values of a molecular test. For example, if a given mutation is extremely rare in the tested population, there is a greater chance that a positive test result may be due to a technical (analytic) FP rather than a TP.

The clinical performance characteristics of a molecular test are intricately related to one another. When the test renders a clinically FN result, it is usually not caused by laboratory errors. Instead, it indicates the presence of other causal factors that may contribute to the development of the interested phenotype, in addition to the specific mutation(s) being tested. When a genetic test produces a FP result, there are two possible explanations. The positive test result may be due to analytic error(s), or it may indicate incomplete penetrance. For instance, a genetic test may correctly identify individuals homozygous for the C282Y mutation in the *HFE* gene; however, they may never develop serious clinical manifestations of iron overload in their lifetime, due to the low clinical penetrance of *HFE* mutations [14]. In addition to penetrance, another relationship between genotype and phenotype needs to be considered. Sometimes, different mutations in the same gene cause different phenotypic effects. In the *DMD* gene, one series of deletions cause Becker muscular dystrophy, while other deletions in the same gene manifest as Duchenne muscular dystrophy. Since this genotype to phenotype relationship (depending on whether the deletion is in-frame or out-of-frame) is highly consistent, some clinicians use this information for prognostic and counseling purposes [15].

Clinical Utility

Clinical utility of a genetic test refers to its ability to influence health outcomes through the adoption of therapeutic or preventive interventions based on test results. Both the risks and benefits of a test's introduction into clinical practice need to be considered. The ACCE framework has formulated a series of questions, namely questions 26 through 41, to facilitate the organization of information regarding clinical utility [2]. Of the four main aspects in the ACCE evaluation process, clinical utility may be considered the most complex component to examine. To properly analyze the clinical utility of a genetic test, one needs to delineate the natural history of the specific clinical disorder, potential risks and benefits, quality assurance of test performance, and associated economic, ethical, legal, social, and policy. Accurate information concerning the natural history of a clinical disorder is important. If the disorder has serious health consequences, the typical age of onset can be utilized to determine the optimal age for either screening or early diagnostic testing. Unfortunately, however, many genetic and neoplastic diseases show wide variation in age of onset. It is important to evaluate the availability and effectiveness of interventions. In the absence of effective interventions, other measurable effects, such as psychological and emotional impact of the information provided by the testing results on the patients, should be considered. When balancing the pros and cons of implementing a new DNA test, health risks need to be considered. Health risks might represent morbidity and mortality associated with subsequent procedures for diagnosis or treatment. They might also encompass less quantifiable risks, such as anxiety and stigmatization. Economic evaluation (including test cost, available CPT codes, insurance coverage, etc.) and resource allocation should also be included in the appraisal of clinical utility.

In order to evaluate the clinical utility of a genetic test, it is necessary to examine the merit and suitability of existing evidence. Similar to the appraisal of analytic and clinical validity, important characteristics that affect the quality of data on clinical utility include the size and selection criteria for the study population, the type of laboratory assay and interventions employed, and the study design [16]. The quantity of data refers to the number of studies and the number of total subjects in the studies. A study that addresses the clinical utility of a molecular test needs to provide a detailed description of the intervention and the context in which the intervention was conducted. The quality of studies depends on their methodology and execution. Randomized controlled trials, cohort, or case-control studies may be employed to evaluate the impact of a molecular test on health outcomes. Of these study methods, randomized controlled trials are believed to offer the most reliable evidence. If the sample size is adequate, randomization ensures equal distribution of both known and unsuspected confounding factors. For instance, cohort studies allow participants to select the desired therapeutic option, and this choice may reflect the test subjects' characteristics, thus introducing confounding factors. Blinding of participants, providers, and investigators further minimizes the likelihood of placebo effects and observational bias. As in studies of clinical validity, meta-analysis of similar studies may be used to estimate the overall consistency of clinical utility.

Formal Assessment of the Clinical Validity of Molecular Tests: Selection of Best Available Evidence and Meta-Analysis

To conduct a formal assessment of the clinical validity of a genetic test, it is imperative to critically appraise the quality and appropriateness of available evidence. Important variables that influence the overall quality of evidence for clinical validity include the number and quality of studies, the size and selection criteria for the study population, the type of assay employed (as well as its analytic validity), and the endpoints measured [16]. The quantity of data pertains to the number of studies and the number of total subjects in the studies. The quality of studies is usually dictated by their designs. For instance, well-designed longitudinal cohort studies usually provide the information necessary to evaluate the strength of association between a genotype or biomarker and a specific phenotype or disorder. Furthermore, meta-analysis of similar studies may be employed to estimate the overall consistency of clinical validity, and to compensate for the small size of individual studies. Since the majority of genetic tests are designed to detect events of relatively low frequency, longitudinal cohort studies are usually not feasible. Thus, case-control and cross-sectional studies can serve as alternative sources of evidence. For currently available genetic tests, their clinical validity may remain uncertain and evolve as evidence accumulates.

Pilot Studies

Often, there is limited or no available information in the literature regarding the potential clinical validity and applicability of a molecular test, and pilot studies are needed to collect data. Even though evidence gathered in pilot studies is not sufficient for clinical application, pilot studies provide valuable information regarding the readiness of a novel molecular test for transition from the lab bench to routine care. They subject the DNA testing process to the daily pressures of clinical testing, thus determining its analytic performance characteristics under real-world conditions. They offer the opportunity to observe and document the test subjects' responses to the testing process. It was through just such a process of pilot studies that the now-accepted universal cystic fibrosis carrier screening program was developed and assessed [17]. Additional information that may be acquired in pilot trials includes patterns of decision-making, economic information, and acceptance rates at various stages of the testing process. Consequently, pilot studies provide the foundation necessary for subsequent clinical trials.

Ethical Issues

In addition to providing diagnostic, prognostic, and therapeutic information, molecular genetics and oncology tests have ethical, legal, and social implications. One of the greatest concerns about genetic testing, especially when performed presymptomatically, involves the potential for insurance or employment discrimination, stigmatization, and long-term psychological harms from testing. Unfortunately, these effects are difficult to study. Since the beginning of the Human Genome Project, genetic discrimination has been a concern of policy-makers, legal scholars, and patients at risk for genetic disorders [18]. In an attempt to prevent genetic discrimination and the misuse of genetic information in employment and health insurance, the Genetic Information Nondiscrimination Act (GINA) was finally passed by the U.S. Congress and signed into law by President G.W. Bush on May 21, 2008 [19]. However, it may take several years before the impact of GINA on the incidence of reported genetic discrimination can be properly evaluated.

Even if the results of genetic testing do not affect clinical management or lead to a measurable effect on health, genetic information can help individual and family decision-making. For highly penetrant, single-gene disorders that lack effective therapy, genetic information provides assistance to inform reproductive or other life decisions. For example, testing for Huntington disease cannot alter the course of this lethal condition, but it allows mutation carriers and noncarriers to prepare for the future with that prognosis in mind. For complex multifactorial illnesses, genetic testing provides information regarding association between genotypic variations and risk of disease. Even though predictive genetic testing can identify individuals at increased risk, it may also cause increased distress and anxiety. Several studies have examined the effects of *BRCA1/2* testing on individuals and their families. The majority of studies have reported no significant change in psychological outcomes among asymptomatic mutation carriers relative to baseline [20]. However, there appear to be short-term increases in anxiety among asymptomatic mutation carriers [21]. It is also important to understand the factors that determine interest in predictive genetic testing. The usefulness and personal value attached to knowledge about genetic disease or cancer risk may vary by age or other personal characteristics. For example, the implications of a positive test for a *BRCA1* or *BRCA2* mutation differ considerably for a woman of child-bearing age compared with a perimenopausal woman, because oophorectomy is an important prevention option for such women. In addition, some testing decisions may be motivated by the desire to help offspring. A female patient with cancer may be more interested in *BRCA1/2* testing if she has daughters who might in turn benefit from the information in terms of their own inherited risk and by making presymptomatic testing in them easier and less expensive since the family's *BRCA* mutation will then be known.

Table 17.1 Critical parameters for determining transition of a research molecular test to a clinical test

Analytic validity
Clinical validity
Clinical utility
Literature review
Meta-analyses
ACCE approach
EGAPP recommendations
Pilot studies
Randomized controlled trials
Professional practice guidelines
Cost and reimbursement policies
Ethical and psychosocial considerations

Real-World Considerations

The experience of predictive testing for mutations in the *BRCA1* and *BRCA2* genes is instructive for our more general discussion of transition of research assays to clinical tests. When those two genes were first discovered in the mid-1990s and their penetrance shown to be appreciably less than 100%, there were some medical ethicists and others who argued that the unknowns were too great to justify clinical mutation testing at that point. Yet, it is only by embarking on widespread testing, even before all the answers were in, that we were able to further refine the genotype–phenotype correlations, predictive value, and clinical penetrance of these mutations. Similarly, testing for K-*ras* mutations in colon cancers, while only modestly predictive of response to anti-EGFR inhibitor therapies, soon led to the revelation that mutation in another gene involved in the same signaling pathway, *BRAF*, could help explain a proportion of the K-*ras*-negative nonresponders. It can be expected that continued testing in the actual clinical setting will reveal other genes and mutations that will steadily raise the predictive value of the molecular tests. Yet another example is the almost overnight and universal adoption of array-comparative genomic hybridization in place of standard karyotype analysis for diagnostic work-up of patients with nonspecific developmental delay, autism, or congenital malformations [22]. Although the approach suffers from the uncertainty produced by the large number of novel deletions and duplications revealed in every human genome, it is only through continued clinical testing, with reporting of such findings in a centralized database, that the true genotype–phenotype relationships will become known and established. Thus, while we have attempted in this chapter to delineate the various parameters and approaches that should be followed in order to make the determination of when a research test is ready for transition to a clinical test (Table 17.1), it is also important to allow some latitude during the phase at which the biology and molecular pathology of these disease processes are still being worked out. And that notion will be even more true in the coming years as we move beyond single-gene molecular tests into whole-genome arrays and next-generation whole-genome sequencing [23].

Conclusions

Molecular pathology presents a particularly difficult challenge to the systematic methodology proposed by evidence-based pathology for the gathering of evidence and classification of such evidence using various evidence level schemes. The rapid developments in the field, complexity of molecular tests, massive quantity of data accrued, and the almost infinite number of analytes addressed by these new technologies render many of the requirements delineated in this chapter – for positive mutation controls, clinical validation, etc. – almost moot. Clearly the genie is out of the bottle, and we have little choice but to move forward thoughtfully, incorporating the approaches we have described when possible, but not adhering to them so rigidly that patients are deprived for too long of their access to these potentially life-saving technologies.

References

1. Khoury MJ, Berg A, Coates R, Evans J, Teutsch SM, Bradley LA. The evidence dilemma in genomic medicine. Health Aff (Millwood). 2008;27(6): 1600–11.
2. Haddow JE, Palomaki GE. ACCE: a model process for evaluating data on emerging genetic tests. In: Khoury MJ, Little J, Burke W, editors. Human genome epidemiology: a scientific foundation for using genetic information to improve health and prevent disease. Oxford: Oxford University Press; 2004. p. 217–33.
3. Eagle A. Seal of approval ACCE rolls out a new certification for clinical engineers. Health Facil Manage. 2004;17(5):30–2, 34.
4. Palomaki GE, Haddow JE, Bradley LA, FitzSimmons SC. Updated assessment of cystic fibrosis mutation frequencies in non-Hispanic Caucasians. Genet Med. 2002;4(2):90–4.
5. Palomaki GE, Bradley LA, Richards CS, Haddow JE. Analytic validity of cystic fibrosis testing: a preliminary estimate. Genet Med. 2003;5(1):15–20.
6. Palomaki GE, Haddow JE, Bradley LA, Richards CS, Stenzel TT, Grody WW. Estimated analytic validity of HFE C282Y mutation testing in population screening: the potential value of confirmatory testing. Genet Med. 2003;5(6):440–3.
7. Gudgeon JM, McClain MR, Palomaki GE, Williams MS. Rapid ACCE: experience with a rapid and structured approach for evaluating gene-based testing. Genet Med. 2007;9(7):473–8.
8. McClain MR, Palomaki GE, Piper M, Haddow JE. A rapid-ACCE review of CYP2C9 and VKORC1 alleles testing to inform warfarin dosing in adults at elevated risk for thrombotic events to avoid serious bleeding. Genet Med. 2008;10(2):89–98.
9. Maddalena A, Bale S, Das S, Grody W, Richards S. Technical standards and guidelines: molecular genetic testing for ultra-rare disorders. Genet Med. 2005; 7(8):571–83.
10. Briss PA, Brownson RC, Fielding JE, Zaza S. Developing and using the guide to community preventive services: lessons learned about evidence-based public health. Annu Rev Public Health. 2004;25:281–302.
11. Teutsch SM, Bradley LA, Palomaki GE, et al. The Evaluation of Genomic Applications in Practice and Prevention (EGAPP) initiative: methods of the EGAPP Working Group. Genet Med. 2009;11(1):3–14.
12. Sequist LV, Lynch TJ. EGFR tyrosine kinase inhibitors in lung cancer: an evolving story. Annu Rev Med. 2008;59:429–42.
13. Whitehall V, Tran K, Umapathy A, et al. A multicenter blinded study to evaluate KRAS mutation testing methodologies in the clinical setting. J Mol Diagn. 2009;11(6):543–52.
14. Rossi E, Jeffrey GP. Clinical penetrance of C282Y homozygous HFE haemochromatosis. Clin Biochem Rev. 2004;25(3):183–90.
15. Bushby KM. Genetic and clinical correlations of Xp21 muscular dystrophy. J Inherit Metab Dis. 1992;15(4):551–64.
16. Little J, Bradley L, Bray MS, et al. Reporting, appraising, and integrating data on genotype prevalence and gene-disease associations. Am J Epidemiol. 2002; 156(4):300–10.
17. Richards CS, Grody WW. Prenatal screening for cystic fibrosis: past, present and future. Expert Rev Mol Diagn. 2004;4(1):49–62.
18. Billings PR, Kohn MA, de Cuevas M, Beckwith J, Alper JS, Natowicz MR. Discrimination as a consequence of genetic testing. Am J Hum Genet. 1992; 50(3):476–82.
19. Erwin C. Legal update: living with the Genetic Information Nondiscrimination Act. Genet Med. 2008;10(12):869–73.
20. Schlich-Bakker KJ, Ausems MG, Schipper M, Ten Kroode HF, Warlam-Rodenhuis CC, van den Bout J. BRCA1/2 mutation testing in breast cancer patients: a prospective study of the long-term psychological impact of approach during adjuvant radiotherapy. Breast Cancer Res Treat. 2008;109(3): 507–14.
21. Meiser B. Psychological impact of genetic testing for cancer susceptibility: an update of the literature. Psychooncology. 2005;14(12):1060–74.
22. Miller DT, Adam MP, Aradhya S, et al. Consensus statement: chromosomal microarray is a first-tier clinical diagnostic test for individuals with developmental disabilities or congenital anomalies. Am J Hum Genet. 2010;86(5):749–64.
23. ten Bosch JR, Grody WW. Keeping up with the next generation: massively parallel sequencing in clinical diagnostics. J Mol Diagn. 2008;10(6):484–92.

18 The Use of Decision Analysis Tools for the Selection of Clinical Laboratory Tests: Developing Diagnostic and Forecasting Models Using Laboratory Evidence

Ji Yeon Kim, Elizabeth M. Van Cott, and Kent B. Lewandrowski

Keywords
Decision support • Medical order entry systems • Laboratory utilization • Evidence-based medicine

Archie Cochrane in his seminal book *Effectiveness and Efficiency* (1972) argued that "health services should be evaluated on the basis of scientific evidence rather than on clinical impression, anecdotal experience, 'expert' opinion or tradition" [1]. This tenet of evidence-based medicine (EBM) [2, 3] has resonated strongly in the ethos of contemporary practice, fueling growth in the number of clinical guidelines and changes in healthcare policy and financing. Further driving the EBM-movement are preventable adverse events related to medical errors, now recognized as a cause of more deaths than those from breast cancer or motor vehicle accidents [4–6]. Recently, the American Recovery and Reinvestment Act of 2009 (ARRA) allocated approximately $19 billion to promote the adoption of electronic health records (EHR), with the idea that such technology can make health care more evidence-based and less error-prone [7, 8].

Despite public enthusiasm for EBM, there has been relatively little change in physician behavior, and in fact, the data shows most physicians have a difficult time following guidelines [9]. Supporting these observations is the striking regional variation in the use of healthcare resources, measured by rates of physician visits, hospitalizations, specialist referrals, laboratory testing, and interventions, which does not correlate with improved quality or access to healthcare, better outcomes, or increased patient satisfaction [10, 11]. In fact, for some measures related to health prevention, such as influenza vaccination rates, increased spending is associated with worse care [10]. This is concerning given that national health spending in the U.S. reached $2.3 trillion in 2008, or 16.2% of the gross domestic product [12].

Laboratory services are particularly vulnerable to potential misuse and overuse [13, 14]. Use of laboratory services can be inflated by public expectations for frequent testing [15] and the practice of "defensive medicine" [16, 17]. Meanwhile, laboratory tests are subject to systemic and random errors, and a "shot-gun" approach to testing increases the potential for false-positive and false-negative results [18]. Operational efficiency in the laboratory and clinical areas can be adversely affected by higher testing volumes from inappropriate and unnecessary orders, compromising turnaround times for laboratory tests with clinical urgency [19]. Downstream, this can directly impact the length of stay for patients, as in the emergency department [20].

K.B. Lewandrowski (✉)
Department of Pathology, Massachusetts General Hospital and Harvard Medical School,
Gray 5–536 Chemistry Massachusetts General Hospital, 55 Fruit Street, Boston, MA 02114, USA
e-mail: Klewandrowski@partners.org

A.M. Marchevsky and M.R. Wick (eds.), *Evidence Based Pathology and Laboratory Medicine*, DOI 10.1007/978-1-4419-1030-1_18,

In terms of financial impact, it has been estimated that eliminating redundant laboratory tests alone would save about $8 billion a year in the U.S. [21], and the burden of ensuring medical necessity for testing is gradually being shifted to the clinical laboratories themselves [22].

With technological advances in laboratory automation and instrumentation greatly reducing analytical errors, more errors now take place outside the laboratory in both test ordering and result interpretation [23–25], with the majority made before the patient specimen reaches the laboratory [26, 27]. At the same time, the information-oriented agenda of EBM has given pathology data an increasingly central role in initiating and coordinating patient care, from diagnosis to treatment decisions to disease monitoring. It is believed that more than half of all medical decisions are influenced by laboratory data [28, 29], with one study demonstrating that 94% of requests to the electronic medical record were for laboratory results alone [30]. Thus, diagnostic errors are of particular concern to both physicians and patients, which is highlighted by the fact that diagnostic errors are the most common reason for medical malpractice claims [31–33].

It has been observed that many physicians have testing- and diagnosis-related questions as they see patients, but are unable to find answers because of lack of time and poor organization of information sources [34, 35]. Hayward has said that "physicians suffer from information hunger in the midst of plenty" [36], which rings particularly true in our internet-based era [37], where online tools such as PubMed currently hosts more than 19 million citations for the biomedical literature (http://www.ncbi.nlm.nih.gov/pubmed; last accessed 12 May 2010). A meta-analysis of various studies has found that diagnosis-related questions comprise, on average, 24% of information need, and another 49% are related to therapy and drug information [38].

In several areas, diagnostic tests are becoming synonymous with targeted therapeutics, inspiring the term "theragnostics" [39]. For example, the Food and Drug Administration (FDA) has recommended that maraviroc, part of a new class of HIV/AIDS drugs that are chemokine coreceptor 5 (CCR5) antagonists, only be used after testing confirms that a patient is infected with a CCR5-tropic viral strain [40, 41]. In cancer, testing for newly identified molecular drivers for lung adenocarcinomas, colorecetal cancer, breast cancer, and oligodendrogliomas, among others, has been critical for establishing patient eligibility for targeted chemotherapy, and for guiding patient management [42–45].

As part of this trend, the number of tests in molecular diagnostics is rapidly expanding, particularly for genetic diseases, infectious diseases, and cancer. In our institution, for tumor diagnostics alone, we currently have 17 distinct assays which cover gene mutations, DNA methylation alterations, microsatellite instability, and diagnostic and prognostic FISH assays, and we are planning on adding five new tests over the next 6 months. In the coagulation laboratory, we have added four new tests over the past 4 months, for a current total of 52 different tests. Our current main reference laboratory catalog lists approximately 7,140 different tests. Both the rate of test menu growth and the sheer number of test options present challenges for clinicians.

Although most specialists are able to stay reasonably current in their narrow area of expertise, the situation for the typical general internist or surgeon is becoming increasingly untenable. Invariably, this leads to an increase in subspecialty consults, with a resulting increase in cost. But these days, even specialists may find it difficult to select or interpret the correct test. Unperceived or unexpressed information needs are difficult to identify [46], but some inappropriate test requests may be due to unacknowledged knowledge gaps. In one example of a routine test, 25-hydroxyvitamin D is the best test to assess vitamin D status under most clinical situations, as opposed to 1-25 dihydroxyvitamin D. At our institution, we noticed that displaying test selection guidelines for vitamin D in a "pop-up reminder" every time a physician requested 1-25 dihydroxyvitamin D caused a 71% reduction in 1,25-$(OH)_2$ vitamin D orders [47]. In virtually every case where the 1,25-$(OH)_2$ vitamin D was not ordered, the user ordered the more appropriate 25-OH vitamin D test.

Laboratory knowledge is specialized and local, and can be difficult to acquire. A laboratory's unique menu of tests and policies may differ from other laboratories. This information may not be readily accessible on global search engines or online references, and is most often maintained internally by the laboratory itself. Thus, local pathologists have an opportunity to play a more proactive role in the total testing process [48].

The entire process of laboratory testing, starting with the decision to order a test, should be evidence-based, and ideally, cost-conscious [49, 50]. There is a need for decision support tools to aid physicians in the selection and interpretation of laboratory tests. Clinical pathologists must also know how to evaluate the clinical context and usefulness of tests in order to make recommendations to hospital administrators and clinicians about adding, replacing, or eliminating tests from the test menu, as well as guiding what defines appropriate testing for specific clinical situations. Pathologists must also consider whether or not studies were carried out in the appropriate populations suspected of the target disease, and not just those with obvious disease compared to healthy controls [51]. With these considerations, a number of statistical tools exist to help evaluate and compare test performance, and some of these will be discussed briefly below.

Statistics

The assumption behind EBM is that there are clinically meaningful subgroups of patients, following a similar disease progression and sharing comparable risks for morbidity and mortality. Identifying a patient as belonging to one of these subgroups allows the clinician to extrapolate treatment and management decisions from the published literature. The ability of a particular test to successfully distinguish subjects in the appropriate diagnostic and prognostic subcategories can be quantified in a number of ways.

With a binary test result (i.e., positive or negative), a 2-by-2 table comparing the test results to true disease status via an independent gold standard (i.e., biopsy) can be used to assess test accuracy (Fig. 18.1). Accuracy can be represented as diagnostic sensitivity (probability of a positive test, given the patient has the disease) and diagnostic specificity (probability of a negative test, given the patient does not have the disease) [52]. The likelihood ratio (LR) combines these two measures, and represents the probability of a test result in the presence vs. absence of disease. For example, the LR for a positive test result (LR(+)) compares the sensitivity, or probability of a positive test result in a disease-positive population, to

	Disease+	**Disease-**	**Total**
Test+	450	50	500
Test-	50	450	500
Total	500	500	1,000

Disease prevalence = 50%

Test performance:
Sensitivity = 90%
Specificity = 90%
PPV = 90%
NPV = 90%

	Disease+	**Disease-**	**Total**
Test+	90	90	180
Test-	10	810	820
Total	100	900	1,000

Disease prevalence = 10%

Test performance:
Sensitivity = 90%
Specificity = 90%
PPV = **50%**
NPV = **98.9%**

Fig. 18.1 Effect of disease prevalence on test performance the false-positive rate, or probability of a positive test result in a disease-negative population. A LR(+) of four means that the positive test is 4 times as likely to occur in patients with disease as in patients without disease, which is not the same as saying that patients with disease are 4 times as likely to have a positive test result when compared to those without disease.

Usually the question is whether or not the patient has the disease, and not about the likelihood of a particular test result. Bayes' theorem allows us to make a statement about the inverse conditional probability, in this case, the probability of disease given a test finding (see Fig. 18.2). This can be reported as the positive predictive value (PPV; probability of disease, given a positive test result) and the negative predictive value (NPV; probability of no disease, given a negative test result), and calculated from the same 2-by-2 table, as long as the total numbers are adjusted to reflect the preexisting disease prevalence in the population (see Fig. 18.1). Both the PPV and NPV are affected by disease prevalence, whereas sensitivity and specificity remain independent of prevalence.

Bayes' theorem can be used to evaluate the clinical utility of a new test. For example, a result of >13 pg/ml for high-sensitivity troponin T (hsTnT) has been reported as a superior marker for acute coronary syndromes (ACS) when compared to a result of >0.03 ng/ml by conventional cardiac troponin T (cTnT), based on improved sensitivity (from 35 to 62%) and a small increase in the area under the ROC curve (see below), although the latter was statistically insignificant

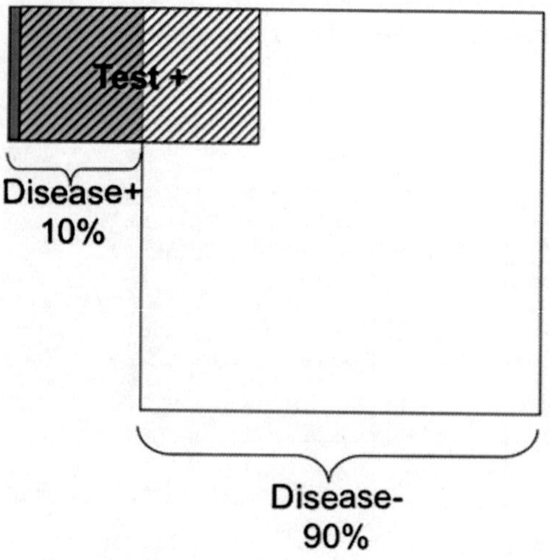

P(T+|D+) = probability of a positive test given disease
= **sensitivity**
= 90%
P(T-|D+) = probability of a negative test given disease
= **false negative rate**
= 1-sensitivity
= 10%
P(T-|D-) = probability of a negative test given no disease
= **specificity**
= 90%
P(T+|D-) = probability of a positive test given no disease
= **false positive rate**
= 1-specificity
= 10%

P(D+) = probability of disease (**prevalence**)
= 10% (grey box)
P(D-) = probability of no disease
= 1-P(D+)
= 90% (white box)
P(T+) = probability of a positive test among all subjects (diseased and non-diseased) (diagonal lines)
= [P(T+|D+)*P(D+)] + [P(T+|D-)*P(D-)]
= [0.9*0.1] + [0.1*0.9]
= 0.18

Bayes' theorem:
P(D+|T+) = probability of disease given a positive test
= **positive predictive value**
= [P(T+|D+)*P(D+)] / [P(T+)]
= [0.9*0.1] / [0.18]
= 50%

Fig. 18.2 Application of Bayes' theorem. P(X) means probability of event X. P(X|Y) means probability of event X, given event Y and the improvement in sensitivity was at the cost of decreased specificity (from 99 to 89%) [53]. When using Bayes' theorem to look at the predictive power of a positive test for ACS, it was demonstrated that even very high values of hsTnT do not establish a diagnosis of ACS if the pretest probability is low [54]. In fact, with a pretest ACS probability of 10%, a positive cTnT is better for predicting ACS (PPV of 80%) than a positive hsTnT (PPV of 39%).

Even so, many test evaluations are reported using sensitivity and specificity assessments, as predictive value estimates require prior knowledge of disease prevalence and outcomes data, which may be difficult to obtain for target patient populations. At the same time, because many tests have results that are on a continuous spectrum, they can exhibit all sensitivity and specificity values (from 0 to 100%) depending on the particular value chosen to represent the "positive" result cutoff (e.g., hsTnT of >13, >14, >15 pg/ml, etc.). Receiver-operating characteristic (ROC) plots are often used to provide a more global view of test performance, as these plots depict all possible sensitivity and specificity pairs for a test [55]. The area under the curve (AUC), also called the c-statistic or c index, can range from 0.5 (no discriminatory ability) to 1.0 (perfect discrimination), and is a summary measure that can also be used to compare whole ROC curves to one another. An alternative is to restrict the area comparisons to a relevant portion of the curve at a desired sensitivity or specificity. The tangent to the ROC curve is equivalent to the LR(+), when that particular test result (with its given sensitivity and specificity) is chosen as the decision threshold.

Given that multiple test values are represented in a ROC plot, a decision threshold must be chosen that incorporates considerations about the relative costs of false-positive and false-negative results, as well as the prevalence of disease in the population being tested. A simplified approach is to calculate a slope using the following equation: m=(false-positive cost/false-negative cost)×((1 − prevalence)/prevalence), and then choose the point on the ROC plot where the tangent has this slope [55].

In practice, calculating the true "cost" of false-positive and false-negative results requires thoughtful conversations between the laboratory and clinicians, and thresholds may change over time. In our hospital, setting notification alarms for critical laboratory values is one such example of this ongoing process, which is negotiated through hospital committee meetings consisting of representatives from the laboratories, clinicians, and hospital administration. Performing callbacks for critical lab values are labor- and time-intensive for the laboratory, and should be limited to those values that are truly dangerous. Using the published literature, consultations with clinicians, and our own internal data on the volume of critical callbacks for each analyte per result value, we made the case for changing the lower limit for glucose callbacks from less than 60 mg/dl (<3.3 mmol/l) to less than 45 mg/dl (<2.5 mmol/l), which has resulted in 2,136 fewer calls per year (reduction of 5.7% for all callbacks) [56].

As previously mentioned, ROC curves classify patients by their likelihood of having a positive test result, but prognostic models evaluate tests for their ability to predict future risk of disease, and may be of greater interest to patients and clinicians [57]. Calibration examines the predictive value of a test result, and compares the observed vs. predicted probabilities of disease within predetermined subgroups of patients sharing similar risks of disease. Risk stratification is initially performed using an existing disease model based on traditional assessment factors, and is compared to a revised stratification scheme including the independent test result. The percent of reclassified patients after the addition of the new test can be used as an indicator of clinical impact. As a result, disease prevalence and the way subgroups are modeled have a major effect on assessments of calibration. The Hosmer-Lemeshow test [58] and the net reclassification index (NRI) [59] are two examples of formal calibration measures.

The ROC curve and the AUC are less sensitive than the NRI when evaluating the addition of new tests/predictors for disease. In particular, the impact on AUC by a new test is blunted when the preexisting model already strongly predicts disease, even if the test is independent from the other predictor variables [57]. For example, among patients with ACS, early stratification helps assign high-risk patients to more aggressive and costly therapies. Patients can be assessed using the clinically robust GRACE (Global Registry of Acute Coronary Events) risk scores [60] to evaluate their risk for mortality and acute myocardial infarction (AMI) events. NT-proBNP (N-terminal pro-B-type natriuretic peptide) has been identified as a biomarker that is useful in patients with AMI [61], and also seems to provide prognostic information for short- and long-term mortality and future MI [62–64]. Investigators examined the effect of adding admission NT-proBNP levels to the GRACE risk score in predicting early and late deaths following ACS [65]. The AUC for 30-day mortality was 0.79 for NT-proBNP, 0.84 for the GRACE risk score, and 0.85 for the combination. The difference between AUC for the combination of predictors vs. the GRACE score alone was not statistically different ($p=0.20$), but the impact on NRI of adding NT-proBNP to the GRACE model was a 24.4% overall improvement ($p<0.001$).

At the same time, when looking at subgroups, the combination of NT-proBNP and GRACE score was better for predicting survivors at 30-days (NRI of 41.4%), and did worse at predicting nonsurvivors [65]. Thus, the clinical utility of NT-proBNP is likely to be poor if it is used to identify patients at high-risk of early events [66]. In considering the NRI, it is therefore important to consider the changes in risk categories for specific outcomes of interest, rather than just the overall score.

Decision Support

EBM attempts to quantify the probabilities associated with medical decisions, and encourages clinicians to face these uncertainties explicitly, rather than relying on personal intuition or expert opinion alone. While laboratory tests are rarely used in isolation, the results are often integrated with medical history, physical examination findings, and imaging studies to assess the likelihood of disease. This complex decision-making process has been difficult to capture, model, and analyze.

Still, a variety of decision support tools are available to assist physicians in the selection and interpretation of laboratory tests (Table 18.1). Specific examples of these tools will be described later in the chapter. In most cases, these tools must be reviewed regularly to ensure the most

Table 18.1 Decision support tools for the selection and interpretation of laboratory tests

Tool	Comment(s)
Diagnostic algorithms	Available in books or online
Published practice standards	Available in books or online
Disease or condition-specific templates	Includes admission, procedure and chemotherapy templates for specific conditions (e.g., heart failure) that specify appropriate tests, medications, and nursing orders. Templates ensure that the correct interventions are accomplished at the appropriate time and standardize care for a specific condition
Interpretive guidelines	Available in books or online. Particularly useful are institution-specific online laboratory handbooks
Consultative interpretive services	Consultative services provided by clinical pathologists to aid in the selection and interpretation of laboratory tests
Computerized provider order entry	Permits real time decision support at the time the test is ordered. Can be used to redirect physicians away from unnecessary tests and suggest more appropriate alternatives
Computer-based decision support	Includes query functions for specific signs, symptoms, or diseases and recommend appropriate tests and their interpretation
Computerized reminder alert systems	Can automatically alert physicians to flagged values or missing/delayed screening or monitoring tests
Online or text handbooks	Describes test performance characteristics, interferences, false-positive and negative results, drug effects and other information

up-to-date content. This is most easily accomplished with online formats, as decision support tools available only in print media usually become obsolete a short time after publication.

To be effective, decision support tools must be used by physicians and the suggested advice acted upon. Physicians are notoriously finicky when it comes to using technologies that will presumably improve their practice. Careful consideration must therefore be given to fitting the tool directly into the physician's regular workflow, as well as to making these systems extremely easy to access and to use [67]. In a study by Bates et al. [68], the authors highlight their "Ten commandments for effective decision support." We strongly recommend this paper for anyone who is designing or planning implementation of a decision support system. The ten key points included the following:

1. Speed is everything
2. Anticipate needs and deliver in real time
3. Fit into the user's workflow
4. Little things can make a big difference
5. Recognize that physicians will strongly resist stopping
6. Changing direction is easier than stopping
7. Simple interventions work best
8. Ask for additional information only when you really need it
9. Monitor impact, get feedback, and respond
10. Manage and maintain your knowledge based systems

An important caveat concerning decision support tools concerns their clinical and scientific reliability. The availability of numerous lay or quasi-professional websites that provide medical advice underscores this growing problem [69–71]. It can be difficult even for experienced physicians to assess the quality of information offered by these websites, especially considering that the physicians may access the site for the very reason that they are unsure about the most appropriate way to proceed. Furthermore, information provided by medical organizations and societies is not *prima fascia* reliable. Contradictions can be easily found when searching different professional websites or publications about the same clinical problem. For these reasons, the physician must approach decision support tools with a degree of healthy skepticism. Careful consideration should be given to the source of the information and how current the information provided is.

Examples of Decision Support Tools

Order Form Design

A simple example of a decision support tool is the laboratory order form. In most cases, whether on paper or a computer screen, the requisition form is the primary and obligatory interface between the clinician and the laboratory. Requisition design has been shown to have a significant impact on ordering practices. Simple changes, such as grouping or separating tests on paper forms or adding or deleting tests from the first-view of a test menu in a computerized order entry system, can change test ordering behaviors dramatically [72–75].

Unfortunately, in many current configurations of order entry systems, user interfaces are not designed to be flexible, and cannot be easily modified or rapidly updated by the laboratory. Most are not designed to interface directly with the laboratory information system (LIS), and their administration is often outside the purview of the laboratory. Going forward, innovative middleware solutions may be able to enhance the flow of information between the local laboratory, LIS, and provider order entry systems [47].

Diagnostic Algorithms

Diagnostic algorithms have been employed for decades in the clinical laboratory to control test utilization and to ensure that the most appropriate tests are selected in the correct sequence. Many algorithms also provide interpretive information to confirm or rule out a specific condition. The classic example is the thyroid reflex algorithm in which the physician requests a "thyroid screen" which enables the laboratory to perform a predetermined sequence of tests (i.e., thyroid-stimulating hormone, if low or high result, follow with thyroid hormone testing).

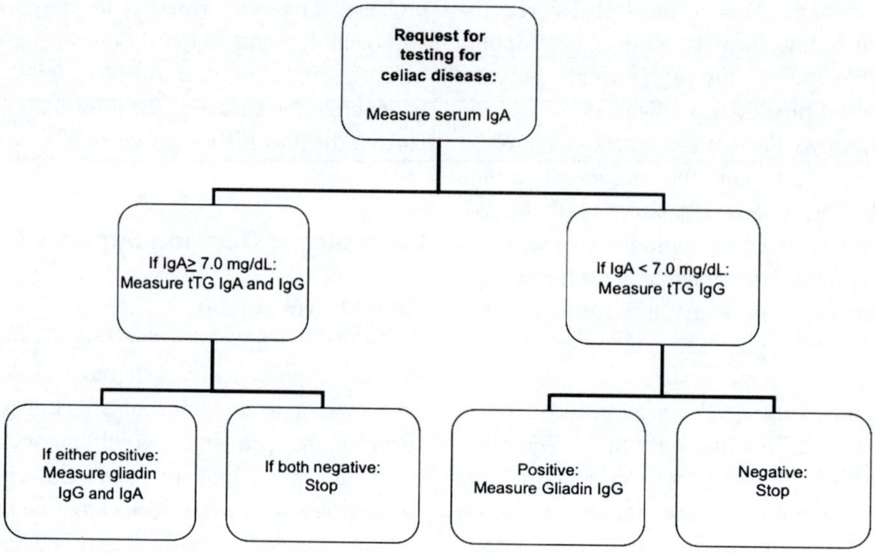

Fig. 18.3 Reflex screening algorithm for celiac disease at the Massachusetts General Hospital *tTG*, tissue transglutaminase

Table 18.2 List of tests for celiac disease that appear on the online laboratory handbook of the Massachusetts general hospital

Test name	Comment(s)
Antitissue transglutaminase IgA	The IgA tissue transglutaminase test is the single most efficient serologic screening test for the diagnosis of celiac disease. The use of antigliadin antibodies as a screening test is no longer recommended
Celiac disease panel	Includes Tissue Transglutaminase IgA and a total IgA level
Endomysial IgA antibody	Note: For initial screening of celiac disease please do not order Endomysial IgA but instead order Tissue Transglutaminase IgA. It is currently recommended in most screening algorithms for celiac disease
Gliadin IgG and IgA antibodies	Note: This test is performed at an external reference lab

Careful consideration should be given to the reflex and diagnostic thresholds chosen, so as to achieve the maximum number of diagnoses for the number of tests performed [76]. As a further example, Fig. 18.3 shows a reflex testing strategy for celiac disease screening that is soon to be in use at the Massachusetts General Hospital. This algorithm was developed because many physicians in our institution were confused about the correct tests to order to evaluate a patient for celiac disease. Available tests on our menu include antitissue transglutaminase IgA and IgG, a celiac disease panel, anti-endomysial IgA and gliadin IgG and IgA. If a physician types "celiac disease" in our online laboratory handbook, a list of tests with recommendations for the most appropriate screening test(s) is displayed, as shown in Table 18.2. If the physician selects the "celiac disease panel," this order will trigger automatic performance of the reflex test panel, shown in Fig. 18.3. Decision support in the case of celiac disease testing therefore occurs on two different levels, one when the physician types in the test request in the online handbook, and the other when they request an approved reflex testing algorithm. Collectively, these interventions assist the physician in test selection, help to eliminate unnecessary tests, and encourage use of the algorithm approved for use in our institution.

Published Practice Standards

Practice standards for the diagnosis and management of various conditions are available from many sources, including textbooks, online publications, and various media produced by medical professional organizations. These standards are intended to give physicians general approaches to specific clinical conditions, although the physician may need to adjust the overall approach to suit the needs of individual patients. For example, the American Diabetes Association (ADA) provides online up-to-date clinical practice recommendations available from the ADA website (http://www.diabetes.org). Taking this approach one step further, some institutions have developed locally approved practice guidelines based on expert review of the available evidence. In some cases, these guidelines are incorporated into the admission or order entry system of the hospital as disease- or condition-specific templates. These templates provide standard orders for pharmacy, nursing care, consultations, and laboratory testing. All that is required is that the ordering physician selects the template, and a standard set of orders is automatically performed efficiently, in a predetermined sequence. In our institution, we employ a large number of admission templates. For example, we have developed a "rule out acute myocardial infarction" template that specifies (among other things) the following set of cardiac marker tests:

1. CPK+CK-MB and Troponin T at 0 h from presentation
2. Troponin T at 8 h from presentation
3. Troponin T at 16 h from presentation
4. ECG at 0, 8 and 16 h from presentation

This testing strategy was developed to standardize test ordering for myocardial infarction and to reduce excess utilization of cardiac markers, including redundant orders, and unnecessary repeat testing for total creatine kinase (CK) and its isoenzyme CK-MB. The template is supplemented with online decision support treatment strategies (Fig. 18.4). Soon we plan to eliminate CK-MB entirely, again reflecting the need to keep decision support tools up-to-date.

Consultative Interpretive Services

Interpretations of laboratory tests, provided by a laboratory pathologist or other qualified expert, can be valuable tools in assisting clinicians. Without an accompanying interpretation, laboratory tests can often be misinterpreted. For example, we encountered a patient who had been misdiagnosed with protein S deficiency, which had led her to abort her pregnancy due to fears of recurrent venous thromboembolism. Neither she nor her physician realized that protein S typically decreases during normal pregnancy. In another case, the diagnosis of von Willebrand disease was missed in a newborn, because the clinicians did not know that von Willebrand factor is typically elevated above a patient's baseline at birth, which can mask the diagnosis. In addition, the newborn was ill from infection and internal bleeding at the time of testing, and acute illness also elevates von Willebrand factor above a patient's baseline. In a third case, an experienced hematologist thought that slightly elevated hemoglobin A2 in a patient with sickle cell trait indicated coexisting beta thalassemia. Fortunately, this third case example occurred at our institution, which provides interpretations by pathologists for hemoglobin electrophoresis and other complex laboratory tests. The interpretation for this patient stated that the results are consistent with sickle cell trait and concomitant alpha thalassemia trait, based on the relatively low percentage of hemoglobin S and the low MCV. Hemoglobin S can falsely elevate hemoglobin A2 due to co-elution, without beta thalassemia. Thus, a misdiagnosis was avoided.

Surveys of physicians receiving pathologist interpretations with their specialized coagulation test results showed that 98% find the interpretations "useful or informative." In addition, responses indicated that 72% of interpretations reduced the number of tests needed to make a diagnosis, 72% helped avoid a misdiagnosis, and 59% shortened the time to diagnosis [77].

Interpretations can also improve physicians' abilities to select the appropriate test(s) needed to reach a diagnosis. Laboratory test ordering

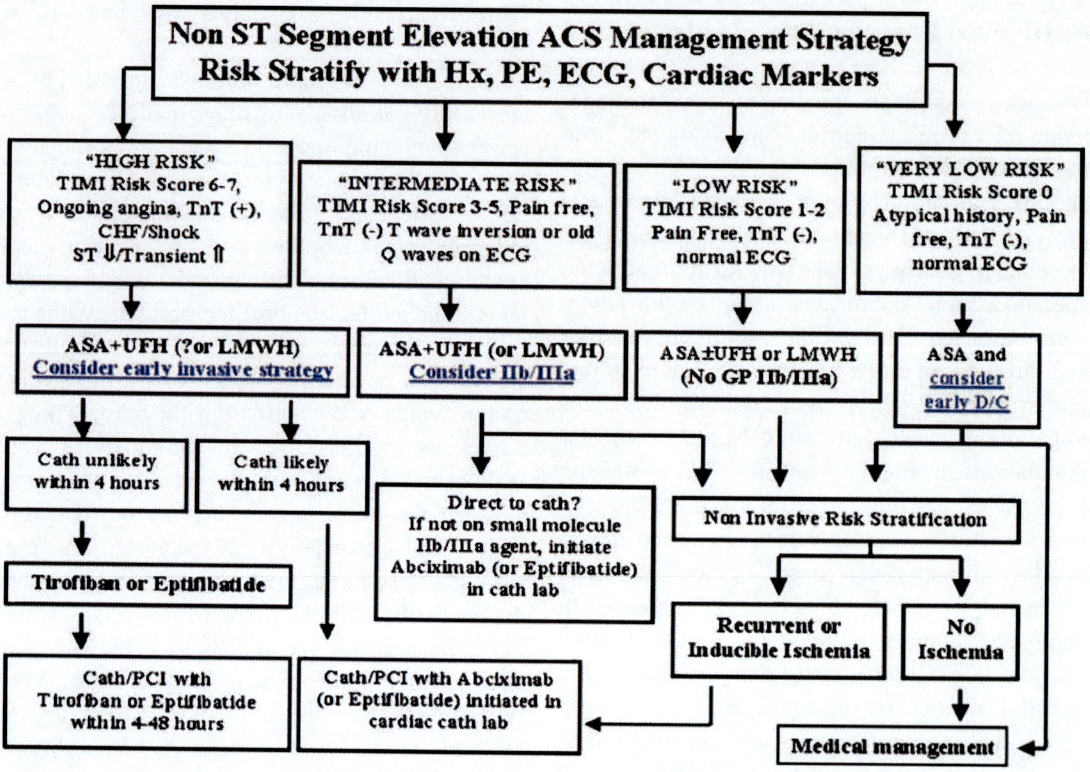

Fig. 18.4 Example of a decision support strategy for non-ST segment elevation acute coronary syndrome at the Massachusetts General Hospital. *Hx* history; *PE* physical examination; *ECG* electrocardiogram; *TIMI* thrombolysis in myocardial infarction; *CHF* congestive heart failure; *Tnt* troponin T; *ASA* aspirin; *UFH* unfractionated heparin; *LMWH* low molecular weight heparin; IIb/IIIa, glycoprotein IIb/IIIa inhibitor; *GP* blycoprotein; D/C, discharge; cath, catheterization; *PCI* percutaneous coronary intervention

patterns were studied immediately after we implemented a coagulation interpretation service for a group of outside hospitals, and the results were compared to ordering patterns after the interpretation service had been in place for 2.5 years. The number of coagulation test ordering errors decreased by nearly two errors per requisition during the study period [77]. Furthermore, initially, over 63% of requisitions had 4 errors, but at the end of the study period, this was reduced to only 10%. For example, clinicians had frequently ordered antigen assays (immunoassays) to assess for protein C, protein S or antithrombin III deficiency, but after receiving interpretations for 2.5 years, they more frequently ordered functional assays, which are the appropriate tests to order. The interpretations include mention that antigen assays are inadequate because they are not able to detect type II (qualitative) deficiencies, as they do not assess protein function. In contrast, functional assays are able to detect both type I (quantitative) and type II deficiencies. The results of this study provided evidence that interpretations can successfully modify physicians' ability to order tests appropriately.

Interpretations are most informative if all the relevant results for a specimen are interpreted together, while also taking into account the patient's medical history. That is to say, patient-specific interpretations are more valuable than generic interpretations. If a patient has low protein C, low protein S, and normal antithrombin III, it is most useful for the interpretation to indicate that the most likely explanation for this combination of findings is warfarin or vitamin K deficiency, rather than list all the possible causes of low protein C, and then separately list all the possible causes of low protein S. Incorporating the normal antithrombin III result into the interpretation allows the exclusion of some other possible causes of low protein C and low protein S, or at least renders them much less likely. The interpretation can also give suggestions for follow-up testing, if appropriate. In the current example, the interpretation would indicate that testing can be repeated any time when the patient has not had warfarin for at least 20 days, because it can take that long for protein S to recover to normal after warfarin discontinuation.

In another example, if a patient on warfarin tests positive for a lupus anticoagulant, the interpretation can notify clinicians that lupus anticoagulants are capable of artifactually prolonging the prothrombin time and international normalized ratio (PT-INR), potentially overestimating the patient's level of warfarin anticoagulation. The interpretation can note that a chromogenic factor X assay can be performed on this specimen if requested, to help determine whether or not the lupus anticoagulant is artifactually prolonging the PT-INR. In an additional example, for a patient with low antithrombin III and 3+ proteinuria on a urinalysis, the interpretation can note that proteinuria can cause an acquired loss of antithrombin III, but other possible causes of low antithrombin III can also be included for completeness. Table 18.3 shows some additional example interpretations.

Table 18.3 Examples of interpretations for the coagulation service at MGH

Scenario	Interpretation
Normal von Willebrand results in the presence of an acute phase reaction	The von Willebrand panel values are normal, however, fibrinogen is elevated at 590 mg/dl. Both fibrinogen and von Willebrand factor are acute phase reactants. Therefore, it is possible that von Willebrand factor is elevated above the patient's true baseline. Taken together, it is not possible to exclude von Willebrand disease with certainty at this time. If a second study has not been performed, a repeat study when the patient is not likely to be in an acute phase reaction (normal value for fibrinogen) may be informative
	The patient is blood type O. Normal blood type O adults have a mean von Willebrand factor level of approximately 75%
Mildly low antithrombin III result in a patient on heparin	Antithrombin III is slightly low. Heparin administration can cause slight decreases in antithrombin within several days, secondary to increased clearance. If hereditary antithrombin deficiency is strongly suspected, the assay may be repeated once the patient has been off heparin for at least 1–2 weeks
	The specimen submitted has prolonged PTT. When the sample was treated with an enzyme that degrades heparin, the PTT corrected into the normal range indicating the prolongation is due to the presence of heparin in the sample

An interpretive service is even more efficient when combined with strategic testing algorithms that simplify the diagnostic process for clinicians. Test requisitions or order entry systems can be simplified to offer the appropriate algorithms. For example, for a patient undergoing evaluation because of a bleeding history, the clinician can order a "prolonged PT and PTT evaluation," and the laboratory will follow an algorithm (Fig. 18.5) to reach the diagnosis on one specimen, without performing any unnecessary tests. The alternative is cumbersome and inefficient, as well as inconvenient for the patient: the clinician waits for the PT or PTT results to come back abnormal, collects another specimen, and tries to remember which coagulation factors to order for which prolongation, and subsequently would need to collect yet another specimen if it turns out that lupus anticoagulant or inhibitor tests are indicated. The clinicians can also order all of these tests up front, but this wastes healthcare resources if the tests turn out to be unnecessary.

Test requisitions or order entry systems can be designed to encourage appropriate test ordering of complex tests by offering these as test algorithms or panels, rather than simply listing all test names individually. For example, most clinicians do not realize that "ristocetin cofactor" is the name of the test for von Willebrand factor activity, so they order "von Willebrand factor antigen"

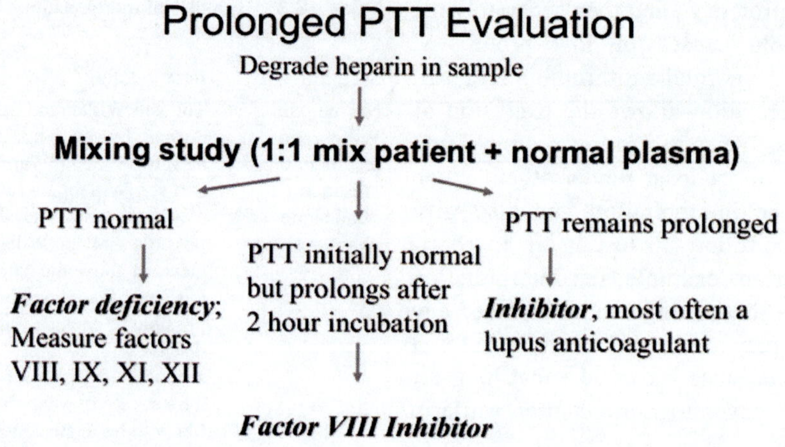

Fig. 18.5 Simplified algorithm for a prolonged PTT evaluation at the Massachusetts General Hospital. An unexplained prolonged PTT with a normal PT is likely to be clinically significant, and an evaluation to determine the etiology of the prolongation is warranted. Even if the evaluation leads to the diagnosis of factor XII deficiency, which does not cause bleeding, the knowledge will spare the patient unnecessary transfusions of fresh frozen plasma. The algorithm shown is highly simplified and the nuances followed by the laboratory are more complex than what is shown. The first step determines whether or not the prolongation is due to heparin, low molecular weight heparin, or fondaparinux anticoagulation. If any of these anticoagulants explains the prolongation, no further testing is performed. If none of these anticoagulants are detected, a mixing study is performed, where the patient's plasma is mixed 1:1 with normal plasma, and the PTT is performed on the mixture both at time 0 and after a 2-hour incubation. Depending on the results, factor assays, lupus anticoagulant tests, and/or Bethesda assays (for a factor inhibitor) may be subsequently performed, until the etiology of the prolongation is determined. *PTT*, partial thromboplastin time; *PT*, prothrombin time

when they see it listed on the requisition or order entry system. By ordering the antigen test without the activity test, type 2 von Willebrand disease could be misdiagnosed as normal. In contrast, if a von Willebrand panel is offered on the requisition or order entry system, the appropriate laboratory tests can be ordered. If panels or algorithms are offered, the requisition or order entry system should explain what tests are or may be included (for example, on the back of the requisition). For hospital laboratories, it is recommended to initially obtain approval from the hospital's medical policy committee for the algorithm (reflex test) protocols that the laboratory would like to use. Clinicians still should have the ability to order a test individually.

Computer-Based Decision Support

Computer-based decision support has been rapidly evolving over the past 10 years. This support can take various forms, such as publicly available online search-capable websites, customized computer programs to aid in specific medical decisions (e.g., pulmonary function tests, electrocardiograms, acid–base disorders) and institution-specific decision support tools provided on the intranet. A number of websites open to physicians and the general public are available to assist in test selection and to provide interpretive information on laboratory testing.

A typical example is "WebMD symptom checker" (http://symptoms.webmd.com). This website allows the user to search by disease, symptom, laboratory test, or other parameters. The site provides general information about laboratory test selection and interpretation within the overall context of the disease or symptom-based search. Other similar web-based tools are available, with the majority of these being not limited to test selection alone.

Another example is "Lab Tests Online" (http://www.labtestsonline.org). On this site, the user can search by test, condition, disease, or screening to access peer-reviewed information on a number of medical topics. Most of these online sites essentially take the place of standard texts in print, where the reader must search the table of contents or index. Online sources are easier to use, are mobile, can be accessed from any computer, and can be updated on a continual basis. To counter this online threat, publishers of established medical textbooks often offer online access and search functions with purchase of the textbook. For example, Cecil Medicine 23rd edition offers an online Expert Consultant with purchase of the book.

Online (or Text) Interpretive Guidelines

Many laboratories provide physicians with online or printed test interpretation guidelines. For example, Mayo Medical Laboratories publishes an annual interpretive handbook. The 2009–2010 edition contains over 800 pages describing the use, interpretation and appropriate cautionary comments for a number of tests on the menu. As one example, under the listing for plasma free metanephrines, the utility of the test is explained, stating that this test is the most sensitive (nearly 100%) test to screen for elevated catecholamines, recommending fractionated 24-h urinary catecholamines as a confirmatory test, and cautioning about specific drugs that may elevate catecholamine levels, producing borderline elevated plasma metanephrine levels. Printed references are very useful, but are not as readily available as online formats. Importantly, many generic online references provide similar information, but the interpretative data is not specific to any laboratory. These generic online sources may yield erroneous recommendations when tests have substantial differences in performance from one laboratory to another. This is particularly true for genetic testing, where different laboratories may test for a varying number of mutations for a given genetic disorder.

Computerized Alerts and Reminders

The amount of individual patient information that the typical physician must be aware of is constantly expanding. Most organizations are attempting to assist the physician in organizing and storing this information in the form of EHR. The EHR is slowly replacing paper-based medical records in hospital and outpatient settings. Beyond simply storing and displaying clinical information in an organized user friendly format, the EHR also permits various alerts and reminders to be incorporated into the physician's regular workflow. This may include reminders to perform screening tests on selected patients, abnormal and critical value alerts and other features, such as disease management protocols to ensure that important tests have been ordered and abnormal results acted upon appropriately.

For example, patients receiving long-term anticoagulation therapy with Coumadin must be monitored at regular intervals using a PT-INR test to ensure adequate anticoagulation therapy. If the patient's PT-INR becomes subtherapeutic, the patient may develop a fatal clot or embolism. Excessive anticoagulation may result in bleeding or hemorrhage. Usually the physician schedules office visits for these patients at various intervals and provides a prescription for outpatient PT-INR testing at more frequent intervals. Once the patient has left the office, the physician has no way to be certain that the patient actually went to the laboratory for the regular PT-INR testing, unless the office staff periodically reviews the patient's records to check for the results of recent testing. Noncompliance on the part of the patient can have potentially catastrophic consequences. On the other hand, if the test orders for PT-INR have been recorded in an order entry system, it is possible to implement an alert system such that the physician is made aware if the patient did not show up for testing within an appropriate time interval. Furthermore, the system could alert the physician of nontherapeutic PT-INR values, thus permitting more timely adjustments to therapy.

Another example is the use of electronic disease management protocols to ensure that important tests and procedures have been performed according to accepted standards of care. For example, patients with diabetes mellitus require regular monitoring of hemoglobin A1c, urinary microalbumnin, lipids, and other parameters. Given the large number of diabetic patients in a typical primary care practice, it is relatively easy for important screening and monitoring tests to be overlooked. Some insurance plans have mandated that testing be performed regularly as part of pay-for-performance incentives. The simplest approach to ensuring that appropriate testing is performed is to use an electronic diabetic patient monitoring template, with automatic reminders when patients have not received recommended testing. A meta-analysis of the effectiveness of computerized decision support systems has found that automatic prompts are associated with improved provider adherence, when compared to systems that required users to activate the system [78].

Decision Analysis and Forecasting Models in the Laboratory

While decision support analysis can be valuable to assist physicians caring for individual patients, these tools can also be applied to populations of patients and to aid in forecasting trends in the clinical laboratory. The capability to aggregate laboratory data across populations of patients presents opportunities to systematically improve medical care on a population-based level. Implementation of electronic medical records facilitates this process by incorporating laboratory data into electronic formats that can be analyzed to detect correlations and trends. The analysis can be performed by the LIS, specialized middleware, or by computer programs that can access the electronic medical record. Examples of specific applications include surveillance for infection control, safety and adverse event analysis, operations and workflow analysis, quality improvement, and forecasting trends in clinical laboratory services.

Surveillance

Figure 18.6 shows quarterly rates of MRSA infection in our hospital tracked over time. As a historical baseline, we had 1.21 infections per 1,000 patients in 2005. The rate has steadily declined, reaching 0.45 infections per 1,000 patients in the most recent quarter. This data is derived by integrating data supplied by the microbiology LIS with clinical electronic medical records. The data could also be analyzed by location, underlying disease or other factors, permitting infection control officers to target specific high-risk areas for further reductions in these infections.

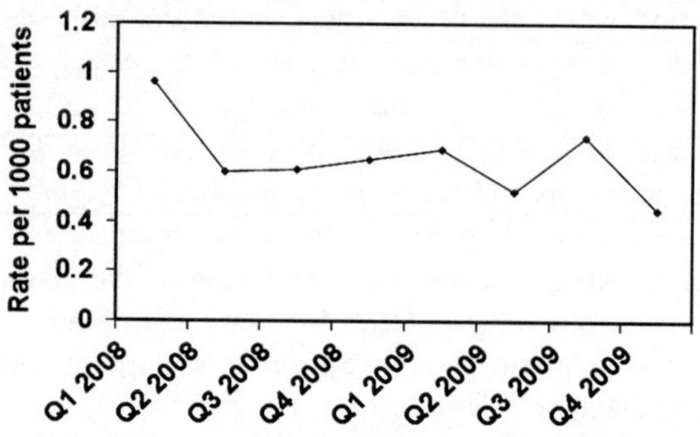

Fig. 18.6 Quarterly rate of methicillin-resistant Staphylococcus aureus (MRSA) infection per 1,000 patients over time. *Q* quarter

Another example of using laboratory data for surveillance in our hospital involves the use of antimicrobial sensitivity data. The microbiology laboratory has implemented a special program that collates sensitivity data for various organisms that is analyzed annually to produce an antibiotic sensitivity profile. This information assists our infectious disease department to produce a list of recommended antibiotics for various infections based on our local antimicrobial sensitivity patterns.

Safety and Adverse Event Analysis

Our hospital utilizes a real time electronic safety reporting system. This system replaced our older paper-based "incident reporting system," that was inefficient and often reported events too long after the incident to permit successful investigation and corrective action. Any employee can file an electronic safety report. The reports are reviewed by the hospital Office of Quality and Safety, and, depending on the location and severity, by the departmental Quality Chair and Quality Manager. Potential outcomes include investigation and/or follow-up of the event, recommendations, implementation of corrective actions, and aggregation of the event data into the quality and safety database. We receive quarterly aggregated reports listing the number of event types (e.g., blood/blood products, diagnosis/treatment, specimen issues), severity levels (e.g., near miss, no harm, temporary minor harm, permanent harm), and aggregated details about events (e.g., number of delayed tests, wrong patient, wrong test, mislabeled specimens, ABO complications). The aggregated data allows us to target quality improvement activities around the most common or high-risk events, and to track the success of our interventions over time.

Forecasting Trends in Clinical Laboratory Services

The clinical laboratory is a service-oriented department that must anticipate and respond to the needs of clinical services. Most laboratory trends occur fairly slowly, and can be monitored by projecting testing requirements and volumes using historical data. However, in some cases hospitals undergo abrupt changes in clinical services that cannot be understood by historical trend data alone. For example, a hospital may open a new oncology or transplant center, merge and consolidate with other area hospitals or start a regional outreach program. These types of events may substantially change the test menu, test volumes, and influence the types of services that must be provided. In some cases, decision support tools can be applied to these types of challenges. For example, predictions of outreach test volumes can be obtained from the expected number of physicians and types of clinical practices, using decision support tools that contain databases of physician test ordering behavior.

Operations and Workflow Analysis

Some consulting companies and vendors of laboratory instrumentation have developed proprietary computer-based systems to aid in operations and workflow analysis. Most of these are based on process flow and lean principles, and are linked to benchmarking databases that allow the laboratory to compare themselves to similar operations. These services are available for a fee or are included as part of a large instrument purchase. There are also inexpensive off-the-shelf decision support programs to aid the laboratory in performing their own operations and workflow analysis. These systems include the basic tools that are required to map operational processes and perform basic analyses based on lean principles.

Decision Support Incorporated into ARRA Legislation and Other Considerations

Beginning in 2011, Medicare physicians who implement and report "meaningful use" of EHR will be eligible for substantial financial incentives approved in the recent ARRA (American Recovery and Reinvestment Act) legislation. The Centers for Medicare & Medicaid Services (CMS) has recently proposed that the "meaningful use" criteria should include the use of "five clinical decision support rules relevant to [each] specialty" [79]. In response, the Meaningful Use Workgroup of the HITPC (Health IT Policy Committee) has recommended that the wording be amended to explicitly require that one of these five clinical decision support rules address efficient diagnostic test ordering [80]. Thus, decision support tools for laboratory test ordering are likely to become a major issue for providers and hospitals going forward.

At the same time, liability issues regarding the dissemination and future use of such tools remain murky [81]. Programs using a "closed-loop" system to make decisions directly controlling a patient's treatment are viewed as medical devices under control of the FDA, but physicians may be held liable when they are making the final assessment for care.

Finally, demonstrations of clinical decision support systems have primarily focused on their effects on practitioner performance [78], and not patient outcomes. Those that have included patient outcomes in evaluations of decision support tools have found inconsistent results; many were hampered by inadequate numbers of patients, and failed to have the statistical power to demonstrate improvements [78]. Particularly when it comes to patient outcomes related to preventative care, studies may have to rely on multicenter cluster-randomized controlled trials [82]. However, given the substantial time and resources required for such collaborations, it is unclear how many such trials will be feasible. Furthermore, it is difficult to imagine having multiple repeated evaluations of a decision support system every time new knowledge is added to the system. The long track record and near ubiquitous use of computers for supporting safety, efficiency, and quality in other nonhealthcare related commercial, industrial, and scientific enterprises suggests that using reasonable proof of effectiveness, rather than imposing onerous requirements, may be the way to move forward.

Conclusion

The number and complexity of available laboratory tests continues to increase at a rapid pace. Staying current with accepted standards for laboratory testing for diagnosis, monitoring and prognosis is extremely challenging, particularly for nonspecialists who see a diverse patient population. Decision support tools to aid physicians in appropriate test selection and interpretation are widely available and will become increasingly important. The most effective and practical decision support tools are developed or selected locally at the institutional level and embedded in the regular workflow of the physician. Many of these tools can be incorporated into the electronic medical record system where they can be easily accessed by any physician while caring for their patients. Careful attention to the "Ten Commandments for effective clinical decision support," described by Bates et al., [68] will enhance the chances for success in the design and implementation of new decision support tools.

References

1. Cochrane AL. Effectiveness and efficiency; random reflections on health services. London]: Nuffield Provincial Hospitals Trust; 1972.
2. Sackett DL, Rosenberg WM, Gray JA, Haynes RB, Richardson WS. Evidence based medicine: what it is and what it isn't. BMJ. 1996;312(7023):71–2.
3. Rosenberg W, Donald A. Evidence based medicine: an approach to clinical problem-solving. BMJ. 1995;310(6987):1122–6.
4. Kohn LT, Corrigan J, Donaldson MS, Institute of Medicine (U.S.). Committee on Quality of Health Care in America.: To err is human: building a safer health system. Washington, D.C: National Academy Press; 2000.
5. Brennan TA, Leape LL, Laird NM, Hebert L, Localio AR, Lawthers AG, et al. Incidence of adverse events and negligence in hospitalized patients. Results of the Harvard Medical Practice Study I. N Engl J Med. 1991;324(6):370–6.
6. Leape LL, Brennan TA, Laird N, Lawthers AG, Localio AR, Barnes BA, et al. The nature of adverse events in hospitalized patients. Results of the Harvard Medical Practice Study II. N Engl J Med. 1991;324(6):377–84.
7. Blumenthal D. Stimulating the adoption of health information technology. N Engl J Med. 2009;360(15): 1477–9.
8. Wilson JF. Making electronic health records meaningful. Ann Intern Med. 2009;151(4):293–6.
9. Timmermans S, Mauck A. The promises and pitfalls of evidence-based medicine. Health Aff (Millwood). 2005;24(1):18–28.
10. Fisher ES, Wennberg DE, Stukel TA, Gottlieb DJ, Lucas FL, Pinder EL. The implications of regional variations in Medicare spending. Part 1: the content, quality, and accessibility of care. Ann Intern Med. 2003;138(4):273–87.
11. Fisher ES, Wennberg DE, Stukel TA, Gottlieb DJ, Lucas FL, Pinder EL. The implications of regional variations in Medicare spending. Part 2: health outcomes and satisfaction with care. Ann Intern Med. 2003;138(4):288–98.
12. Hartman M, Martin A, Nuccio O, Catlin A. Health spending growth at a historic low in 2008. Health Aff (Millwood). 2010;29(1):147–55.
13. Benson ES. Initiatives toward effective decision making and laboratory use. Hum Pathol. 1980;11(5):440–8.
14. Robinson A. Rationale for cost-effective laboratory medicine. Clin Microbiol Rev. 1994;7(2):185–99.
15. van Bokhoven MA, Pleunis-van Empel MC, Koch H, Grol RP, Dinant GJ, van der Weijden T. Why do patients want to have their blood tested? A qualitative study of patient expectations in general practice. BMC Fam Pract. 2006;7:75.
16. Kessler DP, Summerton N, Graham JR. Effects of the medical liability system in Australia, the UK, and the USA. Lancet. 2006;368(9531):240–6.
17. Oboler SK, Prochazka AV, Gonzales R, Xu S, Anderson RJ. Public expectations and attitudes for annual physical examinations and testing. Ann Intern Med. 2002;136(9):652–9.
18. Koch H, van Bokhoven MA, ter Riet G, van Alphen-Jager JT, van der Weijden T, Dinant GJ, et al. Ordering blood tests for patients with unexplained fatigue in

general practice: what does it yield? Results of the VAMPIRE trial. Br J Gen Pract. 2009;59(561): e93–100.
19. Fernandes CM, Worster A, Hill S, McCallum C, Eva K. Root cause analysis of laboratory turnaround times for patients in the emergency department. CJEM. 2004;6(2):116–22.
20. Francis AJ, Ray MJ, Marshall MC. Pathology processes and emergency department length of stay: the impact of change. Med J Aust. 2009;190(12):665–9.
21. Jha AK, Chan DC, Ridgway AB, Franz C, Bates DW. Improving safety and eliminating redundant tests: cutting costs in U.S. hospitals. Health Aff (Millwood). 2009;28(5):1475–84.
22. OIG Compliance Program Guidance for Clinical Laboratories. Fed Regist. 1998;63(163):45076–87.
23. Plebani M. Exploring the iceberg of errors in laboratory medicine. Clin Chim Acta. 2009;404(1):16–23.
24. Howanitz PJ. Errors in laboratory medicine: practical lessons to improve patient safety. Arch Pathol Lab Med. 2005;129(10):1252–61.
25. Plebani M. Errors in clinical laboratories or errors in laboratory medicine? Clin Chem Lab Med. 2006;44(6): 750–9.
26. Plebani M, Carraro P. Mistakes in a stat laboratory: types and frequency. Clin Chem. 1997;43(8 Pt 1):1348–51.
27. Carraro P, Plebani M. Errors in a stat laboratory: types and frequencies 10 years later. Clin Chem. 2007;53(7): 1338–42.
28. Becich MJ. Information management: moving from test results to clinical information. Clin Leadersh Manag Rev. 2000;14(6):296–300.
29. Forsman RW. Why is the laboratory an afterthought for managed care organizations? Clin Chem. 1996;42(5):813–6.
30. Forsman R. The electronic medical record: implications for the laboratory. Clin Leadersh Manag Rev. 2000;14(6):292–5.
31. Holohan TV, Colestro J, Grippi J, Converse J, Hughes M. Analysis of diagnostic error in paid malpractice claims with substandard care in a large healthcare system. South Med J. 2005;98(11):1083–7.
32. Gandhi TK, Kachalia A, Thomas EJ, Puopolo AL, Yoon C, Brennan TA, et al. Missed and delayed diagnoses in the ambulatory setting: a study of closed malpractice claims. Ann Intern Med. 2006;145(7):488–96.
33. Kachalia A, Gandhi TK, Puopolo AL, Yoon C, Thomas EJ, Griffey R, et al. Missed and delayed diagnoses in the emergency department: a study of closed malpractice claims from 4 liability insurers. Ann Emerg Med. 2007;49(2):196–205.
34. Covell DG, Uman GC, Manning PR. Information needs in office practice: are they being met? Ann Intern Med. 1985;103(4):596–9.
35. Ely JW, Osheroff JA, Gorman PN, Ebell MH, Chambliss ML, Pifer EA, et al. A taxonomy of generic clinical questions: classification study. BMJ. 2000; 321(7258):429–32.
36. Hayward R. Clinical decision support tools: do they support clinicians? Fut Pract. 2004:66–68. Available at: http://www.cche.net/about/files/clinical_decision_support_tools.pdf.
37. Hughes B, Joshi I, Lemonde H, Wareham J. Junior physician's use of Web 2.0 for information seeking and medical education: a qualitative study. Int J Med Inform. 2009;78(10):645–55.
38. Davies K. The information-seeking behaviour of doctors: a review of the evidence. Health Info Libr J. 2007;24(2):78–94.
39. Pene F, Courtine E, Cariou A, Mira JP. Toward theragnostics. Crit Care Med. 2009;37(1 Suppl):S50–8.
40. Jones J, Taylor B, Wilkin TJ, Hammer SM. Advances in antiretroviral therapy. Top HIV Med. 2007;15(2):48–82.
41. Mueller MC, Bogner JR. Treatment with CCR5 antagonists: which patient may have a benefit? Eur J Med Res. 2007;12(9):441–52.
42. Ladanyi M, Pao W. Lung adenocarcinoma: guiding EGFR-targeted therapy and beyond. Mod Pathol. 2008;21 Suppl 2:S16–22.
43. Lievre A, Bachet JB, Le Corre D, Boige V, Landi B, Emile JF, et al. KRAS mutation status is predictive of response to cetuximab therapy in colorectal cancer. Cancer Res. 2006;66(8):3992–5.
44. Slamon DJ, Leyland-Jones B, Shak S, Fuchs H, Paton V, Bajamonde A, et al. Use of chemotherapy plus a monoclonal antibody against HER2 for metastatic breast cancer that overexpresses HER2. N Engl J Med. 2001;344(11):783–92.
45. Reifenberger G, Louis DN. Oligodendroglioma: toward molecular definitions in diagnostic neuro-oncology. J Neuropathol Exp Neurol. 2003;62(2):111–26.
46. Buckland MK. Library services in theory and context. 2nd ed. Oxford, New York: Pergamon Press; 1988.
47. Grisson R, Kim JY, Brodsky V, Kamis IK, Singh B, Belkziz SM, et al. A novel class of laboratory middleware. Promoting information flow and improving computerized provider order entry. Am J Clin Pathol. 2010;133(6):860–9.
48. Lewandrowski K. Managing utilization of new diagnostic tests. Clin Leadersh Manag Rev. 2003;17(6):318–24.
49. Mark DB. Decision-making in clinical medicine. In: Fauci AS, Braunwald E, Kasper DL, Hauser SL, Longo DL, Jameson JL, Loscalzo J, editors. Harrison's principles of internal medicine. 17tth ed. New York: McGraw-Hill; 2008. p. 16–23.
50. Cronje RJ, Freeman JR, Williamson OD, Gutsch CJ. Evidence-based medicine: recognizing and managing clinical uncertainty. Lab Med. 2004;35:723–9.
51. Lumbreras B, Parker LA, Porta M, Pollan M, Ioannidis JP, Hernandez-Aguado I. Overinterpretation of clinical applicability in molecular diagnostic research. Clin Chem. 2009;55(4):786–94.
52. Galen RS, Gambino SR. Beyond normality: the predictive value and efficiency of medical diagnoses. New York: Wiley; 1975.
53. Januzzi Jr JL, Bamberg F, Lee H, Truong QA, Nichols JH, Karakas M, et al. High-sensitivity troponin T concentrations in acute chest pain patients evaluated with cardiac computed tomography. Circulation. 2010;121(10):1227–34.

54. Diamond GA, Kaul S. How would the Reverend Bayes interpret high-sensitivity troponin? Circulation. 2010;121(10):1172–5.
55. Zweig MH, Campbell G. Receiver-operating characteristic (ROC) plots: a fundamental evaluation tool in clinical medicine. Clin Chem. 1993;39(4):561–77.
56. Dighe AS, Rao A, Coakley AB, Lewandrowski KB. Analysis of laboratory critical value reporting at a large academic medical center. Am J Clin Pathol. 2006;125(5):758–64.
57. Cook NR. Statistical evaluation of prognostic versus diagnostic models: beyond the ROC curve. Clin Chem. 2008;54(1):17–23.
58. Hosmer DW, Hosmer T, Le Cessie S, Lemeshow S. A comparison of goodness-of-fit tests for the logistic regression model. Stat Med. 1997;16(9):965–80.
59. Pencina MJ, D'Agostino Sr RB, D'Agostino Jr RB, Vasan RS. Evaluating the added predictive ability of a new marker: from area under the ROC curve to reclassification and beyond. Stat Med. 2008;27(2):157–72. discussion 207–212.
60. de Araujo Goncalves P, Ferreira J, Aguiar C, Seabra-Gomes R. TIMI, PURSUIT, and GRACE risk scores: sustained prognostic value and interaction with revascularization in NSTE-ACS. Eur Heart J. 2005;26(9): 865–72.
61. Gill D, Seidler T, Troughton RW, Yandle TG, Frampton CM, Richards M, et al. Vigorous response in plasma N-terminal pro-brain natriuretic peptide (NT-BNP) to acute myocardial infarction. Clin Sci (Lond). 2004;106(2):135–9.
62. Omland T, Aakvaag A, Bonarjee VV, Caidahl K, Lie RT, Nilsen DW, et al. Plasma brain natriuretic peptide as an indicator of left ventricular systolic function and long-term survival after acute myocardial infarction. Comparison with plasma atrial natriuretic peptide and N-terminal proatrial natriuretic peptide. Circulation. 1996;93(11):1963–69.
63. Arakawa N, Nakamura M, Aoki H, Hiramori K. Plasma brain natriuretic peptide concentrations predict survival after acute myocardial infarction. J Am Coll Cardiol. 1996;27(7):1656–61.
64. de Lemos JA, Morrow DA, Bentley JH, Omland T, Sabatine MS, McCabe CH, et al. The prognostic value of B-type natriuretic peptide in patients with acute coronary syndromes. N Engl J Med. 2001;345(14):1014–21.
65. Khan SQ, Narayan H, Ng KH, Dhillon OS, Kelly D, Quinn P, et al. N-terminal pro-B-type natriuretic peptide complements the GRACE risk score in predicting early and late mortality following acute coronary syndrome. Clin Sci (Lond). 2009;117(1):31–9.
66. Rosjo H, Omland T. New statistical methods for the evaluation of cardiovascular risk markers: what the clinician should know. Clin Sci (Lond). 2009;117(1):13–5.
67. Shortliffe EH. Computer programs to support clinical decision making. JAMA. 1987;258(1):61–6.
68. Bates DW, Kuperman GJ, Wang S, Gandhi T, Kittler A, Volk L, et al. Ten commandments for effective clinical decision support: making the practice of evidence-based medicine a reality. J Am Med Inform Assoc. 2003;10(6):523–30.
69. Gottlieb S. Health information on the internet is often unreliable. BMJ. 2000;321(7254):136.
70. Eysenbach G, Powell J, Kuss O, Sa ER. Empirical studies assessing the quality of health information for consumers on the world wide web: a systematic review. JAMA. 2002;287(20):2691–700.
71. Adams SA. Revisiting the online health information reliability debate in the wake of "web 2.0": An inter-disciplinary literature and website review. Int J Med Inform. 2010;79:391–400.
72. Emerson JF, Emerson SS. The impact of requisition design on laboratory utilization. Am J Clin Pathol. 2001;116(6):879–84.
73. Kahan NR, Waitman DA, Vardy DA. Curtailing laboratory test ordering in a managed care setting through redesign of a computerized order form. Am J Manag Care. 2009;15(3):173–6.
74. Shalev V, Chodick G, Heymann AD. Format change of a laboratory test order form affects physician behavior. Int J Med Inform. 2009;78(10):639–44.
75. Westbrook JI, Georgiou A, Dimos A, Germanos T. Computerised pathology test order entry reduces laboratory turnaround times and influences tests ordered by hospital clinicians: a controlled before and after study. J Clin Pathol. 2006;59(5):533–6.
76. Srivastava R, Bartlett WA, Kennedy IM, Hiney A, Fletcher C, Murphy MJ. Reflex and reflective testing: efficiency and effectiveness of adding on laboratory tests. Ann Clin Biochem. 2010;47:223–7.
77. Laposata ME, Laposata M, Van Cott EM, Buchner DS, Kashalo MS, Dighe AS. Physician survey of a laboratory medicine interpretive service and evaluation of the influence of interpretations on laboratory test ordering. Arch Pathol Lab Med. 2004;128(12):1424–7.
78. Garg AX, Adhikari NK, McDonald H, Rosas-Arellano MP, Devereaux PJ, Beyene J, et al. Effects of computerized clinical decision support systems on practitioner performance and patient outcomes: a systematic review. JAMA. 2005;293(10):1223–38.
79. CMS defines 'meaningful use'. Proposed rule outlines requirements for EHR incentive payments. MGMA Connex. 2010;10(3):10–3.
80. Letter to David Blumenthal, MD, MPP, National Coordinator for Health Information Technology [http://healthit.hhs.gov/portal/server.pt/gateway/PTARGS_0_11113_911075_0_0_18/MU%20NPRM%20Recommendations%20Final%20PT_clean.pdf].
81. Miller RA, Schaffner KF, Meisel A. Ethical and legal issues related to the use of computer programs in clinical medicine. Ann Intern Med. 1985;102(4):529–37.
82. Chuang JH, Hripcsak G, Heitjan DF. Design and analysis of controlled trials in naturally clustered environments: implications for medical informatics. J Am Med Inform Assoc. 2002;9(3):230–8.

Implementation and Benefits of Computerized Physician Order Entry and Evidence-Based Clinical Decision Support Systems

19

Stacy E.F. Melanson, Aileen P. Morrison, David W. Bates, and Milenko J. Tanasijevic

Keywords
Evidence-based clinical decision support systems • Computerized physician order entry • Evidence-based medicine • Clinical decision support systems

In the field of clinical pathology and laboratory medicine, test complexity and test menus continue to expand, necessitating that clinicians obtain domain expertise to make the appropriate testing decisions for patients. The efficiency focus is increasingly central because healthcare costs continue to rise and diagnostic testing represents a significant portion of the incremental cost increase [1]. Institutions can no longer afford to diagnose and manage patients without considering the overall cost-benefit impact of laboratory tests. Computerized physician order entry (CPOE) and clinical decision support systems (CDSSs) are one modality through which evidence-based medicine and practice guidelines can be deployed to assist clinicians at the time orders are being placed with the goals of improving the quality of care, decreasing errors, and reducing costs. After a brief introduction to CDSSs, this chapter uses specific examples to illustrate how evidence-based clinical pathology can be used to implement CDSSs and monitor their success through cost-benefit evaluation.

Introduction to Clinical Decision Support Systems

CPOE, which allows physicians to enter orders electronically rather than using paper requisitions, provides the backbone for CDSSs. While the implementation of CPOE requires significant analysis, planning, and resources, the benefits are numerous, including standardization of practice, improved communication, automatic recording of auditing data, and prevention of medication misuse [2].

CDSSs within CPOE are powerful tools with which to influence test ordering behavior. Evidence shows that a substantial portion of diagnostic testing may be unnecessary, that clinicians may be ordering testing inappropriately and that

M.J. Tanasijevic (✉)
Department of Pathology,
Brigham and Women's Hospital,
Harvard Medical School, Boston, MA, USA
e-mail: mtanasijevic@partners.org

A.M. Marchevsky and M.R. Wick (eds.), *Evidence Based Pathology and Laboratory Medicine*,
DOI 10.1007/978-1-4419-1030-1_19,

the cost associated with diagnostic testing is high; making these areas obvious targets for CDSSs. Common strategies include implementing rules-based order entry with reminders, offering testing guidelines and displaying test-specific (e.g., test charges) or patient-specific (e.g., past results, patient medications) information, and using order sentences to promote use of desired tests. In contrast to retrospective reminders and educational sessions, these strategies have generally produced successful results.

Most CDSSs use electronic reminders at the time of ordering, but, importantly, do not dictate how clinical care should be delivered. CDSSs should be designed such that clinicians view these systems as helpful tools instead of nuisances. Moreover, appropriate interventions and guidelines must reach all users of the laboratory, be introduced at the very level of individual decision-making, and be nonintrusive [1].

Basics of CDSS Implementation

The implementation of CDSSs should involve a multidisciplinary team of clinicians, pathologists, hospital administration, and information technology. Pathologists are integral to the process because they understand the technical and clinical aspects of laboratory testing, have multispecialty medical knowledge, are data-oriented, commonly work on multidisciplinary teams, and understand the underlying cost-benefit implications.

Each institution must choose its own strategy and appropriate test(s) to target based on discussion with the multidisciplinary team and audit of current practices. As an example, chart reviews can be performed to assess the degree of inappropriate utilization of laboratory tests based on established or internally derived clinical criteria. Once a target test or group of tests is chosen, a careful design of the intervention is critical for success. It is particularly important that the intervention makes it quick and easy for clinicians to make the correct decision. The effectiveness of a particular intervention should be assessed through a randomized study, including an experimental group that is exposed to the intervention and a control group that is exposed to the current state, which is facilitated by use of the computer system. A reasonable amount of time should also be allowed to measure outcomes in both groups consistent with the learning curve and volume of testing.

Although initial development of the CDSS is important, a committee structure responsible for maintaining and updating the CDSS based on external and internal evidence, literature review, and frequent audits is critical for success, and depending on the size of the institution more than one may be needed. For example, one may handle medication-related issues and another may tackle laboratory issues.

Our group has developed a number of such interventions and randomized studies. Their design and outcomes are described in the following sections to illustrate the general principles described above.

Optimization of Laboratory Test Utilization

Reports have shown that as many as 10% of commonly ordered tests are redundant [3] and at least 30% of arterial blood gases may be unnecessary [4]. Possible explanations for the excessive test ordering include clinicians' difficulty in determining when the most recent test was performed or lacking the knowledge regarding the appropriate testing interval. Redundant testing is not only costly but can also lead to unnecessary interventions or treatments if false-positive results are produced. However, managing test utilization has been difficult and interventions such as feedback, education, rationing, and financial incentives, have shown limited and/or transient reductions in utilization [5–9].

CDSS within CPOE can reduce redundant testing by providing utilization reminders at the time of clinical decision making. Furthermore, CDSSs link the ordering clinicians with the particular order, simplifying utilization audits. These electronic systems also allow outdated tests to be removed from the system.

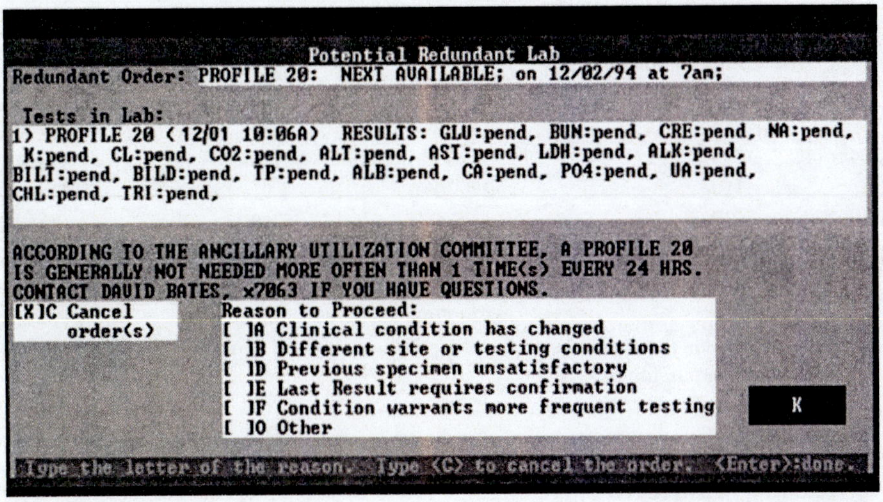

Fig. 19.1 An order for a test can be overridden by providing justification (from Bates et al. [10], with permission of Elsevier)

The published literature shows that well-designed electronic reminders can decrease the number of redundant laboratory tests and decrease the overall number of inappropriate tests performed, thus resulting in improved patient care and cost savings [10–13]. Some successful interventions include displaying the date and the results from the most proximal previous test [13], computerized prediction of abnormal results based on previous results [12], and display of length of stay information based on diagnosis [11]. The selection of appropriate targets for intervention is critical, as either high volume, commonly ordered tests or those with the highest variable cost typically have the highest postinterventional impact. Importantly, these interventions seek to increase the proportion of tests ordered which are appropriate, not merely reduce overall test volume.

In one randomized study at our institution, redundancy checks were triggered when clinicians ordered metabolic profiles, urinalysis, therapeutic drugs, urine cultures, sputum cultures, stool cultures, *Clostridium difficile* cultures, and fibrin split products [10]. In most cases, the interval defining redundancy was <20 h, although the intervals were selected through a review of the available evidence. Tests ordered within the first 24 h of admission were exempted. The default was set to cancel the test order, but the clinician could override the decision support by providing a clinical justification for the override (Fig. 19.1).

Urinalyses, chemistry profiles and urine cultures accounted for a high percentage of redundant orders [10]. Redundancy alerts for these tests were also the most likely to be overridden by the clinician. Some common reasons for a clinician to override a reminder were: (1) condition warrants more frequent testing, (2) clinical condition has changed, (3) last result requires confirmation, (4) previous specimen unsatisfactory, and (5) different site or testing conditions [10]. However, upon reviewing the medical records the override reasons were justified in less than 50% of cases. It was also discovered that many clinicians were never exposed to the electronic reminders because laboratory tests could have been ordered through sets or templates independent to the CDSS [10]. Specimens were also sometimes sent to the laboratory directly without an order being placed, and lab policy at the time required processing such specimens.

Overall, the study found that the CDSS was effective at reducing redundant tests. In the intervention group only 27% of redundant tests were ultimately ordered, while in the control group 51% were ordered (Table 19.1). Importantly, the CDSS in this instance did not have any adverse impact on the quality of patient care, indicating that implementation of similar electronic reminders may be warranted in targeted areas.

Table 19.1 CDSS effectiveness at reducing redundant tests

Test	Intervention ($n=437$) Number ordered	Number performed	Control ($n=502$) Number ordered	Number performed
Urinalysis	136	35 (26%)	185	85 (46%)
Chemistry 20 profile	113	37 (33%)	143	81 (57%)
Urine culture	110	22 (20%)	91	50 (55%)
Sputum culture	39	14 (36%)	28	18 (64%)
Stool culture	15	3 (20%)	14	3 (21%)
Other	24	6 (25%)	41	20 (49%)
Total	437	117 (27%)	502	257 (51%)

[a]The reminders were delivered in the intervention group and triggered, but not delivered, in the control group
From Bates et al. [10], with permission of Elsevier

Antiepileptic Drug Monitoring

Antiepileptic drug monitoring accounts for almost 20% of the therapeutic drug testing performed in clinical laboratories [14]. Our group developed appropriateness criteria for antiepileptic drug monitoring based on evidence-based medicine and expert opinion [14, 15]. These criteria were not developed as extensive guidelines for clinical appropriateness, but instead to provide simple rules with which to evaluate levels. The appropriate indications included suspicion for toxicity or noncompliance, baseline measurement once the patient has reached steady state or a change in dose or clinical condition (Table 19.2). Based on these criteria, a high percentage of antiepileptic drug levels were found to be ordered inappropriately, usually due to routine daily ordering [14]. Furthermore, the inappropriate levels were rarely clinically important.

We next implemented a CDSS to improve the appropriateness of antiepileptic drug level monitoring [16]. For orders which appeared redundant, an automated redundancy reminder was provided (Fig. 19.2a), while nonredundant orders prompted an educational screen with common indications for monitoring and pharmacokinetic parameters of each antiepileptic drug (Fig. 19.2b). These two interventions led to a 27 and 4% order cancellation rate, respectively. Inappropriate test ordering decreased from 54 to 15%. Furthermore, the results were sustainable over a 4-year follow-up period, suggesting that CDSSs can durably affect clinician behavior.

Table 19.2 Appropriateness criteria for antiepileptic drug monitoring

Measuring a serum level is always appropriate
Within 6 h after a seizure recurrence
In the event of suspected dose-related drug toxicity[a]
In the event of suspected patient noncompliance
Measuring a serum level is appropriate only if the blood sample is drawn in steady state conditions, i.e., after 4 half-lives on an unchanged dose regimen[b]
As a baseline measurement after starting antiepileptic drug therapy
As a control measurement after a change in the dose regimen
After adding a second drug with a potential for interaction with the antiepileptic drug[c]
After a change in the patient's liver or gastrointestinal tract function

[a]For phenytoin, nystagmus, ataxia, and drowsiness; for carbamazepine, gastrointestinal symptoms, diplopia, and dizziness; for phenobarbital, sedation, depression, and cognitive decline; and for valproic acide, hepatic dysfunction and tremor
[b]Steady state is assumed to be reached after 6 days for phenytoin, after 3 days for carbamazepine and valproic acid, and after 20 days for phenobarbital
[c]Another antiepileptic drug, warfarin, isoniazid, or rifampicin
From Schoenenberger et al. [14], with permission

Appropriateness of Digoxin Levels

Digoxin levels are commonly performed to assess therapeutic efficacy and compliance as well as evaluate for toxicity. Appropriate timing of levels depends upon many factors including clinical condition, patient status,

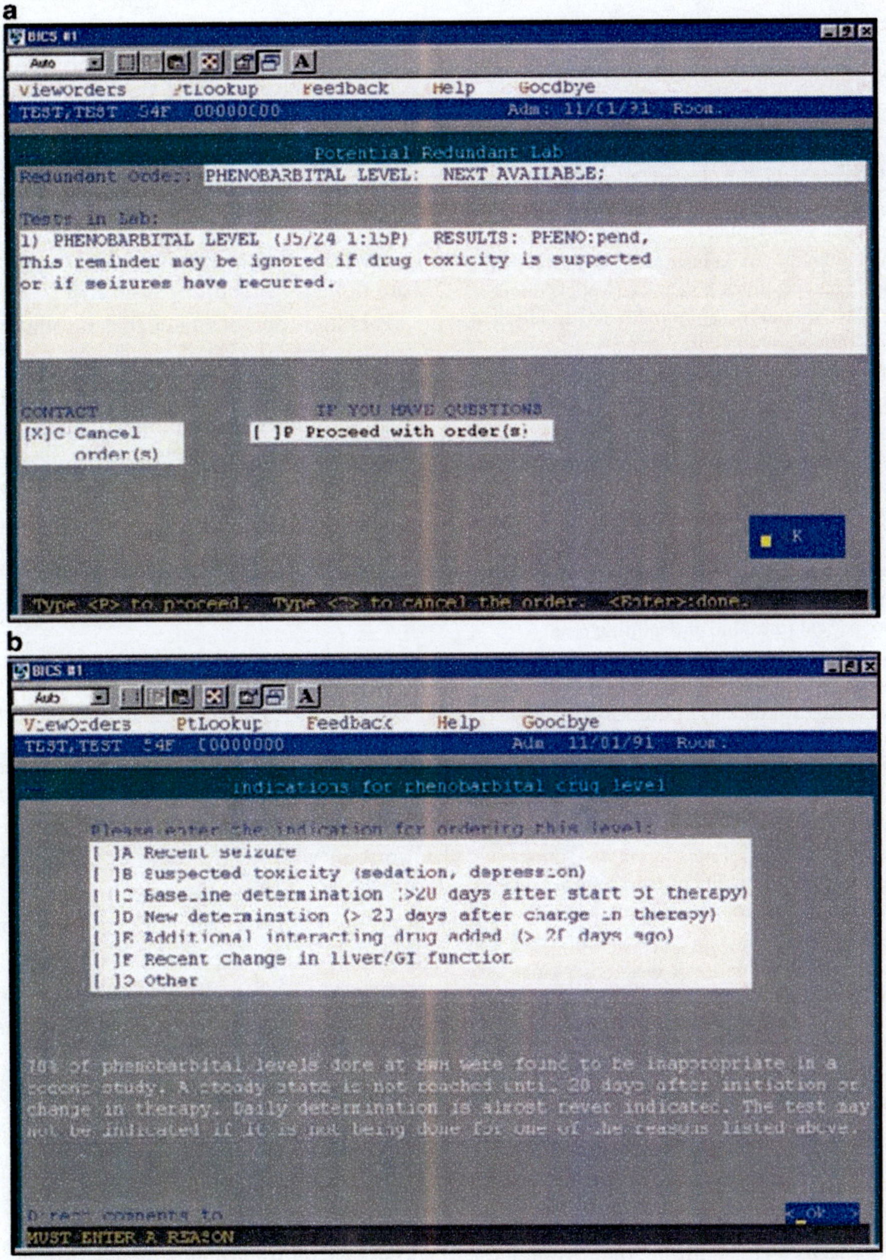

Fig. 19.2 (**a** and **b**) Examples of notes on phenobarbital drug level (from Chen et al. [16], © 2003–2010 American Society for Clinical Pathology; © 2003–2010 American Journal of Clinical Pathology)

pharmacokinetics, and patient location. Clinical criteria to evaluate the appropriateness of digoxin levels are available [17] and can be useful to guide clinicians and reduce the cost and time associated with inappropriate digoxin levels.

Canas et al. [18] used a combination of literature review and expert opinion to develop appropriateness criteria for monitoring digoxin levels (Table 19.3). Appropriate indications included suspected toxicity, high-risk patients, dosage adjustment or monitoring after steady state was

Table 19.3 Appropriateness of serum digoxin level requests

Appropriate if
For both inpatients and outpatients:
1. Subtherapeutic response (either A, B, C, or D) A. No improvement or worsening of congestive heart failure or atrial fibrillation or flutter B. Suspected noncompliance C. Concomitant use of an interacting drug (antacids, a kaolin and pectin combination [Kaopectate], neomycin, quinidine, spironolactone, nifedipine, cholestramine, verapamil) D. Suspected malabsorption
2. Suspected toxicity (either A or B) A. Appearance of arrhythmias suspected to be caused by digoxin (supraventricular tachycardia, atrioventricular conduction defects, multifocal premature ventricular contractions) B. Noncardiac signs or symptoms of digoxin toxicity (visual changes, anorexia, nausea, vomiting, diarrhea, abdominal pain, confusion, headache)
3. High-risk patient (unstable or declining renal function, low serum potassium level, hypoxia, recent increase in diuretic dose)
4. Initiation of digoxin therapy or dosage adjustment after steady state reached (5 half-lives, 10 days)[a]
For inpatients:
5. Admission level for inpatients if no previous digoxin level within last 9 months[b] is available
For outpatients:
6. Routine monitoring annually in outpatients on stable dose of digoxin (inappropriate if level drawn less than every 10 months)[b]

[a] Ten days was chosen in this study as a conservative estimate of the interval required to reach steady state, although some patients may reach steady state in 8 days

[b] Time intervals chosen by consensus of expert opinions

From Canas et al. [18].

achieved, admission levels, serial determinations at least 10 days apart, and yearly routine monitoring in outpatients. The authors determined the number of digoxin levels on both inpatients and outpatients that were drawn appropriately at their institution based on these criteria.

They found that many as 84% of inpatient digoxin levels had no appropriate indication [18]. Most frequently digoxin levels were drawn more often than every 10 days for routine monitoring. In fact, it was common to measure digoxin levels daily in inpatients. The percentage of appropriate levels was higher (52%) in the outpatient population. However, similar to inpatients, the main reason for inappropriate levels was routine or too frequent monitoring. In both the inpatient and outpatient setting the number of toxic levels was low and most likely misleading due to inappropriate ordering of the levels. In one patient, the dose of digoxin was decreased, otherwise no other interventions were done as a result of high levels.

This study demonstrated that introducing CDSSs with simple criteria for appropriate digoxin indications could improve the utilization of digoxin levels without compromising clinical care. Cost savings associated with the CDSS were deemed to be significant. As with antiepileptic drug monitoring, this approach could be taken for other therapeutic drugs, presumably with similar outcomes.

Appropriateness of Prostate-Specific Antigen

Prostate-specific antigen (PSA) testing is relatively costly. Various guidelines are available that indicate clinical scenarios and patient populations in which PSA testing is deemed appropriate [19]. The American Cancer Society recommends providing information about PSA testing to men at average risk for prostate cancer starting at age 50 [20, 21]. PSA testing is also warranted to monitor disease progression and recurrence [22].

Poteat et al. [19] reviewed the available literature at the time of the study and developed a set of appropriateness criteria for PSA (Table 19.4). Testing indications included screening, prostate cancer workup, monitoring for cancer recurrence, and assessing treatment efficacy. Similar to other studies referenced above, the criteria were developed using evidence-based medicine which considers both benefit and cost. Tests with marginal benefits, such as screening patients with a less than 10 year life expectancy, were not considered appropriate. The authors then examined the appropriateness of PSA testing at their institution based on these criteria [19] and developed an algorithm for examining whether clinically relevant new information was obtained from the testing.

Table 19.4 Appropriateness criteria for measuring serum prostate-specific antigen concentration

Appropriateness	Criteria
Appropriate	Assessing prostate cancer progression after therapy
	Evaluating treatment efficacy during therapy
	Monitoring for prostate cancer recurrence 2–4 times per year: patients 1, 2, and 3 years or more after treatment with curative intent receive a PSA assay every 3, 4, and 6 months, respectively
	Diagnostic workup and staging in men with signs or symptoms associated with prostate cancer
	For men with carcinoma of unknown primary site
	Establishing a baseline value before beginning therapy for benign prostatic hypertrophy with a 5 alpha-reductase inhibitor, such as finasteride
Appropriate but debated	As once yearly screening of asymptomatic men aged 50–75 years; screening with PSA should be accompanied by rectal examination
	Screening men with a family history of African-American men aged 40–75 years
	As a staging modality to replace bone scan in selected cases of prostate cancer
Inappropriate	Screening asymptomatic men older than 75 years or asymptomatic patients with less than 10 years of life expectancy
	Screening asymptomatic men with no risk factors younger than 50 years or those with risk factors before age 40 years

From Poteat et al. [19].

The study concluded that most PSA testing was performed on outpatients and approximately one fifth of the orders were considered inappropriate. A CDSS using simple age- and frequency-based criteria could have eliminated most inappropriate test orders without compromising clinical information leading to substantial cost savings in the laboratory.

Effect of Displaying Test Charges

Clinicians are typically unaware of the cost of tests and evidence suggests that displaying lab charges affects clinician behavior and might reduce cost and unnecessary test utilization [1, 23]. Feedback to the clinician regarding charges after they have placed the order, in an attempt to curb future unnecessary orders for expensive tests, has had variable affects [1]. However, displaying charges electronically using CPOE offers the advantage of communicating the information in real time. Furthermore, it is easy, nonintrusive and does not affect quality. Electronic display also provides ongoing reinforcement by displaying the charge each time the clinician attempts to order a test. Previous studies have been performed in the outpatient setting and have shown success using CPOE displays [23, 24].

Our institution performed a randomized controlled trial with over 7,000 patients to determine whether the display of charges for inpatients at the time of ordering affected test utilization and cost, similar to that seen in studies on outpatients [1]. In the intervention group, charges were displayed for nineteen clinical laboratory tests at the time of ordering and the total cost was tallied. The clinical laboratory tests were grouped in two categories: commonly and less commonly ordered. There was no significant difference between groups in the number of tests ordered in either category. In addition, there was no significant decrease in charges or potential cost savings associated with the intervention.

The authors were surprised by the lack of impact from displaying associated inpatient laboratory charges [1]. Possible explanations include the percentage (53%) of orders placed through CPOE, resulting in the number of clinicians exposed to the intervention being smaller than expected. In addition, we displayed laboratory charges as opposed to laboratory costs. The clinicians may have been less sensitive to the former category.

Critical Results

Accrediting organizations such as the Joint Commission and the College of American Pathologists require that the laboratory communicate critical results to a licensed care provider in a timely manner [25, 26]. Critical results, particularly those associated with administering certain medications can also signify worsening clinical conditions. For example, declining platelet counts in the setting of heparin therapy raise the possibility of heparin-induced thrombocytopenia. Many laboratory information systems are not sophisticated enough to flag trends in test results, such as declining values over time or lab test–drug interactions. CDSSs can be designed to alert clinicians when more complex scenarios regarding critical laboratory results or changes in laboratory results are obtained. Furthermore, immediate notification of clinicians can ensure that intervention is performed in a timely manner. Time to intervention is critical as some studies have illustrated that delay in treatment can be significant [27, 28]. Several institutions have implemented CDSSs which page clinicians with results that meet their critical criteria and warrant immediate intervention [29–32].

In a study at our institution, the authors gathered baseline data and investigated the number of critical laboratory results each day, the time it took for a clinician to act on these results and the time it took for the patient's clinical condition to resolve [33]. We evaluated high and low sodium, potassium, and glucose levels, and falling hematocrit. An average of 0.44 of these critical results per patient-day was identified. The median time to treatment was 2.3 h and the median time until the condition was resolved was 14.3 h.

Potential treatment delays associated with the standard, telephone-based critical result reporting prompted the designing, and implementation of a CDSS to help improve the clinical response time [34]. CDSS rules were designed to individualize critical results by accounting for changes in laboratory results over time, and patient–drug interactions (Table 19.5). For example, physicians were paged when the patient's serum potassium was less than 3.3 mEq/L and the patient had an active order for digoxin. Our group also developed criteria to identify appropriate treatments ordered after the critical result, and measured the time to treatment ordered as well as time to critical condition resolved in the control and intervention group. The median time until treatment ordered was significantly shorter for the intervention group vs. control group (1.0 h vs. 1.6 h, $P=0.003$; mean, 4.1 h vs. 4.6 h, $P=0.003$). The time until the critical condition resolved also decreased (median, 8.4 h vs. 8.9 h, $P=0.11$; mean, 14.4 h vs. 20.2 h, $P=0.11$). The studies illustrate a decrease in time to notify the clinicians as well as a decrease in time to take the appropriate action. Physicians were also very satisfied to be paged about these values – 95% of physicians reported a high level of satisfaction with the approach. A key to success was being highly selective regarding which tests physicians were paged directly about.

Cost Benefits

Despite studies that indicate a reduction in medication error rates and improved workflow and test utilization using CPOE and CDSSs [6, 35–37], relatively high costs and limited data on financial benefits may limit their implementation. Appropriate assessment of cost-benefit is difficult to perform since it involves various categories of cost across different hospital departments. Moreover, the cost benefit associated with reduction in high volume automated tests is limited, since a 50% reduction in test utilization may only translate into a disproportionately much smaller savings in the laboratory, which might be only 10–20% [38].

Total system-wide savings may be affected by decreased adverse drug events, improved

Table 19.5 Frequency distribution of alerts

Rule	Alerting criterion	No. (%)[a]
1	Hematocrit has fallen 10% or more since last result and is now less than 26%[b]	38 (19.8)
2	Serum glucose is greater than or equal to 400 mg/dL	34 (17.7)
3	Hematocrit has fallen 6% or more since previous result, and has fallen faster than 0.4% per hour since last result, and is now less than 26% and the patient is not on the cardiac surgery service[b]	32 (16.7)
4	Serum potassium is greater than or equal to 6.0 mEq/L	32 (16.7)
5	Serum potassium has fallen 1.0 mEq/L or more over the last 24 h and is now less than 3.2 mEq/L[c]	29 (15.1)
6	Serum potassium less than 3.3 mEq/L and patient has an active order for digoxin[c]	15 (7.8)
7	Serum sodium is greater than 160 mEq/L	5 (2.6)
8	Serum sodium has fallen 15 mEq/L or more in last 24 h and is now less than 130 mEq/L[d]	4 (2.1)
9	Serum glucose is less than or equal to 40 mg/dL	3 (1.6)
10	Hematocrit is less than or equal to 15%[b]	0 (0)
11	Serum potassium is less than or equal to 2.4 mEq/L[c]	0 (0)
12	Serum sodium is less than or equal to 115 mEq/L[d]	0 (0)
	Total	192 (100)

[a] Combined number of occurrences in control and intervention groups, after exclusions
[b] For low or falling hematocrit, rule 1 takes precedence over rule 3, which takes precedence over rule 10
[c] For low or falling potassium, rule 5 takes precedence over rule 6, which takes precedence over rule 11
[d] For low or falling sodium, rule 8 takes precedence over rule 12
From Kuperman et al. [34], with permission from BMJ Publishing Group Ltd

workflow and efficiency, decreased drug costs, and decreased laboratory and radiological test utilization [35]. Further interventions aimed at reducing hospital length of stay can translate into significant cost savings. For example, a CDSS that provided renal dosing guidance and recommend dose adjustments based on a patient's renal function was shown to decrease length of stay [39].

At our institution, Kaushal et al. [35] demonstrated cumulative savings of $16.7 million over a 10-year period ($2.2 million annualized) following implementation of CPOE and CDSSs. The greatest cumulative savings were renal dosing guidance, nursing time utilization, specific drug guidance, and adverse drug event prevention (Table 19.6).

Key Success Factors

Using experience with CDSSs at our institution, certain patterns emerged that determined the success of our CDSS interventions (Table 19.7) [40]. Most importantly, the applications must not slow down the end user. Even extremely well-documented decision support will fail if it takes too long to place the order. Our end users rated speed as much more important to them than either quality or cost [40]. Next, due to time pressure and performance demands, the information must be available readily when the clinician needs it. If too many interventions are implemented the overall speed of the system can be compromised negating the potential benefits.

CDSSs, rather than simply providing electronic information, should integrate data components such as drug level and abnormal lab and present data that clinicians may miss. In this context, particularly useful are systems which remind clinicians to alter a drug dose based on declining renal function or which suggest a clinical action such as order a trough level based on a medication order for vancomycin; so-called "corollary orders" [40]. These tools should be integrated into clinical workflow such that they are displayed at the time of clinical decision-making. Clinicians should not be able to easily ignore reminders, but in turn, the reminders should be informative and limited in volume.

Table 19.6 Cumulative benefits for clinical decision support system elements at Brigham and Women's Hospital

CDSS element	Method of cost savings	Live dates	Total benefits[a]
Renal dosing guidance	Decreased ADEs: decreased length of stay, decreased ADEs, and increased appropriate prescriptions; 16,470 interventions per year	12/97	6.3
Nurse time utilization	Improved work flow and efficiency: streamlined work flow for nurses particularly by decreasing time to generate a medication administration record	7/93	6.0
Specific or expensive drug guidance (human growth hormone, vancomycin, ceftriaxone, ondansetron, histamine-2 receptor blockers)	Decreased drug costs: decreased use or frequency resulting in decreased doses. For example, 975 interventions per year suggest decreasing frequency of ondansetron use from 4 to 3 times per day, resulting in an overall decrease in frequency from 3.92 to 3.15 does per day; 5,536 vancomycin interventions per year	11/93 10/94 4/98	4.9
Adverse drug event prevention	Decreased ADEs: decreased ADEs through drug dose, route, frequency, allergy, drug interaction, and laboratory warnings	7/95 12/97	3.7
Laboratory charge display and redundant laboratory warnings	Decreased laboratory tests: decreased ordering of laboratory tests. Charges are displayed 10,608 times per year resulting in 4.5% fewer ordered tests. Redundant laboratory warnings are issued 2,817 times per year resulting in cancellation of 69% of suggested tests	5.94 11/94	1.9
Panic laboratory alerting	Decreased ADEs: decreased time to treat ADEs through improved communication; 6,720 alerts are generated each year regarding critical laboratory abnormalities	7/94	1.8
Intravenous to oral guidance	Decreased drug costs: decreased use of intravenous medications by a computerized report that identifies patients on expensive intravenous medications who are taking either oral medications or food; 15,695 alerts are generated per year	2/00	1.1
ADE monitor	Decreased ADEs: decreased ADEs through early physician notification of potential ADEs; generally 230 interventions per year	5/00	1.0
Automated medication summary at hospital discharge	Improved work flow and efficiency: improved information access for patients at time of discharge; decreases staff time otherwise needed to generate a medication list	7/93	0.6
Physician time utilization	Improved work flow and efficiency: streamlined workflow for physicians (e.g., reduced time finding chart or reduce rework with pharmacists)	7/93	0.6
Radiology indications, rule-out, and assistant	Decreased radiological utilization: decreased unnecessary testing and improved documentation; an abdominal (KUB) radiograph assistant generates 2,488 interventions per year to reduce overuse of KUB radiographs	7/97 8/98	0.4
Elderly dosing guidance	Decreased ADEs: decreased ADEs by recommending drug dose reduction in geriatric patients	12/97	0.1
Specific drug level guidance (antiepileptics, rheumatologic tests)	Decreased laboratory tests: approximately 120 rheumatologic test recommendations per year result in fewer tests	3/95 10/96	0.1

ADE adverse drug event; *KUB* kidney, ureter, and bladder

[a]This table depicts the cumulative benefits (in 2002 millions of dollars) from 1992 to 2002 for each element of CDSS at Brigham and Women's Hospital given an 80% prospective reimbursement rate

From Kaushal et al. [35], with permission from BMJ Publishing Group Ltd

Table 19.7 Ten commandments for effective clinical decision support

1. Speed is Everything	User satisfaction depends largely on the speed of the application
2. Anticipate Needs and Deliver in Real Time	Information should be brought to the clinician at the time it is needed
3. Fit into User's Workflow	Guidelines which are available for passive consultation are less effective than those which are built in to the ordering process
4. Little Things Can Make a Big Difference	Screen design and usability can have a big impact and should be carefully attended to
5. Recognize that Physicians Will Strongly Resist Stopping	Clinicians often override suggestions to cancel an order
6. Changing Direction is Easier than Stopping	Changing defaults within the ordering screen or providing alternate suggestions may be an effective way to change physician behavior
7. Simple Interventions Work Best	Reminders should be simplified and fit onto one screen
8. Ask for Additional Information Only When You Really Need It	Requiring physicians to input extra data elements may decrease the success of a computerized guideline
9. Monitor Impact, Get Feedback, and Respond	Recording auditing data and gathering user feedback may help to improve the intervention
10. Manage and Maintain Your Knowledge-based Systems	Systems should be monitored for frequency of alerts, reminders, responses, and overrides

Adapted from Bates et al. [40], with permission from BMJ Publishing Group Ltd

Some systems require clinicians to input a reason why the reminder was overridden. A mechanism should be in place to allow overriding reasons to be tracked and audited.

The CDSS should also be user-friendly by defaulting to the most common decision or by providing drop down menus instead of free text. Importantly, usability testing should be performed by the end users, not the developers or pathologists.

CDSSs that stop clinicians from performing an action, such as ordering a test, should be avoided. Whenever possible an acceptable alternative should be provided. The decision support interventions should be simple and fit on a single screen without extraneous information that may result in clinicians' quitting the ordering session before they reach the intended guideline.

Auditing the impact of the CDSS is also critical as many interventions do not produce the intended results. Feedback from end users is important to determine users' satisfaction and collect valuable suggestions for improvement [40].

Lastly, unanticipated problems should be expected. Our institution implemented a decision support system linked to a specific test, only to find that that test was ordered primarily through order sets and the majority of clinicians were not presented with the support [40]. Therefore, a troubleshooting team should be an integral component of the process.

Future Directions

Review of the literature and data for our own institution illustrate that CDSSs designed using evidence-based medicine are effective at reducing the number of inappropriate laboratory tests and controlling cost. Each institution should determine appropriate target areas for CDSSs that promise to provide the highest impact. Internal audits and evidence-based guidelines are helpful tools in that respect. In our experience, CDSSs targeting test utilization, therapeutic drug monitoring, and critical test result communication are highly effective.

As technology expands and many institutions implement CPOE that communicates bidirectionally with the laboratory and handheld computers to guide specimen collection, the benefits of CDSSs can be magnified. Decision support may be implemented not only at the time of order entry, but also at the time of specimen collection. Some potential benefits include a reduction in the number of "no sample received" and "wrong sample type" errors, which occur when a test is ordered but no sample is drawn, or the wrong type of sample is drawn. Furthermore, such systems in conjunction with barcode technology can prevent specimen labeling errors [41–43]. Automated systems can also be put into place to allow orders to be added to existing specimens in the laboratory, when appropriate, reducing the need for additional phlebotomy. Ultimately, evidence-based practice and CDSSs can capitalize on advances in information technology to improve workflow and quality and safety in healthcare, with the net being substantial improvement in all these areas.

References

1. Bates DW et al. Does the computerized display of charges affect inpatient ancillary test utilization? Arch Intern Med. 1997;157(21):2501–8.
2. Kuperman GJ, Gibson RF. Computer physician order entry: benefits, costs, and issues. Ann Intern Med. 2003;139(1):31–9.
3. Bates DW et al. What proportion of common diagnostic tests appear redundant? Am J Med. 1998;104(4): 361–8.
4. Melanson SE et al. Utilization of arterial blood gas measurements in a large tertiary care hospital. Am J Clin Pathol. 2007;127(4):604–9.
5. Axt-Adam P, van der Wouden JC, van der Does E. Influencing behavior of physicians ordering laboratory tests: a literature study. Med Care. 1993;31(9): 784–94.
6. Bates DW et al. Strategies for physician education in therapeutic drug monitoring. Clin Chem. 1998;44(2):401–7.
7. Harpole LH et al. Automated evidence-based critiquing of orders for abdominal radiographs: impact on utilization and appropriateness. J Am Med Inform Assoc. 1997;4(6):511–21.
8. Solomon DH et al. Techniques to improve physicians' use of diagnostic tests: a new conceptual framework. JAMA. 1998;280(23):2020–7.
9. Lyon AW, Greenway DC, Hindmarsh JT. A strategy to promote rational clinical chemistry test utilization. Am J Clin Pathol. 1995;103(6):718–24.
10. Bates DW et al. A randomized trial of a computer-based intervention to reduce utilization of redundant laboratory tests. Am J Med. 1999;106(2):144–50.
11. Shea S et al. Computer-generated informational messages directed to physicians: effect on length of hospital stay. J Am Med Inform Assoc. 1995;2(1):58–64.
12. Tierney WM et al. Computer predictions of abnormal test results. Effects on outpatient testing. JAMA. 1988;259(8):1194–8.
13. Tierney WM et al. Computerized display of past test results. Effect on outpatient testing. Ann Intern Med. 1987;107(4):569–74.
14. Schoenenberger RA et al. Appropriateness of antiepileptic drug level monitoring. JAMA. 1995;274(20) :1622–6.
15. Tanasijevic MJ, Bates DW. Criteria for appropriate therapeutic monitoring of antiepileptic drugs. In: Therapeutic drug monitoring and toxicology, American Association for Clinical Chemistry, editor. Washington, D.C.; 1997. p. 13–19.
16. Chen P et al. A computer-based intervention for improving the appropriateness of antiepileptic drug level monitoring. Am J Clin Pathol. 2003;119(3):432–8.
17. Michalko KJ, Blain L. An evaluation of a clinical pharmacokinetic service for serum digoxin levels. Ther Drug Monit. 1987;9(3):311–9.
18. Canas F et al. Evaluating the appropriateness of digoxin level monitoring. Arch Intern Med. 1999;159(4):363–8.
19. Poteat HT, et al. Appropriateness of prostate-specific antigen testing. Am J Clin Pathol. 2000;113(3): 421–8.
20. Wolf AM, et al. American Cancer Society guideline for the early detection of prostate cancer: update 2010. CA Cancer J Clin. 2010;60(2):70–98.
21. Smith RA et al. Cancer screening in the United States, 2010: a review of current American Cancer Society guidelines and issues in cancer screening. CA Cancer J Clin. 2010;60(2):99–119.
22. Lieberman R. Evidence-based medical perspectives: the evolving role of PSA for early detection, monitoring of treatment response, and as a surrogate end point of efficacy for interventions in men with different clinical risk states for the prevention and progression of prostate cancer. Am J Ther. 2004;11(6):501–6.
23. Tierney WM, Miller ME, McDonald CJ. The effect on test ordering of informing physicians of the charges for outpatient diagnostic tests. N Engl J Med. 1990;322(21):1499–504.
24. Hampers LC et al. The effect of price information on test-ordering behavior and patient outcomes in a pediatric emergency department. Pediatrics. 1999;103 (4 Pt 2):877–82.
25. College of American Pathologists. Laboratory Accreditation Checklist. [cited 2010 May 28]; Available from: http://www.cap.org/apps/cap.portal.
26. The Joint Commission. 2010 National Patient Safety Goals. [cited 2010 May 28]; Available from: http://www.jointcommission.org/patientsafety/nationalpatientsafetygoals/.
27. Rind DM et al. Effect of computer-based alerts on the treatment and outcomes of hospitalized patients. Arch Intern Med. 1994;154(13):1511–7.
28. Tate KE, Gardner RM, Weaver LK. A computerized laboratory alerting system. MD Comput. 1990;7(5): 296–301.

29. Park HI et al. Evaluating the short message service alerting system for critical value notification via PDA telephones. Ann Clin Lab Sci. 2008;38(2):149–56.
30. Piva E et al. Evaluation of effectiveness of a computerized notification system for reporting critical values. Am J Clin Pathol. 2009;131(3):432–41.
31. Etchells E et al. Real-time clinical alerting: effect of an automated paging system on response time to critical laboratory values–a randomised controlled trial. Qual Saf Health Care. 2010;19(2):99–102.
32. Parl FF et al. Implementation of a closed-loop reporting system for critical values and clinical communication in compliance with goals of the joint commission. Clin Chem. 2010;56(3):417–23.
33. Kuperman GJ et al. How promptly are inpatients treated for critical laboratory results? J Am Med Inform Assoc. 1998;5(1):112–9.
34. Kuperman GJ et al. Improving response to critical laboratory results with automation: results of a randomized controlled trial. J Am Med Inform Assoc. 1999;6(6):512–22.
35. Kaushal R et al. Return on investment for a computerized physician order entry system. J Am Med Inform Assoc. 2006;13(3):261–6.
36. Dexter PR et al. A computerized reminder system to increase the use of preventive care for hospitalized patients. N Engl J Med. 2001;345(13):965–70.
37. Overhage JM et al. A randomized trial of "corollary orders" to prevent errors of omission. J Am Med Inform Assoc. 1997;4(5):364–75.
38. Winkelman JW. Less utilization of the clinical laboratory produces disproportionately small true cost reductions. Hum Pathol. 1984;15(6):499–501.
39. Chertow GM et al. Guided medication dosing for inpatients with renal insufficiency. JAMA. 2001;286(22):2839–44.
40. Bates DW et al. Ten commandments for effective clinical decision support: making the practice of evidence-based medicine a reality. J Am Med Inform Assoc. 2003;10(6):523–30.
41. Hayden RT et al. Computer-assisted bar-coding system significantly reduces clinical laboratory specimen identification errors in a pediatric oncology hospital. J Pediatr. 2008;152(2):219–24.
42. Morrison AP et al. Reduction in specimen labeling errors after implementation of a positive patient identification system in phlebotomy. Am J Clin Pathol. 2010;133(6):870–7.
43. Bologna LJ, Lind C, Riggs RC. Reducing major identification errors within a deployed phlebotomy process. Clin Leadersh Manag Rev. 2002;16(1):22–6.

20 Evidence-Based Pathology and Tort Law: How Do They Compare?

Mark R. Wick and Elliott Foucar

Keywords

Evidence-based pathology • Tort law in medicine • Evidence-based pathology in the legal system • Medical malpractice and evidence-based medicine

"Medical malpractice reform has long been the graveyard for high hopes and good intentions."

– (D. Hyman, JD, Professor, University of Maryland School of Law, 2002) [1]

"Tort reform ...hurts the hapless patients who suffer grievous harm at the hands of incompetent doctors."

– (Editorial opinion, *The New York Times*, January 2005) [2]

"The justice system in America works, and it works very well."

– (Mark Lanier, JD, plaintiffs' attorney, commenting on a $253.5 million jury award based on less than one hour of jury deliberations devoted to the pathogenesis of the cardiac death of the plaintiff's husband. August 2005) [3]

"Jury awards can be ... inexplicable on any basis but caprice or passion."

– (Justice Sandra Day O'Connor, US Supreme Court, commenting on a 1993 9th Circuit Court ruling) [4]

"Tears have always been considered legitimate arguments before a jury. Indeed, if counsel has them at his command, it may be seriously questioned whether it is not his professional duty to shed them whenever proper occasion arises."

– (Proceedings, Tennessee Supreme Court, 1897) [5]

"Tort" (from middle-English, essentially meaning "injury") law is a complex set of procedures for decision-making, the purported goal of which is to use facts to resolve disputes. The problems at issue reflect an allegation – made by the plaintiff(s) – that carelessness has led to a personal injury. The careless, or "tortious" act (in legal parlance, "negligence"), can either be a wrongful deed or the *failure* to do something. Malpractice cases are specialized tort actions that are based on a plaintiff's claim of *professional* negligence (by physicians, dentists, lawyers, architects, engineers, etc.).

The quality of legal decisions in tort law depends on the soundness of the rules on which its procedures are based; the quality of available information; and the skill of ultimate decision-makers in understanding and integrating those

M.R. Wick (✉)
Department of Pathology, University of Virginia Medical School, Charlottesville, VA, USA
e-mail: mrw9c@virginia.edu

A.M. Marchevsky and M.R. Wick (eds.), *Evidence Based Pathology and Laboratory Medicine*,
DOI 10.1007/978-1-4419-1030-1_20,

factors [6, 7]. In medical malpractice cases as well as other kinds of "civil" (noncriminal) suits, "expert" witnesses are often the principal source of technical information that is introduced to the court [8]. Those individuals are usually – but not always – physicians themselves [9]. Lay jurors listen to presentations by the "experts" and the attorneys and are ultimately charged as the "finders of fact." They mix their community values with the evidence presented at trial, under the direction of the trial judge, to reach a legal decision for either the plaintiff or the defendant.

The traditions of English common law have been refined over several centuries, and they are the foundation for administration of the tort system, both conceptually and procedurally. Although many cases that enter the system are "resolved" and never come to trial, negotiations leading to that outcome are dominated by the opponents' opinions of what the outcome *would* be if the case *were* to go to a jury. Early on, it became increasingly apparent that lay jurors would likely require "expert" input to come to rational conclusions concerning technically complicated issues (such as those in the area of medical malpractice). For example, as early as the 1700s, judges opined that medical standards should be "testified-to by the surgeons themselves" [10]. That led to the custom for each party to engage its own "experts." Sheila Jasanoff (John F. Kennedy School of Government, Harvard University) has stated that societies expect "experts" "...to have thought more carefully and responsibly than any of us, as individual citizens, could possibly hope to do" [11]. Whether or not that is always true is open to debate.

Great import has been attached to the ability of juries to deliberate in "good faith" and "good conscience," but much less concern has been expended over the quality of objective data provided to them. Because of the growing technological complexity of society at large, good *information* is every bit as important as "good faith" or "good conscience." Indeed, there is a real risk that, when presented with conflicting opinions on unfamiliar subjects, well-meaning jurors may, in "good faith," be influenced by testimony in the realm of so-called "junk-science" [12].

Recent legal statutes and decisions have aimed to better the quality of tort law decisions by attempting to improve "expert" testimony. However, in analogy to the experience of many physicians with some aspects of "evidence-based medicine," lawyers have found it easier to *describe* ideal scientific evidence than to effectualize it. This is particularly true because the Law has traditionally not been very discerning about scientific rigor. It has instead focused on procedural priorities that are often incompatible with strict scientific standards. In other words, the practice of scientifically-based medicine and the practice of Law can be, and often are, very dissimilar indeed.

This overview examines the American tort system from an evidence-based perspective, with a particular orientation towards medical malpractice actions. It includes a discussion of standards for "outcomes analysis" in the Law; recognition and classification of errors made by the courts; the relationship between medical errors, "negligence," and "standard of care"; and the issue of reconciling plaintiffs' rights with medical–scientific facts. We also consider selected obstacles to developing a system that is capable of reaching evidence-based decisions on complex scientific topics, including the interpretation of tissue specimens by pathologists.

High-Quality Decisions in Tort Law

It is impossible to discuss the importance of "good information" in the courts without first considering how one *recognizes* a high-quality, evidence-based outcome in a tort action. Because the legal process can be said to produce binary results (for or against a plaintiff), an evaluation of its performance can be accomplished using measures that are familiar to pathologists. One such tool is the use of the familiar four-cell table, which compares given test results to accepted standards. This presentation allows for classification of results as "true positives," "true negatives," "false positives," and "false negatives." However, in reference to jury decisions, one could ask what standard of comparison should be used in that process. Many lawyers would say that the jurors' judgment is itself that standard, and therefore only "true-positive" and "true-negative" results are operative in the courts. This viewpoint was apparent in an extreme form when the US Supreme

Court ruled that even the decisions of jurors who were actively using mind-altering drugs during a trial were valid [13].

From a scientific perspective, the approach just described is patently unsound. It is a closed circle that mechanistically compares a result with itself. Moreover, it represents a barrier to *improvement* of the "test." In other words, why study performance when the test is already known to provide the best possible answer?

How does one rectify the problem? The authors believe that when a trial is centered on a putatively erroneous pathologic interpretation, the final jury decision should be compared with the consensus conclusion of a group of knowledgeable and unbiased pathologists (KUPs). Those individuals would *not* be engaged by lawyers for the plaintiff or defense, but rather by the court in general. As such, they would truly constitute a "peer" group with regard to the status of the defendant. A similar paradigm could apply to *all* malpractice actions concerning any professional vocation. Jury pronouncements that departed from the consensus "standard" could then be classified scientifically as "false-positive" or "false-negative" results.

However, pathologists – and physicians in general – must acknowledge that the identification of legal "test"-malfunction is more complicated than finding problems in *medical* validity. Although the courts do make technical information available to jurors, an important basic conceptual difference between the Law and Medicine must be realized – *it is not the primary goal of the tort system to achieve a scientifically correct conclusion, but rather to assure the legal and social rights of the plaintiff.* Because attorneys and judges are educated people, they could certainly design a system intended to mirror the opinions of knowledgeable and unbiased professional "experts." Instead, the existing model simply guarantees the plaintiff a right to bring his or her complaint to the court, and to be adjudicated by a jury of the plaintiff's "peers." As alluded-to earlier, such "peers" are not really "equals" of defendants in proceedings that concern professional and scientific issues. That is especially so because attorneys actually aim to exclude jurors who fit that description.

When a jury trial occurs in the present legal schema, sociopolitical aspects of "peer review" of the plaintiff's complaint are generally met but scientific ones are not [14]. If one accepts the premise that lay jurors will continue to decide the results of professional malpractice cases, efforts at reforming the system must aim to remove personal bias from the testimony of "experts" and assure the validity and strength of their scientific credentials. Panels of court-appointed, unbiased peer-professionals could also be used to provide appropriate counsel to judges.

Trial decisions that differ from the results of scientific analyses can be best understood by dividing them into two categories – (1) technically dissonant and politically consonant, and (2) technically dissonant and politically dissonant.

Type 1 Jury Errors: Technically Dissonant But Politically Consonant

When a type 1 error occurs, the scientific and medical information (SMI) provided to jurors was accurate and complete, but the jurors were unable to understand that information or chose to ignore it. For example, they may have based their group-decision on "community values" (such as feeling sorry for the plaintiff or "liking" the defendant). In other words, the jury members felt that their decision was the "right" (politically consonant) thing to do.

This type of error predictably results from lay-person juries having to make decisions on problems involving complicated scientific issues, or when clinical outcomes produce juror sympathy. Efforts to eliminate this category of jury "malfunction" would require radical changes in the legal system, e.g., removing juries completely from malpractice litigation by invoking the "complexity exemption" in the seventh Amendment to the U.S. Constitution [15]. Realistically, such attempts would undoubtedly face daunting political opposition. Indeed, there is instead an existing social trend in the *opposite* direction, i.e., challenging opinions of the "educated elite" by "democratizing" decisions that concern science and technology [16, 17].

It is discouraging to most physicians and pathologists in particular when valid SMI is ignored, because our focus is on the validity and performance of objective laboratory tests. However, we also accept that "wrong" diagnoses are unavoidable. For example, if one feels that patient welfare is best served by an assay that preferentially produces false-positive results, the test in question is intentionally designed to favor sensitivity over specificity [18].

Even though it is "mixing metaphors," the court consciously weighs "politically-correct" decisions against scientifically valid ones. Furthermore, because tort law is specifically aimed at achieving social–political objectives, the objective scientific integrity of its processes can suffer.

Type 2 Jury Errors: Technically Dissonant and (Therefore) Politically Dissonant

In type 2 errors, at least some SMI provided to the jury did not accurately reflect the reality of medical practice or scientific fact, and the jury apparently relied on that inaccurate testimony to reach a final decision. This form of legal dysfunction is actually amenable to reform.

Accrued evidence supports the idea that most citizens value lay-person "peer" juries, inevitably making the courts vulnerable to type 1 error [19–21]. However, there is no indication that people *want* to be misled scientifically while serving as jurors. Hence, one can conclude that when inaccurate medical testimony produces a verdict that a properly informed jury would not have reached, the legal outcome is both technically flawed and sociopolitically incorrect.

Rights Are Not Equal

Physicians think of laboratory test design in terms of precision and accuracy. They accordingly have trouble understanding a "test" (jury trial) that prioritizes a social goal; namely, the preservation of the plaintiff's rights. As a result, doctors who are sued usually are incensed if a jury reaches a decision that would be contrary to that of their *medical* peers. Indeed, one could justifiably argue that the rights of the *defendant* had been violated in that context.

Doctors – being nonlawyers – must recognize the fact that individual "rights" can conflict with each other and are pragmatically unequal. The courts are focused on deciding which rights take precedence over others. The seventh Amendment assures any defendant the "right" to have a jury of peers in a tort case [22]. Conversely, one has no constitutional right to a jury decision that matches the opinion of unbiased and optimally qualified "experts." No existing statute or judicial decision mandates that professional malpractice defendants have a right to be judged by vocational and educational equals.

The rights of citizen jurors can also be compromised in the courtroom. In their role as consumers, they benefit from legislation aimed to protect against inaccurate information on medications, food, investments, and other tangible life elements [23, 24]. However, as jurors, those same people encounter the rights of plaintiff's and defendant's attorneys to present the "strongest possible case," including the opinions of "experts" for both sides. Lawyers who knowingly use "experts" to misinform juries – a practice that unfortunately is real – are like companies who seek to deceive their consumers [25]. Tort reformers feel that the present system of "expert" testimony is an anachronism that exploits the naivete of lay jurors. Contrarily, defenders of the *status quo* believe that nonprofessional "peer" juries are effective even when presented with "junk" expert testimony.

Adversarial "Experts"

Using physicians to explain pathology-related issues to juries is certainly preferable to using no experts at all, or such "experts" as architects who would likely have no familiarity with the topic at issue. However, one would be incorrect in assuming that every physician specialist reflects the prevailing view of his or her specialty group as a whole. Indeed, some "experts" may hold to opinions that are highly idiosyncratic or even blatantly incorrect. Experience attests to the reality that a medical education does not protect a person against intellectual or ethical failures [26, 27].

It is obvious that the courts do want to know what pathologists think, but it is troubling to see how that information is sometimes obtained. Science holds that in order to draw rational conclusions from a sample of any given population, the sampling must be done systematically [28]. That principle applies to everything from presidential polls to taste-tests of potato chips. One cannot simply have opposing factions report highly select opinions that favor a certain candidate or product. Unfortunately, that basic concept does not have traction in the legal world; the right of lawyers to find "experts" who support their clients' positions supersedes the need for accurate SMI in the courtroom. The selection of "experts" sometimes even ignores the need for specialized training or experience in the pertinent topic. Unlike scientific sampling, legal searches for "experts" are comparable to "comparison-shopping" for predefined items at particular prices. Thus, the jury may hear diametrically opposed "expert" opinions, effectively forcing jurors to rely on factors such as the experts' charisma or lack thereof [29].

Biased selection of "experts" by lawyers is further complicated by the inability of judges to weigh and digest SMI and by personal idiosyncracies of jurists that can be prejudicial [30]. In fact, attorneys recognize that "...the trial judge is hardly a more qualified assessor of scientific credibility than the jury itself" [31]. When the judge fails as a gatekeeper of accurate information, jurors will be faced with apparent uncertainty and disagreement among "experts." In fact, no valid disagreement may exist in the proffered SMI, if testimony were to be evaluated by scientifically adept parties instead of by lay persons.

A quantification of the level of flawed SMI in the courtroom would be helpful in understanding how science affects jurisprudence. However, such data are currently unavailable and will probably continue to be so. Only the most egregious examples of fraudulent (? criminal) scientific testimony have been exposed in public forums, such as the case of a single physician-"expert" who personally certified a diagnosis of asbestosis in >50,000 cases [32].

Scientific Information and Juries

Although the civil court system values social concerns at least as highly as scientific validity, SMI is still a part of malpractice lawsuits. It is germane to ask whether lay jurors can properly digest technical details in cases that involve pathologists or other professional defendants. The process of teaching the intricacies of pathology to residents-in-training takes several years beyond medical school. Hence, as expected, public records reflect the fact that lay juries are often baffled by pathologists' testimony. One juror, who was interviewed after a trial that included pathologic information on coronary arterial thrombosis and myocardial infarction, compared the SMI presented in the courtroom to the inchoate sounds coming from a faceless teacher in a "Charlie Brown" cartoon on television [33]. Nevertheless, most lawyers continue to aver that "expert" testimony can be assimilated successfully by lay jurors. Believing assertions such as that may demand substantial credulity [34].

It would be relatively easy to convene "mock" juries, give them conflicting "expert" medical opinions, and test them to see how much scientific information had been absorbed correctly. That process would provide at least some tangible information on the ability of lay people to digest SMI. Nonetheless, because the legal system lacks even the rudimentary features of an objective, evidence-based mechanism, such tests of procedural validity have never been performed. The effects of professional inertia and self-interest are probably also operative in this problem [35].

Sporadic assertions have been made in the legal literature that a "statistically significant" correlation exists between jury verdicts and "expert" opinions [14]. However, this would only show that jurors do not ignore "expert" opinion. Moreover, physicians who attempt to improve "expert" testimony in the courtroom by publicly challenging the opinions of professional mavericks are in danger of being sued for offenses such as "defamation of character" [36]. Sadly, most physicians and medical specialty organizations have ignored this problem altogether [37].

Two Cultures: Lawyers and Doctors

Lawyers and judges control the legal system, and it would seem rational for physicians to work with these individuals to reduce jury error. Unfortunately, the two parties typically adhere to irreconcilable paradigms in their evaluation of the Law. Physicist and novelist C.P. Snow was famous, in part, for his Cambridge University lectures in 1959, which noted that science and the humanities are populated by people who do not understand each other because they live in different cultures [38–40]. Similarly, the philosophical gap between lawyers and physicians is a sizable one. Each group has its own modes of training, specialized terminologies, professional objectives, ways of evaluating the results of their work, and forums for publication and discussion of professional thought. In the main, these are only marginally related to one another. Consequently, several observers have noted a "rawness" of physician-based antipathy toward attorneys, as well as a "searing distrust" of the courts [41].

Sadly, effective criticism of the use of "experts" who sometimes misinform jurors depends to some extent on the inherently weak foundation of what is known as "argument by incredulity," that is, my view-point is true because I can't imagine it to be false [42]. Physicians may consider it to be simply unacceptable to ever allow the delivery of misinformation to jurors. In contrast, a critical mass of lawyers believes that the opportunity for cross examination of "experts," truthful opposing testimony, and the option to appeal unfavorable verdicts effectively compensates for flaws in "expert" testimony [43, 44]. Physicians are free to consider the latter opinion overtly wrong, but that does not prove that physicians are correct.

Medical Error and "Standard of Care"

There has been widespread, intense pressure to reduce medical error – a laudable goal. With that fact as a background, one might assume that the tort system could be a valuable asset in preventing iatrogenic harm to patients.

In principle, that premise could be true; in actuality, however, it is not. An allegation of medical "negligence" always attends malpractice lawsuits, but many plaintiffs' lawyers try to blur the distinction between *true* negligence – that is, the willful or careless commission of a wrongful act – and simple human or system-based error, or adverse outcomes not due to error. That situation stifles any meaningful input from the courts in estimating the relative weight of those elements as causes of adverse clinical outcome.

In contrast to medical error, which has been studied assiduously over the past decade, departure from "the standard of [medical] care" is a vestigial legalism that has only weak links to medical error analysis. For example, in the Law, it does not matter whether a misdiagnosis stemmed from ambient disturbances in the laboratory, technical problems in the histology laboratory, transposition of specimens before receipt in the pathology suite, or misinterpretation of the disease process by a pathologist. Laboratory directors and practicing pathologists are held personally and globally responsible for all of those factors; they are all subsumed by the phrase "standard of care."

Tort cases involving pathologists depend upon fellow pathologists' perception of standard of care three potential dispositions;

1. No expert can be found to assert that a diagnosis or interpretation fell below the "standard of care," and the plaintiff has no case
2. The mistake is *blatantly* the result of substandard practices or professional incompetence, as judged by unbiased peer-evaluators, and no expert can be found who will testify in favor of the pathologist. The particular details of the error are important only in regard to the award

of damages. The error is so blatant that principles of prevention analysis do not apply

3. "Expert" opinions differ over whether there was a negligent departure from the "standard of care." If the case is not removed from the system by settlement or summary judgment, the conflicting "experts" will address a jury in court. The jury will have to decide which expert opinion reflects practice reality, and then how to integrate this conclusion into a final verdict.

The most valuable information on medical error coming from the courts has been collected by insurance companies, not lawyers, and analyzed by other physicians [45]. However, such data are very incomplete, because many malpractice cases are settled under private terms [46], and details of jury deliberations are not often made available as public information.

Plaintiffs' attorneys aver that they are "fighting medical error" by threatening tort actions against physicians who deliver substandard care [47]. Nonetheless, no credible objective proof has appeared showing that this approach does produce improvement in medical practice or patient welfare. Undeniably, however, it does measurably discourage doctors from practicing in geographic locales where torts are rife. In addition, it has been proven beyond doubt that perceived malpractice risks prompt physicians to over-order tests, medications, and procedures in a defensive posture, elevating the cost and complexity of medical care [48]. The vacuous concept called "standard of care" leads doctors to think increasingly about how lay jurors might respond to each of the many professional decisions that comprise patient care [49]. Typically, that type of rumination is scientifically unproductive, expensive for the medical system, and inefficient.

Is the Professional "Standard of Care" a Valid Concept?

At their extremes, the ideas underlying "standard of care" are straightforward. Everything in-between is a muddle.

One can attempt to resolve this confusion by consulting a legal dictionary, which says that the "standard of [professional] care" is "the average degree of skill, care, and diligence exercised by members of the same profession, practicing in the same or a similar locality, in light of the present state of… science" [50]. That definition is inherently nebulous. In the same dictionary, "average" is defined as "ordinary" or "usual." A meaningful understanding of those words, in turn, requires additional information:

1. Data would have to be gathered on the performance of a representative sample of qualified "local" professionals in a given vocation, regarding the type of case under discussion, plus
2. A reproducible and logical threshold would need to be established to separate "ordinary" from "non-ordinary" performance.

As an example, one might find that unbiased evaluation of a melanocytic lesion by several experienced "local" pathologists resulted in the following diagnoses – Spitz nevus (25%); melanoma (72%); and other lesions (3%). With this information in hand, one could attempt to identify professional conclusions that were "substandard." The process might result in the conclusion that a minority opinion (in this example, "Spitz nevus") did still comport with the "standard of care" [51]. That is particularly true if the recommended *treatment* attached to the latter interpretation did not differ substantially from that used for the preeminent diagnosis. However, the question remains: Is the diagnosis of spitz nevus "average"?

Another challenge to "average" or "ordinary" skill is its unclear relationship to subspecialty training or certification. Indeed, when the latter is required, the advanced certificate-holder would, by definition, be "special" and not "ordinary!" Furthermore, the threshold of "ordinary practice" is not a constant of nature such as the speed of light, and it cannot be identified with precision. In the existing legal system, "ordinary" and "non-ordinary" are completely changeable terms, definitions of which could be chosen arbitrarily to favor a plaintiff, a defendant, or neither party.

As the percentage of pathologists who agree with a given diagnosis becomes lower, the corresponding claim to "ordinariness" becomes less credible. On the other hand, it might theoretically be decided that "ordinary" skill was defined by agreement among ≥95% of reviewing pathologists; that high threshold would inherently produce cases with no standard of care.

Yet another approach to the "ordinary vs. non-ordinary" issue would be to define the most commonly made diagnosis as the proper "standard of care," and all others as "non-ordinary." That model would be regarded as highly illogical and flawed by persons with a scientific background, because the majority of observers can agree on a decision or interpretation that is entirely wrong on objective grounds. Nonetheless, most lay persons are accustomed to separating "winners" from "losers" through majority voting. A review of US Supreme Court decisions shows that 5 to 4 votes are relatively common, but the majority is clearly determinative [52]. On the other hand, majority scientific opinion has definite consequences, but it does not change scientific *reality*. Even if most scientists in the world decided to again assert that the earth was flat, it would still, in truth, be spherical.

Some experienced pathologists who participate in malpractice litigation use self-determined thresholds to identify cases in which they cannot support a defendant as complying with "standard of care" [53]. If, for example, it is concluded that the defendant pathologist has erred, but at least 20% of *all* pathologists would have made the same error, an expert could decide to support the actions of the defendant physician. To date, however, a testable rationale for that approach has not been advanced, nor is there any published proof that a valid method exists for determining how many pathologists would make a certain error. Nevertheless, these issues must be discussed if "standard of care" is to move from the shadows into the realm of evidence-based error analysis.

Applying "Standard of Care" to Features of a Given Case

There is no current administrative legal mechanism for routinely providing judges and juries with information from court-appointed and unbiased "experts." Also, as just discussed, definitions of "ordinary" and "non-ordinary" practice are ethereal.

Peer-reviewed medical publications may proffer general conclusions on diagnostic accuracy and precision, and one might further assume that such information could be used legally to define "standard of practice." For example, published information is available concerning the rate of false-negative interpretation of Papanicolaou (Pap) tests that actually show invasive cervical squamous carcinoma [54]. Nonetheless, those data can be completely irrelevant to allegations of malpractice in a *specific single case* of "missed cancer" using the Pap smear. That is because morphologic findings in a specific case at issue may be (and often are) markedly different from those on which published conclusions were drawn.

The Law invokes the "expert" paradigm to explain how the complex literature should be applied to the case at hand. Theoretically, the "experts" give their views of how the handling of a particular case complied with real-life "standard" practice, and their conflicting conclusions are, in a legal sense, each supposed to be dispositive. However, that construction is ultimately invalid. First of all, none of the "experts" were present in the specific hospital or laboratory on the day a diagnosis was made, and they typically have no detailed knowledge of the circumstances under which the case was evaluated [55]. For example, verbal interchanges of information between pathologists and clinicians are extremely common and very important to patient care, but memories of such communications can be lost or altered with the passage of time if they are not written down in the medical record. The latter fact by no means detracts from the weight they carried in the "here and now." Finally hindsight bias can be almost impossible to eliminate.

Credibility of "Expert" Witnesses

Jurors weigh many factors when coming to their conclusion. In criminal trials, juries have sometimes delivered a verdict of "innocent" when it is obvious that the law has, in fact, been breached [56, 57]. In those instances, one might view the process as defensible because the juries wished to bring their community-based standards to bear against laws that they collectively felt to be unjust. With regard to medical malpractice cases, juries also have determinative latitude. They may base a judgment on the opinion of one "expert," attempt to integrate the assertions of several "experts," or ignore all of them. However, in actual practice, the impact of "expert" testimony on the jury depends on now jurors perceive its credibility, which, of course, derives from jurors perceptions of the people who are offering it [58].

Credibility or "worthiness of belief" is so important that it deserves further evaluation. If trial topics are mainstream and the jury is familiar with them, "credible" testimony must simply meet the test of plausibility. For example, if a witness insists that he saw an accused murderer from a mile away in a dark street on a cloudy night, the jurors' experience and common sense would tell them otherwise. On the other hand, most lay persons charged with assessing the credibility of "expert" testimony in pathology have no familiarity with that topic. They usually search for surrogate indicators of believability, such as the manner of speech and choice of words, style of dress and grooming, respect for the jurors and other people in court, and the perceived strength of the professional credentials of the witness [59].

Problematically, the credibility of an "expert" might be unquestioned in the eyes of a lay jury, whereas medical–scientific authorities would universally judge him or her to be a charlatan. The problem of "pseudo-credible" testimony has, in the past, led to some trial outcomes which departed markedly from those that established SMI would have dictated. This situation threatened the courts with a loss of face and public confidence in the past, and the Supreme Court felt compelled to attempt remedial action in an attempt to salvage the credibility of the legal system [60].

The Daubert Case and Standard of Care

During the 1990s, the US Supreme Court issued several rulings which provided new criteria that judges could apply in performing their "gatekeeper" function regarding "expert" testimony [60–64]. However, one would be mistaken in believing that these rulings are relevant to most current tort cases that involve pathologist defendants [65, 66]. Nevertheless, there are exceptions to that statement. If an "expert" were to assert at deposition that a single physiological mitosis in a melanocytic skin lesion mandated a diagnosis of melanoma on its own weight, that opinion could not possibly be supported by the peer-reviewed literature – a requirement stemming from the case of Daubert v. Merrell-Dow Pharmaceuticals *([92-102], 509 US 579 [1993])*. In some jurisdictions, opposing council would have the option to file a "Daubert challenge" to the testimony. If after reviewing the testimony the case's judge agreed that the testimony was "junk," there would be no need for the attorney filing the challenge to discredit that particular testimony at trial because the testimony would be barred from the courtroom by the judge.

Sadly, that scenario is an idealized one. In real life, things are more complicated. Obfuscating arguments can easily be presented to muddy the medicolegal water over admissibility of "expert" testimony, especially if no literature exists that *exactly* describes the particular case in question. Thus, the "Daubert criteria" are functionally irrelevant in many instances where "expert" testimony is not "expert." The question for the court is not whether the cited literature is valid, or whether it is applicable, but rather whether the *subjective interpretations* of that information by the respective "experts" are valid [62].

With regard to subjective expert opinion, most judges who oversee the admissibility of "expert" medical testimony could only function properly, in a scientific sense, if they sought the advice of unbiased court-appointed authorities. However, there are no mandates, or even procedural provisions, for judges to seek such help, and medical organizations have not offered it to the court spontaneously. Rather than admitting that they are personally unable to evaluate the probative value of scientific-medical testimony, most judges use existing statutes and decisions concerning "expert" witnesses to provide a "preference for admissibility" [67]. Jurors who may have less education than judges are then required to determine the scientific veracity of testimony that is the "admissible truth" rather than the "whole truth" [68].

"Finality" in the Courts vs. "Finality" in Medicine

In addition to bringing values of the community into the legal system, jurors are also charged with ending conflicts between the specific parties at the bar. This process is complicated when credible "experts" disagree, when both the plaintiff and the defendant(s) seem to be worthy people, and when the opposing lawyers present their cases skillfully. Perhaps the testimony of the "experts" indicates that there is genuine disagreement over the crux of the case, but the ultimate scientific validity is not the dominent issue at that moment in time; the needs of the court to resolve the issue before it are more concrete.

Physicians may be offended by this perceived "rush to judgment" in the face of factual uncertainty. Artificial legal "finality" may be contrary to the general principles of science and medicine. Indeed, when one sees dogmatism in the face of uncertain or conflicting objective data, it can generally be surmised that one is dealing with an ingenue or a fraud as a witness.

However, even in the real world of patient care, uncertainty must coexist to some extent with finality. In pathology practice, a low level of disquietude in difficult cases is relatively common, but substantial uncertainty typically stimulates a consultation with medical colleagues. Those helpers may transform what are inherently ambiguous findings into a final diagnosis and plan of action. Similarly, the decisions of juries function to transform medical and legal uncertainties into finalities.

Conclusions

In their role as diagnosticians, pathologists must be able to identify and respond to areas of uncertainty. An evidence-based approach to scientific investigation and medical practice is thought to optimize the specialty's approach to uncertainty. The legal system also must resolve uncertainty, but in many cases, physicians consider the uncertainty surrounding malpractice cases to be artifacts arising out of the scientific weaknesses of the legal system's procedures.

Physicians are one in the view that better scientific presentation in the courtroom is a laudable goal. Moreover, at least some judges would like to improve the quality of SMI offered to lay juries. However, efforts aimed at closing the space between admissible testimony and scientific truth have lacked infrastructural support, and attempts to exclude "outlier" testimony have been largely ineffective [67, 69].

Some medical groups such as the American Association of Neurological Surgeons and the American Association of Radiologists have attempted to improve the quality of "expert" testimony by doing their own peer reviews and imposing sanctions on physicians whose testimony was obviously erroneous [70]. Those efforts are commendable, and they have helped to identify failures of the legal system to control defective "expert" input. Nevertheless, this approach is clearly not the only answer to the problem. Until *all* judges and medical specialty societies cooperate closely to assure the accuracy of "expert" presentations in the courtroom, the legal system will continue to depend on jurors to separate fact from fiction.

Interestingly, the introduction of DNA-based technology into criminal trials has prompted the legal profession itself to question the quality of other forensic evidence that traditionally had been considered to have very high credibility [71]. However, there is currently no indication that the lawyers who control malpractice litigation have identified any reason to re-evaluate their systems or methods. This legal satisfaction with the status quo can be discouraging to pathologists who have had first-hand experience with malpractice litigation, but should not prevent individual pathologists from taking their own small steps to improve the scientific quality of malpractice litigation. First, one must be willing to commit the time and emotional energy required to participate in malpractice litigation as an expert, rather than just complain from the sidelines about tort system deficiencies. As pathologist Richard J. Zarbo observed, "the system only works when good people get involved." Secondly, the pathologist must commit to providing honest, clear, credible, and evidence-based testimony. At that point the pathologist has become a one person force for tort reform.

References

1. Hyman DA. Medical malpractice and the tort system: what do we know and what (if anything) should we do about it? Published as part of a symposium on civil justice in the Texas Law Review, Vol. 80, No. 7, June 2002. Available at http://www.law.umaryland.edu. Accessed 2 Oct 2005.
2. Malpractice mythology (Editorial). The New York Times. January 9, 2005. Available at http://www.nytimes.com. Accessed 9 Jan 2005.
3. Berenson A. Jury finds Merck liable in the Vioxx death and awards $253 million. The New York Times. August 19, 2005. Available at http://www.nytimes.com. Accessed 19 Aug 2005.
4. Olson W. The next Sandra Day. The Wall Street Journal. July 7, 2005. p. A12.
5. Olson W. Justice served, sometimes. The Wall Street Journal. September 8, 2005. p. D10.
6. Wick MR, Adams RK. Medical malpractice actions: procedural elements. Semin Diagn Pathol. 2007;24:60–4.
7. Foucar E, Wick MR. Evidence-based medicine and tort law. Semi Diagn Pathol. 2005;22:167–176.
8. Feld AD, Carey WD. Expert witness malfeasance: how should specialty societies respond? Am J Gastroenterol. 2005;100:991–5.
9. Cecil JS. Ten years of judicial gatekeeping under Daubert. Am J Public Health. 2005;95:S74–80.
10. Rosenbaum S. The impact of United States law on medicine as a profession. JAMA. 2003;289:1546–56.
11. Steinbrook R. Science, politics, and federal advisory committees. N Engl J Med. 2004;350:1454–60.
12. Huber PW. Galileo's revenge: junk science in the courtroom. New York: Basic Books; 1991.
13. U.S. Supreme Court, Tanner v United States, 483 U.S. 107 (1987). Available at http://caselaw.lp.findlaw.com. Accessed 12 Aug 2004.
14. Vidmar N. Expert evidence, the adversarial system, and the jury. Am J Public Health. 2005;95:S137–43.
15. Miller JF. Should juries hear complex cases? Duke Law & Technical Review. April 2, 2004. Available at http://www.law.duke.edu. Accessed 11 Jan 2005.
16. Bal R, Bijker WE, Hendriks R. Democratisation of scientific advice. BMJ. 2004;329:1339–41.
17. Ezrahi Y. Nature as dogma. Book review of: politics of nature: how to bring the sciences into democracy. Bruno Latour. Harvard University Press; 2004. Am Sci. 2005;93:89–90.
18. Foucar E. Diagnostic decision making in anatomic pathology. Am J Clin Pathol. 2001;116(Suppl): S21–33.
19. McDougal L. I trust juries – and Americans like you. Newsweek. December 22, 2003. p. 16.
20. Olson W. Stop the shakedown. The Wall Street Journal. October 29, 2004. p. A14.
21. Mohr JC. American medical malpractice litigation in historical perspective. JAMA. 2000;283:1731–7.
22. Murray I. The malpractice economist: liable to suffer. The American Enterprise. September 2003. p. 50–1.
23. Zhang J. How much soy lecithin is in that cookie? The Wall Street Journal. October 13, 2005. p. D1.
24. Simon R. Payback time for dot-com investors. The Wall Street Journal. February 1, 2005. p. D1.
25. Crossen C. A thirties revelation: rich people who steal are criminals, too. The Wall Street Journal. October 15, 2003. p. B1.
26. Martinson BC, Anderson MS, de Vries R. Scientists behaving badly. Nature. 2005;435:737–8.
27. Saks MJ, Koehler JJ. The coming paradigm shift in forensic identification science. Science. 2005;309: 892–5.
28. Junghans C, Feder G, Hemingway H, Timmis A, Jones M. Recruiting patients to medical research: double blind randomized trial of "opt-in" and "opt-out" strategies. BMJ. 2005;331:940–4.
29. Judge declares mistrial in case of Ohio highway shootings. The Associated Press. May 9, 2005. Available at http://www.nytimes.com. Accessed 9 May 2005.
30. Fridman DS, Janoe JS. Judicial gatekeeping in New Mexico. From The Judicial Gatekeeping Project. 1999. Available at http://cyber.law.harvard.edu/daubert/nm.htm. Accessed 15 June 2005.
31. Michaels D. Scientific evidence and public policy. Am J Public Health. 2005;95:S5–7.
32. Silicosis, Inc. (Editorial). The Wall Street Journal. October 27, 2005. p. A20.

33. Tesoriero HW, Brat I, McWilliams G, Martinez B. Merck loss jolts drug giant, industry. In landmark Vioxx case, jury tuned out science, explored coverup angle. The Wall Street Journal, August 22, 2005. p. A1.
34. Halpern SD. Towards evidence based bioethics. BMJ. 2005;331:901–3.
35. Lipton P. Testing hypotheses: prediction and prejudice. Science. 2005;307:219–21.
36. Albert T. Expert witness sues critics. American Medical News. June 28, 2004. p. 1.
37. Milunsky A. Lies, damned lies, and medical experts: the abrogation of responsibility by specialty organizations and a call for action. J Child Neurol. 2003;18:413–9.
38. Petroski H. Technology and the humanities. American Scientist. 2005;93:304–7.
39. Mawer S. Science in literature. Nature. 2005;434:297–9.
40. Byatt AS. Fiction informed by science. Nature. 2005;434:294–6.
41. Jacobson PD, Bloche MG. Improving relations between attorneys and physicians. JAMA. 2005;294: 2083–5.
42. Andrews M. Making malpractice harder to prove. The New York Times. December 21, 2003. Available at: http://www.nytimes.com. Accessed 21 Dec 2003.
43. Victoroff MS. Peer review of the inexpert witness, or…Do you trust the chickens to guard the coop? Managed Care, September 2002. Available at http://managedcaremag.com. Accessed 7 Aug 2003.
44. Begley S. Ban on "junk science" also keeps jurors from sound evidence. The Wall Street Journal. June 27, 2003. p. B1.
45. Troxel DB. Error in surgical pathology. Am J Surg Pathol. 2004;28:1092–5.
46. Sandlin S. Unser malpractice lawsuit is settled. ABQ Journal.com online edition, October 4, 2005. Available at http://abqjournal.com. Accessed 25 Oct 2005.
47. Hupert N, Lawthers AG, Brennen TA, Peterson LM. Processing the tort deterrent signal: a qualitative study. Soc Sci Med. 1996;43:1–11.
48. Budetti PP. Tort reform and the patient safety movement. Seeking a common ground. JAMA. 2005;293:2660–2.
49. Gold JA. Malpractice. Book review of: Medical malpractice: a physician's source-book. Anderson RE, editors. Humana Press; 2005. JAMA. 2005;293:1393.
50. The Publisher's Editorial Staff, Nolan JR, Nolan-Haley JM. Black's law dictionary (Centennial Edition). 1990. St. Paul: West Group.
51. Reay DT, Davis GJ, and the members of the CAP Forensic Pathology Committee. Legal basis for civil claims (Chapter 6). In: The pathologist in court. A Publication of the College of American Pathologists; 2003. p. 27–33.
52. Sunstein CR. Courting division. The New York Times. October 6, 2005. Available at http://www.nytimes.com. Accessed 6 Oct 2005.
53. Epstein JI. Pathologists and the judicial system: how to avoid it. Am J Surg Pathol. 2001;25:527–37.
54. Rylander E. Negative smears in women developing invasive cervical cancer. Acta Obstet Gynecol Scand. 1977;56:115–8.
55. Wick MR. Medicolegal liability in surgical pathology: a consideration of underlying causes and selected pertinent concepts. Semin Diagn Pathol. 2007;24:89–97.
56. Dalrymple T. Trial by human beings. The jury system and its discontents. Natl Rev. 2005;25:30–1.
57. Balko R. Justice often served by jury nullification. July 28, 2005. Fox News Channel. Available at http://foxnews.com. Accessed 28 July 2005.
58. Be prepared (Professional Issues). Interview with Sara C. Charles and Paul Frisch. American Medical News. July 11, 2005. p. 14–5.
59. Reay DT, Davis GJ, and the members of the CAP Forensic Pathology Committee. Courtroom etiquette (Chapter 11). In: The pathologist in court. College of American Pathologists; 2003. p. 56–9.
60. Petroski H. Daubert and Kumho. American Scientist. 1999;87:402–6.
61. US Supreme Court, 509 U.S. 579. Daubert v Merrell Dow Pharmaceuticals, Inc. 1993. Available at http://supct.law.cornell.edu. Accessed 10 Sep 2003.
62. US Supreme Court, 522 U.S. 136. General Electric Co v Joiner. 1997. Available at http://supct.law.cornell.edu. Accessed 10 Sep 2003.
63. U.S. Supreme Court, 526 U.S. 137. Kumho Tire Company v Patrick Carmichael. 1999. Available at http://supct.law.cornell.edu. Accessed 10 Sept 2003.
64. Jasanoff S. Law's knowledge: science for justice in legal settings. Am J Public Health. 2005;95: S49–58.
65. Faigman DL. Is science different for lawyers? Science. 2002;297:339–40.
66. Foucar E. Pathology expert witness testimony and pathology practice: a tale of two standards. Arch Pathol Lab Med. 2005;129:1268–76.
67. Kassirer JP, Cecil JS. Inconsistency in evidentiary standards for medical testimony. Disorder in the courts. JAMA. 2002;288:1382–7.
68. Gutheil TG, Hauser M, White MS, Spruiell G, Strasburger LH. The "whole truth" versus the "admissible truth": an ethics dilemma for expert witnesses. J Am Acad Psychiatry Law. 2003;31:422–7.
69. Appelbaum PS. Law and psychiatry: policing expert testimony: the role of professional organizations. Psychiatr Serv. 2002;53:389–99.
70. "Expert" witness gets booted from ACR. Diagnostic imaging online. July 8, 2004. Available at http://diagnosticimaging.com. Accessed 31 Oct 2004.
71. Neufeld PJ. The (near) irrelevance of Daubert to criminal justice and some suggestions for reform. Am J Public Health. 2005;95:S107–20.

Index

A.M. Marchevsky and M.R. Wick (eds.), *Evidence Based Pathology and Laboratory Medicine*, DOI 10.1007/978-1-4419-1030-1, © Springer Science+Business Media, LLC 2011

C